FBC
4-
9/72

PSYCHIATRIC APPROACHES TO MENTAL RETARDATION

PSYCHIATRIC APPROACHES TO MENTAL RETARDATION

EDITED BY

Frank J. Menolascino

Basic Books, Inc., Publishers

NEW YORK   LONDON

Second Printing

© 1970 by Basic Books, Inc.
Library of Congress Catalog Card Number: 71-110775
SBN 465–06455–8
Manufactured in the United States of America
DESIGNED BY VINCENT TORRE

This book is dedicated to: (1) The National Association for Retarded Children which was founded nearly twenty years ago. Through the efforts of this organization, the lives of many mentally retarded individuals have been illuminated and made increasingly more relevant; and (2) The past and present members of the helping professions who, in the light of their dedication, faithfully have served their mentally retarded fellow-citizens.

The Authors

RICHARD C. ALLEN LL.D. Professor of Law and Director of the Institute of Law, Psychiatry and Criminology. The George Washington University, Washington, D.C.

EDWARD T. BEITENMAN M.D. Assistant Professor of Child Psychiatry, University of Nebraska Medical Center; Assistant Clinical Professor of Psychiatry and Neurology, Creighton University School of Medicine; Private Practice in Child and Adolescent Psychiatry, Omaha; Consultant, Glenwood State Hospital and School, Glenwood, Iowa.

LAURETTA BENDER M.D. Consultant in Child Psychiatry, New York State Department of Mental Hygiene and former Director of Psychiatric Research, Children's Unit, Creedmoor State Hospital, Queens Village, New York.

NORMAN R. BERNSTEIN M.D. Director of Psychiatric Training Program, Walter E. Fernald State School; Instructor of Psychiatry, Harvard Medical School; Associate Director, Child Psychiatry Unit, Massachusetts General Hospital; and Director of Psychiatry, Shriners Burns Institute.

IRV BIALER Ph.D. Director of Research, Kennedy Child Study Center, New York City; Instructor in Education, School of Education, New York University; and Adjunct Assistant Professor of Special Education, Ferkauf Graduate School, Yeshiva University, New York City.

BURTON BLATT Ed.D. Director and Professor of Special Education, Division of Special Education and Rehabilitation, 805 South Crouse Avenue, Syracuse University, Syracuse, New York.

DOROTHY BROWN A.C.S.S. Preschool Unit, Mental Retardation Center, New York Medical College, Flower and Fifth Avenue Hospitals, New York City.

STELLA CHESS M.D. Associate Professor of Psychiatry at New York University Medical Center where she is responsible for liaison with the Department of Pediatrics; Attending Psychiatrist at Bellevue Hospital and University Hospital, New York City.

EVIS CODA M.D. Director, Saint John's Hospital Community Mental Health Center; Medical Director, Kennedy Child Study Center, Santa Monica, California.

RICHARD L. COHEN M.D. Associate Professor of Child Psychiatry and Director of Training in Child Psychiatry, Department of Psychiatry, University of Pittsburgh School of Medicine; Director, Pittsburgh Child Guidance Center, 201 De Soto Street, Pittsburgh, Pennsylvania.

DOROTHY COLODNY M.D. Assistant Clinical Professor of Pediatric Psychiatry, University of California School of Medicine, San Diego; Psychiatric Consultant to the Department of Pediatrics, University Hospital of San Diego County, San Diego, California.

MILDRED CREAK M.D., F.R.C.P., D.P.M. Honorary Physician to the Hospital for Sick Children, Great Ormond Street, London. Now retired from clinical practice, she was formerly physician in Psychological Medicine at the Hospital for Sick Children, and before that she headed the Children's Department at the Maudsley Hospital.

LEON CYTRYN M.D. Associate Professor of Pediatric Psychiatry, George Washington University Medical School; Research Associate, Children's Hospital of the District of Columbia; Psychiatric Consultant, Jewish Foundation for Retarded Children, Washington, D.C.

GUNNAR DYBWAD J.D. Professor of Human Development, Florence Heller School for Advanced Studies in Social Welfare, Brandeis University, Waltham, Massachusetts.

BARBARA S. FREDERICK A.C.S.W. Department of Social Work, the Neuropsychiatric Institute, University of California at Los Angeles Center for the Health Sciences, Los Angeles, California.

ROGER D. FREEMAN M.D. Director of the Child Psychiatry Clinic, St. Christopher's Hospital for Children; Associate Professor and Head, Section of Child Psychiatry, Department of Psychiatry, Temple University School of Medicine, Philadelphia, Pennsylvania.

WILLIAM I. GARDNER Ph.D. Professor and Chairman, Department of Studies in Behavioral Disabilities, University of Wisconsin; Director, Laboratory of Applied Behavior Analysis and Modification, Training Center in Mental Retardation, Madison, Wisconsin.

NORMA JAFFE M.S.W., A.C.S.S. Psychiatric Social Worker of the Preschool Unit, Mental Retardation Center, New York Medical College, Flower and Fifth Avenue Hospitals, New York City.

LEROY F. KURLANDER M.D. Associate Clinical Professor of Pediatric Psychiatry, University of California School of Medicine, San Diego; Staff Member and Director, Learning Disability Clinic, University Hospital of San Diego County, San Diego, California.

RONALD S. LIPMAN Ph.D. Chief, Clinical Studies Section, Psychopharmacology Research Branch, National Institute of Mental Health, Chevy Chase, Maryland; Assistant Professor of Medical Psychology, Johns Hopkins University, Baltimore, Maryland.

GEORGE LOTT M.D. University Psychiatrist (retired) and Professor (retired), Department of Psychology, Graduate School, Pennsylvania State University. He is currently a Mental Health and Psychiatric Consultant in private practice, and a Child Psychiatrist on the staff of the Mental Health Center, York, Pennsylvania.

MARJORIE C. MACKINNON A.C.S.W. Senior Social Worker in the Social Service Department at the Kennedy Child Study Center of St. John's Hospital in Santa Monica, California.

FRANK J. MENOLASCINO M.D. Associate Professor of Psychiatry and Pediatrics, University of Nebraska Medical Center; Director, Division of Preventive and Social Psychiatry, Nebraska Psychiatric Institute, Omaha, Nebraska.

MARIAN H. MOWATT, Ph.D. Clinical Psychologist in private practice in Seattle, Washington; Consultant to the King County Juvenile Court; Consultant to the Washington State Division of Vocational Rehabilitation; Member of the Faculty, Seattle University.

HOWARD W. POTTER M.D. Emeritus Professor of Psychiatry and former Dean of the State University of New York Downstate Medical Center in Brooklyn, New York. Since his retirement in 1958 he has been Program Director of the Letchworth Village Graduate Course in Mental Retardation, Thiells, New York.

STANLEY E. SLIVKIN M.D. Clinical Instructor in Psychiatry, Tufts University School of Medicine; Staff Psychiatrist, Veteran's Administration Hospital, Boston, Massachusetts; Member, Advisory Committee of the Psychiatric Training Program, Walter E. Fernald State School, Waverly, Massachusetts.

GERALD SOLOMONS M.D. Professor of Pediatrics and Director of the Child Development Clinic of the College of Medicine, University of Iowa, Iowa City, Iowa.

JACK TIZARD Ph.D. Professor of Child Development, University of London Institute of Education, London, England. Recipient, 1968 Kennedy International Award for Research in Mental Retardation.

THOMAS G. WEBSTER M.D. Chief, Continuing Education Branch, Division of Manpower and Training Programs, National Institute of Mental Health, Chevy Chase, Maryland.

WOLF WOLFENSBERGER Ph.D. Associate Professor and Mental Retardation Research Scientist, University of Nebraska Medical Center, Omaha, Nebraska.

KATHARINE F. WOODWARD M.D. Psychiatrist-in-Charge, Preschool Unit, Mental Retardation Center, New York Medical College, New York City. Consulting Pediatric Psychiatrist, Lenox Hill Hospital.

MARGARET M. WRIGHT R.N., M.S. Associate Professor in Nursing, Atlantic Community College, Mays Landing, New Jersey.

Foreword

Howard W. Potter

IN 1962 the report of President Kennedy's Panel on Mental Retardation alerted public officials, professional groups, and the public to the needs of the mentally retarded for a multiplicity of services, many of which were unavailable in most communities. The Panel recommended a national program of action, including mental health services, for the mentally retarded and their families.

Traditionally, mental health has been an immediate concern of psychiatrists. But organized psychiatry, as represented by the American Psychiatric Association (A.P.A.), had done little or nothing for a number of decades to encourage participation of its members in mental retardation and its victims' specific mental health needs. A.P.A. had replaced its section on Mental Deficiency by one on Child Psychiatry. Its programs during its annual meetings had presented but a minimum number of papers on mental retardation. In A.P.A.'s *American Journal of Psychiatry,* articles on mental retardation have been few and far between. Yet, paradoxically, the A.P.A. Council in a position statement it issued on mental retardation in 1963 immodestly claimed mental retardation as a subspecialty of psychiatry! It was this statement that prompted me, in 1965, to write about mental retardation as the Cinderella of Psychiatry.

However, up until the second or third decade of the twentieth century, psychiatry did play a dominant and leading role in mental retardation. Nearly 300 years ago (1672), Sir Thomas Willis, a prominent London neuropsychiatrist, described stupidity (mental retardation) as follows:

Stupidity hath many degrees; for some are accounted unfit or incapable as to all things, and others as to some things only. Some being wholly fools in the learning of letters, or the liberal sciences, are yet able enough for mechanical arts. Others find either of these incapable, yet easily comprehend agriculture, or husbandry and country business. Others unfit almost for all affairs, are only able to learn what belongs to eating or the common means of living. Others merely drivelling fools, scarce understand anything at all, or do anything knowingly.

It was Itard, a pupil of Pinel, who introduced the idiot to the nineteenth-century world. In 1801, he reported on his efforts to make Victor "normal." Victor was a "wild boy," obviously an idiot probably abandoned by his family and left to perish in the forests of the province of Aveyron. Itard devised and vigorously pursued a system of "sensory in-put" and rigorous "habit training." An important ingredient, although perhaps unrecognized, was the interpersonal relationship through which Victor gained enthusiastic support.

Itard's system of sensory input was soon adopted by one of his associates, Edouard Seguin, and had a profound influence on the care and education of the idiot throughout the western world until well up to the close of the nineteenth century. It is perhaps worthy of some note that it was eight psychiatrists who, in 1876, founded the forerunner of the American Association on Mental Deficiency.

In brief, then, nineteenth-century psychiatry described both lunacy and idiocy in psychological and behavioristic terminology, but persistently sought for the ultimate source of these disorders in some structural deviation of the nervous system. Consequently, all psychiatrists in that century knew their neuroanatomy and neuropathology well. Most were as skilled in neurological diagnosis as they were knowledgeable about Kraepelinian symptomatology. Psychiatric treatment embraced the modalities of the moral treatment of the insane and the training of the minds of idiots and imbeciles through an educational system of sensory input and habit indoctrination. Since the all of mental retardation in the nineteenth century comprised mostly a variety of clinical forms of encephalopathy, it naturally commanded the interest of the nineteenth-century neurologically oriented psychiatrist.

Thus, at the turn of the twentieth century and for the next two decades or so, psychiatry had had a dominant and leading role in mental retardation for well over one hundred years. But in a span of twenty years (1915–1935), there occurred a radical shift of psychiatric interest away from mental retardation. Concomitantly, clinical psychiatry was undergoing a phenomenal shift from a biomedical to a psychosocial orientation.

After the first quarter of the twentieth century, American psychiatry rapidly assimilated the dynamic concepts of psychoanalysis into psychiatric evaluation and treatment and, concomitantly, psychiatric training rapidly shifted from a medical-science orientation to a psychosocial orientation. Thus it is that the American psychiatrist of modern times is far more of a behavioral scientist than a medical scientist. Most have had but minimal instruction in the morphology and function of the nervous system, and but a very few have had a minimal training in mental retardation. Most tend to entertain a defect position about all retardation. That 75 to 80 per cent of all retardation is mild retardation and that mildly retarded children have nothing in common with seriously retarded children but much in common with normal children, has escaped them. Nevertheless, the intensive training in adaptational dynamics of the modern psychiatrist and his intimate knowledge of the impacts of constitution and ecology on emotional, intellectual, and social development, admirably prepare him to come to grips with the assessment and treatment of the personality problems and learning impairments of mental retardates.

Although now, in the 1960's, it is clearly recognized that the major problems of over three-quarters of the retarded are psychosocial in kind and thus call for educational and other psychologically based preventative and rehabilitative modalities, these self-same problem morons (mild retardates), newly discovered in 1910 (for example, the Kallikak Family by H. Goddard), were for a number of decades viewed as either sufferers from some attenuated form of idiocy with subclinical encephalopathy or as the product of some kind of vicious heredity. It is to be noted, too, that when emotional and behavioral problems were identified in the moron, these were believed to be additional manifestations of either his vicious heredity, his subclinical encephalopathy, or his stupidity. And above all, since the moron was viewed as a menace to the community, long-term and, in many instances, permanent institutionalization was the policy until shortly before World War I in many states. Strange as it may seem, these views of the mildly retarded are deeply entrenched in some professional disciplines even today.

But the psychodynamic features of retarded children and the phenomenology of psychopathology in association with mental retardation has not gone entirely unrecognized since the first quarter of this century. Even a cursory review of some of the literature on mental retardation over the last thirty years implies that there are many aspects of mental retardation that need serious attention from the modern psychiatrist. For example, the mildly impaired retardates who comprise some 85 per cent of all the retarded, by virtue of their self-image and their unfavorable competitive position in the world about them, are especially prone to anxiety. A large but unknown number or percentage of this group are poorly adjusted. In this group are also found many whose emotional problems contribute significantly to their learning difficulties.

There is indeed much that the modern psychiatrist, with his sophistication about how the human mind works, can do to promote effective adaptive behavior in the mentally retarded. In 1966, the Council of the A.P.A. promulgated an Action Program for Psychiatry in Mental Retardation which, if its twenty principles, propositions, and recommendations become operative, should bring to a close mental retardation's era as the Cinderella of psychiatry. Accordingly, the battle to bring psychiatric services to the retarded has been officially joined by the A.P.A. through its already mentioned Action Program. But the battle has yet to be won. Whether it will be, or how soon it will be won, will depend upon how rapidly psychiatry can acquire the kind of manpower so essential for engineering and participating in mental health services for the retarded and their families.

To what extent and how soon the A.P.A.'s Action Program becomes operative will depend in part upon how many chairmen of medical college departments of psychiatry will stir themselves to provide a sophisticated and imaginative program of instruction and supervised experience for their respective residents in psychiatry. Unfortunately, more likely than not there still are a few professors of psychiatry who believe the psychiatric resident can learn all he needs to know about mental retardation by sending him out on a "walkie-talkie" tour through the nearest in-service mental retardation center.

In contrast, we should facilitate the training of mental health personnel to take their place on the multidisciplinary professional teams so essential in providing the many different services necessary in any meaningful program for the mentally retarded.

It is indeed a privilege to have the opportunity to prepare the Preface for this book on psychiatric approaches to mental retardation. It is edited by a psychiatrist whose involvement with mental retardation had its beginnings in a course ("The Letchworth Village Graduate Course in Mental Retardation") he took under my tutelage in the spring of 1961.

Preface

THERE has been a recent renaissance of interest in the behavioral dimensions of mental retardation, and psychiatrists have actively participated in this new wave of professional involvement and activities. Yet many of the written signposts of both past and current psychiatric contributions are diffusely distributed in the professional literature. Indeed, at a recent psychiatric conference, a number of my colleagues asked, "How *do* we summarize current psychiatric efforts in mental retardation—for our trainees, colleagues in other fields, even for ourselves?" The inspiration for this volume came from repeated such experiences wherein there was an expressed need for a summarization of contemporary psychiatric viewpoints and techniques in the area of mental retardation. It is the editor's opinion that a book is needed which will literally corral some major representatives of the current psychiatric ferment and activity in the area of mental retardation.

This book is intended to serve only as an introduction to the psychiatric aspects of mental retardation, not as an introductory text for mental retardation. I believe the psychiatrist would be well advised to complement the reading of this book by a study of the general aspects of the field of mental retardation. I suggest that this particular body of knowledge can be reviewed by close attention to the following texts: (1) Clarke, A. M., and Clarke, A. D. B. (Eds.), *Mental deficiency: The changing outlook* (2nd ed.). New York: Free Press, 1965; (2) Robinson, H. B., and Robinson, N. M., *The mentally retarded child: A psychological approach.* New York: McGraw-Hill, 1965; and (3) Baumeister, A. A. (Ed.), *Mental retardation: Appraisal, education, and rehabilitation.* Chicago, Ill.: Aldine, 1967.

The focus of this collaborative work is to present, in both general and specific coverage, an overview of major areas of psychiatric involvement in mental retardation. The general focus is achieved by both the structure of the book's format (from general to specific aspects of a problem or area) and the continuity of flow between major divisions of the book. The specific foci highlight recurrent diagnostic and treatment problems and challenges. A conscious attempt has been made to balance the general and specific contributions.

The book also serves as a current assessment of psychiatric involvement in mental retardation—particularly in the closing section of the volume. It should be noted that the majority of the chapters were written expressly for this book. The few chapters that are based on previously published material have been updated, expanded, and adapted to the format of this book.

My overriding concern as the editor has been that the book be aimed at the level of the psychiatric practitioner. There is, however, a common core of interest between us and many of our colleagues in closely allied fields of endeavor. It is anticipated that individuals who can profit from this work will also include those with training in the clinical aspects of personality, its developmental aspects, and its disorders. Accordingly, it is hoped that the book will be of value to colleagues in psychology, social work, nursing, education, child development, and vocational rehabilitation.

Part One initially presents general considerations concerning the psychopathology of mental retardation, followed by selective emphasis on symptoms and syndromes therein. Part Two, by its composite approach to available treatment modalities, samples the wide diversity of techniques and methods that are likely to be both of interest and of help to psychiatrically trained practitioners. Again, general presentations are followed by more specific approaches. Part Three focuses on the challenges in current service systems; both relatively new and future challenges are embraced in the chapters therein. Part Four encompasses a trio of chapters which underscores one of our major future routes for change. Part Five presents both general and specific viewpoints concerning psychiatric research in mental retardation. Lastly, Part Six is a summation of perspectives on the psychiatrist's past, current, and future roles in the field of mental retardation.

It is anticipated that this book will fill the need for a contemporary repository of work in the psychiatric aspects of mental retardation and a sharing of ideas and guideposts that will accurately transmit our current progress and illuminate the road ahead.

I especially want to thank Dr. Robert Kugel, Dean of the University of Nebraska Medical Center, and Dr. Wolf Wolfensberger, Mental Retardation Research Scientist, for their inspiration and assistance in the preparation of this book. As significant contributors to the field of mental retardation, their encouragement has been invaluable to me.

Also, I thank the many people who have worked on the secretarial and technical aspects of publication, particularly my research assistants Miss Rosemary Fogarty and Mrs. Myra Robinson.

Omaha, Nebraska/September, 1970   *Frank J. Menolascino*

Contents

PART ONE
Psychopathological Problems in Mental Retardation

[A] GENERAL CONSIDERATIONS
  1: *Unique Aspects of Emotional Development in Mentally Retarded Children*   3
       Thomas G. Webster
  2: *Emotional Problems in Mentally Retarded Children*   55
       Stella Chess
  3: *Emotional Disturbance and Mental Retardation: Etiologic and Conceptual Relationships*   68
       Irv Bialer

[B] SYNDROMES AND SYMPTOMS
  4: *Apparent and Relative Mental Retardation: Their Challenges to Psychiatric Treatment*   91
       Norman R. Bernstein and Frank J. Menolascino
  5: *Infantile Autism: Descriptive and Diagnostic Relationships to Mental Retardation*   115
       Frank J. Menolascino
  6: *Diagnostic and Treatment Variations in Child Psychoses and Mental Retardation*   140
       Mildred Creak
  7: *The Life Course of Children with Autism and Mental Retardation*   149
       Lauretta Bender
  8: *Down's Syndrome: Clinical and Psychiatric Findings in an Institutionalized Sample*   191
       Frank J. Menolascino
  9: *Rumination, Mental Retardation, and Interventive Therapeutic Nursing*   205
       Margaret M. Wright and Frank J. Menolascino

PART TWO
Treatment Approaches

[A] INDIVIDUAL APPROACHES

10: *Psychotherapy of the Mentally Retarded: Values and Cautions* 227
George Lott

11: *Use of Behavior Therapy with the Mentally Retarded* 250
William I. Gardner

12: *Early Psychiatric Intervention for Young Mentally Retarded Children* 276
Katharine F. Woodward, Norma Jaffe, and Dorothy Brown

[B] PSYCHOPHARMACOLOGICAL APPROACHES AND ISSUES

13: *Psychopharmacology and the Retarded Child* 294
Roger D. Freeman

14: *Psychopharmacology as a Treatment Adjunct for the Mentally Retarded: Problems and Issues* 368
Dorothy Colodny and LeRoy F. Kurlander

15: *The Use of Psychopharmacological Agents in Residential Facilities for the Retarded* 387
Ronald S. Lipman

16: *Methodological Considerations in Evaluating the Intelligence-Enhancing Properties of Drugs* 399
Wolf Wolfensberger and Frank J. Menolascino

[C] GROUP APPROACHES

17: *Group Therapy Approach to Emotional Conflicts of the Mentally Retarded and Their Parents* 422
Marian H. Mowatt

18: *Group Approaches to Treating Retarded Adolescents* 435
Stanley E. Slivkin and Norman R. Bernstein

[D] FAMILY DIMENSIONS

19: *Counseling Parents of the Retarded: The Interpretation Interview* 455
Gerald Solomons

20: *A Theoretical Framework for the Management of
Parents of the Mentally Retarded*   475
   Wolf Wolfensberger and Frank J. Menolascino

21: *A Shift of Emphasis for Psychiatric Social Work
in Mental Retardation*   493
   Marjorie C. Mackinnon and Barbara S. Frederick

PART THREE
Challenges to the Psychiatrist in Current Service Systems

[A] CHALLENGES IN COMMUNITY SERVICES
   22: *Community Psychiatry and Mental Retardation*   507
      Evis Coda

[B] CHALLENGES IN RESIDENTIAL SERVICES
   23: *The Psychiatric Consultant in a Residential
   Facility for the Mentally Retarded*   527
      Edward T. Beitenman

   24: *Empty Revolution beyond the Mental*   542
      Burton Blatt

   25: *Roadblocks to Renewal of Residential Care*   552
      Gunnar Dybwad

   26: *Human Values as Guides to the Administration of
   Residential Facilities for the Mentally Retarded*   575
      Howard W. Potter

[C] CHALLENGES IN THE LEGAL SPHERE
   27: *Law and the Mentally Retarded*   585
      Richard C. Allen

PART FOUR
Training

28: *Mental Retardation and Child Psychiatry*   615
   Jack Tizard

29: *Experiences of Pregnancy: Some Relationships to
the Syndrome of Mental Retardation*   633
   Richard L. Cohen

30: *The Training of Pediatricians and Psychiatrists in
Mental Retardation*   651
   Leon Cytryn

PART FIVE
Research Viewpoints

31: *Facilitation of Psychiatric Research in Mental
     Retardation*   663
        Wolf Wolfensberger
32: *The Research Challenge of Delineating Psychiatric
     Syndromes in Mental Retardation*   690
        Frank J. Menolascino

PART SIX
A Perspective

33: *Psychiatry's Past, Current and Future Role
     in Mental Retardation*   **709**
        Frank J. Menolascino

     Index   **745**

PART ONE

===

Psychopathological Problems in Mental Retardation

[A]

GENERAL CONSIDERATIONS

: 1 :

Unique Aspects of Emotional Development in Mentally Retarded Children

Thomas G. Webster

INTRODUCTION

WHAT is unique in the personality development of mentally retarded children?[1] What is "normal" or optimal emotional development for a retarded child? If we can establish more clearly those qualities of emotional development which are uniquely associated with mental retardation, as distinguished from characteristics that are not unique to mental retardation, then we can provide the diagnostician with a clearer baseline from which to assess other factors in a given case. We can also provide professional persons and others who work with retarded children with a better understanding and less stereotyped thinking about what sort of people mentally retarded children are as against that which is characteristic of only certain types of retardation and that which is unique in each individual. At the same time we can provide parents with a more realistic appreciation of those qualities about their child which are, in contrast to qualities that are not, part and parcel of the child's mentally retarded condition. Lastly, a clearer specification of emotional characteristics most uniquely associated with mental retardation can help guide clinical and basic research into the etiology, prevention, and treatment of mental retardation.

The determination of unique features without fostering inappropriate stereotypes is a difficult task requiring thoughtful definition, description, and clarification, because a wide variety of conditions are included under the term "mental retardation." Variations in emotional development are at least as great as the variations in etiology, brain pathology, and intellectual functions. What, then, is unique to mental retardation and to the personality of mentally retarded children? Despite the great complexity of the problem, there are some relatively simple features that can be defined and described.

First, the criteria for defining "uniqueness" can be specified as follows. The characteristic features of social-adaptive and intellectual ability which are *unique* to mentally retarded children should, by definition, characterize all retarded children and not be limited to subgroups or individual variations. Also by definition, these features should characterize mentally retarded children more specifically than any comparable group of the population. Further, the unique features should have prominence or intensity roughly proportional to the degree of mental retardation which is present. The unique features should be evident in mentally retarded children of all ages, though specific developmental features may be more easily distinguished at one age than another.

Second, we must remind ourselves what mental retardation is and what it is not. Mental retardation is a clinical developmental syndrome. Three basic features of this syndrome which have implications for personality development are: an intellectual impairment or specific learning difficulty which is associated with a unique type of intellectual growth; a slow rate of development; and characteristic qualities in emotional growth, social adaptation, and personality traits.

A later section of this chapter will expand on these three basic features, but first I want to underscore what the mental-retardation syndrome is *not*. Mental retardation is not a brain condition except in the very broadest sense; it is not etiology; and it is neither an intellectual deficit, a cultural condition, nor an emotional disturbance as such. Mental retardation is definitely a handicap in a developmental and adaptational sense, but it is not a "defect" in the sense of certain stereotyped attitudes which that term frequently evokes. An IQ or developmental quotient below 70 is in general usage the most distinguishing sign of the mental-retardation syndrome, but intellectual functioning is only one element in the mental-retardation syndrome.

Professional workers as well as families of retarded children are apt to jump to false conclusions or engage in stereotyped thinking because of the tendency to equate a given etiologic diagnosis, a given brain condition, an IQ, or an emotional disturbance with the mental-retardation syndrome. Unfortunately, an image of a permanent, concrete, organic defect is then too often applied to "explain" many other aspects of the retarded child's behavior. A thorough diagnostic assessment of the mentally retarded child should include relatively independent assessment of etiology, brain function, intellectual function, and emotional development so as to avoid this stereotyping tendency and arrive at a more accurate composite picture of a child's assets and limitations.

One manifestation of these problems is a tendency for clinical investigators to exclude cases of organic brain disorder and psychosis from clinical studies of the emotional aspects of mental retardation. While this is an understandable effort to obtain cases in more "pure culture," the investigator might just as rationally exclude cases with known separation from the mother during infancy, or cases with known environmental deprivation. The relative role of a brain disease as compared to other factors in the emotional development of retarded children can best be put in perspective by clinicians when all major varieties of the mental-retardation syndrome are studied. The relation of a known central-nervous-system (CNS) lesion to the mental-retardation syndrome is no more specific, and is at least as complex psychologically, as the relation of maternal deprivation to the mental-retardation syndrome. The same may be said of cultural deprivation.

Another example of an oversimplified assumption occurred in my own experience. I began my work with retarded children with the rather naïve hope of finding a child who was "simply retarded" for purposes of comparison with patients with various neurological and emotional complications. After a series of 159 cases, I still had not found a retarded child who was "simply retarded" in the sense that his emotional development was truly comparable to a nonretarded child of the same mental age. Still another example is the tendency of child psychiatrists to move too readily to etiologic inferences when emotional disturbance is found associated with mental retardation—invoking thereby sometimes a premature implication of psychogenesis or pseudoretardation.

The main body of the present chapter will present a review of the literature and a clinical study, with an attempt to distinguish unique features of emotional development in the mental-retardation syndrome within the context of many other factors that commonly confront clinicians who work with mentally retarded children. The clinical study elaborates on the many associated factors, but focuses on the unique features, termed "primary psychopathology." The concluding section will focus on general implications, stereotypes, problems of terminology, and research relevant to the unique features of emotional development in retarded children.

REVIEW OF THE LITERATURE

Anyone who has worked with or lived with retarded persons is aware of how frequently their lives are complicated by their emotional problems. Psychiatrists, psychologists, and educators have emphasized the great significance of social and emotional factors in the mentally retarded. The fact that mental retardation (or subnormality) includes an adaptational behavioral handicap as well as subaverage intelligence has been emphasized in modern definitions, such as those of the World Health Organization Expert Committee on the Mentally Subnormal Child (1954), the President's Panel on Mental Retardation (1962), the American Association on Mental Deficiency (Heber, 1958), and by authors of modern textbooks such as Stevens and Heber (1964), Tredgold and Soddy (1963), Kanner (1957), and Robinson and Robinson (1965). Eisenberg (1958) was representative of many authors when he emphasized, "The interdependence of emotion and intelligence is a fundamental fact of human behavior, at the psychological and the biological levels of integration."

A review of the classic texts on mental retardation revealed that Tredgold and Soddy (1963) gave perhaps the most detailed attention to emotional development. They devoted sections to subjects such as the subnormal mind, disorders of relationship formation, and mental deficiency and behavior disorders. Their efforts to interweave psychoanalytic concepts of child development with more traditional concepts of mental deficiency were at times confusing, but they provided some valuable descriptive passages and many case illustrations. Their textbooks and other writings over the years have represented an admirable attempt to introduce consideration of emotional development into the traditional coverage of mental deficiency. Asperger (1960) emphasized the behavioral problems associated with mental retardation and used concepts such as "erethism" (a surplus of impulses).

Recent textbooks, monographs, and reports of symposia in the United States have devoted increased attention to behavioral and emotional problems. However, the integration of concepts of child psychiatry with those from psychology and education is still at an early stage. There has been valuable work in fields closely related to emotional development by clinical psychologists and educators. Masland et al. (1958), Stevens and Heber (1964), and Robinson and Robinson (1965) have reviewed past and recent research in this area. Educators also have long been interested in the special problems of the mentally retarded. Kirk (1958) and Blatt (1966) are among those who have placed an emphasis on the importance of personality and behavioral aspects in the education of retarded children.

Heber (1964, p. 169) summarized his comprehensive review of experimental research in personality of retarded persons as follows:

The extreme paucity of experimental data bearing on the relationship between personality variables and behavioral efficiency of the retarded person is indeed remarkable in view of the generally acknowledged importance of personality factors in problem solving. Textbooks are replete with statements describing the retarded as passive, impulsive, rigid, suggestible, lacking in persistence, immature, and withdrawn, and as having a low frustration tolerance and an unrealistic self-concept and level of aspiration. Yet, not one of these purported attributes can be either substantiated or refuted on the basis of available research data.

It is apparent that the mentally retarded and particularly those who are institutionalized have a substantially higher prevalence of psychotic and psychoneurotic disorders than the general population. . . . The few striking and consistent findings from the meager investment in "personality research" with the retarded converge in highlighting the importance of motivational variables. Even severely retarded persons appear to be responsive to variations in incentive conditions; social reinforcement in the form of verbal praise and encouragement or just simple attention appears to be at least as effective as with normal persons. There is a strong suggestion that the performance of retardates may be depressed as a function of generalized expectations of failure and that proportionately more retarded than normals may respond to the threat of failure with decreased rather than increased effort.

Some of our greatest insights into understanding the emotional problems of any medical or psychiatric patient have come from a dynamic psychiatry through which the physician could enter empathetically into the patient while maintaining an objectivity of observation. Until recent years, this type of contribution was conspicuously rare in the efforts to understand the mentally retarded child. Potter (1927) wrote of the possibility that "an overwhelming narcissism" in some retarded infants might interfere with "the outflow of libidinal urge" needed for the development of intelligence. Clark (1933) stated, "There is found in all mental defectives a weak ego structure in association with an impounding of libido within the personality and an inbinding of primary narcissism, thus limiting the psychic energy available for object relationships, which in turn dilutes the motivation for learning or acquisition."

Studies by Spitz (1945, 1946), Skeels (1966), and others have called attention to the impact that early deprivation and loss can have in retarding development, sometimes producing irreversible mental retardation. Mahler-Schoenberger (1942) and many more recent authors have described pseudoretardation [2] in which the psychopathology is rooted in later developmental levels and in which the retardation is partial, superficial, and sometimes modifiable by treatment. Kanner (1944), Bender (1955), Rank (1949), and Putnam (1955) have enhanced our knowledge of childhood psychosis, autism, or atypical development which are often associated with mental retardation. Jervis (1959) estimated that one-third of the patients with childhood psychosis are also mentally retarded.

Organic brain syndromes have features that overlap with problems of retardation and childhood psychosis. For example, Karelitz et al. (1960) demonstrated the difference in infant vocalizations between brain-defective children and normal youngsters and noted that the lessened development of the cry as a means of expression could present implications for early emotional development. Bender (1956) has been a fundamental contributor to the assessment of characteristic psychopathology in children with organic brain disorders. Rank (1949 a, b), Rappaport (1961), and Sarvis (1960) pointed out the poor integration in early ego development—particularly in the handling of aggression—which characterized individual children with organic deficits. The clarification by these authors of the functions of specific organic lesions in the psychic life of the child was a major advance beyond the traditional tendencies to attribute certain behavioral disturbances and retardation directly to "organic brain disease," without specificity as to either the nature of the lesion or the ego functions which are affected. They also clarified in each case those aspects of the emotional disturbance which were related to the early mother-child relation, and they demonstrated the improvement that was possible by means of intensive psychotherapy.

The retarded child's later development may suffer from the impact of the conscious and unconscious resentment, depreciation, overprotection, rejection, and unsuccessful competition he experiences first in his family and later in the community. An early theoretical contribution in this regard was that of Pearson (1957). He described an "ego defect," a subsequent "superego defect," and the deep sense of worthlessness of the retarded child. Such problems are more apt to occur when the retarded child is an obvious deviant in his family and community, which is often the case with children seen by child psychiatrists and private physicians. A series of reports by the Committee on Mental Retardation of the Group for the Advancement of Psychiatry (1959, 1963, 1967) elaborate on these and other emotional and social problems of the mentally retarded.

Of direct relevance to the clinical study in the present chapter are the findings from psychotherapeutic work with retarded children, such as the work edited by Stacey and DeMartino (1957), which included early contributions from Ackerman and Menninger and Chidester and Menninger. In a more recent work, Woodward et al. (1958) reported on their psychiatric work with nine preschool retarded children who were without evidence of organic brain disease. They found that "in spite of efforts to exclude clear-cut cases of schizophrenia, all but one child in the group revealed some schizoid characteristics . . . withdrawal and preoccupation . . . mildly bizarre mannerisms or gestures. . . ." The one exception was a child with marked compulsive and perseverative traits. Most of these children showed a partial ability to relate to adults but related less warmly than normal children the same age. Fears and overcautiousness were common. Improvement over a two-year period was accompanied by a great increase in activity, aggressiveness, and the quality of group play.

Chess (1966) reported on the first forty cases from a study in progress of fifty retarded children, five to eleven years old, with an IQ range of 50 to 75, excluding children with a degree of motoric disturbance "which could interfere sufficiently with motor functioning to influence level of competence and self-care play, etc." She reported that "70 per cent of the first forty children in the sample were found to show significant behavior disorders on psychiatric evaluation." The other 30 per cent she found "without significant behavior disorders." She wrote: "In our experience a significant minority of retarded children (30 per cent) do show emotional development comparable to nonretarded youngsters of the same mental age." Of the 70 per cent (28) with significant behavioral disturbances, 45 per cent (18) had "reactive behavior disorder," 5 per cent (2) had "neurotic behavior disorder," 17.5 per cent (7) had "behavioral dysfunction due to brain damage," and 2.5 per cent (1) had psychosis.

Chess went on to say that "a striking finding has been the frequency with which professional workers whom the families had consulted have avoided the diagnosis of mental retardation." She decried such tendencies of psychiatrically oriented professionals who use the diagnosis of "pseudoretardation" and unintentionally induce increased guilt and misunderstanding in the parents. In another section of her report she maintained that it would "appear self-evident that the degree of intellectual retardation is a significant factor in determining the child's adaptive capacities and potential for coping with the demands of his environment." She also emphasizes the "attribute of temperament . . . a child's characteristic style of reaction," which in interaction with environmental stresses played a significant role in the development of behavioral disturbances in her series of cases.

Philips (1966) reported on 170 families with children who were referred to the Langley Porter Neuropsychiatric Institute for evaluation of retardation. The children, whose ages ranged from nine months through adolescence, included "all degrees of severity of mental retardation."

At the beginning of our program, we hoped to see retarded children whose intellectual deficit was not complicated by emotional disorder. We contacted pediatric, public health, social welfare, and psychiatric facilities to request referral of children who were mentally retarded but had no emotional disorder. . . . We did see a few children who were making an adequate adjustment and whose parents only wished help with future plans and someone with whom to discuss current problems. . . . It was uncommon, however, to see a retarded child who presented no emotional maladjustment of moderate to severe degree as part of his clinical picture.

Philip's report included clinical impressions, discussion, and case illustrations to clarify the variety of emotional problems and influences in retarded children and their families. Statistical data on clinical types were not included. He emphasized that the emotional problems of retarded children, as of all children, are greatly influenced by interpersonal relations and the total life experience. He also stated that the emotional symptoms may be influenced by constitutional endowment, the retardation, and the "special vulnerability of retarded children to problems in personality development."

Menolascino (1965, 1966) reported initially on a series of 616 children evaluated at the Nebraska Psychiatric Institute. All children had been referred with "a suspicion of mental retardation," ranged in age from seven days to eight years, and were mainly outpatients. Of the 616 children, 191 (31 per cent) "displayed prominent psychiatric problems . . . of a nature and extent to warrant a formal AAMD and/or APA diagnosis." Of the 191 cases, "40 were considered to have primary emotional disturbances without mental retardation, and 151 (33 per cent of the total 576, excluding the 40 cases not retarded) were considered to be both emotionally disturbed and mentally retarded."

Menolascino (1968) later reported on 1,025 young children of which 153 boys and 103 girls, whose ages ranged from 1.6 to 14.2 years, were diagnosed "emotionally disturbed and mentally retarded." In this report, Menolascino classified the four most frequent types of emotional disturbance in these 256 retarded children as follows: "Chronic brain syndromes with behavioral and/or psychotic reactions (117 cases), functional psychosis (8 cases), adjustment reactions of childhood (39 cases) and psychiatric disturbance not otherwise specified (11 cases)." The fourth group were all in the moderate range of retardation and "commonly displayed frequent periods of general irritability against a personality backdrop of passivity, inflexibility and personal immaturity." He elaborated on descriptive features and differential diagnosis of the emotional disturbances, clarifying the interplay of different influences on development and describing management of the different types of disorders.

In a subsequent personal communication, Menolascino stated that his studies did not include specific efforts to determine common emotional characteristics in the more than 700 retarded children who were not diagnosed as emotionally disturbed, and that the observations and impressions of his evaluation team were consistent with the description of primary psychopathology given by Webster (1963) and in the present chapter. He further noted that retarded children have a high frequency of special sensory and integrative disturbances, such as visual and motor problems, and that these problems obviously influence the capacity of these youngsters to use play as a means for emotional problem solving. Menolascino also raised the possibility that sensory and integrative disturbances alter the children's view of reality and their own body image, which could have implication for their unique personality development. He pointed out that many external factors, not just the physical condition of the child, lead to sensory or emotional deprivation, particularly those that affect the early mother-child relationships. Lastly, he observed that in school situations retarded children tend to demonstrate less humor, less creativity, less interest in language, and reduced ability to abstract, all of which tends to alter their play patterns markedly.

A CLINICAL STUDY OF
YOUNG RETARDED CHILDREN

After an initial review of methodology, this report of a clinical study (reported in part, previously, Webster, 1963), will approach the problems of emotional development in retarded children through the following four perspectives: a review of 159 cases of young retarded children for the purpose of noting any gross trends in medical diagnosis, degree of retardation, severity of demonstrable brain disease, and severity of emotional disturbance; a description (with case illustrations) of what appeared to be the primary psychopathology of the mental-retardation syndrome; a description of secondary influences that commonly complicated emotional development in the retarded children studied; and a description of moderate and severe emotional disturbances that were commonly observed in our series of children.

Methods of the Study

The 159 cases of this study included all those children who came for intake interviews in their application for the nursery schools of the Boston Preschool Retarded Children's Program [3] during the first three years of operation, 1958–1961. To be accepted for intake interviews, the child had to (1) be between three and six years old, (2) live with his parents in the greater Boston area and with parents who could arrange transportation to a nursery school in their vicinity, (3) have had a previous medical examination with reports available to us, (4) have had reasonable evidence of mental retardation, and (5) be ambulatory. Only one child who met the above criteria was excluded from the study. His application was withdrawn before sufficient data could be obtained on him.

The basis of this study was a review by the author of the 159 case records, which included a copy of the hospital birth record, all available medical and hospital records, interviews with parents, psychiatric diagnostic interviews, psychological tests, reports of the nursery teachers, and reports of case conferences. In some cases the reports were not complete, but for each child there was sufficiently detailed information for the author to feel able to make the gross clinical judgments used in the present study. We are indebted to the hospitals and neurologists who were our major source of referrals and medical data.[4] Children for whom further neurological examination, electroencephalogram (EEG), or laboratory studies were indicated were referred for such evaluation and reports were obtained. The rating of the degree of mental retardation was based primarily on psychological testing by means of the Stanford-Binet Test, the Merrill-Palmer Test, the Cattell Infant Intelligence Scale, and the Vineland Social Maturity Scale, but other tests, separately or in addition to the foregoing, were given in individual cases. Where there had been more than one psychological evaluation over the years, the estimate used was based on what seemed the most reliable testing, which often presented also the highest performance of the child. In a majority of cases the psychologist had to utilize his or her clinical judgment in arriving at an estimate based upon a variety of tests and performance factors. In this respect we were pleased that most of the testing was done by psychologists [5] who were trained in this complex task under Dr. Edith Meyer Taylor at the Children's Medical Center of Boston. A monograph by Dr. Taylor (1959) describes her methods for psychological appraisal of children with cerebral defects.

Those cases in which the psychologist felt the least reliability in estimating intellectual ability were apt to be also the cases in which the psychiatrists found moderate or severe disturbances in emotional development. In addition, they were apt to be also the cases in which there were wide variations in the way the child was perceived in the independent views of the neurologist, psychologist, psychiatrist, social worker, and teacher. Another source of difference in independent opinions occurred when clinicians and teachers were misled in their estimate of the degree of retardation by a child's winning ways in social functioning. The psychological testing then provided reliable evidence of more limited intellectual capacity than others had surmised.

It was out of these experiences with 159 cases that we all gradually became more sophisticated in our understanding of young retarded children. Gradually the author became better able to sort out those emotional characteristics which seemed most closely associated with the degree of mental retardation. These characteristics are later presented as part of the "primary psychopathology of the mental-retardation syndrome."

The ratings of the severity of emotional disturbance represent clinical estimates made by the author at the time of reviewing all relevant material in the 159 case records. The basis for the ratings (+ to + + +) is evident in the clinical descriptions. These ratings and the clinical descriptions are based on observations by the author in individual psychiatric diagnostic sessions with eighty-six of the children. Most of the other seventy-three children were either observed by the author in the nurseries, or had psychiatric evaluation by other examiners in the same agency or elsewhere, and some underwent both. Weekly consultations with one or more teachers during the three-year period and multiple psychiatric interviews with a few of the children also familiarized the author with the children on a continuing longitudinal basis.

The emphasis of the present report is on the clinical observations and discussion, especially the sections on primary psychopathology, secondary influences complicating emotional development, and moderate and severe disturbances in emotional development. The last of these sections and Table 1–1 also present background information and orientation to the other two sections. It should be kept in mind that the basic nature of the entire study was an exploratory one based on many clinical observations and judgments. Anyone who has attempted to evaluate such young retarded children, whether neurologically, psychologically, or psychiatrically, can appreciate the many difficulties involved. Hence, the categories in Table 1–1 and in the section on moderate and severe disturbances in emotional development are necessarily rather gross and the ratings are at times arbitrary. An attempt at finer distinctions would convey a false sense of precision in this complex clinical task.

Review of 159 Cases, Statistical Trends

Characteristics of the Sample

The data in Table 1–1 can first be reviewed with questions as to the nature of the group of children as a whole.

What sort of retarded children show up for a community preschool program such as this? What sort of children form the basis for the clinical observations to be described later?

WIDE VARIETY OF DIAGNOSTIC TYPES

An initial inspection of Table 1–1 reveals the great variety of cases. Despite the restrictions imposed by the method of their selection, these 159 children provide a roughly representative sample of young retarded children, missing mainly the familial cases and milder varieties that do not appear until a later age. Thus, every major clinical type of retarded child and several of the rarer types are represented. All the degrees of retardation from severe to borderline also are included, but no extreme cases with IQ's below 20 or cases that are clearly above the borderline range. Finally, many different types of emotional disturbance with varying degrees of severity also appear in the table.

TABLE 1–1

Distribution of the Severity of Three Handicaps
According to Medical Diagnosis

		DEGREE OF RETARDATION	SEVERITY OF BRAIN DISEASE	SEVERITY OF EMOTIONAL DISTURBANCE
Mongoloid (N=39)	+	4 (borderline)	8 (mild)	29 (mild)
	+ +	24 (IQ 50–69)	31 (moderate)	10 (moderate)
	+ + +	11 (IQ 20–49)	0 (severe)	0 (severe)
Metabolic disorder	+	0	0	2
(N=4)	+ +	2	3	2
	+ + +	2	1	0
Organic brain disorder, other types:				
Prenatal with skull	+	2	9	7
anomaly (N=24)	+ +	11	11	15
	+ + +	11	4	2
Prenatal, other	+	1	2	2
(N=8)	+ +	2	5	5
	+ + +	5	1	1
Perinatal (N=14)	+	0	3	5
	+ +	6	6	7
	+ + +	8	5	2
Postnatal (N=9)	+	2	1	1
	+ +	3	5	7
	+ + +	4	3	1
Undetermined	+	3	15	4
origin (N=22)	+ +	13	7	15
	+ + +	6	0	3
Familial (N=6)	0	—	3	—
	+	1	3	1
	+ +	3	0	4
	+ + +	2	0	1
Childhood psychosis,	0	—	14	—
functional (N=16)	+	4	2	0
	+ +	8	0	2
	+ + +	4	0	14
Etiology undetermined	0	—	10	—
(N=16)	+	4	7	5
	+ +	8	0	9
	+ + +	5	0	3
	0	—	28	—
	+	21	49	56
Totals	+ +	80	68	76
(N=159)	+ + +	58	14	27
		159	159	159

The socioeconomic spectrum of participating families varied from minority group families in urban poverty areas with mothers on Aid to Dependent Children to professional families living in suburban areas. The majority of nursery classes were located in or near poverty areas, and many of the children came from poverty areas, but the average socioeconomic level of all families served exceeded that of poverty areas.

A group of children who were missed by this program were the type who are unlikely to appear for special medical and educational help until after they have started to attend regular school. Presumably, they would include many familial cases and many children who are mildly retarded. They would be likely to have a lower prevalence of organic brain disease and less evidence of emotional disturbance than the children in our series. However, we are guarded in making diagnostic assumptions about children we did not see. For example, our experiences with "familial" cases raised some doubts about the assumptions that usually accompany such a diagnosis. Of the children in our series whom we could regard as "familial," several were classified in other categories on the basis of demonstrable brain disease. The remainder were classified as familial, and there was moderate or severe emotional disturbance in all but one of them.

Some of the children who later show up as retarded in regular school might function above the retarded range during the preschool period. A preschool child who functioned with an IQ in the 80's was rarely referred to our program. Most such children are kept at home or can be referred to a normal nursery school elsewhere in the community.

We would like to emphasize that, whatever the nature of the many cases that were missed by our program, the absent cases represent a large and fertile field for early diagnosis and help. Most of these particular children are not likely to receive attention during the preschool period without the development of special case-finding methods. Fortunately, subsequent to our study Operation Headstart was initiated and now reaches many of the types of children of which we had only a small sample.

PROMINENCE OF BRAIN DISEASE,
MODERATELY SEVERE RETARDATION,
AND EMOTIONAL DISTURBANCE

As might be anticipated in such a community program, the children who show up at this early age include a relatively high proportion of cases with organic brain disease. Roughly five out of six demonstrated fairly clear evidence of organic brain disease. We could conservatively say that well over half the children had unquestionable evidence of brain disease. A finding that does not appear in Table 1–1 was that thirty out of the eighty-two children with "organic brain disease, other types" had convulsive disorders.

Included also was a relatively high proportion of the more severely retarded children. Over one-third of them had an estimated IQ or developmental quotient below 50. This is twice the proportion usually estimated for the total population of retardates.

Another characteristic of the present series was the frequency of moderate or severe disturbances in emotional development. In our series of children, 17 per cent were rated as severely disturbed (psychotic) and 48 per cent were moderately disturbed. Other psychiatric studies, such as those mentioned in the review of the literature earlier in this chapter, are consistent in finding large proportions with moderate or severe disturbances.

NONE WERE "SIMPLY RETARDED"

Efforts to find a child who was simply retarded, one who was developing just like other children except more slowly, were in vain. Even those retarded children who showed the best emotional development were not comparable to nonretarded children of the same mental age. The author believes that, if the emotional development of retarded children differs in quality from that of nonretarded children, an effort should be made to define the unique qualities that are fundamental to retarded development. In the section on primary psychopathology, this unique variety of emotional development is defined and illustrated as a component of primary psychopathology of this mental-retardation syndrome. The definition and description are based particularly, but not exclusively, on observations of the retarded children who demonstrated the mildest degrees of disturbance in emotional development for their respective degrees of retardation.

MEDICAL DIAGNOSIS FREQUENTLY DIFFICULT,
ETIOLOGY OFTEN OBSCURE

A final point that comes to mind while viewing the group of children as a whole is the problem of accurate medical diagnosis. Even with relatively thorough and competent evaluations, there were still approximately 25 per cent of the cases, those listed in the two categories of undetermined etiology, which could not be easily classified in even the gross categories used. In most of these cases there were factors that might lead the casual observer to jump to conclusions, such as family history or suggestive findings, but they would not hold up convincingly under closer scrutiny.

Trends According to Three Medical Diagnostic Subgroups

A breakdown of the data according to medical diagnosis reveals three basic types of diagnostic clusters:

The first cluster is that seen in the mongoloids and in those with metabolic disorders. These groups of children have moderate amounts of demonstrable brain disease, relatively mild degrees of emotional disturbance, and an absence of severe emotional disturbance.

The second diagnostic type is seen rather consistently in the five categories of "organic brain disease, other types." These categories contain all but one of the severe cases of demonstrable brain disease and a preponderance of moderate brain disease. (The cases of brain disease of undetermined origin are an exception in that they have a preponderance of mild brain disease.) In each of these five categories there is a characteristic distribution of emotional disturbance; that is, a preponderance of moderate disturbance with comparatively smaller proportions of mild and severe disturbances.

The third diagnostic type is seen in the last three diagnostic categories: familial, functional childhood psychosis, and etiology undetermined. In these categories there was an absence (or at most a questionable, mild degree) of demonstrable brain disease and few cases of mild emotional disturbance, but a preponderance of moderate or severe emotional disturbance. A subcategory of this third type of diagnostic cluster involves the "familial" and "etiology undetermined" categories. While they most resemble functional childhood psychosis in the relative absence of demonstrable brain disease, they more nearly resemble the "organic brain diseases, other types" in the distribution of emotional disturbance.

A question is raised as to whether these three different diagnostic clusters have any relation to the severity of retardation. For example, might the third type, which has the least brain disease and the most emotional disturbance, contain the milder cases of retardation? The interesting fact is that each of these three clusters contains roughly the same distribution of ratings as far as the severity of retardation is concerned: approximately 15 per cent borderline retardation, 50 per cent with an IQ of 50 to 69, and 35 per cent with an IQ below 50. There is a tendency for those of the third diagnostic type to be less retarded and for those of the second type to be more retarded, but this slight difference is unimpressive. The most remarkable fact is that there is so little difference in the degrees of retardation between these two groups, considering they have a marked difference in the amount of brain disease.

The comparison between the first and third groups is also remarkable. For example: a sample of retarded children from the community, such as those applying for a public nursery, can be broken down into one group that is primarily composed of mongoloids and a second group primarily composed of all the children with no demonstrable brain disease. One might expect that the latter group would tend to include the more mildly retarded, for example, the "familial or physiological" cases, and that the mongoloid group would tend to contain the more severe degrees of retardation. In point of fact, the two groups show essentially the same degrees of retardation; however, they do differ markedly in the degrees of emotional disturbance.

The term "mongolian idiot," commonly used in earlier years and in England, implied that an extreme degree of retardation was quite directly associated with mongolism. The mongoloid children of this study included no idiots (IQ less than 25) and tended to have lesser degrees of retardation than is usually found in institutional reports. For example, twenty-three of thirty-nine have IQ's above 50. This is consistent with a clinical impression of Benda (1960) that mongoloid children reared at home tend to show lesser degrees of retardation than mongoloids in institutions.

A second interesting feature of the mongoloid children was their notable absence of severe emotional disturbance.[6] There was also a notably high proportion of mongoloids with only mild emotional disturbance. Some relevant factors in the parent-child relations of mongoloids will be brought out in later discussion, but the author does not presume to explain these striking findings in solely environmental terms.

Implications

The three broad diagnostic clusters are useful for clarifying trends. However, the categories are too broad to make any specific etiologic inferences, except in the case of mongolism. One must also bear in mind the method of case selection. For example, the fact that 153 of 159 cases had either demonstrable brain disease or moderately severe emotional disturbance certainly raises questions regarding the actual prevalence of uncomplicated "familial" or "physiological" retardation. But in this particular series, such a phenomenon could merely indicate that retarded children do not show up for preschool nurseries unless they have organic brain disease or serious emotional complications. By the same token, the mongoloid children who appear for nurseries may include an unusually high proportion of all mongoloid cases in the community owing to the obvious stigmata by which they are identified at an early age. This factor of selection could partially account for the higher proportion of mongoloids with mild retardation and optimal emotional development. That is, had such a child no stigmata, his parents would be less likely to seek help while he is of preschool age. A similarly selective factor could be significant in determining whether a child is institutionalized. Hence one cannot use the limited data of the present study to make an inference such as, for example, mongoloid children will not become so retarded if they are kept out of institutions, even though the inference may be true. On the other hand, the diagnostic data of this study do refute certain stereotypes and raise new questions regarding mongolism.

The tabulated data of Table 1−1 merit more detailed breakdown. A number of interesting questions are raised which would require a separate and more detailed study of the available data. Only the gross trends have been described, because they are most germane to the present report on emotional development of mentally retarded children.

The gross statistical trends have been useful in clarifying the relationship of four major variables including medical diagnosis, intellectual functions, brain disease, and emotional development in mental retardation, thereby challenging some of the assumptions which are sometimes made in clinical evaluations of individual children. Perhaps equally striking is the fact that such statistical trends are not more prominent, that there are so many exceptions. The exceptions point up the degree to which these four major factors are somewhat independent of each other and merit separate evaluation in each individual case. A fourfold diagnosis is of great value in understanding a retarded child in these various perspectives and is especially helpful in consultations with teachers and in efforts to help parents gain an understanding of the child as a unique individual. In spite of the usefulness of the study of certain trends in a large series of retarded children, there is much that remains to be understood only by means of a thorough study of individual cases.

The diagnostic findings in this heterogeneous series of retarded children brought emphasis to the fact that mental retardation is in its nature a clinical syndrome; it cannot be equated with an intellectual defect, a metabolic defect, or a brain disease as such. Nor can it be regarded simply as a slower version of normal development. The syndrome can best be understood in dynamic developmental terms, regardless of the specific etiologic factors contributing to it. To emphasize that mental retardation is a syndrome need not detract from the obvious relevance of understanding the various intellectual and etiologic factors with greater specificity. The emphasis on the syndrome can, however, combat certain stereotypes and open new areas to investigation.

The mental-retardation syndrome regularly includes disturbances in emotional development which only recently have become generally recognized and are still not very clearly defined in much of the literature on mental retardation. An awareness of the type of diagnostic data herein described should reduce the tendency in a given case to maintain a concrete concept of a direct relation between the emotional disorder, the brain disease, and the retardation instead of appreciating the dynamic developmental processes that are involved. Some characteristics of the disturbances in the developmental process will be described in the sections on primary psychopathology, secondary influences complicating emotional development, and moderate and severe disturbances in emotional development. There is still so much uncertainty and controversy in the literature on the relation between organic brain disease, childhood psychosis, and mental retardation, that it is useful to define more clearly the specific features that are most unique to the mental-retardation syndrome, as distinguished from other emotional complications commonly observed in children with either mental retardation, organic brain disease, or both.

Primary Psychopathology of the Mental-Retardation Syndrome

In this study, psychological characteristics that were more consistently associated with the degree of retardation than with any other diagnostic factor are termed the "primary psychopathology of the mental-retardation syndrome." Primary psychopathology refers only to basic clinical features and to the disturbance in emotional development and neither to primary etiology nor to underlying neuropathology.

Since the primary psychopathology includes only features that, in our series, were observed to be roughly proportional to the degree of retardation, the manifestations were mild in mildly retarded children. In some mildly retarded children with relatively optimal emotional development and in children with moderate or severe emotional disturbance, these behavioral features of primary psychopathology were sometimes sufficiently subtle or clouded by other traits so that they were not necessarily the personality characteristics that came most readily to the attention of individual examiners, teachers, or the parents of a particular child. However, in a retrospective review of the records and further confirmatory observations of children still in the nurseries, we were unable to find cases in which features of primary psychopathology were definitely lacking. Furthermore, in moderately and severely retarded children these features appeared commonly and often prominently in the recorded descriptions of the children. Naturally, the "textbook case" with all features prominent and clear of other complications was the exception rather than the rule.

There are three basic features in the primary psychopathology. The first two features are generally recognized and will not receive elaboration here: they are the intellectual impairment or specific learning difficulty and the slow rate of development. Less generally recognized is the third feature, the disturbance in the quality of emotional development. That feature includes developmental disturbance with impairment in the differentiation of ego functions. The slow and incomplete unfolding of the personality is associated with partial fixations, which result in an infantile or immature personality structure. This particular style of ego development is accompanied by special descriptive features: a nonpsychotic autism, repetitiousness, inflexibility, passivity, and simplicity in emotional life.

The Developmental Disturbance

Despite the fact that there was sufficient growth and ego differentiation to pass developmental milestones at a rather consistent rate, close observation revealed that in many ways there was only a superficial resemblance to normal emotional development. The advancing phases of ego differentiation involved a lesser segment of the ego and differed in quality from the maturation of a nonretarded child. Some of this impairment in ego function was concealed from the casual observer by virtue of functions that were imitative in nature or were learned by rote conditioning. For example, a six-year-old retarded child with a mental age of three had six years to learn certain behavior patterns that resembled, or even exceeded, those of a nonretarded three-year-old. However, a quite different emotional foundation underlies such functions. This poor differentiation of ego functions was observed in a variety of areas: modification of instinctual impulses, reality orientation, object relations, and the achievement of autonomy. Practically all retarded children we observed showed poor development in their capacity to make emotionally significant distinctions between the familiar and the unfamiliar, between friends and strangers, between persons and places, and between persons and inanimate objects.

The retarded child's emotional development is impaired by a difficulty in finding new solutions for old conflicts and frustrations. We noted an impairment in the capacity for spontaneous displacement of drives to new interests. Rather than seeking them spontaneously, the children often had to be led into new interests. There was a tendency toward repetition and inflexibility in solving emotional problems just as in other functions.

The following four case vignettes illustrate the primary psychopathology in four of the children who showed some of the least disturbance in emotional development and the best integration of ego functions.

Rod was a 6-year-old mongoloid boy with a mental age of approximately 4 years. He displayed a wider range of emotional expression than most of the children in the nursery and was pleasant, sociable, and a cooperative participant in most of the nursery routines. He had a close companionship with a younger brother at home. In the nursery he was for a while attached to one of the other boys whom he seemed to miss when the other boy was absent. In his individual diagnostic sessions his initial greetings to the psychologist and the psychiatrist were the same as to his mother, his teachers, and often to other children, i.e., a hug and a kiss with mild but genuine pleasure. During his psychiatric session he demonstrated some phallic interests in guns, table legs, a chimney, etc., all of which is common in 4-year-old boys but quite uncommon in the children in our series. He was unfamiliar with the punching bag, but after brief instructions and an invitation to hit it he gave it a slap. He then stepped back and said with genuine apology to the punching bag, "I'm sorry." While initially somewhat reluctant to leave his mother and go with the doctor, he immediately acquiesced as soon as the doctor took his hand, and did not show direct signs of missing his mother until late in the interview. Throughout the session he kept in close verbal and physical contact with the doctor, seemingly not so much because of the threat a stranger imposed, but as a source of comfort and satisfaction. At the end of the session he spontaneously extended his hand to shake farewell, as though well trained in proper behavior, then offered another kiss. During his first year in nursery school he functioned well in all types of activities, but he did not progress as rapidly as the teacher expected on the basis of his behavior and apparent ease in handling the routines. The teacher commented, "Rod seems to have little inner motivation of his own, but he follows along compliantly and seems to enjoy himself." His teacher also noted that despite his sociability and cooperativeness, if left unstimulated he would continue in isolated activity indefinitely. "If left alone, Rod would spend the day playacting in a little dream world of his own."

Archie was a 5-year-old boy with mild cerebral palsy. On verbal tasks he functioned slightly above the 3-year level, on motor performance tasks at about the 2½-year level. He was warm and friendly, more so with adults than with children. He was especially close to his mother after three deaths in the family, and the separation process in the nursery was a protracted one. However, his moments of tears and asking for his mother seemed to represent unusually advanced object relations as we observed him gradually deal with the separation. He took to nursery routines quite well and with apparent enjoyment, though the first month he had to be led by the hand through all routines. The teacher commented that if not interrupted by other children, "he would ride the truck the entire morning." His mother first stayed in the nursery room, then outside in the hall where Archie could go to reassure himself when he needed to. One day Archie began crying as though missing his mother, went to the door, and—to the teacher's concern—found no mother in the hall. Archie turned around smiling and comforted as usual, and thereafter a trip to the hallway was all it took to console him whether mother was present or not.

Martha, a child with cretinism, was referred to us at the age of 5½. She was one of the most advanced in emotional development among our most severely retarded children. When she first was hospitalized for evaluation at the age of 10 months, her parents described her as a "good baby" who practically never fussed or cried. But she was a poor feeder, and they were concerned about her slow development. She was started on thyroid at that time, with dramatic improvement within forty-eight hours. When seen by us four years later, she was still severely retarded with a mental age under 2 years and a developmental quotient of around 30. She was still in diapers, walked with an unsteady toddler's gait, was below the third percentile in height and weight. Though her affect was flat, she was capable of more intense affect than most children who are so severely retarded. She had a mild smile, a tense excitement, and a frightened tearless cry. She took more interest in her environment than is usually seen in severely retarded children. Still, the nature of her activity was very monotonous and repetitious. When she had a bowel movement during the middle of her psychiatric session, she showed not the slightest trace of concern and did not seem to understand the doctor's reference to it or why she was taken to her father. Though she had shown no concern for her father during the earlier part of the interview, when it was later made clear that her father was in the room next door, she began going back and forth from one room to the other. In doing this she paid attention neither to her father nor the doctor, and she seemed to show no preference for one room over the other, being easily led in either direction if the doctor intervened. She discovered there was a telephone in each room and began going back and forth from one phone to the other, with increasing signs of satisfaction and a relaxation of an earlier underlying tension.

Freddy, a 5-year-old mongoloid boy, was unimpressed when a nun came to visit the nursery. She was introduced as Sister Mary Theresa. Freddy showed none of the curiosity and awe many 3- and 4-year olds would show if they were not very familiar with nuns. Neither did he show any of the special reactions of a child who was familiar with a nun as a special sort of person. When about an hour later the teacher and some of the children were saying goodby to "Sister," Freddy looked up from his play long enough to wave and exclaim, "So long, Mary!"

In any single one of the preceding incidents one could find a number of ways to explain the child's reaction. One might have thought nothing of Freddy's remark to the nun except to assume it was one of those cute remarks young children can make with such simplicity and directness. Or it could be assumed that Freddy's inexperience and limited intellect prevented him from perceiving anything unusual about a nun. With Rod one could have assumed that he was apologizing to the doctor for having hit the punching bag. One might have been impressed with Archie's ability to substitute a ritual for his missing mother. One might think that Martha was able to use the telephones as symbolic representations of persons and thus achieve a solution to her separation anxieties. All these explanations may be true to some degree, but after getting to know many such children and observing many such incidents, we became increasingly impressed with the relatively primitive ego functions that underlie such behavior. In a very real and direct manner Rod was making a sincere apology to the punching bag, not to the doctor. Archie's instantaneous substitution of the doorway ritual and the view of the hallway for his missing mother involved a more primitive process and much less differentiation of his mother as an object than one might suppose from other features of his separation reaction. The difficulty in making emotionally significant distinctions between objects is a characteristic of basic ego function, not merely an intellectual limitation.

The poorly differentiated ego functions that underlie superficially normal behavior were observed in the separation reactions of the children at the beginning and end of their clinic sessions. They displayed much the same variety of separation reactions as can be observed in nonretarded children, but the retarded children's reactions tended to be less intense and less definite. They were less apt to show a specific sign of relief and pleasure in viewing or rejoining their mothers after an initial interview. Often it seemed almost by accident that the child happened to return to the same room as the parent, and he was just as apt to wander on or take a mild interest in something on the social worker's desk as he was to show signs of recognizing his mother. This is not to say the mother was not meaningful. Some such reactions presumably involved a resentful ignoring of the mother, as is often observed in young children who are reunited after a separation. But the source and nature of the anxiety of the children studied were apparently not nearly so specific in their minds as one might at first suppose. As experience with such children accumulated, the child psychiatrist developed the impression that he had been overinterpreting certain behavior on the basis of his experience with nonretarded children. For example, he was inclined to assume too readily that some aimless wandering past the mother was "separation anxiety."

In the nurseries there were many instances of poorly differentiated ego functions. For example, our teachers observed that these children were not so likely to have special school behavior compared to home behavior as nonretarded nursery children.

Special Descriptive Features

There was an *autism* in each child's emotional life despite a capacity for social responsiveness and warm object relations. People were important, but to some degree these children could take them or leave them. Sometimes the autism was obscured by a symbiotic mother-child relation or by a child's impulsive hyperactive behavior, either of which tended to keep him in contact with others. However, if left unstimulated, practically all our retarded children could settle rather readily into contented isolated activity (like Rod's "dream world of his own"). The hazy boundaries of the retarded child's private world seemed to be defined by his own restricted attention rather than by a defensive barrier. The child's private world could be entered or left with remarkable ease. Apparently this was due to his passive responsiveness and to the concrete superficial quality of the relation he established. The more retarded the child the less personal was the quality of this contact.

Repetitiousness was observed in many areas of the child's functioning. In his emotional life there was a tendency to repeat the familiar, which usually involved an element of pleasure seeking and contentment, such as Archie's "riding the truck the entire morning" if not interrupted. He did not exclude the unfamiliar, he just had no interest in it.

The tendency to repeat the familiar apparently contributed to an *inflexibility* that was commonly observed in our series of retarded children. The inflexibility was distinguished from repetitiousness in that the latter seemed more closely related to motivational drive. The inflexibility was also distinguished from negativism and compulsive traits (to be discussed shortly) which are not part of the primary psychopathology. However, inflexibility commonly reinforces these latter traits.

The monotony and boredom one associates with the repetitious activity of retarded children seemed more a reaction of the observer than of the child. However, dullness or flatness of affect was common, and the most notable exceptions to this were among the mildly retarded. Is emotional flatness a part of the primary psychopathology? In our observations, the intensity of affect was so variable and so obviously related to other factors that the author regarded flattened affect as a secondary complication.

Closely related to other primary traits was the *passivity* of the retarded children. They were responsive if stimulated, but they did not tend to seek external objects except in terms of some rather immediate direct gratification. They could enjoy and enter into new worldly experience if led by the hand until conditioned to it. But there was relatively little spontaneous reaching out into the outer world or fascination with the new. The hyperactive and aggressive impulsiveness of some retarded children was easily confused with an active interest in the world about them. Sometimes the teachers described a child as curious or exploring, but closer observation revealed that such activity had a driven quality about it. The child had been taken over by his own impulses, and the drive tended to lack a more purposive investigative quality. The motor activity did not yet function in the service of the ego. The activity had not yet been integrated with those pleasure-seeking drives by which a child can gain satisfaction from exploring. Neither had the activity been integrated with aggressive drives in the form of a specific move to eliminate a specific threat or frustration.

Another trait was the *simplicity of emotional life* of the retarded children. As a descriptive trait, such simplicity is common knowledge to all who know retarded individuals. In the developmental perspective the simplicity is one more manifestation of the undifferentiated ego. For example, there was a tendency for simple direct expression of basic instinctual drives, although this was sometimes obscured by secondary emotional complications, such as deeply established inhibitions.

Differential Diagnosis

The autism or isolation of mental retardation differed from the autism of *psychotic children* in that the autism of the retarded (1) was not such a prominent feature, except when the retardation was severe; (2) was not so highly developed as a defense that actively excluded the outer world, (3) tended not to involve as much fragmentation of ego functions with its associated distortions and bizarreness, and (4) coexisted with a more consistent, harmonious, appropriate responsiveness to stimuli. The autism of mental retardation is perhaps a more truly *infantile* autism than the condition to which Kanner (1957) gave the term, for the former more nearly resembles the undifferentiated early infantile ego. One may well imagine that this infantile aspect is a predisposing factor to the higher incidence of psychotic autism among retarded children. The close association of the two types of autism was also evident in our observation that in the most severely retarded children there was greater difficulty in the differential diagnosis between retardation and psychotic autism.

The repetitiousness and inflexibility were partially related to *perseveration* as described by psychologist-examiners and as commonly found in organic brain syndromes. However, perseveration is of a slightly different nature and not so closely related to the degree of retardation. Perseveration could be observed as a purely intellectual function in psychological testing, and it could sometimes function as a security operation in the face of anxiety. The repetitiousness of the primary psychopathology, on the other hand, was more closely associated with pleasure seeking. It is common knowledge that retarded children can find pleasure in activities that become boring and monotonous for others.

Negativism and compulsive traits were commonly observed. However, since they were not so closely related to the degree of retardation and were secondary to other factors, they could be distinguished from the primary psychopathology. Negativism partly represents a phase of ego maturation, and some of the more severely retarded children had not achieved much of this stage. The retarded child's negativism contained a lesser element of self-assertion than that seen in most two-year olds, thus reflecting his basic passivity. Also, there was a tendency to acquiesce if firmly pressed. In children we observed over a period of two years we noted that this negativism, which is partly a step toward greater autonomy, did not develop into self-sufficiency comparable to the transition in nonretarded children.

Negativism and compulsive traits were commonly exaggerated by virtue of the tug-of-war to which the retarded child and his mother were predisposed, particularly if the child's condition and abilities were still uncertain. The more extreme degrees were often due to a specific mother-child relation of the same type that is seen in negativistic or compulsive nonretarded children.

The inflexibility differed from compulsiveness in that the inflexibility was related to the degree of retardation and functioned with a complacency or a paucity of available responses. Repetitiousness was associated with a drive that tended to repeat the familiar. Compulsions, on the other hand, had a more forceful defensive quality, with ambivalence and a defensive posture against aggression. The latter were associated with the same classical emotional conflicts found in any compulsive child. The inflexibility and repetitiousness appeared to be strong predisposing factors in the development of compulsive defenses. In severely retarded children the inflexibility and repetitiousness were so prominent, and the capacity for object relations was so limited, that it was at times difficult to distinguish true compulsive defenses from the primary psychopathology.

Discussion of Primary Psychopathology

In attempting to describe primary psychopathology on the basis of observations of this particular series of children, one must have some reservations because of the selection of cases studied. Since there was such a preponderance of cases studied with organic brain disease, might these observations have been more specific for organic brain disease than for mental retardation? May there be many children in the community who are mildly retarded but who do not have the features that are here described as part of the primary psychopathology? May the primary psychopathology be partially a manifestation of the deprivation that is so common in the early experience of many retarded children?

Regarding the first question, there was no clinical evidence in this series of children that the features described as primary psychopathology had any consistent or prominent relation with the type or degree of brain pathology. On the contrary, it was difficult to identify any single emotional feature that was consistently related to brain disease unless one became more specific as to which type of brain disease. Also, the primary psychopathology was observed in the cases without demonstrable brain disease and had a rather consistent relation to the severity of retardation.

The second question certainly merits a more complete sampling and psychiatric study of mildly retarded children in the community.

However, on the basis of the data we have, of clinical descriptions in the literature, and of our theoretical knowledge, we would be surprised to find retarded children who were free of the disturbance in emotional development which has been described. The exceptions would likely be *not* retarded children with optimal emotional development, but some type of pseudoretardation.

The third question is intriguing. Deprivation in the more extreme sense in which that term usually is used in studies of early child development is sufficiently rare and variable so that it definitely was not responsible for all the primary psychopathology in our series of children. However, special types of sensory deprivation based largely on the infant's condition (and partially on the mother's response in some cases) could conceivably be almost universal among retarded children. Close observations of the infancy of potentially retarded children are indicated to clarify whether some special types of deprivation during early development may be very crucial experiences by which brain pathology, sensory pathology, metabolic deficiencies, and environmental deprivation act in combinations that produce the syndrome of mental retardation.

Secondary Influences That Commonly Complicate Emotional Development

Retarded children are subjected to an unusual number of complicating influences other than their retarded state. Naturally, they are subject to the usual varieties of complications that can affect both retarded and nonretarded children, but they also have a high liability for special complications. Brain disease, sensory impairment, physical handicaps, illnesses, and other sources of emotional trauma or deprivation were observed with great frequency in our series of children. The response of mother, family and others to the child's condition also brought complications. This section of the chapter deals with complications in emotional development which were associated with these secondary influences. Such complications were more variable and not so intimately related to the degree of retardation as in the case of the primary psychopathology. However, the complications due to secondary influences were more closely related to the *child's condition* than were emotional complications that had more obvious relation to the unique emotional problems of individual parents.

"Primary" and "secondary" as used in this report refer to the degree of association with the mental-retardation syndrome, not to either etiology or the relative prominence of different clinical features in individual cases. For example, a "secondary" influence or complication for purposes of the present report may, in fact, have been a primary factor in the assessment of an individual case.

Deprivation

The first secondary influence is deprivation with its aftermath of flattened affect, disturbed ego development, and widespread effects on physical and psychological development. In our observations the amount of deprivation varied rather widely, but we were impressed with how very common it was for this feature to be present to some degree in the great majority of cases. Deprivation is used here in the broad sense of the term to include all types of sensory and perceptual deprivation from whatever cause, of which a real lack of consistent affectionate mothering is only one variety.

Some degree of deprivation is closely associated with the retarded state, regardless of how and when the retardation begins. The tendency toward isolation, the tendency to repeat the familiar and to leave the unfamiliar unexplored, and the impairment in sensory and perceptual capacities all contribute to a relative deprivation of the retarded child's sensory experience. In many of the retarded children in our series the deprivation was also fostered by a placid state that did not demand or stimulate the attention of others. Even in the children who were very warm, responsive, and outgoing, there was underlying primary psychopathology, which contributed to a type of deprivation. Perhaps equally relevant is the fact that the tendency for repetitiousness and the prolonged infancy provide a strong reinforcement of certain primitive sensory experiences. These primitive sensory experiences arise predominantly from the infant's own body, both as inner sensation and as an object for exploration with hand or mouth. By the age of one the retarded infant has had an impoverished contact with the external world; he also has had an unusual amount of repeated experience with certain primitive infantile sensory processes.

Consistent with the foregoing factors, retarded children are less apt than nonretarded children to have instinctual tensions relieved, or wishes gratified, in the intimate presence of another human being. They have a proportionately much greater experience with autoeroticism, touch of self, touch of inanimate objects, and staring at the ceiling. This apparently has an impact on early ego development, contributing to the self-contained world and undifferentiated object relations. We also wondered while observing a retarded child standing and staring out of the window for long periods, or manipulating inanimate objects with hand or mouth, how much such behavior developed as a derivative of early instinctual experience. In this sense the child manifested not only a relative lack of ego differentiation, but a special style of ego differentiation. Unfortunately, such instinctual development further reinforces a barren existence as compared to normal human relations, for there is no genuine counterstimulation, only a very meager and monotonous one.

In cases where the child was comparatively placid or made relatively little demand for attention, we could appreciate that the mother on her part experienced a type of deprivation, namely, deprivation of her maternal interests. Often the children in our series were described as infants who lacked vigor in their sucking. There were also many other ways in which they did not stimulate maternal interest. Since mothers often had many other interests, they usually did not describe this as a deprivation. More commonly they referred to what a good baby the child was, "never any trouble." In addition there was the rejection that could arise from the mother's individual reaction to her retarded child. In some families this was more the mother's distraction or discouragement with the many other demands upon her rather than direct rejection of the child we happened to see. All such features of the mother's experience have their impact on the mother-child relation, thus reinforcing the deprivation the child suffers. A cyclic process is thus set up, *a vicious circle of deprivation.* The tendency toward deprivation is all the more important when one appreciates that, at least after infancy, the attentive care of most retarded children takes an unusual amount of patience and love—day after day and month after month.

In our observations there were two factors (in addition to natural maternal interest) that would reduce the deprivation process. The first was when there was some characteristic of the child which either won or demanded attention, such as appealing appearance or mannerism. In other instances there was something about the child's physical condition or behavior which elicited attention. Paradoxically, we found that some children with physical complications and multiple hospitalizations that demanded much attention and concern seemed to have prospered better in their emotional development than some "good babies" who were never any trouble to anybody.

A second factor we found to ameliorate the deprivation process was when the parents or other members of the family had a lot of affection available in a form that did not require much response from the baby for them to maintain their interest. In such cases the child was likely to be regarded as a doll or a pet and was thus lavished with a lot of interest and affection. Interestingly, many mongoloid children qualified in both respects. They were cute and appealing, and it was easy for the families to think of them as special children in which the families did not have the same expectations as with other children. Our social worker, Miss Virginia Cook, was impressed with how frequently the parents of mongoloid children referred to their child in terms such as "my pet" or "my little monkey," rather than by name.

Regardless of the source and nature of maternal interest, there were many cases in which a warm and affectionate mother-child relation existed. In such cases the child was responsive and stimulated further interest, a reversal of the deprivation cycle. However, even under optimal circumstances the autism and poor ego differentiation of the primary psychopathology were in evidence in the children we observed. This raises a perplexing question: In our usual understanding of early emotional development, an affectionate mother-child relation—one even less optimal than that we observed in several of our cases— would avoid the autism and impaired ego development of the mental-retardation syndrome. Could it be that in such cases, in spite of a rather optimal mother-child relation, some of the maternal stimuli do not "get through" to the child? One is reminded of the decreased sensory capacity for tactile discrimination which has been found in mongoloid children. One is also reminded of the finding that brain-defective infants required a greater stimulus in order to elicit a cry. Can such sensory and perceptual deficits be responsible for a relative deprivation in even the most warm and responsive mother-child relation we have observed? Studies that begin with close observation from the very time of birth can help sort out the potentially retarded infants who from the beginning make relatively little appeal to the mother from those who become listless or placid only after much experience with unanswered pleas or inconsistent mothering as well as sort them out from those who develop the retardation syndrome in spite of a warm responsive interchange between mother and child.

Overstimulation

Less common than deprivation were cases of overstimulation. Some of the children in our series manifested the anxieties that come from overstimulation. This usually occurred at later stages of development, and it can occur even in the presence of a more basic deprivation. In one such case where the child showed clinical evidence of excessive erotic stimulation, we later learned that at the age of seven she was still playing a "hugging game," rolling around with her father before he got out of bed each morning. Such cases remind one of the "pseudoimbecility" described by Mahler-Schoenberger (1942), in which the child's imbecility becomes a "magic cap of invisibility." Parents grant many erotically stimulating privileges by rationalizing that the child "doesn't understand anyway."

Confused Expectations

A third type of secondary influence was that which occurred because of confused expectations on the part of the parents. Misguided expectations led to a push-and-pull struggle between parent and child and to alternating periods of expecting too much and then giving up in despair. One of the effects was an increase in the negativism and compulsive traits of the child. There was also an obvious effect on the emotional relation between parent and child and there were secondary complications in other family relations. Not infrequently, the result was that the parent could not anticipate very accurately what the child was ready to learn, which is an important factor in normal development. Thus the confused expectations can interfere in several ways with learning and development.

Parents' Partial Decathexis of the Child

A fourth type of secondary influence was observed in cases where the parents were still in the midst of the process of accepting a more realistic view of their child's handicap. This is often a gradual process that can go on over a period of years as new evidence is forthcoming or as the parents' intellectual knowledge takes root at deeper levels. At times a fresh awareness of the handicap occurred suddenly with an element of stunned shock on the part of the mother, which led to grief and partial decathexis or withdrawal of emotional investment from the child. Such a process has been observed prior to a decision for institutionalization or following an especially strong confrontation with the fact of the child's handicap. For instance, a child in our nursery was observed to go through a period of prolonged crying spells and then a gradual withdrawal with flattening of affect during the period immediately after a shocking confrontation his mother had experienced at the hands of the mother of an older child with the same condition. The parents assumed that this change in the child was due to a sudden advancement in his Hurler's disease. When the mother was interviewed, she was found to be in a state of tearful grief with mixed feelings that alternated between clasping the child closer and giving him up. First she said that now she loved the child all the more, yet a few minutes later she asked if it were all right to hit him more to discipline him.

One of the prominent differences between the mongoloid cases and most of the other cases was the fact that the mongolism was usually known from shortly after birth, and that it was well defined as an entity to which the parents could adjust. The parents' initial shock was of course great, but they usually had good access to information and displayed good acceptance of the reality because of the child's observable stigmata.

Fusion of Defective Parental Self-Image with the Child's Image

Another common influence on the child's development was the tendency of parents to fuse their image of the child with their own partial image of themselves as defective persons. All the reactions and defenses relevant to their own defective image come into play in their relation with the child and their efforts to gain (or avoid) a realistic understanding of the child's condition. Some parent groups express this by referring to themselves as "EDP's" (emotionally disturbed parents). Counselors of parents must be guarded in overinterpreting the parents' emotional problems, for the parents are reacting in part to an external reality, and a counselor can increase the stress upon parents by unintentionally fostering the image of their own defectiveness. Often when parents pressed us with the question, "Is it (the child's difficulty) emotional?" they seemed to be asking, "Am I to blame?"

Family Reinforcement of Infantilization

A sixth secondary influence was reinforcement by the family of the infantilization of the child. In addition to the immaturity that is part of the primary psychopathology of the retarded child, a more exaggerated infantilization can be fostered by an attitude on the part of the parents which tends to keep the child a perpetual infant. Infantilization is especially likely to happen when the child is the youngest of the mother's children. While we were at first dismayed with how commonly this occurs, we gradually came to the opinion that infantilization is not the worst of solutions, especially during the early developmental years. For all its disadvantages, infantilization or "babying" does at least permit a continuing affectionate parental relation with the child as a separate person, and it does not have the more serious effect on emotional development that we observed with deprivation, decathexis, or fusion of the child with the mother's defective image of herself. Nor does it give rise to the frustrations and resentment caused by an overexpectation and an effort to push the child too fast. Infantilization can also make it more possible for the mother to enjoy the child during the early formative years. On the other hand, one can imagine that this solution leads to special complications as the child gets older.

Frequent, Multiple Emotional Traumata

A seventh common influence on emotional development was the frequent occurrence of emotional traumata. Physical illness was common, and hospitalizations and surgery were not infrequent. Physical handicaps, seizures, and the fact of being different from other children were but some of the factors that increased the stress on the child and the incidence of emotional trauma.

Organic Brain Disease

Last but not least, organic brain disease exerted a major influence on emotional development in a variety of ways in addition to its contribution to the development of a mental-retardation syndrome. A point of interest in the present study was the difficulty we found in generalizing about organic brain disease when we were dealing with such different clinical conditions as mongolism, birth injuries, and postnatal meningitis. In the section that follows, brain disease with relation to disorders of impulse and behavior will be discussed, and it will be seen that seizures are one factor in cases with excessive fears and inhibitions.

Moderate and Severe Disturbances in Emotional Development

In our series of 18 children, 48 per cent were rated as moderately and 18 per cent as severely disturbed in their emotional development. Such children had the primary psychopathology described in an earlier section of this chapter, though this was sometimes obscured or confused by the presence of other characteristics such as impulse disorders or psychosis. Secondary influences (also dealt with previously) were present in one form or another. Factors more specific to individual mothers and homes also figured prominently in many of the moderate and severe disturbances. Because these disturbances were so individualized, the present discussion can only attempt to list some of the major types of disturbance we observed and to describe some of the associated factors involved.

Disorders of Impulse and Behavior

First were the disorders of impulse and behavior. Sometimes we had to draw a rather arbitrary line between impulsive behavior, such as kissing, biting, or hitting, which we regarded as a manifestation of the immature modification of instinctual impulses characteristic of all retarded children, and the more serious disorders of impulse control which were manifestations of either abnormal brain discharges, poor ego control of impulses, or both. In either case the poorly modified impulses had an inevitable impact on emotional development, both in terms of the child's inner experience and in terms of the reactions of others.

In individual cases it was by no means easy to estimate to what degree the impulse was due to the brain disorder as such, for example, an abnormal focus of discharges, and to what degree the impulse was due to the disturbance in the child's ego development. Severe impulse disorders sometimes appeared due to an unusual amount of aggression. In any event, there was certainly a special problem in handling aggression. In comparing our observations with much of the literature on the behavioral manifestations of brain damage, we were struck by the tendency to ascribe a rather direct relation between the behavior disorder and the demonstrable brain disease. We were impressed with the importance of the child's ego development as a factor in his ability to cope with such impulses and with the role parents and teachers could play in helping the child to modify his aggressive impulses. This view is consistent with the psychoanalytic observations regarding two children with organic handicaps as reported by Rank (1949) and Rappaport (1961).

One observation of interest was that despite the hyperactivity, impulsiveness, and strong drives manifested by such children in our study, they were also apt to have periods of the same placidity, passivity, autism, repetitiousness, and lack of truly exploratory interest as have been described under primary psychopathology.

We reviewed our cases of brain damage to see what common behavioral characteristics, if any, such children might have. There were exceptions to every behavior pattern, but the term that seemed best to characterize the behavior of the brain-damaged children was that they were "erratic." Many tended to show impulsive or hyperactive behavior at times. However, the specific pattern this might take, the ego capacity for modifying the impulse and the responsiveness to intervention varied widely. In all these respects it was not possible to distinguish them as a group from some other children with impulse disorders and no evidence of brain damage.

Excessive Shyness, Fears, and Inhibitions

Another type of emotional disturbance of moderate degree occurred in the form of excessive shyness, fears, and inhibitions. While at
times we loosely referred to such children as "phobic," this was only a
partially correct usage of the term. Their anxiety was of a more diffuse immature nature, and their poor development of object relations
did not permit a focusing of the anxiety on a specific object. Sometimes there were special factors, such as a convulsive disorder, which
increased the anxiety. Some of these fearful children were the ones
who responded most favorably to the nursery school experience.
Teachers and parents were often very gratified to see the developmental progress that accompanied the emotional blossoming of such children. However, parents and teachers were not always so pleased with
some of the aggression that accompanied the blossoming. The favorable response to the nursery school was of special interest, because
sometimes the parents of such a fearful, immature child had been cautioned by physicians or other advisors against nursery school for fear
that the child might find it too overwhelming. These observations regarding fears and a favorable response to nursery school were similar
to the findings of Woodward et al. (1958), except that children with
such fears were not so predominant in our series as in their more
highly selected group of nine.

In some retarded children, just as in nonretarded children with
whom the author was familiar at the James Jackson Putnam Children's Center, we found severe degrees of inhibitions that operated at
such deep levels that the child was seen not as frightened, but as an
atypical or psychotic child. Such children sometimes are referred to as
having "borderline atypical development" or "borderline psychosis."
The prognosis for improvement in their mild psychotic features is apt
to be fairly good.

Reaction to Loss

A third type of moderate emotional disturbance was reaction to
loss. The most obvious reactions to loss were those in which we observed the child to be in a dejected state of mind in which tears came
readily and in which there was reasonable evidence of a recent loss,
either through separation or through emotional withdrawal of the parent. When we saw such a grief reaction in our young retarded children,
we tended to feel encouraged to see that the child had a sufficient object relation to be capable of such a reaction. When we saw the child
later brighten up and recover from this state, we regarded the reaction

as a successful grief reaction rather than as a pathological reaction to loss.

When we pursued the more complex forms of loss reaction and depression we experienced greater uncertainty, both in our clinical observations and in our understanding of what was happening. When the loss was not so clearly in evidence and when the observed reaction was not one of active grief, we found the clinical picture of withdrawal, flattened affect, lack of vitality, regression, and listlessness, all of which are so commonly observed in retarded children. There were times when it seemed that the majority of our retarded children were in some such state of reaction to loss or deprivation. Spitz (1946), Rochlin (1961), and others have pointed out that depression in the sense in which we usually use the term cannot occur in such young children, for they do not have the superego and other personality development that are essential for an adult depressive reaction. Some of the literature on reactions to deprivation does not distinguish clearly between a primary sensory and emotional deprivation as compared to rejection-frustration or to loss of the mother or other primary figure through separation. We hope that longitudinal studies of infancy and early childhood will help clarify this significant area of early child development which is so relevant to the problems of the mentally retarded.

Exaggerated Negativism and Compulsiveness

A fourth type of moderate emotional disturbance was an exaggerated state of negativism, compulsiveness, or both. Negativism is often a prominent part of the maturational phase which one would expect to find in preschool retarded children. Negativism and compulsiveness were regarded as a moderate emotional disturbance only in certain exaggerated cases—usually cases in which the child was being pushed for performance or was under pressure to maintain tight control of impulses for other reasons. As was discussed in the section on primary psychopathology, the repetitiousness and inflexibility as well as some of the driven quality of the impulse disorders sometimes resembled compulsive behavior. However, these "compulsions" did not always serve the same defensive functions as compulsiveness in a more technical sense. Some of the "training" routines to which retarded children often respond quite well appear to reinforce certain compulsive traits, sometimes at the expense of maturation. The latter hazard presented a real dilemma for the teacher who wished to foster intellectual development while training the child in the rudiments of socially acceptable behavior.

Immaturity

Another type of disturbance in emotional development was a greater degree of immaturity than would be expected simply from the degree of retardation. When the immaturity was not associated with a comparable degree of autism, we usually found an exaggerated tendency toward infantilization of the child by the mother or another parent figure. Sometimes we also observed exaggerated immaturity in cases where there was a rather symbiotic relation between mother and child.

Regression

Some retarded children had a greater than usual tendency for regression. This could involve a temporary loss of any previously acquired function, including toilet training, clear speech, or social skill. When the regression was more prolonged it sometimes produced the picture of pseudoretardation.

Precocious Sociability and Social Talent

A seventh type of emotional disturbance, which we found was not usually appreciated as pathologic during the preschool period, was a type of precocious sociability and social talent which exceeded most other levels of development and often led to an overestimation of the child's intellectual capacity. Naturally, precocious social ability can occur on more than one basis, and it is not necessarily pathologic. There were a few socially precocious children in our nursery whom we regarded as predelinquent in their evolving character structures. There were some children who used their superficial social talents in such a way that they did not receive recognition or help for some of their more pressing needs, because the parents and teachers tended to accept them as contented and competent. These were often the children who did not progress as expected in the nursery. Rod was a mild example. He was also an example of a certain type of excessive stimulation that can induce precocious social development. His mother called him "da biggest freshie."

Childhood Psychosis, Infantile Autism, or Atypical Development

The last type of disturbance to be discussed is the most severe disturbance: childhood psychosis, infantile autism, or atypical development. This complex subject has had more attention from child psychiatrists than most of the other emotional problems of retarded children. In our series of cases, this severe emotional disturbance was no respecter of medical diagnosis or brain disease, except for its notable absence among the mongoloid children. At least one case of psychosis appeared in every major category of medical diagnosis except mongolism and metabolic disorders (see Table 1–1). In cases where demonstrable brain disease was also present, we became quite guarded in making assumptions as to just what part the brain pathology played in the psychosis. In describing the primary psychopathology and secondary complications, we have attempted to clarify certain characteristics of the child and of the parent-child relation which predispose retarded children to psychosis. We have also elaborated on the distinction between the autism of mental retardation and the ego pathology of atypical or psychotic children.

DISCUSSION

The present discussion will first elaborate on implications for unique personality development which go beyond the aspects of primary psychopathology described in the clinical study. Unique considerations of emotional development in mentally retarded children will then be discussed to clarify concepts and problems of terminology and to place the author's clinical study in perspective with the work of other authors and to spell out the implications for future research.

Unique Personality Development

Intellectual impairment or specific learning difficulty was listed as the first feature of primary psychopathology of the mental-retardation syndrome. The reported clinical study did not elaborate on this first feature, but several implications for unique emotional development should be mentioned.

In addition to the obvious implications for a cumulative impact on intellectual development, the intellectual difficulty has a number of implications for handling the problem solving of emotional and social problems just as in other learning. Limitations in abstraction are closely associated with limitations in language development, symbol formation, and imaginary play. This impairment not only interferes with problem solving at early crucial stages of emotional development, but also has a cumulative effect in that it places the retarded child further and further behind his peers in the growth of his problem-solving capacity with each advancing year. Furthermore, this growth of problem-solving capacity has a time limit, so that after a certain age (for example, seventeen years) he has also lost the theoretical potential for catching up. While the potential for social and emotional growth continues into adult life, the development of the basic problem-solving equipment ends at roughly the same chronological age as for his nonretarded peers.

On the brighter side potentially, the retarded child often has not had the help he *can* utilize in order to make greater use of his own problem-solving equipment for the solution of his own emotional problems. For this reason, if he is helped to conceptualize in simple terms his emotional problems the therapeutic results can often be even more dramatic than with some of his nonretarded peers. Every psychotherapist knows the problems of the highly intellectualized patient who has difficulty learning something really new about his own emotional life. The intellectual prowess of the therapist who can talk in simple terms can often be teamed up with the special attributes of the retarded person to make a very productive therapeutic team as compared to two persons who both major in intellectual defenses. A similar collaborative "therapeutic team" can capitalize on current developments in operant conditioning and behavior therapy, which utilize methods of focused intensive conditioning that can help compensate for the retarded child's limitations in his capacity for spontaneous problem solving.

The slow rate of development, the second feature of primary psychopathology, also has a number of implications for unique personality development which were not elaborated in the clinical report. The retarded child experiences differences in the pacing and timing of intellectual, as compared to both emotional and physical, growth and development. While there are delays in some aspects of motor and other physical development, generally speaking the retarded child is not as prepared mentally to cope with and integrate his own growing size and biological milestones when compared to a nonretarded child. There are further complications in that his size and biological maturation carry him into social situations which he is not so well prepared to meet. Part of the solution is for him to restrict his own activity or to be restricted by others, often for his own protection. Because his emotional maturation is retarded he must cope with biological milestones with relatively less mature defenses and thus be that much less prepared for each succeeding milestone. All of these factors in timing and pacing of emotional development associated with the slow rate of development have many secondary implications for the personality development of the retarded child. Such differences in the developmental pattern of retarded children as compared to nonretarded children should not be regarded as necessarily pathological, for in many ways they merely represent differences in patterns of growth and in personality development which, nonetheless, are integrated for adaptive purposes in the best interests of the retarded individual. Whatever the disadvantages in being mentally retarded, not all processes associated with the slow rate of development are maladaptive or pathological.

The third basic feature of primary psychopathology and a major part of the unique emotional development in retarded children includes those qualities of emotional development and descriptive personality traits described in the section on primary psychopathology. To recapitulate, these include the disturbance in emotional development (immature elements in the personality maturation process), "nonpsychotic autism" (or personal withdrawal and isolation), repetitiousness, inflexibility, passivity, and simplicity in emotional life.

A variety of later external influences contribute to the relatively unique development of school-age retarded children. These influences include the reactions of peers and teachers, the many experiences at failure or unfavorable comparisons, the tendency to be easily led, and limitations in social judgment. These later influences and their impact on personality are commonly described in clinical-descriptive psychiatric and educational literature on mental retardation. Interestingly, Heber's careful review (1964) of experimental research led him to emphasize similar "motivational" and "social reinforcement" variables as the most striking and consistent findings that distinguished retarded from nonretarded subjects.

Consideration of older retarded children calls attention to the importance of age level in any attempt to define the unique emotional development of retarded children. Differences in individual and environmental circumstances tend to bring added complexity and individualized overlying factors with each advancing year. For example, features that significantly distinguished retarded children from nonretarded children in some controlled experimental studies were complicated by the fact that the retarded subjects were in residential schools for the retarded while the nonretarded subjects were not. I am not aware of descriptive studies of emotional development in large heterogeneous series of school-age retarded children, adult retardates, or infants with later confirmed retardation which have attempted to identify unique features that are more intimately and commonly associated with the degree of mental retardation than with any other diagnostic factor.

On the basis of available studies and theoretical considerations, the following comments may be made on unique emotional development of retarded children. The most universally unique features may be expected to be rooted at the same early developmental age and arise from similar varieties of etiologic factors as the intellectual handicap in mental retardation. For purposes of later personality development this means the unique features tend to be rather elemental in basic character structure, which may be overlaid with a wide variety of psychological defenses and individualized development with each advancing year. Particularly in the older and mildly retarded, these unique aspects may be so subtle and complicated by other personality factors that their manifestation is sometimes partially obscured and relatively insignificant in the total assessment of a particular child's adjustment. On the other hand, even with wide variations in environment, the mental-retardation syndrome elicits sufficiently common reactions from home, school, and community environments to make certain "socially reinforced" traits extremely common, although not entirely unique.

The clinical study herein reported provides supportive evidence that emotional characteristics that are most unique to the degree of mental retardation are not necessarily the most prominent or striking features associated with individual cases of retardation in children. Nor are the most unique features the same as certain diagnostic and descriptive terms commonly used and based on subtypes, such as "brain defect," "poor impulse control," "happy," "dull," "rigid," "anxious," "affectionate," or "defective delinquent." Rather, the most unique features are basic qualities of personality which are persistently present or recurrent but not necessarily most impressive, particularly on brief acquaintance. They are more like the tide than either a surface storm or a placid sea. Naturally, the more retarded the child, the more prominent is the primary psychopathology.

Problems of Terminology

In view of the accumulation of experimental, educational, and clinical literature on the behavioral aspects of mental retardation, particularly during the past ten years, why do the unique aspects of emotional development remain relatively so unrefined as to permit arguments among highly trained professionals as to whether a retarded child can indeed have emotional development comparable to a nonretarded child of the same mental age? There are some quite understandable reasons for this, and they reflect the state of the field and the problems of terminology.

Most clinical descriptive studies of emotional characteristics in large series of retarded children tend to focus on the moderate and severe emotional disturbances, not on retarded children with "mild disturbance" or optimal emotional development. On the other hand, most experimental studies do not include psychiatric assessment, and they require such finely controlled behavioral variables that it becomes difficult to generalize the findings—even though statistically significant—from the behavioral element measured to more complex emotional development and personality traits. Similarly, experimental feasibility usually limits the number and variety of retarded subjects. Hence, valid generalization as to uniqueness for all retarded persons must be guarded.

In the past, relatively few child psychiatrists have devoted time to the mentally retarded. In studies that include large series of retarded children it is most natural for the investigators to direct their attention to the emotional disturbances most relevant to clinical services rather than to basic research on personality development. There is also the further complication of a lack of commonly utilized nomenclature for childhood emotional disorders, as well as for common patterns of "nondisturbed" emotional development. This problem is reflected in the varieties of diagnostic types used by different authors in psychiatric studies cited in the present chapter. A significant effort to establish more useful common diagnostic nomenclature by the G.A.P. Committee on Child Psychiatry (1966) holds greater hope for the future, although there would still be problems in adapting to A.P.A. and A.A.M.D. nomenclature which serves a broader professional field.

Use of the terms "primary" psychopathology and "secondary" influences for purposes of the clinical study herein reported should not be confused with either primary and secondary etiology or the relative prominence of primary psychopathology in individual cases. For example, in a given child the "secondary influence" may be a more significant factor in emotional development than is the mental retardation or primary psychopathology. "Primary" as used in medical nomenclature sometimes refers to primary etiology, although the term is also used to refer to symptom complexes for which no other etiologic factor is evident. An example would be "primary behavior disorder," which is used in some classifications of childhood disorders and explained as "not secondary to other groups in this classification (of childhood disorders)."

Child psychiatrists have been even less concerned with rating the severity of emotional disturbance than they have been with diagnostic nomenclature. Tizard (1966) pointed out that in child psychiatry "few attempts are made to assess the severity of any condition," whereas "in mental deficiency practice the rating of severity or grade of mental deficiency has proved indispensable." Tizard perhaps overstates the case, for the gross clinical judgments in the several psychiatric studies cited in the present chapter (Woodward et al., 1958; Philips, 1966; Chess, 1966; Menolascino, 1965, 1966, 1968; and Webster, 1963) probably are very much in agreement as to differentiating between moderate and severe disturbances. However, this is a personal impression, and there is an obvious need for more specific criteria as to the severity of the emotional disturbance.

An area of even greater ambiguity and semantic difficulty is the terminology used for "mild emotional disturbance," "without significant behavior disorder," "normal," "healthy," or "optimal emotional development." The problem exists in almost any psychiatric clinical discussion and is accentuated in considerations of emotional development of retarded children. In the psychiatric studies cited, each author handled the potential issue of mild or minimal emotional disturbances differently; that is, children in their series who were not "moderately," "severely," or "significantly" emotionally disturbed. It must be remembered that the first four authors (Woodward, Philips, Chess, and Menolascino) neither intended nor attempted to focus particularly on the emotional characteristics of retarded children with minimal emotional disturbance, or on optimal emotional development in moderately and severely retarded children.

Woodward reported on only nine children, who were selected to avoid obvious cases of schizophrenia and organic brain disease. Her observations were consistent with those of the present author, but she understandably made no attempt to generalize as to mild or minimal emotional problems of retarded children; in fact, she implied a mild or moderate degree of disturbance by her clinical descriptions. Philips gave two case illustrations of children with minimal problems, that is, "making an adequate adjustment," but he did not attempt to elaborate on the criteria or general traits in a larger number of such children. Chess distinguished 30 per cent "without significant behavior disorder," but did not provide additional clinical descriptions or criteria. Menolascino did not address himself to this group, except in the personal communication quoted.

The present author rated 34 per cent of cases "mild emotional disturbance," which was related to but not identical with his description of "primary psychopathology of the mental-retardation syndrome." The present author, in the clinical study reported, sometimes used the phrase "optimal emotional development" to refer to retarded children with "mild emotional disturbance," thereby attempting to convey that a borderland exists and that one may choose to focus on either the emotional problems or the healthy aspects.

The issues can be usefully clarified in the context of an apparent disagreement between the reports of Chess and the present author. Naturally, some of the differences may be associated with real differences between the two samples of retarded children studied, but this difference appears minor compared to the differences in terminology, concept, and clinical descriptive work reported. Chess reported that 70 per cent of the children in her series were found to show "significant behavior disorders on psychiatric evaluation." Her finding of the other 30 per cent "without significant behavior disorder" may at first glance seem inconsistent with what the present author described in an earlier report and in the present chapter.

The difference is probably more apparent than real. In other writings, Chess places strong emphasis on assessing the healthy as well as the pathological aspects of emotional development in children and decries the tendency of professional persons to emphasize pathology. This writer heartily concurs in her refreshing emphasis and cannot help but agree that many of the children whom he categorized as "mild disturbance in emotional development" or with "optimal emotional development" for the degree of retardation could for some purposes be regarded as "without significant behavior disorder"— particularly some of the children with only mild or borderline degrees of retardation. In some respects the references to emotional problems of retarded children might better use some term other than "psychopathology," even though a definite adaptive handicap indeed exists. Chess also stated: "In our experience a significant minority of retarded children (30 per cent) do show emotional development comparable to nonretarded youngsters of the same mental age." While she may thus make a valuable emphasis to counteract the tendency of our profession to overemphasize pathology, this writer doubts Dr. Chess would differ strongly with the technical point that has been elaborated in the present chapter. In fact, she has stated that it would "appear to be self-evident that the degree of intellectual retardation is a significant factor in determining the child's adaptive capacities and potential for coping with the demands of his environment." One could add that it also appears self-evident that a child of the chronological age of six and the mental age of four cannot possibly have an emotional development truly comparable to that of a nonretarded child of the age of four. Naturally, in children with mild or borderline retardation the unique features of personality development may sometimes be so subtle that many other factors would weigh more heavily in the overall clinical assessment of individual cases.

In these types of semantic problems, which are not uncommon in the field of mental retardation, we can only hope to be as clear as possible as to what we mean in our choice of words and to give each other the benefit of the doubt. As the field gradually advances, new technical terminology will also evolve and find more commonly agreed usage. Hazards lie in opposite directions. At one extreme, in discussing psychopathology or characteristics unique to mentally retarded children, there is a danger of giving an overly pathological view and reinforcing common images of defectiveness and hopelessness concerning retarded children. At the other extreme, we may lean over backwards with statements such as "a retarded child is just like any other child except a little slower," which fail to make a realistic assessment of the special problems confronting the retarded child. Both these extremes are familiar to us as we have seen parents struggling to gain a realistic view of their own child's handicap. Another important dimension which has not been given sufficient attention in the field in general is more careful descriptive work regarding the special strengths and resources that are successfully employed by retarded children in the course of their development.

Implications for Future Research

Future research on the unique aspects of emotional development in retarded children should go far beyond the exploratory study herein described. Larger representative samples, nonretarded controls, trained observers with clearly defined criteria for complex clinical ratings, pretests of interrater reliability, longitudinal studies, and other clinical research methods should be employed. Neither experimental methods with highly isolated behavioral samples that lack the integrative skill of trained clinicians, nor usual clinical diagnostic methods not subjected to more disciplined criteria and methods, are likely to push back the frontiers very far.

Both child psychiatrists and research psychologists will have a better opportunity to realize their potential contributions if a coordinated effort to achieve a common language is actualized and a common basis of understanding is effected.

SUMMARY

A clearer specification of those qualities of emotional development which are uniquely associated with the mental-retardation syndrome and are roughly proportional to the degree of retardation, would be useful to diagnosticians, research workers, parents, and all others who work with retarded children. The benefit to retarded individuals would be even more significant if the above persons and the general public were also aware of the many qualities that are *not* necessarily part of the mental-retardation syndrome. Present knowledge is too incomplete to make such distinctions with precision, but much can be done to reduce present stereotypes and point the way toward better understanding.

The present chapter has sought to clarify this complex issue by means of a review of the literature, a report of a clinical study of 159 preschool retarded children, and a clarification of terminology and concepts that sometimes confuse the picture or permit inappropriate stereotypes. The review of the literature and the clinical study give attention to the variety of emotional problems found in retarded children—mainly from a clinical child psychiatry perspective—and a special effort was made to distinguish features most unique to the mental-retardation syndrome as compared to the many other complications encountered in certain subgroups or individual cases of retarded children.

A series of 159 preschool retarded children, applicants for a nursery school program who were still living at home, were reviewed with clinical ratings as to medical diagnosis, severity of retardation, severity of brain disease, and severity of emotional disturbance. All major diagnostic subgroups of mental retardation were represented, although not in the same proportions as in the total population of retarded children.

Five out of six of these children had at least strongly suggestive evidence of brain disease. Close to half (48 per cent) were rated as moderately emotionally disturbed, and 18 per cent were rated as severely disturbed (childhood psychosis). All the children had some disturbance in emotional development compared to normal children of the same mental age, even though some had relatively optimal emotional development.

It was emphasized that mental retardation is a clinical syndrome that can best be understood in dynamic developmental terms, regard-

less of the specific etiologic factors contributing to it. Also emphasized was the fact that one can find individual exceptions to almost
every statistical trend. Therefore, each child should have careful evaluation of each of the four basic diagnostic factors: namely, medical or
etiologic diagnosis, brain disease, intellectual functions, and emotional
development. Assumptions should not be made on the basis of one or
two of the factors. Much is left to be understood in terms of the
uniqueness of each child.

Primary psychopathology of the mental-retardation syndrome was
described and illustrated in an effort to clarify the disturbance in emotional development which in our series of children appeared to be a
fundamental part of the mental-retardation syndrome. In addition to
the intellectual deficit and the slow rate of development, there was a
difference in the quality of emotional development as compared to
nonretarded children. There were infantilization or immaturity of the
evolving character structure, poor differentiation of ego functions,
and some special descriptive characteristics. The latter included
nonpsychotic autism, repetitiousness, inflexibility, passivity, and simplicity of emotional life.

Complications in emotional development associated with the intellectual handicap and slow rate of development were discussed as features closely associated with the degree of retardation. Limitations in
abstraction, language development, symbol formation, and imaginary
play interfere with the emotional problem-solving capacity at early
crucial stages of development and also have a cumulative effect that
places the retarded child further and further behind his peers in the
growth of his problem-solving capacity with each advancing year.
However, the child can sometimes benefit greatly by therapeutic assistance in the endeavor to make greater use of his own problem-solving
capacity for the solution of his own emotional problems. The slow
rate of development contributes to his unique emotional development
via factors such as the differences in pacing and timing of intellectual,
emotional, and physical milestones.

Secondary influences commonly complicated emotional development in the series of children studied. Brain disease, sensory impairment, physical handicaps, seizures, illnesses, and emotional traumata
were frequent. Deprivation was one of the most prominent secondary
influences. Overstimulation occurred occasionally. Other complicating
influences included confused expectations on the part of the parents,
partial decathexis of the child by the parents, the tendency of parents
to fuse their image of the child with an image of their own defectiveness,
and parental tendencies to reinforce the infantilization of the child.

These secondary influences were described as directly related to the child's condition and thus were distinguished from major external influences by individual parental psychopathology, family pathology, and sociocultural factors. This distinction was understandably of a gross nature because of the continuous interrelation and impact of child, family, and community upon one another.

Retarded children are subject to the usual varieties of emotional disturbance which can affect any child, even though retarded children also have some special vulnerabilities. *Moderate disturbances* in emotional development which were common in our series of children, but which were not uniquely associated with the degree of retardation, included: disturbances in impulse and behavior, excessive fears and inhibitions, grief and loss reactions, exaggerated negativism and compulsive traits, exaggerated immaturities, and exaggerated or prolonged regressions. The twenty-seven children with *severe disturbances* (psychoses) included eleven with demonstrable brain disease. Only in the most severely retarded was there difficulty in the differential diagnosis between psychosis and the primary psychopathology that appeared uniquely associated with the mental-retardation syndrome.

The most universally unique features of the emotional development of retarded children, basic features of the mental-retardation syndrome which are roughly comparable to the degree of retardation, appear to be rooted at the same early developmental age and arise from similar varieties of etiologic factors as the children's intellectual retardation. For purposes of later personality development, this means the unique features are rather elemental in basic character structure and may be overlaid with a wide variety of psychological defenses and individualized development with each advancing year. Particularly in the older and mildly retarded, these unique considerations may be so subtle and so complicated by other personality factors that their manifestation may be obscure or relatively insignificant in the total assessment of a particular child's adjustment. On the other hand, even with wide variations in environment, the mental-retardation syndrome elicits sufficiently common reactions from the home, school, and community environments to make "socially reinforced" traits extremely common, although not entirely unique, as described in both experimental and clinical descriptive studies.

The exploratory nature of the present study, problems in concepts and terminology, and the need to combine careful clinical descriptive studies with experimental research on retarded children with optimal emotional development all were discussed. In considering concepts and terminology for unique emotional development of retarded chil-

dren, a plea was made to avoid the hazards of giving an overly pathological view and thereby reinforce common images of defectiveness
and hopelessness. On the other hand, we should not lean over back-
wards and fail to make a realistic assessment of the special problems
confronting the retarded child.

NOTES

1. Mental retardation is used synonymously with mental subnormality as defined
by the World Health Organization (1954).

2. In general usage "pseudoretardation" is a broad term used somewhat synonymously with "mental retardation" (as compared to "subnormality") as defined by
W.H.O. Some authors (for example, Mahler-Schoenberger, 1942), use pseudoretardation or pseudoimbecility to refer to more specific syndromes.

3. This is an agency of the Massachusetts Department of Mental Health, Division
of Mental Hygiene, in cooperation with the Boston Association for Retarded Children. The nurseries are part of a statewide nursery clinic program. The Boston Preschool Retarded Children's Program (PRCP) was set up with the guidance of the
Child Psychiatry Clinic of the Massachusetts General Hospital and the James Jackson Putnam Children's Center. It was established for the purpose of diagnostic evaluation and placement of children in the nurseries, consultation to the nursery teachers, social casework with parents, referrals for other services as indicated, and the
development of research and training in this field.

4. The author is especially indebted to the PRCP Mental Health Coordinator,
Miss Virginia Cook, a psychiatric social worker who obtained detailed histories from
parents, pursued medical records and referrals with diligence, and was the clinical
mainstay of our program because of her work with parents and her maintenance of
liaison between the various elements of the program.

We are equally indebted to the Children's Medical Center of Boston, our major
source of referral, for their medical and neurological evaluations. Other frequent resources included Joseph P. Kennedy, Jr., Memorial Hospital, Massachusetts General
Hospital, Boston City Hospital, Walter E. Fernald State School, and the James Jackson
Putnam Children's Center.

5. The psychologists who did examinations for the PRCP were Dr. Donald Wes-
ton, Dr. Selma Rappaport and Mrs. Iris Fodor. We are also indebted to psychologists of referring agencies.

6. Dr. Peter Bowman, discussant of the earlier report of this study at the meeting
of the American Psychiatric Association in 1962 (1963), reported that he found 3
psychotic mongoloid children, ages 7 to 19, among the resident population of 94
mongoloids (ages 5 to 58 years) at Pineland Hospital and Training Center (Pownal,
Maine).

REFERENCES

Ackerman, N. W., & Menninger, C. F. Treatment techniques for mental retarda-
tion in a school for personality disorders in children. In C. L. Stacey & M. E.
DeMartino (Eds.), *Counseling and psychotherapy with the mentally retarded.* Glencoe,
Ill.: The Free Press, 1957.

Asperger, Hans. Behavior problems and mental retardation. In P. W. Bowman
(Ed.), *Mental retardation.* New York: Grune & Stratton, 1960.

Benda, C. E. *The child with mongolism.* New York: Grune & Stratton, 1960.

Bender, L. Twenty years of clinical research on schizophrenic children, with special reference to those under 6 years of age. In G. Caplan (Ed.), *Emotional problems of early childhood.* New York: Basic Books, 1955.

————. *Psychopathology of children with organic brain disorders.* Springfield, Ill.: Charles C Thomas, 1956.

Blatt, B. *The intellectually disfranchised, impoverished learners and their teachers.* Community Mental Health Monograph Series, 1966, No. 1.

Chess, S. Psychiatric aspects of mental retardation. Presented at the Conference on Mental Retardation for Physicians, San Francisco, Feb., 1966.

Chidester, L., & Menninger, K. A. The application of psychoanalytic methods to the study of mental retardation. In C. L. Stacey & M. E. DeMartino (Eds.), *Counseling and psychotherapy with the mentally retarded.* Glencoe, Ill.: The Free Press, 1957.

Clark, L. P. *The nature and treatment of amentia.* New York: William Wood & Co., 1933.

Eisenberg, L. Emotional determinants of mental deficiency. *A. M. A. Arch. Neurol. & Psychiat.,* 1958, *80*(1).

Farrell, M. Mental deficiency. In Ewalt, Strecker, & Ebaugh (Eds.), *Practical clinical psychology* (8th ed.). New York: McGraw-Hill, 1957.

Goldfarb, W. The effects of early institutional care on adolescent personality. *J. Exp. Educ.,* 1946, *12,* 96.

Group for the Advancement of Psychiatry. *Basic considerations in mental retardation.* Report No. 43. New York, 1959.

————. *Mental retardation: A family crisis—the therapeutic role of the physician.* Report No. 56. New York, 1963.

————. *Psychopathological disorder in childhood: Theoretical considerations and a proposed classification.* Report No. 62. New York, 1966.

————. *Mild mental retardation: A growing challenge to the physicians.* Report No. 66. New York, 1967.

Heber, R. A manual on terminology and classification in mental retardation. *Amer. J. Ment. Defic.,* 1958, *64* (Monogr. Suppl. 2).

————. Personality. In H. Stevens & R. Heber (Eds.), *Mental retardation, a review of research.* Chicago: University of Chicago Press, 1964.

Jervis, G. The mental deficiencies. In S. Arieti (Ed.), *The American handbook of psychiatry,* Vol. 1. New York: Basic Books, 1959.

Kanner, L. Early infantile autism. *J. Pediat.,* 1944, *25,* 211.

————. *Child psychiatry.* Springfield, Ill.: Charles C Thomas, 1957.

Karelitz, S., Karelitz, R. F., & Rosenfeld, L. S. Infants' vocalizations and their significance. In P. W. Bowman (Ed.), *Mental retardation.* New York: Grune & Stratton, 1960.

Kirk, S. A. *Early education of the mentally retarded.* Urbana, Ill.: University of Illinois Press, 1958.

Mahler-Schoenberger, M. Pseudoimbecility: A magic cap of invisibility. *Psychoanal. Quart.,* 1942, *11,* 149.

Masland, R. L., Sarason, S. B., & Gladwin, T. *Mental subnormality.* New York: Basic Books, 1958.

Menolascino, F. J. Emotional disturbance and mental retardation. *Amer. J. Ment. Defic.,* 1965, *70*(2), 248–256.

————. The facade of mental retardation: Its challenge to child psychiatry. *Amer. J. Psychiat.,* 1966, *122* (11), 1227–1235.

————. Four common behavioral reactions in mentally retarded children. Presented at the Annual Meeting of the American Psychiatric Association. Boston, May, 1968.

Pearson, G. H. J. Psychopathology of mental defect. In C. L. Stacey & M. E. DeMartino (Eds.), *Counseling and psychotherapy with the mentally retarded.* Glencoe, Ill.: The Free Press, 1957.

Philips, I. Children, mental retardation, and emotional disorder. In I. Philips (Ed.), *Prevention and treatment of mental retardation.* New York: Basic Books, 1966.

Potter, H. W. Mental deficiency and the psychiatrist. *Amer. J. Psychiat.*, 1927, *33*, 67.

The President's Panel on Mental Retardation. *Report to the President. A proposed program for national action to combat mental retardation.* Washington, D.C.: U.S. Government Printing Office, 1962.

Putnam, M. Some observations on psychosis in early childhood. In G. Caplan (Ed.), *Emotional problems of early childhood.* New York: Basic Books, 1955.

Rank, B. Adaptation of the psychoanalytic technique for the treatment of young children with atypical development. *Amer. J. Orthopsychiat.*, 1949, *19*, 130. (*a*)

———. *Psychoanalytic study of the child,* Vols. 3, 4. Aggression. New York: International Universities Press, 1949. (*b*)

Rappaport, S. *Psychoanalytic study of the child,* Vol. 16. Behavior disorder and ego development in a brain injured child. New York: International Universities Press, 1961.

Robinson, H. B., & Robinson, N. M. *The mentally retarded child, a psychological approach.* New York: McGraw-Hill, 1965.

Rochlin, G. *Psychoanalytic study of the child,* Vol. 16. The dread of abandonment; a contribution to the etiology of the loss complex and to depression. New York: International Universities Press, 1961.

Sarvis, M. A. *Psychoanalytic study of the child,* Vol. 15. Psychiatric implications of temporal lobe damage. New York: International Universities Press, 1960.

Skeels, H. M. Adult status of children with contrasting early life experiences. *Monogr. Soc. Res. Child Devel.*, 1966, *31* (3, whole no. 105).

Spitz, R. *Psychoanalytic study of the child,* Vol. 1. Hospitalism. New York: International Universities Press, 1945.

———. *Psychoanalytic study of the child,* Vol. 2. Hospitalism. New York: International Universities Press, 1946.

Stacy, C. E. & DeMartino, M. (Eds.), *Counseling and psychotherapy with the mentally retarded.* Glencoe, Ill.: The Free Press, 1957.

Stevens, H., & Heber, R. *Mental retardation, a review of research.* Chicago: University of Chicago Press, 1964.

Taylor, E. M. *Psychological appraisal of children with cerebral defects.* Cambridge, Mass.: Harvard University Press, 1959.

Tizard, J. Mental subnormality and child psychiatry. *J. Child Psychol. & Psychiat.*, 1966, *7*, 1–15.

Tredgold, R. F., & Soddy, K. *A textbook on mental deficiency* (9th ed.). Baltimore: Williams & Wilkins, 1963.

Webster, T. G. Problems of emotional development in young retarded children. *Amer. J. Psychiat.*, 1963, *120*(1), 37–43.

Woodward, K. F., Siegel, M. G., & Eustis, M. J. Psychiatric study of mentally retarded children of pre-school age. Report on first and second years of a three-year project. *Amer. J. Orthopsychiat.*, 1958, *28*, 376.

World Health Organization. *Report of expert committee on the mentally subnormal child.* Geneva, 1954.

: 2 :

Emotional Problems in
Mentally Retarded Children

Stella Chess

INTRODUCTION

THE mentally retarded child is highly vulnerable to stresses from an environment organized primarily for youngsters of average intelligence. Long before his retardation has been accurately identified, the child experiences a host of inappropriate demands for levels of performance, judgment, and impulse control that are beyond his capacity. Even after his defective development has been recognized, he continues to be thrust into situations where he is expected to function in accord with his chronological age. His inability to do so evokes disapproval and ridicule, particularly after he reaches school age.

As a result of such interpersonal stresses, the retarded child may be considered at risk for the development of behavior disorders. Most psychiatric studies agree that emotional disturbances are proportionately more frequent among mentally retarded children than in the general population of children. However, there is a marked difference of opinion about the actual incidence. While a few investigators find that all retardates suffer from some degrees of emotional disorder, others tend to minimize the psychiatric differences between this group of children and children of normal intellectual capacity.

Coexistence of Emotional Problems and Mental Retardation

Webster (1963, p. 38) reports that in a group of 159 retardates three to six years old, not one child was "simply retarded." He concludes that "the slow and incomplete unfolding of the personality is associated with partial fixations that result in an infantile or immature character structure. This particular style of ego development is accompanied by special descriptive features: a nonpsychotic autism, rep-

55

etitiousness, inflexibility, passivity, and simplicity in emotional life."
On the other hand, Shaw (1966) observes that "the majority of high-
level retarded children, if their family environment is reasonably
healthy, do not evidence emotional disturbances in their earlier years.
The major difficulties begin as the child grows older and gets out
among other children." While some studies assign a risk of psychotic
illness as high as 40 per cent, Cytryn and Lourie (1967) find that "it
is possible for the vast majority of the retarded to develop personality
patterns as normal as compatible with their level of mental functioning."

Unfortunately, we do not have nearly enough systematic information on either the prevalence or specific etiology of behavioral disturbances in retarded children. Many authors have discussed, often
speculatively, the influence of emotional factors on intellectual functioning. However, very little work has been done on the possible effects of retardation upon psychological functioning and personality
development.

To be sure, there has been an abundance of glittering generalizations. These usually rest on a basic fallacy: they ignore the extreme
heterogeneity of the mentally retarded as a group, whether considered
in terms of etiology, degree of defect, individual temperament, or environmental setting. Moreover, many conclusions are built on studies
of patients in psychiatric hospitals or residential centers where the
proportion of disturbed children is relatively high. In private practice,
too, the children who come to psychiatric notice are likely to be those
whose behavior has been sufficiently troublesome to make a referral
necessary.

In my own clinical and research experiences, I have been unable to
identify any emotional or behavioral characteristics that are peculiarly
and invariably associated with mentally retarded children. Not all retardates have emotional disturbances. And among those who do, not
all exhibit the same symptoms. These observations are supported by
other recent studies. For example Philips (1967), in a review of 227
cases seen over a seven-year period at the Langley Porter Neuropsychiatric Institute, disputes the "common misconception" that maladaptive behavior in a retarded child is a function of his retardation
rather than of his interpersonal relationships. He also rejects the
widely held view that emotional disorder in the retardate is different
in kind from that in the child who is not mentally deficient.

In attempting to appraise the retarded child's behavior, it is essential to examine his interaction with a specific environment, particularly the significant persons around him. Discordances in the child-en-

vironment interaction especially in view of the retarded youngster's vulnerability, generate and prolong emotional disturbances. Therapeutic intervention, to be effective, cannot deal with the child alone or the environment alone, but must focus on modifying the abrasive interaction.

"*The Emotional Block*"

To clear the way for such an approach, it is necessary to emphasize that the coexistence of mental subnormality and behavioral abnormality does not necessarily imply that the emotional disorder is primary and the retardation secondary and, hence, reversible. The concept of "emotional block" has itself blocked a realistic understanding of the retarded child's emotions.

As Kanner (1956, p. 181) noted, "Somewhere along the line, the term 'emotional block' was coined to indicate the masking of innate intellectual assets by psychotic or near-psychotic disturbances." It is of course true that IQ scores can be negatively influenced by emotional factors such as anxious perfectionism, just as test results can be affected by visual, auditory, or neuro-orthopedic handicaps. But some professional persons, Kanner (p. 182) adds,

. . . have gone to the extreme of ascribing primary emotional etiology to children who, by all standards, were, are, and will remain defective in the sense of an inherent minus. It has come to a point when some parents' advisers have become reluctant to acknowledge the fact of innate intellectual retardation as such and see in any malfunctioning child evidences of the working of an "emotional block." Any bit of odd behavior, such as waving the hands, manipulating a string, or grimacing, is viewed as "proof."

All too often, parents are advised that both the child and they require intensive psychotherapy in order to "unblock" the emotional difficulty. "This not only calls for backbreaking financial expenditure but has convinced many parents that it was their attitudinal outlook and resulting relationship with the child which brought about his failure to develop. There is no excuse for thus adding insult to injury."

The concept of "emotional block" is closely linked to the theory of "pseudoretardation," a label that has been indiscriminately applied to children whose deficiency was presumed to be secondary to an emotional disorder. Many psychiatrists formerly believed (perhaps some still do) that their main responsibility was to distinguish "pseudoretardation" from "true retardation." Once the judgment was made, the psychiatrist went on to diagnose and treat the emotional disturbance, often without reference to the cognitive issues, which were considered to be the province of a special school or institution. If the diagnosis was "true retardation," unrelated to emotional disturbance, the psychiatrist often considered his responsibility fulfilled when he recommended an appropriate school or institutional placement.

DIFFERENTIAL DIAGNOSIS

General Considerations

The approach toward an "emotional block" was hardly calculated to encourage systematic study of the dynamics of behavioral organization in retarded children. Clearly, the diagnosis of retardation is only the beginning of psychiatric exploration, not the end. Once the diagnosis has been established, the psychiatrist has to make a behavioral assessment of the child. He must determine how the fact of retardation is related to the youngster's overall adaptation.

In making this assessment, the experienced clinician is on guard against certain pitfalls. It is all too easy to arrive at judgments of pathology based on fragmentary, out-of-context observations of deviant behavior. Patterns of behavior in a mentally retarded child differ significantly from those observed in normal children of the same age. A deviant behavioral expression is not necessarily a sign of emotional disturbance. One must consider various explanations. It is possible that the behavior, while inappropriate for the child's chronological age, may be quite in keeping with his mental age. In that case, there would be no reason to assume that a pathological condition exists. Or the behavior may represent attempts at adaptation to or defense against unreasonable environmental demands. This would suggest the need to change the pressuring environment. It is also possible, of course, that the deviant behavior represents an underlying psychological disorder, which must then be dealt with as such.

To reach a differential diagnosis, one must keep in mind a number of basic considerations. It is essential, for example, to distinguish between a child's habitual level of functioning and his maximum capacity. Very often, there is a gap between a child's routine performance and his sporadic demonstration of ability under optimal conditions. This gap does not invariably reflect an emotional problem that is impairing performance. For example, a parent may report that her retarded child can dress himself completely, whereas the child's teacher maintains that he always needs help at school. It is tempting to jump to the conclusion that there is an emotional or motivational component in the discrepant behavior. But it may be that for this child the act of dressing is not a routine accomplishment, but is possible only under optimum conditions at home. At school, faced with many distractions and noise, he requires help.

Confusing a child's maximum and habitual levels of functioning may result in emotional problems, since overestimation of his capacities leads to excessive expectations and demands. On the other hand, exclusive attention to routine abilities may lead to an underestimation of the child's capacities and the setting of inadequate goals. It is unfortunate that the differentiation between habitual functioning and optimal capacity is not made in the performance scales currently in use, such as the Vineland Social Maturity Scale.

The developmental history also requires close study. While most retarded children are slow from birth onward, others begin life normally. They manifest intellectual retardation only after some traumatic event, such as infection, inflammation, or degenerative neurologic disease affecting the brain. A child who has always been slower than average will not face the same demands as one who has functioned normally for a number of years and only then begun to display a lag. For this child, as well as for his parents, emotional difficulties may be acute.

Contributing Factors

A significant factor in determining the child's capacity for coping with environmental pressures is the degree of mental retardation. This would appear to be self-evident, but it is too often overlooked. The stresses and tensions of attempting to function with normal children and adults will be more difficult for the child with an IQ of 50 than the one with an IQ of 75. In addition, the specific aspects of cognitive functioning, such as retentive memory and imitative ability, may be influential in determining the child's adaptive abilities.

Because retarded children are repeatedly confronted with tasks that they are intellectually ill-equipped to handle, they build up a higher expectancy of failure than other children. The emotional significance of this fact has been noted by Zigler (1967, p. 298), who points out that the retarded child tends to distrust his own solutions and to seek guidance from others. These emotional factors may lead to less effective behavior than the child's mental capacity permits. Many of the reported behavior differences between normals and retardates, Zigler

suggests, may be viewed as ". . . products of motivational and experiential differences between these groups, rather than as the result of
any inherent deficiency in the retardates." From another angle, Rosenthal and Jacobson (1968) report that teacher expectations of poor
results may affect the performance not only of children of average intelligence, but also of a group of retarded boys, within the limits of
their capacity.

Temperament

A most important factor entering into the child-environment interactional process is the attribute of temperament. From early infancy,
children manifest striking differences in their characteristic reactions
to the varied stimuli and demands of day-to-day living. The individual
behavioral style of children has been systematically studied in terms
of such primary characteristics as rhythmicity of biological functions,
general activity level, positive or negative responses to new situations
(approach/withdrawal), sensory threshold, quality of mood, intensity
of reactions, persistence in ongoing activities, and distractibility and attention span (Thomas et al., 1963). These temperamental qualities significantly affect the normal child's responses to childcare practices
and to intrafamilial and extrafamilial demands. Certain patterns of
temperament combined with environmental stress may lead to disturbances in behavioral development (Thomas et al., 1968).

These findings apply to retarded children as well. In a psychiatric
study (discussed in detail in the section on the coexistence of emotional problems and mental retardation of this chapter) of fifty-two retarded youngsters between the ages of five and twelve whose mental
ages ranged from four to six years, this writer was able to identify a relationship between temperament and the retarded child's capacity to
perform adaptive functions in ordinary daily life (Chess, 1970a). Children who are more positive in mood and more mild in their reactions
tend to be those with higher performance levels. Rejection of aid, often
with overt anger, is also related to temperament. Such rejection of proffered assistance tends to occur among children who are less positive
in mood, more intense in their reactions, and more distractible.

Awareness of temperamental qualities is essential for evaluating behavior, as well as for proper management. One child in our study had
frequent tantrums that expressed her negative response to new and unfamiliar experiences. Each time a new food or a new toy was introduced, the child seemed to respond with anger. The parents dealt with

this problem by shielding her from new experiences. She had fewer tantrums, but the lack of new stimuli and learning experiences resulted in a stagnation of her level of functioning below her potential capacity. The parents were advised to expose the child to selected new situations gradually and gently, and to expect tantrums the first few times. With this appropriate management, the child was given a learning atmosphere that corresponded to her temperament and intellectual level. The tantrums subsided. Had the temperamental factor not been recognized, it would have been easy to interpret the tantrums as an inherent emotional problem. Mishandling might well have created an emotional disorder.

Another child, on the other hand, adapted quickly to new situations, but was extremely persistent. His persistence, combined with his retarded level of functioning, resulted in his sticking to a difficult task in a perseverative, repetitive fashion without mastery. His IQ level decreased as his perseverative habits became more pronounced. But it was possible to interrupt this cycle by adopting a special approach to the child. Each new task was divided into small sequential fragments, each of which he could master in turn. The child could then pass on to the next segment.

A BRIEF REVIEW OF A PSYCHIATRIC STUDY OF RETARDED CHILDREN

In the study of fifty-two retarded children, a detailed behavioral and language analysis was made (Chess and Hassibi, 1970*b*). Of the entire group, all of whom came from middle-class families and were living at home from birth, thirty were diagnosed as having a behavior disorder.

Behavioral Patterns

A high proportion of the children exhibited bizarre behaviors such as are often associated with childhood schizophrenia and other psychoses. A number of children engaged in activity that was apparently aimless, including jumping, rocking, flapping of the arms, and eye blinking. Many interrupted their routine of eating, dressing, or watching television to perform these activities. Other children engaged in stereotyped play activity, using toys or other objects in a rigidly unmodified way. About one-third of the children manifested an unusual seeking of sensory experiences. Others insisted on the repetition of certain environmental conditions. In some children this insistence was limited to a particular ritual; they were fairly flexible in other respects.

Such stereotyped and repetitive activities are often assumed to be pathognomonic of schizophrenia in a child whose general behavior is incongruent with his chronological age. Yet basically, these children function in an organized way at their intellectual level. They follow an orderly routine in the home, dress themselves, keep their toys in designated places, and help with household chores. Living at home, they are able to participate in many acts of daily life that are not experienced by institutionalized youngsters with the same degree of retardation. It is hardly surprising, therefore, that studies of institutionalized children have often been unable to discern their capacities to develop appropriate social manners, discriminating affective behaviors, and mastery of complex sequences of action in the context of siblings, neighborhood activities, and school.

In the fifty-two children of our study, there was little correlation between unusual behaviors and the psychiatric findings. Aberrant actions may exist side by side with well-related and adaptive behavior. One of the children accumulated index cards with street names on them. This might appear to be unrelated stereotyped behavior. But in this instance, it was the reflection in a mentally limited child of an activity that seemed to him part of the life around him. Few observers would consider a child's repetitive behavior unusual if it has some ideational content. The boy who collects stamps or rocks and is always looking for these objects is not judged to be disturbed. If similar behavior lacks ideational content in a retarded child, may this not be seen as part of the syndrome of retardation rather than as a sign of emotional disturbance?

Language Patterns

Language patterns, too, were repetitive, perseverative, and stereotyped in many of the children. Such verbal indices are often used to diagnose emotional disturbance and autism. It is, therefore, important to note their presence in psychiatrically normal but mentally retarded children. To assume automatically that such speech characteristics are signs of emotional disorder or disorganization of thought process is to invite trouble. It is hardly wise to arrange for psychiatric treatment of a child who really needs an effective educational and management program.

Coexistence of Emotional Disturbance and Mental Retardation

But what of the child who does have a significant emotional disturbance? Of the thirty youngsters in our study who were diagnosed as having a behavior problem, ten had difficulties that were direct symptoms of brain damage, eighteen had reactive behavior disorders, one had a neurotic behavior disorder, and one was psychotic. Inaccuracies are inherent in any classification that subdivides so heterogeneous a group as the mentally retarded. But it is convenient to discuss the disorders under these headings.

Behavior Disorder Due to Brain Damage

While brain damage in itself does not necessarily result in disordered behavior, the direct symptoms of organic dysfunction may include hypermotility or hypomotility, brevity or excessive length of attention span, high distractibility, lability or monotonous sameness of mood, difficulty in shifting direction of thought or activity, excessive dependence on people or inappropriate independence. One may also see obsessive thought and compulsive behaviors in brain-damaged retarded children, manifested in repetitive questions or statements, stereotyped gestures, or rhythmic body movements. Forced laughter or crying is sometimes found or stereotyped self-mutilation, such as picking at sores or biting a thumb or wrist to the point of maceration and infection.

Some of these symptoms can be modified by drug therapy. But for the most part, treatment of organically determined symptoms requires changes in the child's milieu. It is necessary to organize a way of life, a set of attitudes, and a level of demands and expectations that take into account the child's vulnerabilities as well as his abilities. This applies to all aspects of the youngster's life—home, school, playground. The hyperirritable child needs to be shielded from harsh scolding; the hypoactive child needs intense stimulation; the child with short attention span must be presented with new demands in brief teaching episodes.

Reactive Behavior Disorder

With poor handling, intellectually handicapped children may develop reactive patterns of aggressive activity, overdependence, or fearfulness. Old stereotypes like "the quiet and contented mongoloid" have long ago been demolished as crude distortions. Retarded children, like all others, may be happy or sad, assertive or docile, adventurous or timid. What is true is that an unhealthy interaction between child and environment can distort feelings, turning happiness into clowning, sadness into depression. Glaser (1967, p. 572) notes that children and adolescents with mild-to-moderate degrees of mental retardation often recognize the overt or covert rejection by peers and elders: "The feelings of inadequacy, hopelessness, as well as rejection may find their expression in overt symptoms of depression; very often, however, these feelings produce anger against the environment, especially when superiority of siblings, schoolmates, and friends is obvious, and this anger is then expressed in acting-out behavior."

Neurotic Behavior Disorder

While reactive behavior disorders are reversible, given appropriate changes in environmental organization, retarded children with neurotic behavior disorders may exhibit more firmly fixed patterns. Neurotic manifestations may reflect anxieties or defenses against anxiety. The child may have phobic reactions unrelated to the intentions or actions of the persons around him.

Mental Retardation with Psychosis

When subnormal intellectual functioning coexists with childhood psychosis, the decision as to which is to be considered primary is often purely semantic and nondeterminative of treatment plans. For the youngster with affective disorder of the autistic type one may postulate that increased awareness of the people and activities around him would result in better cognitive function. An attempt should be made to stimulate the child through a recreation group, speech or music therapy, specified parental interaction, or a trial at direct psychotherapy. But the degree of achievement, so far as we can now determine, will depend on the severity and reversibility of the psychopathology.

In each of the four categories just summarized, the treatment modality will vary. In none of the categories is there any justification for a do-nothing approach.

Treatment Considerations

For certain types of disturbances, particularly neurotic behavior disorder, direct psychotherapy may be advisable. In a previous report (Chess, 1962), I described the results of an experimental program at a clinic for retarded children. While it is hazardous to generalize the aims and approaches of this experience with twenty-nine children, a measure of success can be noted. To a large extent, the child's intellectual level determined whether it was possible to reach him on a conceptual level, or whether relationship therapy or the establishment of new patterns of behavior by conditioning was to be most effective. The experiment indicated that some gains in at least alleviating anxiety and fear may be possible with any child, no matter how limited his intelligence. Clinical experience has confirmed that psychotherapy can lead to the inclusion of a defective child in some approximation of a normal family in cases where this had before seemed impossible.

Of course, the techniques of psychotherapy with normal children need modification when applied to retarded youngsters. The goals of such treatment must be individualized, with full recognition that the child will continue to function on a retarded level, though hopefully on a higher one.

Some children, notably those with psychoses, may require treatment designed to give them maximum superimposition of structure in order to limit their wandering flights of thought and activity. In other instances it may be necessary to focus on alleviating a fear of authority figures, a damaging degree of competitiveness, or an overwhelming sense of inferority engendered by comparison with a sibling who is extremely bright and alert.

A basic technique of psychotherapy is parent guidance, which should have an important place in psychiatric treatment of the mentally retarded child. The prevention and treatment of emotional problems in the youngster requires an orientation toward using the parent as a colleague.

This approach, it should be emphasized, is quite different from the traditional one that concentrates on helping parents "accept" their retarded child. While it is true that parental love and acceptance are essential for healthy psychological development, it does not follow that warmth of feeling can alone overcome the stressful effects of the retarded child's world.

Parent guidance implies a concrete program of altered parental function designed to help the retarded child cope with the special stresses and demands in his life. As a basis for achieving this, it is desirable to make a detailed inventory of the data available for the child. This inventory should include (1) IQ level and any special characteristics of perceptual and cognitive functioning revealed by psychometric testing; (2) the level of functioning in activities of daily life—both the maximum and habitual level; (3) temperamental characteristics; (4) learning patterns, including the child's response to correction by others; (5) patterns of parental practices in dealing with the child's problems; (6) special intra- or extrafamilial stresses; and (7) relevant features of medical, neurological, and psychiatric examinations.

The interrelationship of these factors provides the basis for evaluating the child's emotional problems. The discussion with the parents focuses on making them aware of the demands that are easy, difficult, or impossible for the child to master. A program of activity is then laid out with the aim of removing, so far as feasible, the impossible expectations and of increasing the child's ability to master difficult demands.

Overwhelmed as the parents are by the multiplicity of daily as well as long-range concerns, they need an objective program in which priorities are designated and some idea of the time required for results is estimated. Indeed, the parallel might well be drawn with muscular defect in which the physician would assume that his medical management must include a plan of exercises, a listing of incapacities, and rules for participation in and restriction of activities. Such guidance has proved to be an effective therapeutic tool. It is an essential technique for helping to prevent emotional problems in the retarded child, whose world is so often structured on false assumptions about his abilities.

SUMMARY

Because of their greater vulnerability to environmental stresses, mentally retarded children are more likely than other children to develop emotional disturbances. This does not mean, however, that all retarded children are disturbed or that they manifest a special set of emotional characteristics. In making a behavioral assessment, it is essential to study the child as an individual, focusing on his specific developmental history, degree of retardation, habitual level of functioning, environmental setting, and temperamental characteristics. To make a valid identification of emotional disorder, the diagnostician must avoid the assumption that unusual behaviors reflecting the fact of retardation are pathological.

Among retarded children with emotional disturbances, it is convenient to distinguish four categories: (1) difficulties due to brain damage, (2) reactive disorders, (3) neurotic behavior disorders, and (4) psychoses. Treatment modalities are varied and depend on the specific nature of the disorder. Parent guidance, based on a concrete program of altered parental function, is an effective technique for preventing and treating emotional problems in retarded children. The parent is enlisted as a colleague to help improve the child-environment interaction by modifying inappropriate demands, adapting such demands to the child's capacities and temperament.

REFERENCES

Chess, S. Psychiatric treatment of the mentally retarded child with behavior problems. *Amer. J. Orthopsychiat.,* 1962, *32,* 863–869.

———. Temperament and levels of functioning in mentally retarded children, 1970. (*a*)

Chess, S., & Hassibi, S. Behavior and language in mentally retarded children living at home, 1970. (*b*)

Cytryn, L., & Lourie, R. S. Mental retardation. In A. M. Freedman and H. I. Kaplan (Eds.), *Comprehensive textbook of psychiatry.* Baltimore: Williams & Wilkins, 1967.

Glaser, K. Masked depression in children and adolescents. *Amer. J. Psychother.,* 1967, *26,* 565–574.

Kanner, L. The "emotional block." *Amer. J. Psychiat.,* 1956, *113,* 181–182.

Philips, I. Psychopathology and mental retardation. *Amer. J. Psychiat.,* 1967, *124,* 29–35.

Rosenberg, R., & Jacobson, L. *Pygmalion in the classroom: Teacher expectation and pupils' intellectual development,* New York: Holt, Rinehart & Winston, 1968.

Shaw, C. R. *The psychiatric disorders of children.* New York: Appleton-Century-Crofts, 1966.

Thomas, A., Chess, S., Birch, H. G., Hertzig, M. E., & Korn, S. *Behavioral individuality in early childhood.* New York: New York University Press, 1963.

Thomas, A., Chess, S., & Birch, H. G. *Temperament and behavior disorders in children.* New York: New York University Press, 1968.

Webster, T. G. Problems of emotional development in young retarded children. *Amer. J. Psychiat.,* 1963, *120,* 37–42.

Zigler, E. Familial mental retardation: A continuing dilemma. *Science,* 1967, *155,* 292–298.

Emotional Disturbance and Mental Retardation: Etiologic and Conceptual Relationships

Irv Bialer

INTRODUCTION

THE diagnostic constructs "emotional disturbance" and "mental retardation" may be considered as being basically independent to the extent that one of these pathological conditions may manifest itself without the other, and that each has a body of theory and practice which is capable of standing on its own and which sets it apart as a professional area. Nevertheless, there is a good deal of concern among both theoreticians and practitioners in each area regarding the extent to which the two overlap, and many of these concerns have been expressed by other contributors to the present volume, as well as by this author in another context (Bialer, 1970).

This chapter will attempt to focus on those relationships among the given constructs which bear on etiologic and diagnostic considerations in mental retardation and on a meaningful conceptualization of the roles played by certain social-cultural variables in personality development among retardates.

To avoid semantic stumbling blocks to effective communication, let us begin with brief definitions of the two concepts under consideration.

The current American Association on Mental Deficiency (A.A.M.D.) manual on terminology and classification (Heber, 1961) provides our definition of the term *mental retardation*. Accordingly, "mental retardation refers to subaverage general intellectual functioning, which originates during the developmental period and is associated with impairment in adaptive behavior" (Heber, 1961, p. 3). Thus, an individual may be considered to be mentally retarded if he meets all of the following criteria: (1) on a test of general intelligence he has attained a score (usually IQ score) that is more than one standard deviation below the norm (usually 100) for that test; (2) the causative agent was effective before the age of sixteen; (3) he is deficient in either maturation, learning, or social adjustment, or a combination of these when compared·to his age-mates.

In discussing problems inherent in arriving at a comprehensive description of children who may be classified under the rubric "emotionally disturbed," Bialer (1970) has pointed out that no authoritative source has yet come up with what seems to be a generally acceptable delineation of the concept *emotional disturbance*. Hence, we shall provide our own less dogmatic frame of reference for that construct. As used in the present essay, the term refers to any significant emotional deviation that causes the retardate to have difficulty in meeting or adjusting to the demands of his culture, or in achieving an effective relationship with the environment in which he finds himself. The emotional states involved may range from severe tension to outright psychotic behavior, but for our purposes the definition is not intended to cover those pathological behaviors which are subsumed by the terms "sociopathy," "delinquency," or "criminality."

ETIOLOGIC AND DIAGNOSTIC CONSIDERATIONS

A common frame of reference for discussion of the diagnostic and etiologic relationships between mental retardation and emotional disturbance is provided by the current classification schema of the A.A.M.D. (Heber, 1961). More specifically, Category VIII of that system is intended for the classification of those cases where it has been determined that there is no reasonable evidence of central-nervous-system (CNS) pathology which could justifiably underlie the behavioral retardation. Thus, that category addresses itself to mental retardation that is due to presumed psychogenic or psychosocial factors. Two of the five subunits or "codes" comprising Category VIII are particularly pertinent to our present deliberation. Their purposes are as follows:

Code 83: "Psychogenic mental retardation associated with emotional disturbance" was purportedly designed to subtend cases with histories of prolonged and extremely severe *neurotic* disturbance dating from early childhood.

Code 84: "Mental retardation associated with *psychotic* (or major personality) disorder" provides for retardation concomitant with histories of such personality deviations or psychotic states as "autism" or "childhood schizophrenia."

Etiologic connections among the variables under consideration may be seen as falling into any one of the following four conformations. Mental retardation is consequent to (that is, results from) emotional disorder. Mental retardation is antecedent to (that is, leads to) emotional disturbance. Mental retardation and emotional deviation—when they coexist in a given individual—are both consequent to a common etiologic factor such as CNS dysfunction. And, mental retardation and emotional problems are (presumably) independent of each other.

The need for taking note of each of the foregoing alternatives before a definitive diagnostic statement can be formulated in any given case has confronted the theoretician, researcher, and practitioner with two crucial issues. The first issue is that of the validity of the concept of "pseudofeeblemindedness"—or "pseudoretardation"—as a diagnostic construct. The second issue is the problem of differential diagnosis. Let us examine these questions more closely.

Pseudoretardation

Over a period spanning at least fifteen years, a number of writers, including the present author, have put forth cogent arguments to the effect that, since the concept of "pseudoretardation" has been assigned a multiplicity of meanings, it lacks both clarity and utility and that it therefore adds nothing to understanding or enhancement of the etiologic, diagnostic, or therapeutic aspects of mental retardation. Consequently, the following authors have strongly advocated that the concept be eliminated: Beier (1964); Benton (1956, 1962, 1964); Bialer (1966a, 1966b, 1970); Cantor (1955); Clarke and Clarke (1955); Papageorgis (1963). For the same reason, it was also a major intent of Category VIII of the A.A.M.D. classification system to render the construct unnecessary (Heber, 1962). That intent is furthered on the one hand by the A.A.M.D. position that complete emphasis must be placed on the *current* functional level of the individual, and on the other hand by the provision of a broad schema that applies to those cases which would not be considered "truly" retarded from some other point of reference.

In spite of these attempts, use of the term "pseudoretardation" has persisted under a plethora of referents throughout the world (as exemplified briefly in Table 3–1). By perpetuating a scientifically questionable construct in an assortment of languages, such persistence has surely tended to deter productive communication among international workers in the field of mental retardation.

TABLE 3–1

Examples of International Referents for the Term "Pseudoretardation"

SOURCE	REFERENTS
Austria Schmuttermeier (1963)	Intellectually, physiologically, academically *"normal."* There is an "impression" of mental defect based on "autistic" behavior.
England Kratter (1959)	Intellectual and academic performance *subnormal* due to lag in physical or emotional development which is based on either functional or organic pathology.
France Heuyer (1963)	*Reversibility is the prime criterion.* Academic achievement and IQ level below "potential" because of emotional problems, sensory deficiencies and/or glandular dysfunction.
Girard (1967)	Retardation of moderate or mild degree without "organic brain damage." School achievement inhibited by "psychosensory anomalies."
Israel Frankenstein (1958)	"Potential" intelligence is not attained owing to emotional "preoccupation," sensory deficiency, neurological or endocrine dysfunction, or physical weakness.
Japan Makita et al. (1964)	Subnormal intellectual function that is based on emotional disturbance and is reversible through psychotherapy.
Netherlands Grewel & Van den Horst (1959)	Subnormal level of intelligence resulting from auditory defect.
United States Markenson & Read (1965)	Learning problems evidenced by marked underachievement despite "adequate intellectual potential," which is indicated by absence of "psychosis" or "brain damage" with psychomotor defects and "impression" of average IQ.
Richardson & Normanly (1965)	Learning disability due to emotional, sensory, linguistic, or speech problems, or to minimal cerebral dysfunction, *with or without normal intelligence.*

SOURCE: Adapted from I. Bialer, 1970. (See references.)

In the following paragraphs we shall, therefore, once more attempt to make a case for the universal abandonment of the notion of "pseudoretardation" as a diagnostic construct.

Historically, the major referents of the construct have been related to diagnosis, prognosis, and etiology (Benton, 1956, 1962, 1964; Heber, 1962). Under the first rubric, the concept has been used to denote an erroneous original diagnosis based on inadequate or inappropriate procedures in gathering or interpreting the assessment data. Benton (1956, 1962) has held that competent assessment is the responsibility of the clinician, and that diagnostic errors based on data that are invalid or unreliable should not be accorded the status of bona fide clinical entity. The present writer is of course in complete agreement with that point of view.

The prognostic aspect of pseudoretardation has been tied to the concepts of genetic "capacity" or "potential" and to the related criterion of "incurability" as necessary for the understanding of course and outcome in mental retardation (Heber, 1962). From that standpoint, an individual who demonstrated either competent intellectual behavior, competent social behavior, or both subsequent to an original diagnosis of retardation was judged post hoc to have been not "really" retarded to begin with. In addition, strict theoretical adherence to these concepts and criteria would make it impossible to derive a definitive diagnosis until the subject had died. The A.A.M.D. schema, which stresses *present* behavior, ignores the untenable concepts "constitutional origin," "capacity," or "incurability."

The third and most widely used sense in which the notion of pseudoretardation has been and continues to be employed has rested on the implication that "true" or "real" mental retardation can be etiologically rooted only in neuropathology. Benton (1962, p. 86) has suggested that from this viewpoint, "Pseudofeeblemindedness may be said to represent mental deficiency of atypical etiology," and that such etiology may be subclassified into broad groups of determinants which include sensory deprivation, motor deficit, cultural deprivation, and emotional disturbance.

Within the context of atypical etiology, the label "pseudoretarded" implies that the observed behavioral retardation represents a "true" defect state—one that differs from that based on CNS pathology only with respect to etiologic considerations (Benton, 1956, 1962). If the observed characteristics represent an accurate reflection of the individual's functional ability at the time they are diagnosed, it seems legitimate and appropriate to include them within a broad classification system as cases of mental retardation with specific etiologic elements. We can then consider the possibility of future development or improvement of the given individual as matters for empirical consideration. The A.A.M.D. classification system, in following that logic, seems to have rendered the term "pseudoretardation" completely meaningless as a diagnostic construct. It is apparent that discarding the concept altogether would be in the interests of all concerned.

Differential Diagnosis

The issue of differential diagnosis is primarily concerned with the attempt to isolate and identify all relevant factors in the case of a given individual who is functioning as a retardate, so as to enable the most effective treatment planning and disposition for that individual. From that viewpoint, how crucial or useful is the diagnostic decision as to whether we have on hand a severely disturbed child whose emotional disorder has significantly depressed his behavioral efficiency so that his functional level has been assessed as falling within the range of mental retardation, as opposed to whether we are faced with a retarded child who shows a severe emotional problem?

If we assume that such definitive differentiation is possible, the importance of the different diagnostic decisions may be manifested in several directions. For one thing, our own expectations as to the outcome of a certain therapeutic or educational program may be determined by the specific decision. For example, one implication of the first alternative in the foregoing question is that, with the amelioration of the emotional problem, the given child might eventually function at a nonretarded level. Thus, in the case of the hypothetical severely disturbed child who is "functionally" retarded, it might be expected that psychotherapy would lead to the attenuation of the intellectual deficiency—perhaps in direct proportion to the restoration of emotional stability. However, if the second alternative is emphasized, the primary focus would be on treating the personality problem in an individual who is behaviorally retarded for any reason. Here, any observed increase in measured intelligence would be considered incidental to the alleviation of behavioral and emotional distress.

Another, and probably more crucial, consequence of a differential diagnostic decision may be the nature of the facility to which the given child is assigned for treatment or programming. Unfortunately, admission to specific facilities or programs is too often determined by the diagnostic category into which the child has been relegated. Where the diagnostic label rather than the child's needs is the determining factor in his disposition, it may lead to that child's being tossed back and forth between a state school and a state hospital, or between agencies serving the disturbed and those serving the mentally retarded, each claiming the responsibility rests with the other.

Withal, one aspect of the complex situation appears painfully obvious: it is extremely difficult (if not virtually impossible) to make a clear-cut delineation of the exact etiologic connection between the deficiency in intellectual functioning and problems in emotional adjustment which may exist in a given case. Therefore, we are evidently enjoined to pay less attention to the manifestly sterile distinctions that have been sought up to now and to direct our diagnostic endeavors toward assessing the major strengths and most urgent needs of the multiply affected child, so as to enable the assignment of that child to the most appropriate or feasible program that may be available.

Postulates and Hypotheses

The literature bearing on the relationship of mental retardation to emotional disturbance discloses a number of additional issues and controversies that demand consideration and point toward some provocative and explorable hypotheses. These also will be discussed within the framework of Category VIII.

Code 84 specifies that cases may be included therein only when they satisfy the necessary developmental and behavioral criteria along with the absence of reasonable evidence of CNS pathology. In that regard, a growing body of literature presents data that seem to necessitate reconsideration of the categorization of "major personality disorders" among children as significant social-cultural precursors of mental retardation. Pertinent findings pointing to such reconsideration seem to lead to the following four conclusions:

1. Conditions such as "autism" or "childhood schizophrenia" seem to be very strongly (if not invariably) associated with neuropathology. For example, Hertzig and Birch (1966) found that neurological abnormality was significantly more frequent in adolescent female patients diagnosed as schizophrenic than in those classified otherwise. They noted that these results suggested that primary neurological dysfunction was a major etiologic factor in the development of schizophrenia in children and early adolescents. A more recent study by Gittelman and Birch (1967) supported and expanded those findings and led to the conclusion by those investigators that (1) their results did not support the concept of psychogenic etiology of childhood psychosis and (2) their results did support the view that early CNS pathology may characterize an extensive group of noninstitutionalized children who have been diagnosed as schizophrenic. On another front, Rimland (1964) has presented extensive physiological evidence to the effect that defects in the reticular system of the brain stem may underlie what has been described as "autistic behavior" in children. The general conclusions reached by Birch and his associates and by Rimland have been supported by other workers (for example, Rutter, 1965; Schain and Yannet, 1960; Wing, 1966).

2. The symptomatology of "childhood schizophrenia" is not identical with that which characterizes schizophrenic states that become apparent in late adolescence and adulthood. This seems to be a fairly general conclusion that is upheld by a number of sources (among

them Goldberg and Soper, 1963; Hutt and Gibby, 1965, Chapter viii; Pollack, 1958, 1967; Rutter, 1965, 1966).

3. When "autistic behavior" and "childhood schizophrenia" appear in association with mental retardation, both the emotional disorder and the intellectual deficiency are due to CNS dysfunction. After extensive and analytical reviews of the literature, Pollack (1958, 1967) came to the conclusion that where "childhood schizophrenia" and mental retardation coexist, the emotional and intellectual impairment are both manifestations of neurological damage that has had its origin during either the prenatal or the paranatal period. This reasoning is supported by other recent works (for example, Gittelman and Birch, 1967; Hinton, 1963; Marzani and Paracchi, 1967; Menolascino and Eaton, 1967).

4. Evidence for the untenability of severe neurotic disturbance as a precursor to behavioral retardation (Code 83) is less marked. Nevertheless, some indication exists that this relationship may also be called into question. Beier's (1964, pp. 479–480) conclusion from a survey of the literature is typical: "In terms of the psychoneuroses [and their relationship to mental retardation] . . . , the research does not demonstrate any causal . . . connections." In view of the latter conclusion, let us postulate that any relationship between mental retardation and deviant emotional states of relatively less severity than psychoses may be conceptualized as the retardate's defensive reaction to factors that bear directly on his intellectual and social subnormality. These variables might include either such environmentally imposed external stresses as severely frustrating situations, rejection, and stigma; such subjective factors as feelings of anxiety, failure, low self-esteem, incompetence, and insecurity; or two or more of these external and subjective stresses combined.

Let us further postulate that any given pathological condition based on the aforementioned variables would rarely lead to distortions of reality severe enough to be characterized as a psychotic condition. This postulate appears to be bolstered by a stand such as that of Wolfensberger (1960, p. 706) to the effect that what appear to be delusional systems in retardates actually represent "forced attempts to make sense out of events they cannot otherwise explain, rather than being secondary symptoms of a schizophrenic process."

In consideration of the foregoing findings and conclusions, tentative hypotheses such as the following have been advanced by the present writer (Bialer, 1970) with regard to the relationship between emotional disturbance and mental retardation:

Hypothesis I: The notion that antecedent psychotic states are etiologic to mental retardation no longer serves a useful purpose. The given diagnostic entities should be seen as related only insofar as both conditions are consequent to CNS damage.

Hypothesis II: The only significant causal connection between mental retardation and emotional disturbance of lesser degree is that where the personality deviation is related to antecedent affective variables that may be directly associated with the retardation.

Pursuant to the philosophical position expressed in the above hypotheses, we shall address ourselves, in the section that follows, to the viewpoint that a consideration of the etiologic and conceptual relationships between mental retardation and emotional deviation should "focus on those aspects of the life experience of a retarded . . . [person] which may be expected to produce deficits in personality development" (Heber, 1964, p. 170).

SIGNIFICANT FACTORS IN PERSONALITY DEVELOPMENT

Some of the behavioral and situational factors which seem especially pertinent may be grouped under two major rubrics. These rubrics are *motivational variables,* namely, those aspects of the person—or of the task he is required to undertake—which may influence a given individual's performance in specific settings or situations; and *phenomenological variables,* that is, variables that bear on the extent to which the retarded person's behavior is determined by his perception of himself and of the world around him as well as by the world's perception of him as an individual.

Motivational Variables

Anxiety

The general literature seems to uphold the proposition that on a variety of measures, retardates as a group show higher levels of manifest anxiety than do comparable normal subjects.

If we grant this proposition, the question still faces us whether this finding invariably reflects a characteristic that is disadvantageous to the retarded individual. It has become generally accepted that, under some conditions, certain levels of anxiety may facilitate a person's accomplishments and that, under other circumstances, anxiety may be debilitating. Hence we might expect that in retarded populations, level of manifest anxiety does not necessarily show a negative correlation with performance. A fairly large body of research aimed at exploring that expectation has substantially confirmed it (Bialer, 1970).

On the basis of an exhaustive analysis of the research on the relationship of anxiety to intelligent behavior in general, Butterfield (1970) has reached the following two conclusions. First, anxiety is not a chronic state, but appears in response to specific situations. Thus, test anxiety, which may be either facilitating or debilitating, reflects a specific response to a given situation. Second, it is expected that test anxiety measures response tendencies in life situations generally only insofar as those situations are test-like.

Applying these views to the mentally retarded, we might expect that to the extent that the retardate perceives each circumstance as a challenge or a test, his test-anxiety scores may well mirror his response tendencies in real-life situations. Consequently, it is conceivable that given life conditions may evoke anxieties that will serve to either raise or lower the level of performance in the retardate.

Success and Failure

In an earlier study, this writer (Bialer, 1960, 1961) advanced (and validated) the proposition that among both retarded and normal children, the subjective experience of success and failure depends primarily upon the individual's capacity to conceptualize the relationship between his own ability and the outcome of his goal-directed behavior, and that the given capacity is a developmental phenomenon that is related primarily to mental age. Results of that study also suggested that in the subjective awareness of success and failure, retarded children are chronologically older than their normal counterparts at any given stage of development.

On another track, early research (Cromwell, 1963, 1967) had proceeded on the assumption that, as opposed to normal children, retarded individuals showed a prolonged history of failure. That assumption generated the predictions that, after a failure experience, normal children would tend to increase effort, but that comparable retardates would show decreased effort. Research based on those predictions (Cromwell, 1963, 1967) has shown convincingly that while normals respond to failure with increased effort more than do retardates, failure may also be motivating for the latter under certain conditions.

Attempts at circumscribing parameters of failure as motivation with retardates have pinpointed at least four major determinants that need not be considered as independent. These parameters are (1) the

child's developmental level as determined primarily by his mental age
(Bialer, 1960, 1961; Bialer and Cromwell, 1960); (2) the collateral
ability to recognize and experience success and failure subjectively
(Bialer, 1960, 1961; Bialer and Cromwell, 1965); (3) a tendency toward success-striving (SS) versus failure-avoiding (FA) behavior as a
general personality construct (Bialer and Cromwell, 1965); and
(4) motivation to seek and respond to adult approval (Butterfield
and Zigler, 1965; Lingren, 1967).

Internal-External Dimensions of Motivation

In the field of mental retardation, these facets of behavior have
been studied from three primary standpoints. The construct *locus of
control,* first applied to retarded children by the present writer (Bialer,
1960, 1961) emphasizes differential tendencies toward assignment of
responsibility to self (internal locus of control) or nonself (external
locus of control) for the outcome of events. The apparent tendency
for retardates to be more externally controlled than are normals has
not been significant. The dimension *inner directed versus outer directed,* developed and explored by Zigler and his students (Zigler,
1966a, 1966b), is concerned with differential orientation of the subject
toward the utilization of cues in problem-solving behavior. Research
to date has consistently found retardates to be more outer-directed
than are normal subjects. The concept *motivator-hygiene,* contributed
to the field of mental retardation by Haywood (1964), stresses individual orientation toward either intrinsic or extrinsic incentives or reinforcements. The motivating properties of the given orientations on
specific tasks has been demonstrated among retardates as well as
among normal individuals (Haywood, 1967).

The parameters of the various constructs just outlined still await
sharper delineation and call for definitive research.

Phenomenological Variables

Conception of Self

Exhaustive surveys of relevant issues and of research encompassing
those issues among children in general have been provided in an extensive literature (Wylie, 1961, among others). Yet such research with
retardates is not only in a notable minority, but what there is of it
does not provide sufficient answers to many of the relevant questions.
Nevertheless, perusal of available sources from the world literature indicates that some directions and relationships are emerging. These
may be summarized as follows:

1. The self-conception of retardates cannot inevitably be characterized by a single set of patterns. Whereas some retarded individuals show extremely positive attitudes toward themselves, others view themselves as worthless, weak, and undeserving (Guthrie et al., 1961).

2. There is a consistently positive connection between level of intelligence and the direction of self-appraisal. This is true both *within groups of retarded subjects* (see Gorlow et al., 1963) and *among subjects* who range from retarded to superior in intellect (see Curtis, 1964).

3. There is a significantly positive association between self-attitude and school achievement among both normal and retarded boys (Marasciullo, 1968). That this association seems to be independent of IQ has been indicated by research with retarded females (Gorlow et al., 1963).

4. There appears to be a general tendency for retarded subjects to overrate themselves on measures of self-estimation of either current or future performance as compared to average or bright children. This tendency has been found with estimates of academic achievement, physical skill, and intellectual level (Brengelmann, 1967; Fine and Caldwell, 1967; Merlet, 1964; Perron and Pecheux, 1964; Ringness, 1961).

Conception of Others

The retardate's view of the world around him may be conceptualized as involving (1) his perception of other retarded individuals, (2) his concepts concerning nonretarded peers, and (3) his perception of "significant others" in his environs. Following is a brief overview of selected findings of pertinent sociometric research.

PERCEPTION OF OTHER RETARDATES

One basis for judging the behavior of others is the retardate's concept of himself; that is, the retarded individual often sees the world in his own image (Gladstone and McAfee, 1960). There seems to be a significant correlation between motor ability and peer acceptance among mentally retarded children (Smith and Hurst, 1961). However, in one French study which held CA and IQ constant, the more physically developed retardates were adjudged less intelligent by their peers than were the relatively underdeveloped subjects (Perron, 1965). Whereas mental ability is positively and significantly associated with sociometric choice status, rejection scores are inversely related to IQ (Dentler and Mackler, 1962; Merini et al., 1967). An attempt to determine the effect of specific environmental conditions on social status (Dentler and Mackler, 1964) found that such status was progressively associated with the degree of individual compliance to institutional norms. Another French study (Merlet, 1962) indicated that "popular" retardates were consistently characterized by positive traits, but that "rejected" subjects were seen in a negative light by their peers. Finally, special school retardates in West Germany showed general dissatisfaction with their own group by assigning relatively more negative than positive traits to their subnormal peers (Von Bracken, 1967a, 1967b).

An obvious direction for future research seems to be further investigation of the possibility that sociometric status may be highly dependent upon specific characteristics of both the individual and the situation within which the ratings are made.

PERCEPTION OF NONRETARDED PEERS

Only a single study of the retardate's perception of his nonretarded peers has come to this author's attention; namely, the study by Von Bracken (1967a, 1967b) in West Germany. His special-school retardates assigned more positive traits to normal children of a regular elementary school than they did to students of their own school. Von Bracken concluded that such retardates consider themselves "inferior" to their nonretarded age-mates.

The severe dearth of research on this particular phenomenological dimension seems to emphasize a vacuum that demands filling. That also appears to be true of the following dimension.

PERCEPTION OF "SIGNIFICANT OTHERS"

The values and expectations of "significant others" would seem to have a good deal of significance for and influence on the retardate in various social interactions.

Nevertheless, reports of investigations concerning the retardate's view of "significant others" are notably lacking. An interesting, though relatively minor, exception is the study by Towne and Joiner (1966). Their data showed that "significant others" and "academic significant others" named by adolescent educable mentally retarded students did not differ from those of comparable normals. Much more research along these lines seems imperative, as are efforts to determine more precisely *how* the child perceives the "others" whom he names as well as to what degree his behavior is determined by theirs in a variety of interactions.

Attitudes

An extremely crucial phenomenological factor in the retardate's behavior is how he is perceived by the world.

Guskin's review (1963) of the stereotypical thinking of community, family, and peer groups which goes into the formation of their attitudes toward the retardate has been amplified by more recent work (for example, Efron and Efron, 1967; Fine, 1967; Wolfensberger, 1967*a*, 1967*b*). The following four points, which Guskin in 1963 proposed as "approaches and hypotheses," now seem to have attained a status of more defensible conclusions:

1. Within a normal group, the retardate is likely to be viewed as deviant in ability—and to be held in a low status role generally.
2. A retarded child in the family may lead to breakdown in family relationships as well as to unfavorable attitudes toward the subnormal individual by parents and siblings alike.
3. The behavior of individuals who are interacting with a retardate may be determined by their expectations concerning the behavior of the retarded person as well as by the actual behavior of the latter in the given situation. Conversely, the behavior of the mentally retarded individual may be greatly determined by the consistent expectations held by others concerning such behavior.
4. Popular attitudes and stereotypes may have great bearing on the manner in which the subnormal person is evaluated by others in his milieu.

The preceding conclusions suggest two major problems for research: (1) investigation of the extent to which the retardate's self-concept is congruent with the manner in which the world perceives him; and (2) exploration of the probability that there might be some common factors in attitudes manifested toward other "exceptionalities," various ethnic, religious, and socioeconomic groups, and the retarded. To this writer's knowledge, no research has been specifically oriented toward exploring either of those issues, although Von Bracken's work (1967*a*, 1967*b*) touches on the first and the study by Chesler (1965) bears on the second issue.

Projected Self-Percept

A further phenomenological variable that has undergone extremely sparse experimental exploration is the retardate's view of how the world perceives him. There appear to be only two minor reported investigations along those lines.

Clark and Ozehosky (1965) found that more than 50 per cent of the perceptions of the special class subjects as to their acceptance or rejection by normal peers were validated by the latter. Von Bracken (1967a, 1967b) found that special-school retardates (realistically) considered themselves to be very negatively regarded by their normal peers.

Disability Versus Handicap

Consideration of the phenomenological aspects of adjustment must also take into account the disability–handicap dichotomy. Briefly, *disability* circumscribes the intellectual or physical deficit; *handicap* includes the deficit along with its psychosocial ramifications. By that token, if society construes an individual's behavior as defective or aberrant, but does not give him special treatment as a consequence of such construction, this individual cannot be viewed as sociologically handicapped. Conversely, if an individual perceives his defect realistically, but does not behave as if that deficit is severely limiting to his effective social interaction, he cannot be considered personally handicapped. Possible application of these concepts—and their theoretical underpinnings (for example, Meyerson, 1963b)—to the understanding (and possible prevention) of emotional problems among retardates is readily perceptible.

A SUGGESTED THEORETICAL APPROACH TO ADJUSTMENT PROBLEMS OF THE RETARDED

Certain aspects of the Lewinian Field Theory, as expanded and applied to the social psychology of adjustment to physical disability (see Barker, 1948; Barker et al., 1953; Meyerson, 1963a, 1963b) offer an exciting conceptual framework for discussing some aspects of adjustment problems among the retarded. A major construct of the approach advocated by those authors has been the theory of a somatopsychological relationship between physique and behavior.[1] In applying somatopsychological principles to the adjustment problems of the physically deviant, Meyerson (1963a, 1963b) has emphasized that the latter tend to have more numerous and more severe problems of adjustment because they are more often subjected to either new psychological situations, overlapping psychological situations (or roles), or both. Interestingly enough, these two concepts readily lend themselves to an understanding of some adjustment difficulties in the mentally retarded. This may be illustrated briefly.

New Psychological Situations

New psychological situations are those in which the individual has not yet learned the proper sequence of behavior which will enable him to achieve a specific goal (Barker, 1948; Barker et al., 1953). The location of the goal and the means for reaching it are not immediately obvious. When placed in such a situation, the person is likely to manifest unstable, trial-and-error behavior—behavior that may lead to frustration and conflict, with resulting emotionality and behavioral disruption. To prevent the emotional upheaval that may result from being exposed to such new situations before the individual has developed the necessary coping mechanisms, Meyerson (1963b) has suggested that the "newness" of life experiences must be reduced for the physically disabled. That such situations may operate in the case of the retardate is evident when we note that the traditional stand of special educators has been to give the retarded child only total (if artificial) success experiences in the special class and to protect him from failure at all costs. In keeping with this philosophy, there seems to have been a conspiracy on the part of society in general to render all situations "old" by offering the retarded child minimal exposure to experiences that were not already within his behavioral repertoire, or to structure novel situations so rigidly that pathways to goals were very sharply delineated and mobility was possible only in specific directions. Such an approach operates to inhibit the child's learning how to seek and reach positive goals, and how to recognize and avoid negative contingencies. Thus, when the inevitable social and vocational problems arise after the child has left school, they tend to become "new" situations that he cannot handle effectively and that may generate emotional problems in him. It has been suggested elsewhere by the present writer (Bialer, 1964) that reduction in the "newness" of such situations is partially dependent upon acknowledgment by society that the retardate has the ability to tolerate and to be motivated by challenge and failure. Such recognition should be followed by the introduction of realistically stressful materials and procedures into the curriculum of the special class. Such stress has been considered as motivation for learning and as preparation for the expected hardships of life after leaving school (Bialer, 1964).

Overlapping Psychological Situations

Overlapping psychological situations, or roles, are those in which the individual must respond according to the demands made by two or more contrasting configurations of social and psychological forces which impinge upon him at the same time (Barker et al., 1953). By way of illustration, the world in which the retarded person lives specifies competence and interaction as minimal prerequisites for social status and self-esteem. Yet the retardate is simultaneously confronted by his comparative incompetence and is frequently denied opportunities for social and vocational participation (Edgerton, 1967). Both of these contingencies have a debilitating effect on the retardate's status and self-attitudes. They also render him visible and vulnerable, which often leads to emotional distress. The alleviation of adjustment problems that may be consequent to the foregoing contingencies might be fostered by society's recognition of and emphasis upon the retardate's abilities rather than by focusing upon his inabilities and incompetencies. Along with that emphasis, the individual should be directed toward recognizing and using those abilities he possesses, with the prospect that this will serve to develop in him positive attitudes toward self and society.

RAMIFICATIONS OF THE FIELD-THEORETICAL POSITION

The preceding conceptual framework presents an intriguing opportunity to speculate on the application of an ecological approach to assessment and treatment of personality and adjustment difficulties among the mentally retarded.

Assessment

In the assessment of personality variables, adequate evaluation of the role played by the interaction of situational, phenomenological, and motivational factors is very difficult unless the forces impinging on the person in his life space can be delineated in specific detail. That is the task and aim of ecological research with a field-theoretical orientation.

Standard paper and pencil measuring devices are usually designed to predict single criteria. In addition, they often rely too heavily on verbal or reading facility for adequate use with retardates.

Picture selection or arrangement techniques (see Pauker et al., 1967) or miniature situation procedures (see Santostefano, 1962) are closer to "real life," but they cannot reveal behavior in its somatopsychological setting.

Observational techniques seem to offer the best approach consistent with an ecological philosophy. However, observational inventories in general usually give only a molecular description of the behavior under immediate consideration. Global observation techniques that are consistent with a field-theoretical ecological approach are exemplified by the well-known work of Barker and his associates (1955) and Wright (1967), who are the prime exponents of ecological investigation in social psychology, as well as by the tangentially related contributions of Stevenson and his group (1961). Extension of those techniques to retarded populations holds promise of significant developments in the field.

Treatment

One interesting possibility in the treatment of emotional problems is that, with ecological behavior analysis yielding specific data as to the personal and environmental dynamics that are basic to any given pathological behavior pattern, while helping to bring into clear focus those behavior units which require alteration, behavior-modification techniques based on operant-conditioning principles—that is, "behavior therapy"—might be employed most effectively with disturbed retardates.

SUMMARY

In exploring etiologic and conceptual relationships between emotional disturbance and mental retardation within the frameworks of the A.A.M.D. classification system and certain aspects of the Lewinian Field Theory, this essay has attempted to stress the following five points:

1. For a number of reasons, the concept of "pseudoretardation" is meaningless for diagnostic and descriptive purposes and should be discarded as a scientific construct.

2. In the realm of differential diagnosis, past attempts at distinguishing between the "emotionally disturbed retarded child" and the "child who is retarded because he is disturbed" have been essentially futile. What we must emphasize is the child's abilities and strengths—rather than a particular diagnostic category—in treatment and program planning for that child.

3. Consideration of issues related to the foregoing suggests at least

two provocative and explorable hypotheses concerning etiologic relationships between mental retardation and emotional deviation of any
degree of severity.

4. Significant behavioral and situational factors in personality development among retardates include those which may be classed
under the headings of *motivational* and *phenomenological* variables.
Areas of needed research concerning these critical variables were outlined.

5. Some constructs based on the Lewinian Field Theory, specifically those of *new* and *overlapping psychological situations* and of the
ecological approach to social psychological research, are applicable to
assessment, understanding, and treatment of adjustment problems in
the mentally retarded.

In conclusion, this chapter has served as a forum for the advancement of some ideas deliberately designed to generate conjecture and
discussion among all concerned. It is hoped that the results of this endeavor will be both edifying and heuristic.

NOTES

1. Somatopsychological theory derives from the fundamental formula advanced by
Lewinian Field Theory to the effect that *behavior is a function of the individual interacting with his psychological environment* and thus holds that "variations in physique . . . [may] affect the psychological situation of a person by influencing the
effectiveness of his body as a tool for action or by serving as a stimulus to himself
and others" (Barker et al., 1953, p. 1).

REFERENCES

Barker, R. G. The social psychology of physical disability. *J. Social Issues,*
    1948, *4*(4), 28–38.
Barker, R. G., Schoggen, M. F., & Barker, L. S. Hemerography of Mary
    Ennis. In A. Burton & R. E. Harris (Eds.), *Clinical studies of personality.*
    New York: Harper, 1955, pp. 768–808.
Barker, R. G., Wright, B. A., Meyerson, L., & Gonick, M. R. *Adjustment to
    physical handicap and illness: A survey of the social psychology of physique
    and disability* (rev. ed.). New York: Social Science Research Council, 1953.
Beier, D. C. Behavioral disturbances in the mentally retarded. In H. A. Ste-
    vens & R. Heber (Eds.), *Mental retardation: A review of research.* Chicago:
    University of Chicago Press, 1964, pp. 454–487.
Benton, A. L. The concept of pseudofeeblemindedness. *A.M.A. Arch. Neurol.
    & Psychiat.,* 1956, *75,* 379–388. Also reprinted in E. P. Trapp & P. Himmel-
    stein (Eds.), *Readings on the exceptional child: Research and theory.* New York:
    Appleton-Century-Crofts, 1962, pp. 82–95.

————. Psychological evaluation and differential diagnosis. In H. A. Stevens & R. Heber (Eds.), *Mental retardation: A review of research.* Chicago: University of Chicago Press, 1964, pp. 16–56.

Bialer, I. Conceptualization of success and failure in mentally retarded and normal children. (Doctoral dissertation, George Peabody College.) Ann Arbor, Mich.: University Microfilms, 1960, No. 60–5859.

————. Conceptualization of success and failure in mentally retarded and normal children. *J. Pers.,* 1961, *29,* 303–320.

————. Enhancing prospects for personal and social mobility in the mentally retarded. In M. B. Miller (Chm.), *Enhancing prospects for mobility in the mentally retarded.* Symposium presented at the Eastern Regional Conference of the Council for Exceptional Children, Washington, D.C., December, 1964.

————. Intellectual functioning and social adaptation. In E. Benjamin (Chm.), *How retarded are the mentally retarded? A P.I.E. approach to clinical assessment of adaptive behavior of the retarded individual as a member of society.* Symposium presented at the meeting of the Northeast Region, American Association on Mental Deficiency, Manchester, Vt., October, 1966. (*a*)

————. Psychological determinants in mental retardation: The functional reaction alone manifest. In B. Nagler (Chm.), *Organicity versus non-organicity revisited as determinant in mental retardation.* Symposium presented at the American Academy on Mental Retardation, Chicago, May, 1966. (*b*)

————. Relationship of mental retardation to emotional disturbance and physical disability. In H. C. Haywood (Ed.), *Social-cultural aspects of mental retardation.* New York: Appleton-Century-Crofts, 1970.

Bialer, I., & Cromwell, R. L. Task repetition in mental defectives as a function of chronological and mental age. *Amer. J. Ment. Defic.,* 1960, *65,* 265–268.

Bialer, I., & Cromwell, R. L. Failure as motivation with mentally retarded children. *Amer. J. Ment. Defic.,* 1965, *69,* 680–684.

Brengelmann, J. C. Die untersuchung der persönlichkeit des retardierten (Investigating the personality of the retarded). In F. Merz (Ed.), *Reports of the 25th Congress of the German Society for Psychology.* Göttingen, Germany: C. J. Hogrefe, 1967, pp. 474–478.

Butterfield, E. C. The roles of motivation and personality in the development and expression of intelligent behavior. In H. C. Haywood (Ed.), *Psychometric intelligence.* New York: Appleton-Century-Crofts, 1970.

Butterfield, E. C., & Zigler, E. The effects of success and failure on the discrimination learning of normal and retarded children. *J. Abnorm. Psychol.* 1965, *70,* 25–31.

Cantor, G. N. On the incurability of mental deficiency. *Amer. J. Ment. Defic.,* 1955, *60,* 362–365.

Chesler, M. A. Ethnocentrism and attitudes toward the physically disabled. *J. Pers. & Soc. Psychol.,* 1965, *2,* 877–882.

Clark, E. T., & Ozehosky, R. J. Veridicality and stability of retarded adolescents' perceptions of normals' acceptance and rejection. *Percept. & Motor Skills,* 1965, *21,* 775–778.

Clarke, A. D. B., & Clarke, A. M. Pseudofeeblemindedness—some implications. *Amer. J. Ment. Defic.,* 1955, *59,* 505–509.

Cromwell, R. L. A social learning approach to mental retardation. In N. R. Ellis (Ed.), *Handbook of mental deficiency: Psychological theory and research.* New York: McGraw-Hill, 1963, pp. 41–91.

————. Success-failure reactions in mentally retarded children. In J. Zubin & G. A. Jervis (Eds.), *Psychopathology of mental development.* New York: Grune & Stratton, 1967, pp. 345–356.

Curtis, L. T. A comparative analysis of the self-concept of the adolescent mentally retarded in relation to certain groups of adolescents. *Dissert. Abstr.,* 1964, *25,* 2846–2847.

Dentler, R. A., & Mackler, B. Mental ability and sociometric status among retarded children. *Psychol. Bull.,* 1962, *59,* 273–283.

————. Effects on sociometric status of institutional pressure to adjust among retarded children. *Brit. J. Soc. & Clin. Psychol.,* 1964, *3,* 81–89.

Edgerton, R. B. *The cloak of competence: Stigma in the lives of the mentally retarded.* Berkeley, Calif.: University of California Press, 1967.

Efron, R. E., & Efron, H. Y. Measurement of attitudes toward the retarded and an application with educators. *Amer. J. Ment. Defic.,* 1967, *72,* 100–107.

Fine, M. J. Attitudes of regular and special class teachers toward the educable mentally retarded child. *Except. Child.,* 1967, *33,* 429–430.

Fine, M. J., & Caldwell, T. E. Self evaluation of school related behavior of educable retarded children—a preliminary report. *Except. Child.,* 1967, *33,* 324.

Frankenstein, C. Low level of intellectual functioning and dissocial behaviour in children. *Amer. J. Ment. Defic.,* 1958, *63,* 294–303.

Girard, J. Problemes etiologiques et fausse debilite (Etiological problems and pseudofeeblemindedness). Presented at the meeting of the 1st Congress of the International Association for the Scientific Study of Mental Deficiency, Montpellier, France, September, 1967.

Gittelman, M., & Birch, H. G. Childhood schizophrenia: Intellect, neurologic status, perinatal risk, prognosis, and family pathology. *Arch. Gen. Psychiat.,* 1967, *17,* 16–25.

Gladstone, R., & McAfee, R. O. The relationship between self-concept and others-concept in mental retardates with IQ's between 50–75. *Proc. Oklahoma Acad. Sci.,* 1960, *40,* 85–88.

Goldberg, B., & Soper, H. Childhood psychosis or mental retardation: A diagnostic dilemma. In Psychiatric and psychological aspects. *Canad. Med. Assoc. J.,* 1963, *89,* 1015–1019.

Gorlow, L., Butler, A., & Guthrie, G. M. Correlates of self-attitudes of retardates. *Amer. J. Ment. Defic.,* 1963, *67,* 549–555.

Grewel, F., & Van den Horst, A. P. J. M. Pseudo-imbecillitas door gehoorstoornissen (Pseudoimbecility due to defective hearing). *Nederlands Tijdschrift voor Geneeskunde* (Amsterdam), 1959, *103*(34), 1716–1719. See also *Amer. J. Ment. Defic.,* 1960, *65,* Select. Abstr., No. 1840.

Guskin, S. Social psychologies of mental deficiency. In N. R. Ellis (Ed.), *Handbook of mental deficiency: Psychological theory and research.* New York: McGraw-Hill, 1963, pp. 325–352.

Guthrie, G. M., Butler, A., & Gorlow, L. Patterns of self-attitudes of retardates. *Amer. J. Ment. Defic.,* 1961, *66,* 222–229.

Haywood, H. C. A psychodynamic model with relevance to mental retardation. Presented at the meeting of the American Association on Mental Deficiency, Kansas City, Mo., May, 1964.

———. Experiential factors in intellectual development: The concept of dynamic intelligence. In J. Zubin & G. A. Jervis (Eds.), *Psychopathology of mental development.* New York: Grune & Stratton, 1967, pp. 69–104.

Heber, R. (Ed.). A manual on terminology and classification in mental retardation (2nd ed.). *Amer. J. Ment. Defic.,* Monogr. Suppl., 1961.

———. Mental retardation: Concept and classification. In E. P. Trapp & P. Himmelstein (Eds.), *Readings on the exceptional child: Research and theory.* New York: Appleton-Century-Crofts, 1962, pp. 69–81.

———. Personality. In H. A. Stevens & R. Heber (Eds.), *Mental retardation: A review of research.* Chicago: University of Chicago Press, 1964, pp. 143–174.

Hertzig, M. E., & Birch, H. G. Neurologic organization in psychiatrically disturbed adolescent girls. *Arch. Gen. Psychiat.,* 1966, *15,* 590–598.

Heuyer, G. Les fausses arrierations mentales (States of pseudo mental retardation). In O. Stur (Ed.), *Proceedings of the Second International Congress on Mental Retardation* (Vienna, 1961), Part II. Basel, Switzerland: S. Karger, 1963, pp. 222–245.

Hinton, G. Childhood psychosis or mental retardation: A diagnostic dilemma. II. Pediatric and neurological aspects. *Canad. Med. Assoc. J.,* 1963, *89,* 1020–1024.

Hutt, M. L., & Gibby, R. G. *The mentally retarded child: Development, education, and treatment* (2nd ed.). Boston: Allyn & Bacon, 1965.

Kratter, F. E. The pseudo-mental deficiency syndrome. *J. Ment. Sci.,* 1959, *105,* 406–420.

Lingren, R. H. Anxiety, praise, and reproof: Their effect upon learning and recall of MR boys. *Amer. J. Ment. Defic.,* 1967, *72,* 468–472.

Makita, K., Okonogi, I., Iwasaki, T., Nanbo, M., & Katayama, T. Therapeutic process and psychodynamics of pseudofeebleminded children. *Jap. J. Child Psychiat.,* 1964, 5(3), 52–57. See also *Ment. Retard. Abstr.,* 1965, *2,* No. 301.

Marasciullo, D. L. The self-perception of deviate boys in special public school classes and its relationship to their achievement and adjustment. Unpublished doctoral dissertation, St. John's University, New York City, 1968.

Markenson, D. J., & Read, F. E. Some dynamic factors in clinically diagnosed pseudo-mental retardation. Presented at the meeting of the American Orthopsychiatric Association, New York City, March, 1965.

Marzani, C., & Paracchi, G. Psychotic manifestations and mental deficiency in children: Some diagnostic and pathodynamic aspects. Paper presented at the meeting of the 1st Congress of the International Association for the Scientific Study of Mental Deficiency, Montpellier, France, September, 1967.

Menolascino, F. J., & Eaton, L. Psychoses of childhood: A five year follow-up study of experiences in a mental retardation clinic. *Amer. J. Ment. Defic.,* 1967, *72,* 370–380.

Merini, A., Loperfido, E., & Bolko, M. Studio di una communita di insufficienti mentali attraverso il reattivo sociometrico di Moreno. (A study of a community of mentally retarded children through Moreno's sociometric method). *Psichiatria Generale e Dell'eta Evolutiva,* 1967, Anno V., N. 3, 321–356.

Merlet, L. Perception d'autrui et structures sociometriques chez les adolescents debiles mentaux (Perception of others and sociometric structures in mentally retarded adolescents). *Enfance,* 1962, No. 3, 303–308.

———. Perception de soi et statut sociometrique chez les adolescents debiles mentaux (Perception of self and sociometric status in mentally retarded adolescents). In J. Oster (Ed.), *Proceedings of the International Copenhagen Congress on the Scientific Study of Mental Retardation,* Vol. 2. Copenhagen: Det Berlingske Bogtrykkeri, 1964, pp. 709–710.

Meyerson, L. A psychology of impaired hearing. In W. M. Cruickshank (Ed.), *Psychology of exceptional children and youth* (2nd ed.). Englewood Cliffs, N.J.: Prentice-Hall, 1963, pp. 118–191. (a)

———. Somatopsychology of physical disability. In W. M. Cruickshank (Ed.), *Psychology of exceptional children and youth* (2nd ed.). Englewood Cliffs, N.J.: Prentice-Hall, 1963, pp. 1–52. (b)

Papageorgis, D. Pseudo-feeblemindedness and the concept of mental retardation. *Amer. J. Ment. Defic.,* 1963, *68,* 340–344.

Pauker, J. D., Sines, J. O., & Sines, L. K. The Missouri Children's Picture Series: A non-verbal, objective test of personality for use with mentally retarded children. Presented at the meeting of the 1st Congress of the International Association for the Scientific Study of Mental Deficiency, Montpellier, France, September, 1967.

Perron, R. Les problemes d'insuffisance personelle chez les adolescents, debiles mentaux: Influence des statuts et des roles de debile (Problems of personal inadequacy in adolescent retardates: The influence of status and roles). *Enfance,* 1965, Nos. 4–5, 469–482.

Perron, R., & Pecheux, M. G. Les debiles mentaux percoivent-ils leur handicap? Donnees experimentales sur l'autoestimation de l'equipment personnel. (Are the mentally retarded aware of their handicap? Experimental data on the self-estimation of personal ability). In J. Oster (Ed.), *Proceedings of the International Copenhagen Congress on the Scientific Study of Mental Retardation,* Vol. 2. Copenhagen: Det Berlingske Bogtrykkeri, 1964, pp. 620–622.

Pollack, M. Brain damage, mental retardation and childhood schizophrenia. *Amer. J. Psychiat.,* 1958, *115,* 422–428.

———. Mental subnormality and childhood schizophrenia. In J. Zubin & G. A. Jervis (Eds.), *Psychopathology of mental development.* New York: Grune & Stratton, 1967, pp. 460–471.

Richardson, S. O., & Normanly, J. Incidence of pseudoretardation in a clinic population. *Amer. J. Dis. Child.,* 1965, *109,* 432–435.

Rimland, B. *Infantile autism.* New York: Appleton-Century-Crofts, 1964.

Ringness, T. A. Self concept of children of low, average, and high intelligence. *Amer. J. Ment. Defic.,* 1961, *65,* 453–461.

Rutter, M. The influence of organic and emotional factors on the origins, nature, and outcome of childhood psychosis. *Devel. Med. & Child Neurol.,* 1965, *7,* 518–529.

————. Behavioural and cognitive characteristics of a series of psychotic children. In J. K. Wing (Ed.), *Early childhood autism: Clinical, educational, and social aspects.* London: Pergamon Press, 1966, pp. 51–81.

Santostefano, S. Miniature situation tests as a way of interviewing children. *Merrill-Palmer Quart.,* 1962, *8,* 261–269.

Schain, R. J., & Yannet, H. Infantile autism. *J. Pediat.,* 1960, *57,* 560–567.

Schmuttermeier, E. Zur phenomenologie der pseudodebilitat (Toward a phenomenology of pseudofeeblemindedness). In O. Stur (Ed.), *Proceedings of the Second International Congress on Mental Retardation* (Vienna, 1961), Part II. Basel, Switzerland: S. Karger, 1963, pp. 246–248.

Smith, J. R., & Hurst, J. G. The relationship of motor abilities and peer acceptance of mentally retarded children. *Amer. J. Ment. Defic.,* 1961, *66,* 81–85.

Stevenson, H. W., & Stevenson, N. G. A method for simultaneous observation and analysis of children's behavior. *J. Genet. Psychol.,* 1961, *99,* 253–260.

Towne, R. C., & Joiner, L. M. *The effects of special class placement on the self-concept-of-ability of the educable mentally retarded child.* East Lansing, Mich.: Michigan State University, 1966.

Von Bracken, H. Attitudes concerning mentally retarded children. Presented at the meeting of the 1st Congress of the International Association for the Scientific Study of Mental Deficiency, Montpellier, France, September, 1967. (*a*)

————. Behinderte kinder in der sicht ihrer mitmenschen (Retarded children as viewed by the world). In F. Merz (Ed.), *Reports of the 25th Congress of the German Society for Psychology.* Göttingen, Germany: C. J. Hogrefe, 1967, pp. 489–493. (*b*)

Wing, J. K. Diagnosis, epidemiology, aetiology. In J. K. Wing (Ed.), *Early childhood autism: Clinical, educational, and social aspects.* London: Pergamon Press, 1966, pp. 3–49.

Wolfensberger, W. Schizophrenia in mental retardates: Three hypotheses. *Amer. J. Ment. Defic.,* 1960, *64,* 704–706.

————. Counseling the parents of the retarded. In A. A. Baumeister (Ed.), *Mental retardation: Appraisal, education and rehabilitation.* Chicago: Aldine, 1967, pp. 329–400. (*a*)

————. Vocational preparation and occupation. In A. A. Baumeister (Ed.), *Mental retardation: Appraisal, education and rehabilitation.* Chicago: Aldine, 1967, pp. 232–273. (*b*)

Wright, H. F. *Recording and analyzing child behavior: With ecological data from an American town.* New York: Harper & Row, 1967.

Wylie, R. C. *The self concept: A critical survey of pertinent research literature.* Lincoln, Nebr.: University of Nebraska Press, 1961.

Zigler, E. Research on personality structure in the retardate. In N. R. Ellis (Ed.), *International review of research in mental retardation,* Vol. 1. New York: Academic Press, 1966, pp. 77–108. (*a*)

————. Mental retardation: Current issues and approaches. In L. W. Hoffman & M. L. Hoffman (Eds.), *Review of child development research.* Vol. 2. New York: Russell Sage Foundation, 1966, pp. 107–168. (*b*)

[B]

SYNDROMES AND SYMPTOMS

: 4 :

Apparent and Relative Mental Retardation: Their Challenges to Psychiatric Treatment

Norman R. Bernstein and Frank J. Menolascino

INTRODUCTION

KANNER (1948) classified the possible symptomatic manifestations of mental retardation as "absolute," "relative," and "apparent."[1] He used the term "absolute" to encompass those disease processes which profoundly alter a child's ability to respond to the outside world. Anencephaly and untreated cretinism represent such disease processes. The extent of the child's handicaps may necessitate custodial care throughout his life.

By "relative" mental retardation, Kanner means those instances in which a child's mild cognitive handicaps become magnified by adverse social-cultural-economic factors and by limited opportunities to employ his albeit minimally impaired adaptive equipment for successful adjustment. Rather than intrinsically determined limits to adaptability (as in "absolute" mental retardation), the crucial determining factors here are the relative availability of an extrinsic support system for the child to overcome his mild adaptive difficulties. Second, by "apparent" mental retardation Kanner refers to those cases in which a child who appears to be mentally retarded at the time of diagnostic evaluation is not mentally retarded at other times and under different circumstances (or after effective removal of the cause). Major emotional disturbances (for example, childhood psychoses) and special disabilities such as childhood aphasia can be mistaken for poor general ability and are examples of "apparent" mental retardation.

Kessler (1966) stressed the same theme of relativity as to the heterogeneous diagnostic disease categories that can produce the symptom of mental retardation. She underlines the common denominator of slowness to learn in the various categories that can produce the symptom of mental retardation and suggested that, rather than a fixed characteristic, "We are really discussing a variety of social, organic, cultural, familial, psychogenic, and ego-developmental syndromes." More specifically, Garrard and Richmond (1965) have noted that mental retardation has been observed as a symptom of at least 240 different disorders, and that this etiologic spectrum ranges over a wide variety of models of disease.

Clinical vignettes will be used to illustrate and then discuss some of the frequently recurring psychiatric dilemmas of "apparent" and "relative" manifestations of mental retardation in young children. The importance of these considerations for ongoing psychiatric programs to aid children with such developmental disturbances will be underscored. Lastly, we shall stress the need to realign the role of the psychiatrist in view of new knowledge and current approaches to such children and their families in the community.

"APPARENT" MANIFESTATIONS OF MENTAL RETARDATION

Psychotic reactions of childhood and associated major psychosocial deprivation syndromes are commonly noted in children who display indices of "apparent" mental retardation. Each of these groups of disorders can profoundly alter the child's adaptive capacity and motivations for responding to external interpersonal-social-educational expectations. We shall not focus on illustrations of socioeconomic and cultural-familial instances of "relative" mental retardation, since these dimensions have been rather extensively reviewed elsewhere (see Menolascino, 1966).

The psychotic reactions of childhood, though heatedly debated as to their ultimate origins and specific clinical manifestations, comprise classic examples of major obstacles to the utilization of native intellectual abilities. Whether viewed as major "emotional block" to cognitive functioning, as a restructuring of personality involvements in external versus internal orientation and goals, or as manifestations of an intrinsic dysfunction, these disorders *all* have the common clinical denominator of atypical or deficient responses to the environment with associated descriptive findings that suggest "apparent" mental retardation. The following three case vignettes review representative instances of childhood psychoses that can mimic as "apparent" mental retardation.

Illustrative Cases

Early Infantile Autism

D. N. first was referred to us at the age of 19 months, with a history of withdrawn behavior, uncommunicativeness, intense insistence on sameness in her environment, and verbalization consisting primarily of grunts. Historical review of the pregnancy, birth, and neonatal periods was essentially normal. In the early weeks of life, she was described as having been an extremely passive child who would rarely smile, and by the end of the first year "She would not smile at all, didn't seem to care who was around, she seemed to be in a world all her own" (mother's statement). She showed little anticipatory pleasure at being picked up and appeared to draw back when held—first with her mother, later with babysitters. In early life she did not follow her mother with her eyes and did not seem alert to, nor interested in, any facets of her environment. Toward the end of the first year of life, D. N. was observed to do much rocking—especially to music. From the age of 10 months onward, she employed grunting as her major form of speech. At the age of 11 months she said "Mama," but her mother reported "I never knew if she meant the word for me or for anybody or anything, she just said it." Prior to one year of age, the child was very selective as to what foods she would eat. The remainder of the developmental timetable, except for speech, was within normal limits.

Shortly after an initial outpatient evaluation, D. N. was admitted to the hospital for further evaluation at the age of 21 months. On admission she was unresponsive, displayed severe temper tantrums when her solitary play patterns were disturbed, and rejected both emotional and physical attempts at contact. She communicated her demands by guiding the therapist over to the objects she wanted. Interaction on any other levels was not noted. Physical, neurological, and laboratory examinations—including an EEG —were all within normal limits. Psychometric examination revealed an atypical pattern of mild mental retardation, with some successes in a few tasks (nonverbal) near her age level.

The family history revealed no instances of emotional or hereditary-degenerative disorders. The patient's mother, who was 24 years old, had been a teacher throughout the child's first 16 months of life. The mother is described as a very insecure person who was in competition with her teacher-husband intellectually and in conflict with him over who should take care of the physical needs of the child, do the housework, etc. After surgical removal of a tubal pregnancy, when D. N. was 17 months old, the mother recuperated at home. She stated: "I suddenly realized how much I had left her by herself. . . . I've tried to make it up to her." D. N.'s father, a 30-year-old high school mathematics teacher, was continuously enrolled in correspondence courses at a local university, in an effort to obtain a postgraduate degree. He confessed he had not wanted children before completion of his advanced studies. He appeared only peripherally involved in the functions of the home, and, referring to the child's problem, he felt she "would grow out of it." The couple had no other children.

During her six-month stay in the hospital, where she had play therapy five times a week, the child made increasing affective contact, expressed herself more intelligibly with vocalization of words, and became more responsive toward her parents when they came to visit (and for collateral, individual —and later—group therapy). Three periodic six-month follow-up examinations, in conjunction with ongoing outpatient treatments, have revealed a consistent improvement in all of D. N.'s behavioral and intellectual dimensions.

COMMENT

This child clearly has a capacity to respond to the people around her and fits into the group that Kanner (1943) initially described as "early infantile autism." Emotional deprivation and inhibited intellectual and personality development appear to be based on psychogenic factors. This does not deny the special sensitivities of children to their environments. The reports on parents of such children remain difficult to assess. Some authors stress the normality of parents who have psychotic children (Bender, 1955), while others (Garner and Wenar, 1959) have pointed out that the parents of a severely disturbed child frequently distort the most critical data of the history concerning their relations with their child. The case of D. N. clearly shows that other such children, who might on casual evaluation be dismissed as "apparently just retarded," are in fact suffering from a reversible and treatable psychogenic syndrome that can be clearly differentiated.

Childhood Schizophrenia

S. L. was a 7-year-old boy who was brought for psychiatric evaluation because of the parents' difficulties in finding a school for him. He was hyperactive; preoccupied with manipulating his body, squirming, and hitting his left index finger with his right hand; and compulsively uttering the words "kill, kill!" and "cut, cut!" He had no friends and kept himself occupied mainly with his toys (a few trucks and cars) and the furniture in his room. His parents were middle-class, educated people with one other child (a normal girl three years younger than the patient). A maternal aunt and one of his grandmothers had been mentally ill. Psychiatric evaluation of the aunt had eventuated in a diagnosis of chronic undifferentiated schizophrenic reaction.

Historical review of the pregnancy, birth, and neonatal periods was essentially normal. However, S. L. was noted to be colicky in the first few months of life and to sleep irregularly. During regular visits to the pediatrician during the first two years of the boy's life, there were repeated questions of "soft signs" in the physical examination (for example, generalized hypotonia), but no distinct neurological diagnosis was made. He sat at 9 months, never crawled, and did not walk until the age of 27 months. He started to employ language at this time, but not complete sentences, and he did not use the pronoun "I" until he was almost 5 years old. His hyperactivity mounted; he was not interested in toilet training, and was destructive to diapers and furniture for the period between 3 and 5 years that his toilet training entailed. Also at the age of 5 years he began compulsively to stomp and to hit doorways and windowsills, calling repeatedly "out, out," and he would do this as often as twenty to thirty times a day. Initial evaluation, when S. L. was 5 years old, eventuated in the diagnostic impression of mental retardation with an associated behavioral reaction.

Shortly thereafter, the family moved to another part of the country, and when they inquired about school possibilities for him, the entire family unit was reevaluated. The atypical nature of his past developmental profile and the current behavioral findings strongly suggested the diagnosis of a schizophrenic reaction of childhood. Psychological assessment revealed a very uneven pattern of responses, with an operational intellectual assessment of 70 on the Stanford-Binet. Both parents were noted to be perplexed, embroiled in their own marital dissatisfactions, and only minimally interested in considerations of ongoing child care.

Intensive psychotherapy was commenced with the boy, and he was admitted to a special education class for the emotionally disturbed; casework with the parents also was initiated. During two and one-half years of active treatment, S. L. showed slow but progressive improvement. His more determined rituals had abated, and he adapted in a rather withdrawn and contained way to his environment. He was able to attend a regular education class. Repeat psychological testing eventuated in a rather uniform test response, with a global intellectual score of 100.

COMMENT

Atypical early developmental patterns are frequently noted in children who thereafter slowly manifest increasingly severe behavioral problems. Though this combined pattern of physical-emotional developmental difficulties has been interpreted by some investigators as the clinical manifestations of an intrinsic general maturational deficit (Bender, 1955), it has also been viewed as stemming from severe problems in the early mother-child interactional unit (Reiser, 1963). Unfortunately, once again we note the medical emphasis on diagnosis instead of on early psychiatric intervention. The quality and quantity of S. L.'s major behavioral problems from the age 2 years onward suggests that we should energetically attempt to intervene therapeutically as early as possible, instead of passively documenting the destruction of personality which is occurring. In these instances, "apparent" mental retardation masks an insidious process that eventually may make the child retarded in the sense of his later social adaptive abilities.

Childhood Psychosis and Atypical Developmental Profile

S. K. was a 5-year-old boy who was referred both because of his marked "shyness," his difficulty in relating to his peers and his family members, and his parents' concern about the refusal of the local school to admit him to kindergarten in view of his "immaturity and fearfulness around people." Historical review of the past clinical history revealed that he was born four weeks prematurely (birth weight: three pounds and eleven ounces). He remained three extra weeks in the nursery for the newborn. When brought home, S. K. was described by his mother as an "ideal" child, because he slept throughout the night and was generally very quiet. At two months of age, he made tracking movements with his eyes, according to the parents, and began to respond sedately to their cuddling and ministrations. His father (a salesman) was athletically inclined, competitive, and eager to have a vigorous son; he prided himself on every noise the child made. In contrast, the wife was relieved about the calm pace of the child's development. However, the child did not sit up until he was 8 months old, and, though he ate well, his weight gain was slow. At the age of 15 months he was not crawling, but worked himself around on the floor by squirming, and played with toys and had a shy smile. S. K. rarely cried or made loud noises and no words were noted. He responded to music by repetitive rhythmic movements with his trunk. He was regularly seen by a pediatrician who informed the parents of his continuing concern about their child's progress as manifested by his unreactiveness and slow motor development. When the child was seen by a pediatric neurologist at the age of 24 months, nothing specific was noted, and the parents were told that he had "loose ligaments in his legs and feet and seems to be slow."

S. K. began to walk at the age of 30 months, with very little prior standing or apparent experimentation. Words were slow to come even in the third year of his life. Behaviorally he was noted to abruptly cease contact with people when he had a toy to cuddle, when there were loud noises, and when his father exuberantly tried to get him to play. With mounting discomfort the parents took their child to a succession of specialists who noted no specific organic disease and continued to suggest general mental retardation. Psychological evaluation when he had reached the age of 3.5 years indicated borderline mental retardation. However, a repeat psychological evaluation when he was 5 years old reported that he was functioning in the normal range of intelligence. Psychiatric examination at this time (the age of 5 years) revealed a child who presented a delicate, fearful facade; very tentative reactions to peers and strangers; and a definite tendency to engage in autistic play whenever left alone. He was interested in music and quick to respond with humming or bodily movements to accompany the music. When given sufficient time and encouragement, he could pick out letters and draw diagrams and figures in a manner appropriate to his age. No specific neurological deficits were defined, though he was mildly incoordinate and frequently tended to stumble. Family study revealed that his mother was perplexed as to how she should relate to him. His father couldn't contain his eagerness to keep his child in action. He kept after the boy to *do* physical things, to which the child reacted by freezing.

COMMENT

S. K. represents a mixed picture of autistic behavior and slowness of intellectual maturation. However, the expectations of the environment, particularly those of the father, had a jarring impact upon this little boy. Both parents naturally were shocked and saddened by the idea that he might be retarded. However, the father, who so hungered for an active, aggressive son, had the greater difficulty accepting the quiet, placid quality of his child. Webster (1963) pointed out that retarded children have an autistic quality as part of their retardation. He felt that this differed from the autism of psychotic children in that it was milder and could readily be arrested by the stimulation that is provided when people care for such a child. In all children there is a point at which the stimulation from the environment ceases to be a challenge to be mastered and becomes a threat which the child fearfully evades through ego constriction or other inhibitory mechanisms. When incoming stimuli are shut off, learning inevitably suffers.

The pattern of shopping for help in this family also illustrates the need for less diagnostic focus and more attention to family support and counseling in conjunction with specific interventive tactics (Call, 1963) with such children (for example, public health nurse visits, nursery school placement, and so forth).

"RELATIVE" MENTAL RETARDATION

Both quantitative and qualitative factors of a child's developmental timetable can frequently tip the scales of his potentials for personality and intellectual growth toward progressively fewer opportunities for successful adaptation. The large group of disorders that can produce "relative" mental retardation encompasses a wide variety of factors that can also impair a child's ability to adjust to his environment. The etiologic spectrum ranges from intrinsic vulnerabilities to extremely adverse external interpersonal environments for growth. Further, we note here factors such as disruptive crises at vulnerable points of the developmental timetable (for example, parental divorce just as a mildly handicapped child is beginning to master early ego defects), fixed professional attitudes toward *possible* mental retardation (as in the following case vignette on the Apert-Park-Powers Syndrome), and negative expectancy "sets" in the socioeconomic milieu which condition a child to give up trying to achieve higher cognitive potentials (Zigler et al., 1958).

Illustrative Cases

Central Language Disorder (Childhood Aphasia)

S. N., a girl who was 3 years and 11 months old, initially was evaluated because of severely delayed speech and language development. On evaluation, her level of language development was one year. Her vocabulary consisted of the words "no," "cow," "tag," and "ow." She often mouthed her words without using voice and expressed wants through jargon and gesturing. She followed simple commands only when they were accompanied by a gesture. Her motor skills appeared to be essentially at her age level. In informal testing of hearing, she turned to noise makers on initial presentation, but made no response to verbal stimuli even when her name was used. A tentative clinical diagnosis of a central language disorder was accomplished.

Shortly thereafter, S. N. was admitted to the hospital for more complex diagnostic assessments. Psychiatric examination revealed a young girl child who initially was rather passive and fearful of the examiner; however, with support she took part in the play situation quite actively. No structured speech was noted during attempts at speech stimulation such as asking her to name a toy, objects in the room, etc. Her nonverbal level of interaction appeared to be within normal range, conforming to the usual chronological developmental expectations. No major elements of hyperactivity, impulsiveness, shortened attention span, or personality immaturity were noted. Good affective contact with the child could be established. The general impression was that of a child with a central language disorder who had marked difficulty in deciphering the verbal signals that were being asked of her at any given time in the interview situation.

Further observation, psychological test results, and experimental evaluation of this child's parents suggested individuals who were very empathic toward their daughter's problems, but at a loss as to how to communicate with her. They were also worried about the child's future education. In regard to the latter, they stated that they had made tentative plans to have her enrolled in an opportunity school (for the retarded), with associated special speech instruction. These parents described their child as having many self-help skills: getting her own breakfast, gathering the eggs, and going down to the mailbox (more than three blocks away) on her tricycle. We had the general impression of parents who, though perplexed by their child's developmental difficulties, were very much involved in and with her in a most supportive way with regard to her general developmental and personality needs.

It quickly became apparent that S. N. was in need of special educational procedures rather than of specific psychiatric care. After twelve speech-therapy sessions, the patient exhibited the ability to imitate six sounds, would say, "m-m-m-m" for the sound a car makes, and could use the words "bye-bye," "yellow," and "umbrella" appropriately.

Interviews with the parents focused on resolving their perplexity about their child's developmental problems. We were able to communicate our diagnostic and therapeutic recommendations effectively to both the parents and the special education teacher in their school district (a district that operated a therapeutic nursery school program with emphasis on speech therapy). With clarification of and attention to their daughter's special therapeutic needs, the parents were able to focus more directly on her emotional needs as a child.

COMMENT

Although mutism (central language disorder) may mimic autism, scrupulous observation of such children in a number of settings will usually distinguish the quality and quantity of attention to the environment (since this particular dimension is most aberrant in the autistic child). Similarly, secondary emotional factors in children with central language disorder can mask themselves as lack of motivation and as fear of interpersonal involvements (social and educational). Their families tend to categorize these children as "different," "stubborn," or "retarded." Labeled as cases of "relative" retardation, such children may continue to follow an aberrant pattern of developmental expectations on this basis.

Childhood aphasia (or central language disorder) is generally viewed as the inability to either express or understand language symbols, or both. This condition results from some defect in the central nervous system rather than from a defect in the peripheral speech mechanism, a defective ear or auditory nerve, low general intelligence, or severe emotional disturbance. While the primary problem of the aphasic child involves a disturbance in symbolic language formulation, he may also have other disturbances. Not uncommon are failure on tasks involving organization, distractibility, perseveration, inconsistent and infrequent response to sound, and periodic temper tantrums.

Aphasia is relatively infrequent in childhood (Brain, 1963), but it can be shattering to the sequence of development when it does occur. The use of psychic energy to compensate for being unable to express what one thinks directly into words is an exhausting effort. Terman and Merrill (1937) noted, "Language essentially is the shorthand of the higher thought processes, and the level at which this shorthand functions is one of the most important determinants of the level of the processes themselves." Some children electively withhold words and communicate by other signals and acts (elective mutism). This can be a rewarding game, enabling the child to hold his parents' attention and to express anger. However, these very interpersonal tactics do not effectively help him to learn or mature. When a child is unable to communicate, he quickly notes that other people respond to this differently, and the whole style of his relations becomes frustrating on both sides. Parents of such children often try to smother their anger when the child does not speak readily, but this tactic imposes a constant drain on their equilibrium since it is words that convey not only thought but much of the affection between parents and children.

Minimal Cerebral Dysfunction (Two Cases)

K. M., when seen at the age of 4 years, was an attractive boy who was described as "into everything and constantly on the go." His parents were worried about how to cope with their son's aimless hyperactivity. On psychiatric examination, his general behavior was observed to be very hyperkinetic and impulsive. Physical and neurological examinations were within normal limits, except for general awkwardness and mildly delayed development of finer hand movements. His short attention span notwithstanding, psychological examination revealed the boy to have average intelligence and only a suggestion of mild visual-motor problems.

Initially, the chief therapeutic focus was behavioral, with secondary attention directed toward a combination of remedial educational and structured environmental experiences in the home. A trial of a psychotropic drug was made; noticeable benefit was obtained. Nursery school entry was then suggested to help in stabilization of behavior as well as to provide early sensory-perceptual training and give additional stimulation and opportunity for use of large and small muscles in an effort to improve coordination as well as develop motor skills. Suggestions were made for home recreational activities which would supplement these areas.

By the age of 7, the boy's hyperactivity was sufficiently decreasing to permit withdrawal of medication while some attention to moderate structuring of the environment continued. He was more sociable, but was more easily distracted than his peers. He was having mild problems in both reading and arithmetic. The chief therapeutic focus at this time became special education for the "brain injured child," with structuring of the environment at school and, to a limited extent at home.

When he reached the age of 11 years, K. M. had profited sufficiently from his special education and other environmental supports to be returned to a regular classroom. By this time his coordination was average for his age, as was his general behavior. Mild visual-motor problems remained for which he was learning to compensate to a large degree. Supplemental tutoring in reading was the only special help he still needed.

COMMENT

The necessity for an open-minded approach is underscored in this case as one considers what might have happened if our original therapeutic emphasis had been directed toward the upset parents who were seen when K. M. was four on the assumption that, since there was no positive history of "brain damage," this must be hyperkinesis on an emotional basis. It was amply demonstrated, as we followed this boy, that the parental behavior observed in the early visits was secondary to their perplexity and frustrations over how to cope effectively with (and help) this difficult hyperactive son. These parents need support from the outset; and they respond to it more promptly than neurotic couples. Again in follow-up, had not our approach remained as unbiased as possible, this child might still be in a special educational classroom since the epithet "brain injured" had been applied. One must remain as inquiring and flexible as possible for the optimal treatment of such children, lest their "relative" intellectual-learning-behavioral problems become "absolute" developmental handicaps.

M. M., a girl of 1 year and 11 months, was evaluated because of her parents' complaint that "She has been termed mentally retarded by two doctors; we are wondering how retarded she is now." Review of the clinical history revealed that this was the second of three children born to a 24-year-old mother. While pregnant with M. M., this mother had periodic bleeding during the first trimester, for which she took progesterone; had an episode of pleurisy during the fourth month of pregnancy; and at seven months was exposed to rubella, although she did not develop overt signs of the disease. She had had three miscarriages (all during the first trimester) prior to the pregnancy with M. M.

While M. M. was in the nursery for the newborn, torticollis (of unknown etiology) was noted on the right. This was corrected by regularly scheduled physical stretching. The child's developmental milestones were relatively slow: she sat at 8 months, crawled at 12 months, and walked at 22 months. However, her language development commenced with "mama" and "dada" at 9 to 10 months and rather rapidly evolved from then onward so that she had a vocabulary of fifteen words and employed two-word sentences at the time of our initial examination (when she was 23 months).

Evaluation of M. M. at one year had reported slow motor development and mild skull asymmetry. These findings were apparently the reasons for the clinical diagnosis of mental retardation by the previous examiners. Relevant family factors included the mother's guilt about the events of this pregnancy, her concern about the child's physical findings (the torticollis at birth and the skull asymmetry) and slow motor development, and the parents' reaction to the dire developmental prognosis previously obtained. The parents were perplexed and seeking developmental guidelines and expectations.

Physical examination of M. M. was normal except for mild skull asymmetry (prominent right occipital and left frontal regions); skull circumference was within normal limits. Neurological examination revealed that the child had a wide-based gait with generalized mild hypotonia and hyperextensibility; an equivocal Babinski response on the left and negative Babinski on the right were noted. The laboratory studies, including an EEG, were normal. Psychological testing eventuated in an overall level of functioning at 21 months (chronological age, 23 months). On speech-pathology evaluation, speech and language development was adjudged within the normal range.

Parental supportive counseling was instituted in conjunction with a preschool program for the child. Regularly scheduled conferences between the parents, the preschool staff, and members of our staff have served to keep the communication channels open and to document this child's excellent developmental progress.

COMMENT

Parents hear so many things about minimal cerebral dysfunction that it is very difficult for them to avoid confusion. There are a variety of syndromes under this rubric, many of them not clearly defined. Physicians are trained to believe that a diagnosis implies a cause and a mode of therapy and, when they make a diagnosis of minimal brain damage, often assume they have a "solid" diagnosis. However, this is clearly not the case and the parents quickly feel the ambiguities that are imposed on them. They become upset and irritated by the scattered terminology that is pressed upon them, which putatively explains the condition but does not appreciably help their child while at the same time implying a prognosis that frightens them. It is not unusual for a mother to comment, "I was in pieces after he read me that report." All physicians working with such children should take into account the inevitable need of parents to have time to accept the idea that there is something astray with the synchrony of their child's central nervous system, that this problem is difficult to define, troublesome to treat, and hard to prophesy about. The variety of consultants —neurological, psychological, psychiatric, and educational—all tend to use slightly different words which often serve only to make the parents more confused. As the ambiguities of such a diagnostic label are discussed with parents, they should be given as much support as possible from the physician.

Diagnostic "Label" Equated with "Absolute" Mental Retardation

When initially evaluated at the age of 12 months, this boy displayed the classical manifestations of an Apert-Park-Powers Syndrome (craniostenosis with associated facial dysostosis, fusion of the digits of the hands and feet, etc.). The parents were understandably concerned about their son's prognosis for general development, educational expectations, and allied psychosocial issues. Since the disorder had been apparent at birth, they had been counseled to expect retarded physical and intellectual development in their child. When first interviewed by us, the parents were literally looking for "any signs that show whether he's coming along or not—or what can we expect." They had just moved to the area prior to our first evaluation. Neurological and neurosurgical assessments eventuated in the recommendation that the child should undergo a surgical procedure for the stenosis of his coronal suture (there were indices of increased intercranial pressure with resultant visual and auditory impairments). The need for such surgery was discussed with the parents with the emphasis on preventative dimensions. A similar tactic was taken in regard to a second suggested surgical procedure: separation of the thumb-forefinger mass so as to allow pincer grasp for future training in self-help skills (holding a spoon, buttoning, etc.). The stress on continuing family counseling had three major goals: support, removing the aura of mystery from their child's disorder, and attention to ongoing parental instructions for approaching the psychosocial-development of their child.

The results of the conference that followed the second evaluation (when the boy was 36 months) suggested that the developmental timetable was within normal limits. Early entry into nursery school was suggested and effected. Both parents have been empathic with their son's difficulties and most cooperative in following through on our recommendations.

Recent reevaluation, when the boy was 5 years old and had completed his second year in nursery school, revealed the physical stigmata of Apert-Park-Powers Syndrome, an articulatory speech problem, and good general health. Language assessment revealed that his language development was in the low normal range, with a developmental level of 4 years and six months. His hearing sensitivity for speech and pure tones appeared within normal limits in the left ear, but mildly depressed in the right ear. Speech therapy was recommended for his articulatory-hypernasality status. Psychological testing eventuated in the impression that he was currently functioning in the average intellectual range with a mental age of 5 years 2 months. Significantly, since the time of his last psychological testing (18 months earlier) the boy had gained 30 months in overall development. We felt that the boy was capable of entering kindergarten and made appropriate recommendations as to the need for collateral speech therapy.

The family milieu is both supportive of the child's special developmental needs and complex in regard to overdetermined considerations. There is one sibling in the family, a 10-year-old boy who is doing very well scholastically. The parents are very aware of their afflicted child's cosmetic problems (in having to face neighbors, his peer group, his teachers, etc.), and are worried about his future developmental and psychosocial hurdles: "Will he continue to develop as nicely as he has, or will he level off? Will he continue to be as happy and carefree as he is now, or will he sense that he is different? Will people continue to be as nice and helpful to him as they have been in the past, or will they look at what he has rather than what he is?" These concerns, which have added a fascinating dimension to the ongoing family counseling, have taken on new urgency as the child is now ready to enter a kindergarten class.

COMMENT

The Apert-Park-Powers Syndrome is an excellent example of the frequent medical blindspot of *ipso facto* equating diagnosis with prognosis. Since the disorder is obvious at birth, the parents' hopeful expectations for a normal child are literally shattered. Yet, the physician often compounds this parental existential crisis by prognosticating for children with this syndrome as a group, instead of basing the prognosis on the merits of the individual case. Reference to textbooks on mental retardation (Tredgold and Soddy, 1963; Penrose, 1963; Hilliard and Kirman, 1957) reveals a striking vagueness as to etiology, treatment, and developmental expectations. Although most of the textbooks on the subject suggest that mental retardation is *not* an automatic accompaniment of this syndrome, and that when present it is most commonly of mild degree, there is a continuing negative professional posture toward treatment intervention for such children. Yet, there is much that can be accomplished for these children (neurosurgical correction of their craniostenosis, family counseling, attention to their high frequency hearing loss, assessment and surgical correction of their syndactyly so as to expedite the acquisition of finer hand movements as a prerequisite for self-help training, among others). The lack of such intervention can obviously convert a "relative" predisposition to retarded development into an "absolute" one. Thus, this can become an exemplary, albeit tragic, instance of treating the diagnosis rather than the patient.

Early and long-term family support and guidance are of crucial importance. Further, the cosmetic (appearance) the child displays may be a more damaging factor to his development and social acceptance than his physical impediments. Born with major anomalies into a family whose hope for a normal child has been crushed, and into a society that too readily labels "differentness" as "abnormality," the child may be irreparably damaged by rejection, isolation, and deprivation. How many such children have been assessed "unsalvageable" at birth and left to the ravages of slowly increasing intracranial pressure, of visual and auditory impairment, and to profound aloneness? The repercussions of these physical anomalies on the evolving personality functioning and structure of these children can provide fertile ground for extending our knowledge of personality development in the handicapped.

In treating a child with the Apert-Park-Powers Syndrome, the physician must clearly go beyond merely presenting the family with the medical-physical problems confronting them. The physician must make an alliance with the family if he plans to continue to help them manage their child. When parents are subjected to this kind of disaster they feel depressed, helpless, and angry. This anger often erupts as criticism of the physicians and other care-taking people. It is important for the physician to be able to perceive bitter parental complaints as sadness rather than actual attacks on the doctor and his skill. Counter-hostility from the physician does not help these people and may impair the child's chances for effective long-term help and management.

Hypsarrhythmia and Infantile Spasms: A Developmental Prognostic Paradox of "Relative" Mental Retardation

A 16-month-old girl was evaluated prior to being committed to a state home for the retarded. The clinical history revealed that she was the second child born to a 20-year-old mother; the first child died of viral pneumonia when she was 4 months. The second pregnancy and the birth history of the child under treatment were not remarkable. There was apparently normal development in the early neonatal period. At 4 months of age, the child began to have infantile spasms, as many as sixteen to twenty a day. Medical evaluation at that time (hospitalization and full clinical assessment with EEG) eventuated in the diagnostic impression of "infantile spasms, cause unknown." Steroids were employed in an attempt to control the seizures; the child did not respond favorably to this treatment regime. She was placed on Dilantin and phenobarbital, which produced only fair seizure control. Developmental assessment of the child at 11 months of age (with strong emphasis on the previous clinical history and the continuing seizures) had eventuated in the overall medical impression of severe mental retardation, with the recommendation to the parents to seek early institutionalization for their child. This turn of events and resultant recommendation apparently precipitated emotional changes in the father (acute alcoholism and marital infidelity) and plans by the mother to seek vocational training to prepare herself for her own needs after a contemplated divorce (and institutionalization of the child). The parents were separated and the child stayed with maternal grandparents while awaiting admission to a facility for the mentally retarded.

When she was examined at the age of 16 months, it became apparent that this child was *not* mentally retarded. She had essentially normal results on physical, developmental, and neurological examination, and her EEG was compatible with a seizure disorder, showing polyspike and wave with slow wave focus over the right anterior temporal area. The overt clinical seizure disorder was psychomotor in type, and the child responded favorably to primidone (Mysoline). Formal psychological testing placed her tentatively in the borderline to low average range of intellectual functioning. Accordingly, plans were quickly instituted for rescinding the commitment plans for this child and concerted efforts were made to reintegrate the family unit in intensive family counseling.

Reevaluation when she was 3 years and 4 months old revealed an alert child whose language development was normal for her age, and formal psychological assessment placed her in the low average range (with some signs of organicity). Infrequently she had two or three seizures a week while on anticonvulsant medications, but these are only partial seizure phenomena at this time. Both parents have shown growth during ongoing family therapy since the last evaluation. Interestingly, the mother had equated the loss of her first child with impending "loss" of this child and, in seeking vocational rehabilitation, had "wanted to forget forever the idea that I was able to have or care for children who could grow normally . . ." The relationships between such crises and the destruction of the maternal and other portions of the self-concept would be interesting to study.

COMMENT

Countertransference usually refers to the unconscious attitudes psychotherapists have toward their patients, but we can broaden this to include the conscious attitudes of physicians as well. With a vague diagnosis such as infantile spasms, some physicians often feel uncomfortable about guiding parents. The experienced physician knows that the more often he has given explicit prognoses, the more often he has been wrong. What the parents need is a general expectation for the future and categorical acceptance by the doctor. In his social study of medical school education, Becker (1961) stresses how much of the physician's training serves to help him handle uncertainty about illness. Nevertheless, with vague diseases that carry the social stigma of mental retardation, it is harder for physicians to console parents about the uncertainties of the future. In the last century Breuer and Freud (1893) complained that they could not make truly "scientific" formulations in psychiatry, and that they were sometimes forced to write like novelists when they described people's life problems. Lowrey (1950) pointed out an antidiagnostic attitude in psychiatry, a "tendency to treat first and then inquire what was the matter."

Physicians need to travel between rigid categorization—which makes them feel better, but limits the outlook for patients—and casual vagueness—which can prevent the application of essential specific treatments. Parents pick up the attitudes of their physicians, and patients often react to the style of the physician and seek another one who suits their own tolerances (Aldrich, 1955). It well behooves the physician to know his style and what he expects from his patients if he wants to help the widest spectrum of patients.

DISCUSSION

In 1919 a book by Rogers and Merrill entitled *Dwellers in the Vale of Siddem* was published. It became one of the classic studies of socially and intellectually inadequate families which were so often quoted to document the familial, hereditary, and hopeless aspects of mental retardation. However, forty years later a follow-up study on one of the Vale of Siddem families, namely the Glade family, was published by Reed and Phillips (1959). All of the Glade family descendants were found and studied. Contrary to the pessimistic prognoses that were usually made for such families, the Glade family had moved considerably toward the socioeconomic norm. Their intelligence levels and social adequacies had improved considerably. All members of the Glade family had emancipated themselves from their miserable habitat in a ravine, and most of them had "made good" in society. A high percentage of their descendants were intellectually normal, a few of them bright. One girl, whose father had an IQ of 77, had an IQ of 160.

This particular family is presented more for symbolic than didactic reasons. The improvements perhaps were due partially to faulty original estimates and partially to mating with genetically better stock. That environment interacting with heredity contributes substantially to intellectual development is now beyond doubt. However, the changes would remain almost unexplainable unless a great share of the Glade family underwent environmental changes and improved education. It is obvious that a deeper understanding of this interaction between environment and heredity is needed. We must also attempt to define the exact psychosocial mechanisms that may produce mental retardation—thereby distinguishing "absolute" mental retardation from the "relative" and "apparent" forms of this syndrome (Kanner, 1948). We would like to briefly review some of these pychosocial parameters.

Dexter (1964) has described the struggles of the family of middle-class socioeconomic status to educate the retarded child and has dwelt on their long-range concerns and problems in rearing such a child. In contrast, families from a lower socioeconomic status are less worried about the ultimate future of the retarded child, but are more burdened with the challenges of taking care of his immediate problems. Accordingly, mental retardation is a phenomenon that shows itself more in certain situations than in others. Mental retardation now presents a more frequent clinical challenge, because changes in transportation and technology have made the retarded individual relatively more conspicuous. Further, socioeconomic class aspirations lead to considerable differences in how such children are demarcated as retarded. In formal learning situations, children with learning handicaps show up in greater numbers while many retarded people can live and work comfortably in agricultural jobs in rural sections of our country without ever being designated as "retarded." Within such settings they have been termed "invisible retardates." Dybwad (1967) reported recent studies in England which attempted to find the predicted prevalence rate of mental retardation of 3 per cent, but turned up only 1 per cent. He feels this is due to the fact that many more individuals with learning handicaps adjust well in society than has been predicted. Indeed, these considerations strongly suggest that there are many more invisible retardates than is commonly suspected.

Similar considerations are relevant to the consideration of the concept of "relative" mental retardation. Bowlby (1951) and Spitz (1951) have shown the influence of institutionalization in limiting early intellectual development, while Provence and Lipton (1963) and Goldfarb (1945) have confirmed the specific impairment of general personality development which occurs during institutional care. Fixation on a psychogenic level, regression, and inhibition of learning in the retardate all have been further defined and distinguished (Eisenberg, 1958). Dexter (1964) reported on the diminished progress of children who are expected to do poorly, while Goffman (1963) expatiated upon the results of stigmatizing individuals with attitudes that lead to poor performance. Zigler and his associates (1958) underscored the extrinsic source of the poor motivation of retarded children in learning situations. In studying psychosomatic disease in children, Blom and Whipple (1959) developed the "special child" concept, according to which a particular role within the family is assigned to a particular child—be he sickly, aggressive, truculent, or otherwise "different"—which then leads to a special set of reverberations and internalized attitudes on the part of the child. A similar conflict of role expectancy is often unwittingly accomplished by the family unit of a retarded child.

All of these observations converge upon the conclusion that the intellectual and motor functioning of young children are markedly influenced by the handling they receive in their early development. Once parents hear that their child may have "something wrong" it is difficult for them to forget it. Pincus and Glasser (1966) observed:

Recognition of the organic nature of the disorder rests largely upon a history of events known to produce or to be associated with brain damage, the presence of major or minor neurologic signs, electroencephalographic changes, and characteristic abnormalities on psychologic tests. The basic etiology of behavioral symptoms associated with brain damage is not known but is probably related to a combination of environmental and organic factors. The natural history of the syndrome also is not entirely known, but acute symptomatology seems to decrease with age though intellectual deficits remain. Therapy is largely symptomatic . . .

Unfortunately, "symptomatic" therapy leads us to the predicament wherein soft signs, incomplete knowledge, and pessimistic prognoses eventuate in "hard" conclusions that may destroy the lives of children for no necessary reason.

Bourne (1955), in a study of perverted rearing and mental dwarfism, discusses the clinical picture of psychogenic defectiveness and stressed its importance as a condition that appeared to produce about 10 per cent of the mentally retarded patients in his study. He documents the opinions of many that retardation can be induced in a large number of children by poor environmental conditions within the family. Bourne concludes that "the understanding of ego psychopathology is impeded by the unnatural divorce of mental deficiency from other branches of psychiatry; for there are pathogenic processes common to all."

Bearing in mind all the factors previously reviewed, it seems clear that "undistorted mental retardation" probably does not occur. The retarded child by his very nature appears to have a quality of autism described by Webster (1963) and is frequently in a situation with psychopathological consequences. His pediatrician looks at him peculiarly; his parents with despair; his sibling with a mixture of shame, competitiveness, manipulativeness, and affection. His parents also possess special attitudes and responses toward him. His peers and his "special" class all shape his personal identity, motivational stance, and access to stimulation and satisfaction. Korner and Opscig (1966) have substantiated earlier studies (for example, Anna Freud, 1945) that indicate that arrest in one segment of development often spreads to other segments, and that this process can become very crippling and leave an imprint on all future development. Korner and Opscig describe these phenomena in neurotic children, in whom curiosity is stunted, or acquisitiveness is inhibited, when new experiences are avoided for the sake of internal security. These writers also state that innate ego variations or deficits color and distort each new developmental acquisition. Nowhere is this clearer than in the maldevelopment of the speech function, as language is such a fundamental organizer of the psyche and the main instrumentality of interpersonal communication.

Poor coordination in athletically interested families, late speech in academically oriented homes, a dependent manner in children whose mothers cannot tolerate this, inattentiveness in the children of parents who demand prompt obedience—all of these situations can feed into the selective developmental delays, with growing anger from the parents and anxious inhibition in the children.

Nonetheless, it appears that children with poor "equipment" have been handicapped by the negative conditioning of their parents, physicians, and teachers as well as by the surrounding society of their peers and relatives, to the point where they do not employ the natural yearning for learning to the fullest.

Such extrinsic-experiential dimensions may tip the scales toward "absolute" mental retardation, where relative and reversible factors had originally been present. As Bruner (1966) noted,

. . . the single most characteristic thing about human beings is that they learn. Learning is so deeply ingrained in man that it is almost involuntary, and thoughtful students of human behavior have speculated that our specialization as a species is a specialization for learning. For, by comparison with organisms lower in the animal kingdom, we are ill-equipped with prepared reflex mechanism. William James said, decades ago, that even our instinctive behavior occurs only once, thereafter being modified by experience. With half a century's perspective of the discoveries of Pavlov, we know that man not only is conditioned by his environment, but may be so conditioned even against his will.

All of these considerations are pertinent to the growing clinical impression that the bulk of the children presently designated as "mildly retarded" are not fixed at this level of intellectual functioning (Cantor, 1955; Potter, 1964). These clinical and theoretical contributions suggest that a large proportion of the mildly mentally retarded group probably consists of two major clusters: (1) There are children who were subjected to severe and prolonged psychotoxic experiences in early childhood, with resultant relative fixation of intellectual growth. Lacking definitive psychiatric care, their relative fixation may have become permanent. (2) There are children who have minimal cerebral-dysfunction syndromes within the context of adverse sociocultural and economic factors. These children probably could have profited from specific psychiatric and educational programs at the prekindergarten level, but without these therapeutic-educational interventions, the full repertoire of intellectual growth was not consummated. Thus, in the near future, this large group of children who are presently categorized as "mild mentally retarded" may become amenable to treatment and educational approaches that—hopefully—can lead to programs of prevention. Because of its wide personal, social, educational, and vocational repercussions, this facade of mental retardation has priority in its continuing challenge to the child psychiatrist.

We have attempted to review some of the present clinical and theoretical parameters of that general group of the child population which Kanner (1948) referred to as the "apparent" and "relative" forms of the syndrome of mental retardation. We are continuing to explore the challenge to the child psychiatrist which he outlined at that time as follows:

This Journal issue [on mental retardation] is a logical outgrowth of a development which has tended to make the study of "feeblemindedness" and its ramifications an important, instructive, and inseparable part of the field of Child Psychiatry. Nothing has contributed to this trend more potently than the work that has been done in the area, covered by the term and concept of "Pseudo-feeblemindedness."

From the dire prognostic overtones of the initial study on the dwellers in the Vale of Siddem to Kanner's more optimistic "progress" note to the present social-cultural-economic experiment of Project Headstart—we note continuing interest and empathy, both lay and professional, for those factors and conditions that may eventuate in a facade of mental retardation.

Professional feelings and treatment postures often suggest that neurological disorders are hopeless and untreatable. The pediatric and psychiatric community is very much involved with finding patients with whom they can continue to work and is concerned to provide services that are helpful. But with too many demands on their time that they cannot meet, they tend to seek hopeful situations in which to work. Professional people share the prejudice of the public against the retarded and define mental retardation in nonmedical and prejudged patterns (Dexter, 1964). Fortunately, such attitudes can be changed, as Philips (1966) and others have reported. We need further definition not only of the syndromes of mental retardation, but of our biases. As Burtt (1965) observed, "Facts of observation do not always speak an unambiguous message with a clear voice," but calling people "retarded" is no more specific and helpful than calling people "disturbed."

The role of the psychiatrist is changing in regard to mental retardation; he needs to recast his thinking and be aware of new knowledge and new models of patient and family care. Both psychiatry and mental retardation have lost by so much separation, and the way toward active reintegration involves careful rethinking of many traditional attitudes (Menolascino, 1967). Many types of behavioral disturbance which have been viewed as "unchangeable" (autism, childhood schizophrenia, mixed psychotic and neurological pictures, mutism, and minimal cerebral dysfunction among them) appear to be positively modifiable by the psychological treatment and management they receive. It has become clear that psychiatrists have a new potential for helping to improve this situation. With increased awareness, there is a new responsibility to take up the challenge.

━━━━━━━━

NOTE

1. This investigation was supported by research grant No. HD–00370 from the National Institute of Child Health and Human Development and Project No. 405 from the Children's Bureau, Dept. of Health, Education, and Welfare, and National Institute of Mental Health Grant No. 5 Tl MH–5331–15.

REFERENCES

Albee, G. W. Needed—A revolution in caring for the retarded. *Trans-action, 1,* 1967, 37–42.

Aldrich, C. K. *Psychiatry for the family physician.* New York: McGraw-Hill, 1955.

Becker, H. *Boys in white: Student culture in medical school.* Chicago: University of Chicago Press, 1961.

Bender, L. Twenty years of clinical research on schizophrenic children with special reference to those under six years of age. In G. Caplan (Ed.), *Emotional problems of early childhood.* New York: Basic Books, 1955.

Breuer, J., & Freud, S. *Studies on hysteria* (Standard ed., 1893), Vol. 2, trans. James Strachey. London: Hogarth Press, 1955.

Blom, G. E. D., & Whipple, B. A method of studying emotional factors in children with rheumatoid arthritis. In Lucie Jessner & Eleanor Pavenstedt (Eds.), *A dynamic psychopathology of childhood.* New York: Grune & Stratton, 1959.

Bourne, Harold. Protophrenia: A study of perverted rearing and mental dwarfism. 1955, *2,* 1156–1165.

Bowlby, J. *Maternal care and mental health.* Geneva: World Health Organization, 1951.

Brain, R. The languages of psychiatry. *Brit. J. Psychiat., 109,* 1963, 4–11.

Bruner, J. *Toward a theory of instruction.* Cambridge, Mass.: Harvard University Press, 1966.

Burtt, E. A. *In search of philosophical understanding.* New York: New American Library, 1965.

Call, J. Prevention of autism in a young infant in a well-baby clinic. *Amer. Acad. Child Psychiat.,* 1963, *2,* 451–459.

Cantor, G. N. On the incurability of mental deficiency. *Amer. J. Ment. Defic.,* 1955, *60,* 362–365.

Dexter, L. A. *The tyranny of schooling.* New York: Basic Books, 1964.

Dybwad, G. Who are the mentally retarded? Paper presented at the Summer Institute on Social Work in the Rehabilitation of Mentally Retarded Persons, Teacher's College, Columbia University, New York City, July, 1967.

Eisenberg, L. Emotional determinants of mental deficiency. A.M.A. *Arch. Neurol. & Psychiat.,* 1958, *130,* 114–122.

Freud, A. *Psychoanalytic study child,* Vol. 1. New York: Basic Books, 1945.

Garner, A., & Wenar, C. *Mother-child interaction in psychosomatic disorders.* Urbana, Ill.: University of Illinois Press, 1959.

Garrard, S. D., & Richmond, J. B. Diagnosis in mental retardation. In C. C. Carter (Ed.), *Medical aspects of mental retardation.* Springfield, Ill.: Charles C Thomas, 1965, pp. 3–31.

Goffman, Erving. *Stigma: Notes on the management of spoiled identity.* Englewood Cliffs, N.J.: Prentice-Hall, 1963.

Goldfarb, W. Psychological privation in infancy and subsequent adjustment. *Amer. J. Orthopsychiat.,* 1945, *15,* 247–255.

Hilliard, L. T., & Kirman, B. H. *Mental deficiency.* London: J. & A. Churchill, 1957.

Kanner, L. Autistic disturbances of affective contact. *Nerv. Child.*, 1943, *2*, 217–250.

———. Feeblemindedness: Absolute, relative and apparent. *Nerv. Child.*, 1948, *7*, 365–397.

Kessler, J. W. *Psychopathology in childhood.* Englewood Cliffs, N.J.: Prentice Hall, 1966.

Korner, M., & Opscig, S. J. Developmental considerations in diagnosis and treatment: A case illustration. *J. Amer. Acad. Child. Psych.*, 1966, *5*, 594–616.

Lowrey, L. G. Training in the field of orthopsychiatry. *Amer. J. Orthopsychiat.*, 1950, *20*, 667–672.

Menolascino, F. J. The facade of mental retardation: Its challenge to child psychiatry. *Amer. J. Psychiat.*, 1966, *122*, 1227–1235.

———. Mental retardation and comprehensive training in psychiatry. *Amer. J. Psychiat.*, 1967, *124*, 45–52.

Ornitz, E. N., & Ritvo, E. R. Perceptual inconstancy in the syndrome of early infantile autism and its variants. *Arch. Gen. Psychiat.*, 1968, *18*, 76–98.

Penrose, L. *The biology of mental defect.* New York: Grune & Stratton, 1963.

Philips, I. Teaching mental retardation to medical students in the psychiatric curriculum. *J. Med. Educ.*, 1966, *40*, 1170–1172.

Pincus, J. H., & Glasser, G. H. The syndrome of "minimal brain damage" in childhood. *New England J. Med.*, 1966, *275*, 27–35.

Potter, H. Some considerations of the causative role of narcissism in mental retardation. *Psychiat. Quart.*, 1964, *38*, 627–634.

Provence, S., & Lipton, R. *Infants in institutions.* New York: International Universities Press, 1963.

Reed, E. W., & Phillips, V. P. The Vale of Siddem revisited, *Amer. J. Ment. Defic.*, 1959, *63*, 699–702.

Reiser, D. E. Psychosis of infancy and early childhood, as manifested by children with atypical development, *New England J. Med.*, 1963, *269*, 790–798, 844–850.

Rogers, A. C., & Merrill, M. A. *Dwellers in the Vale of Siddem.* Boston: Gorham Press, 1919.

Spitz, R. The psychogenic diseases in infancy. *Psychoanal. Study Child*, 1951, *6*, 255–275.

Terman, L. M., & Merrill, M. A. *Measuring intelligence.* Boston: Houghton, 1937.

Tredgold, R. F., & Soddy, K. *Textbook of mental deficiency (subnormality).* Baltimore: Williams & Wilkins, 1963.

Webster, T. G. Problems of emotional development in young retarded children. *Amer. J. Psychiat.*, 1963, *120*, 37–43.

Zigler, E. F., Hodgden, L., & Stevenson, H. W. The effect of support on the performance of normal and feebleminded children. *J. Personal.*, 1958, *26*, 106–122.

Infantile Autism: Descriptive and Diagnostic Relationships to Mental Retardation

Frank J. Menolascino

INTRODUCTION

THIS chapter on infantile autism will focus on three important facets of this problem: the relationship of infantile autism to related disorders; issues in clinical diagnosis; and classification—the problems it poses and the guidelines that should be established. Finally, the general topic of the autistic child and his family matrix will be intertwined with these topics and also briefly reviewed.[1]

In a number of papers, I have reported the psychiatric findings of a multidisciplinary mental retardation clinic for the evaluation of young children (Menolascino, 1965; 1966; 1967). This clinic, at the Nebraska Psychiatric Institute in Omaha, had the opportunity to assess 1,025 young children who had one feature in common: a clinical suspicion of mental retardation. From this series of experiences, I had the opportunity to closely approximate the clinical matrix wherein Dr. Leo Kanner had initially reported his sample of eleven young children whom he believed to present a new and unique syndrome—"early infantile autism" (Kanner, 1943). We have specifically focused on our experiences with psychotic reactions of childhood within this clinic's sample, including a five-year follow-up study of a sample of such children, with and without treatment (Eaton and Menolascino, 1967).

THE RELATIONSHIP OF INFANTILE AUTISM TO RELATED DISORDERS

Our experiences with the original (Kanner, 1943) and expanded (Rimland, 1964) diagnostic criteria for the syndrome of "early infantile autism" has not approximated the diagnostic clarity and the prognostic overtones reported in the last review of this syndrome by Kanner (1965). In that report, Kanner rather tenaciously held to his view that "early infantile autism" was still a unique syndrome, and that it should continue to be studied as a separate entity from the diagnostic syndromes of childhood schizophrenia and mental retardation. Recent reviews (Wing, 1966; Creak, 1967; O'Gorman, 1967) suggest caution as to the inferred uniqueness of the syndrome of early infantile autism.

The term "autism" is frequently employed in the differential diagnosis of severe emotional disturbances in infancy and early childhood. However, to label a child "autistic" presents some formidable problems in regard to definition of the term, specific etiologic-diagnostic implications, and treatment considerations for any given child so designated. Benda (1952) has noted that the term "idiocy" has the same derivation from the Greek that "autism" has from the Latin, both signifying the condition of a person who lives in his own world. As Benda (p. 11) stated, "Applying psychiatric standards to behavioral patterns, the idiot is almost by definition an 'autistic child.' " Too often the word is used as if it were a diagnosis ("autistic child"), a synonym of "childhood schizophrenia," or an abbreviation for "early infantile autism." Such usage is obviously imprecise and contributes further to the diagnostic confusion that abounds in the literature on childhood psychosis.

Thus, having been employed in various contexts, the term "autism" at times loses its original definition (Bleuler, 1911) and is employed as the description of a stage of personality development, a type of thinking disorder, a group of behavioral symptomatology, or a specific nosological entity. Bleuler (1911), in his classical reevaluation of dementia praecox, referred to autism as a primary symptom in the "group of schizophrenias." He viewed autism as a disturbance of consciousness in which there is detachment from reality, with predominance of the inner life. It must be stressed that Bleuler sharply limited his concept of autism to the formal thinking processes, whereas many of the current concepts of autism include both thinking and particular types of behavioral relationships (especially withdrawal). In my opinion, the more recent, rather liberal definition of the term "autism" is crucial to an understanding of Kanner's concept of "early infantile autism" and of some of the problems that continue to arise in considering its possible relationship(s) to other disorders. Currently, "autistic behavior" is characterized in the literature by reference to extreme preoccupation, a highly personalized and stereotyped approach to inanimate objects, and unrelatedness to people (Rimland, 1964). In Kanner's initial descriptive study of "early infantile autism" (1943), he felt his sample of eleven children presented two major primary symptoms: extreme interpersonal aloneness and a marked desire for the preservation of sameness. On the basis of these specific diagnostic guidelines, a wide number of clinical disorders that display autistic reactions in young children have been reported. The range of these clinical disorders, as reported by numerous researchers, is shown in Table 5–1.

TABLE 5–1

Etiologic Variables Reported in Autistic Reactions of Childhood

Acute situational stress reactions (Boyer, 1956; Sarvis & Garcia, 1961).
Central language disorders (Ingram, T. S., 1959; West, 1962).
Childhood schizophrenia (Ekstein et al., 1959; Goldfarb, 1963).
Chronic brain syndromes of diverse etiologies (Pollack, 1958; Bender, 1959; Creak, 1963).
Constitutional factors (Bergman & Escalona, 1949; Mahler & Gosliner, 1955).
Convulsive disorders (Grunberg & Pond, 1957; Sarvis, 1960).
Deafness (Anthony, 1958; Bruner, 1959).
Deprivation: maternal, sensory, affective, etc. (Goldfarb, 1943; Spitz & Wolf, 1946; Bowlby, 1951).
Early infantile autism (Kanner, 1943; Rimland, 1964).
Idiot savant (Goldstein, 1959; Anastasi & Levee, 1960).
Parental overprotection with infantilization (Boyer, 1956; Sarvis & Garcia, 1961).
Mental retardation (Tredgold & Soddy, 1956; Schain & Yannet, 1960; Webster, 1963).
Multifactorial etiologies (Grunberg & Pond, 1957; Wing, 1963).
Precipitate of severe parental psychopathology (Boatmen & Szurek, 1960; Sarvis & Garcia, 1961).

Table 5–1 strongly suggests that the two primary signs (extreme aloneness and a desire for preservation of sameness) of "early infantile autism" as described by Kanner have been noted in a variety of other disorders, rather than only in "early infantile autism" as a singular or unique descriptive diagnostic or etiologic entity.

We have had extended experience with these and similar diagnostic considerations. This included the opportunity to treat and follow a group of thirty-four young children who presented autistic reactions of childhood (Menolascino, 1966). We noted seven distinct diagnostic categories in this particular sample of young children with autistic behavioral pictures, and these are reviewed in Table 5–2.

Perusal of Table 5–2 reveals that cases 1, 9, 10, 11, 13, 16, 17, 19, and 20 fulfill the two basic diagnostic criteria of Kanner (1943) concerning "early infantile autism." Further, the speech characteristics of cases 9 and 19 were consistent with those reported for this disorder. However, close attention to clinical-historical considerations (for example, time of onset, associated examination findings, and so forth) resulted in only two cases that we thought could be classified as

T A B L E 5-2
Follow-up Study of Autistic Children

CASE NO.	SEX M	SEX F	PHYS. EXAM	NEUROL. EXAM	AB-NORMAL EEG	SPEECH RETARDATION MILD	MOD.	SEV.	DEGREE OF MENTAL RETARDATION NONE	MILD	MOD.	SEV.	INDET.	FINAL DIAGNOSIS (AFTER FURTHER EVALUATION OR TREATMENT)
1	x							x					x	Early infantile autism
2		x						x		x				Childhood schizophrenia
3	x		x	x	x			x		x				
4	x							x	x					
5	x			x							x			
6		x						x					x	
7	x								x					
8		x											x	
9	x		x	x		x				x				Encephalopathy of unknown or uncertain cause with the structural reaction alone manifest; with associated psychotic reaction
10	x				x			x				x		
11	x		x					x		x				
12	x			x				x					x	
13	x			x	x			x				x		
14	x							x				x		
15	x		x	x	x			x			x			
16	x		x	x	x			x			x			
17		x	x	x	x			x				x		
18		x	x	x	x			x				x		
19	x		x			x			x					
20	x			x				x				x		

T A B L E 5–2
(continued)

CASE NO.	SEX M	SEX F	PHYS. EXAM	NEUROL. EXAM	AB-NORMAL EEG	SPEECH RETARDATION MILD	MOD.	SEV.	DEGREE OF MENTAL RETARDATION NONE	MILD	MOD.	SEV.	INDET.	FINAL DIAGNOSIS (AFTER FURTHER EVALUATION OR TREATMENT)
21	x							x	x					Central language disorder; with associated adjustment reaction of childhood
22	x				x			x	x					
23	x							x	x					
24	x							x	x					
25		x							x					Acute situational stress reaction
26	x								x					
27	x		x	x				x		x				Encephalopathy due to unknown prenatal influence; with behavioral reaction
28	x		x					x				x		
29		x	x	x				x			x			
30	x		x	x	x	x				x				
31	x			x			x				x			Encephalopathy due to unknown or uncertain causes with the functional reaction alone manifest; with psychotic reaction
32	x								x					
33	x		x					x			x			
34	x		x	x				x			x			Encephalopathy due to postnatal infection; with psychotic reaction
TOTALS	24	10	12	15	9	2	1	24	10	6	7	7	4	

early infantile autism. The general diagnostic impressions noted in Table 5–2 would tend to confirm the emerging spectrum of reported etiologic variables in these autistic disorders which are given in Table 5–1. It is of interest that many of the children reviewed in Table 5–2 are not psychotic,[2] and this suggests that the symptomatic picture in these particular autistic reactions is not predicated upon the degree of personality disturbances usually suggested by the rubric "early infantile autism."

An excellent example of the explicit application of Kanner's diagnostic criteria (1943) to a group of severely retarded young children was reported by Schain and Yannet (1960). Although the fifty children studied by these investigators fulfilled Kanner's criteria for descriptive clinical diagnosis exactly, the etiologic determinants suggested a far different conceptualization of both treatment expectations and prognosis. This particular study underscores some of the recurrent problems that one encounters in attempting to delineate a "unique" syndrome of "early infantile autism."

In summary, the problem of the nosological relationship of "early infantile autism" to the severe emotional disturbances of early childhood is not one of a unique syndrome versus a heterogeneous grouping of syndromes, but rather—in my opinion—the far too frequent loose use of the symptom of autism as a descriptive label that takes on syndromic implications for a wide spectrum of behaviors that emanate from a variety of young children with handicaps (emotional, physical, neurological, special sensory, combined problems, and so forth). Further, we have noted a number of children who had prominent autistic behavioral pictures, but were not psychotic according to either the previous definition given herein or their future clinical course.

ISSUES IN CLINICAL DIAGNOSIS

At this point, I believe that a brief discussion of the concept of psychotic reactions in childhood is necessary, since this is probably at the core of most of the continuing discussions concerning infantile autism and its possible relationship to other disorders.

Considerations Pertinent to the Concept of
Psychosis in Childhood

The literature tends to refer to childhood psychoses, central-nervous-system (CNS) disorders with associated emotional disturbance, childhood schizophrenia, atypical children (Rank, 1949), and "early infantile autism" almost interchangeably. It would appear that the theoretical inclination of the given investigator rather than the behavior of the child may determine to which factor (or factors) the primary etiologic diagnosis is attributed. The descriptive-diagnostic aspects also present formidable problems, since, it must be stressed, many reports of clinical cases raise the question as to why the designation "psychosis" has been employed. As previously reviewed, we have noticed autistic behavioral pictures in children who are not psychotic. Further, we have observed many "mixed" clinical pictures (that is, etiologic-diagnostic considerations suggesting two, three, and more primary or secondary diagnoses), and relatively few unitary etiologic diagnoses that aptly encompass the given clinical picture.

These considerations emphasize the need for an initial formalized and thorough developmental history on these children. The recognition of this need appears to be only a recent occurrence in many of the clinical approaches to this problem. Too often the approach has been, "If the parents talk long enough, things will become clear." The necessity for thinking developmentally encompasses the approach to the child, to his parents, to the particular social-cultural-economic factors operating, and any recent reactive elements (for example, a crisis situation). A developmental approach also emphasizes the close relationships between the emotional aspects of delayed personality unfolding in the young mentally retarded child (Webster, 1963) and the autistic stage of normal early personality formation. Piaget (1952, 1954), in his monumental studies concerning the origins and growth of cognitive facilities in children, described autistic thinking as non-goal-directed subconscious ideation. He thought this form of thinking typified the very young child and was thus an initial stage in normal personality development. Interestingly, he also held that further development (to egocentric status) was dependent on the intactness of the specific sense organs.

Piaget's developmental findings are crucial, in my opinion, to understanding some of the past and current divergent conceptualizations of etiologies in childhood psychoses. Many clinicians seemingly dismiss this crucial need for an intact "set" of intrinsic CNS "equipment" for further personality growth. For example, Bettleheim (1967) avoids this area by making an unwarranted conceptual jump to wholly extrinsic factors as the "reason" autistic children have arrested personality development. Likewise, Weiland and Rudnik (1961) avoid the same developmental problem by overemphasizing the nature and quality of early extrinsic interpersonal programming in line with the thought of Harlow (1959).

These considerations seem particularly pertinent to some of the cases reported in the literature, wherein mental retardation, chronic brain syndromes, and central language disturbances are present in conjunction with symptoms of infantile autism. The associated autistic reactions in these children may reflect delayed global personality development secondary to limited intellectual capacities, the specific behavioral response to CNS insult from a variety of causes, the modification of personality development in relation to altered modes of sensory reception, the emotional repercussions from disturbed interpersonal interactions, and possible combinations of any of these (and other) factors.

In many of these children we noted that temporal factors such as developmental timing and stages are operative and important, since they may markedly alter the clinical picture observed at any given point of time. This awareness of the multi-factorial nature of some of these clinical problems also allows for tentative initial impressions that can be more fully explored during further observation and study of the child. Thus, the initial clinical examination on an acutely disturbed child can be validated after he is in a more supportive setting, wherein periodic controlled observations can be obtained. In this regard, one seriously wonders if the diagnosis of "early infantile autism" can be accomplished (and confirmed) on an outpatient basis. It would be equally hazardous in sound medical practice to diagnose bronchiectasis during an initial bronchitic episode, or to designate that the patient had a "steppage gait," without further evaluating him for the etiology of his foot drop. These considerations are most relevant to some of the basic questions concerning a methodological approach to ascertaining the primary or secondary role of autistic behavior in any given child. Is the child reacting to his deficits by withdrawal? Or is his withdrawal a primary and chronic interpersonal coping device? Have the parents insisted that the child *must* change, or are they more inclined to be less rigid? Needless to say, these considerations demand a comprehensive approach to the total clinical picture—past and present.

Descriptive Diagnostic Dimensions

Current viewpoints concerning the "raw ingredients" of the descriptive diagnosis of psychotic reactions in childhood embrace three major trends: the behavioral dimensions, the clinical encounter with the child, and mannerisms and motor phenomena.

The *behavioral dimensions* that are stressed repeatedly are (1) bizarreness of manner, gesture, or posture; (2) uncommunicative speech; (3) no discrimination between animate and inanimate objects (this is felt to be one of the primary signs of such descriptive designations); (4) the child tends to identify excessively with inanimate objects; and (5) deviant affective expressions.

In the *clinical encounter with the child,* most commonly reported are absent or sparse reciprocal interpersonal relationships manifested by (1) lack of eye contact; (2) minimal, if any, response to structured play sequences; and (3) markedly diminished spontaneous identification interchange with the examiner. These descriptive signs and symptoms from the clinical encounter with the child tend to strongly suggest psychosis if they prevent any meaningful interaction with the child during the interview situation. Additional descriptive features frequently noted in the clinical encounter with this child include the language of such children: the voice tone is described as monotonous, speech is halting or stilted, and echolalia without change of affective stress (for example, repeating TV commercials such as "Mr. Clean will clean it"; or "You must have patience with the mentally ill"; or, when you push the inhibited patient to be aggressive, he responds with "I hope that this is helping me."). Also, in the area of language production one notes pronoun reversals such as the "I-you" problem in a child with well-established speech development.

Mannerisms and motor phenomena that are frequently reported are repetitive and preoccupied manipulation of light switches, doors, and small electric appliances and motor phenomena such as persistent unusual posturing (for example, tip-toe walking or hand flapping).

These three current viewpoints of the "raw ingredients" of the descriptive diagnostic approach to symptoms of childhood psychoses are usually followed by an assessment of the differential diagnostic "weights" of these symptoms. The next step is to literally marshal the descriptive symptoms into discrete disorders or syndromes, which is our next topic.

SYNDROMIC APPROACHES TO DIAGNOSIS

In many ways, the term "infantile autism" probably suggests a syndromic (derived from the Greek, meaning different entities running together) approach to all psychotic disorders in early childhood, since it encompasses "early infantile autism," childhood schizophrenia, the "atypical child," childhood psychosis, and the mentally retarded child with psychotic reactions. In the past I was of the opinion that there were distinct diagnostic categories of "early infantile autism," chronic brain syndrome with psychotic reactions, and schizophrenic reactions of childhood within the syndrome of "childhood psychosis." Indeed, these three categories appeared to have the clearest descriptive criteria for diagnosis according to our past studies in this area (Menolascino, 1965; Eaton and Menolascino, 1966). At the time of our initial studies, we thought our data helped lend clinical discreteness to these three major categories of psychosis in childhood. Our recent follow-up studies (Eaton and Menolascino, 1967) demonstrated that our sample typified recurring problems in the diagnosis of psychotic reactions of childhood since no consistent relationships were noted between types of psychosis, types and lengths of treatment in relation to improvement, and the clinical behavioral status on five-year follow-up study.

At this time, it appears questionable to us that childhood psychosis is a different process as such in the infant and in the two- and three-year-old child. We suspect the chief reason childhood psychosis has appeared sufficiently different in infancy to achieve a separate name (such as "early infantile autism") is related primarily to the infant's maturational level at onset, his constitutional endowment (including reactivity, alertness, and intelligence), and his interactions with parents who may be pathogenic in themselves or reactive to a nonresponsive or "difficult" infant. The psychoses seen in neurologically impaired children appeared to show greater variety, perhaps because all of the variables mentioned tend to be operating as well as the neurological impairment, the manifestations of which vary greatly depending on location and degree of insult, age and developmental level of the child at the time of the cerebral insult, and the manner in which these handicaps are handled by parents and others in the environment.

The nature of the process producing the clinical picture of psychosis, be it something that reduces integrative capacities,[3] or something that intervenes with a previous level of integration, we believe to be the same. If this is true, one would expect a similar clinical picture to appear in infants who are prevented from normal integration irrespective of etiology. Regression could then be viewed as interruption of integrative patterns, with return to a more comfortable level of functioning. In other cases where the psychotic process is less marked, the child does not regress, but integration is interfered with so that a lack of progression (either a psychological or developmental fixation, or both) occurs.

On the basis of these observations and deductions, we now consider that childhood psychosis is a syndrome, and that the clinical subgroups mentioned in the literature depend on the age and stage of development of the child at onset of psychosis, on his underlying protoplasmic endowment, and on the nature of the interpersonal environment in which he finds himself. In brief, a variety of etiologic factors eventuating in one final common pathway (Bellak, 1958) that becomes clinically apparent as a common syndrome of childhood psychosis is more consistent with our experiences than the concept of "unique etiology equals unique syndrome."

It is questionable that either diagnostic criteria or concepts of therapy are clearly enough defined to make valid comparisons at this time of studies made by different investigators. In reading other studies, one feels critical at the grouping of what appears to be described as a child with brain damage with those considered to have "early infantile autism." It does not seem logical to compare treatment data and prognosis in youngsters in whom the psychotic process may be the same, but in whom the psychological, biological, physiological, and other genetically determined substrata are so different. It also seems illogical to compare a child with a central language disorder who has a superimposed psychosis with a child who has lost speech as a part of the disintegrative process of his psychosis. Another problem in making comparisons is introduced by studies that include children whose psychosis began in the preadolescent years. Children who have matured psychologically and physically in a relatively normal way but become psychotic as preadolescents probably have different prognoses (with the same treatment) from those who have histories of borderline or erratic psychological and physiological development prior to onset of the psychosis. One would expect greater variability in outcome in cases in which cerebral dysfunction is known to be present, or in which retardation without specific known cause is a factor. Such considerations are cited to highlight our questions concerning the need for increased attention to definition of terms and syndromes in both diagnostic and treatment dimensions.

Another syndromic approach to childhood psychosis focuses on the clinical gestalten one obtains from the full evaluation of the child. This particular syndromic approach is well illustrated by the work of Dr. Mildred Creak and her colleagues (1961) on the delineation of nine criteria of the "schizophrenic syndrome in childhood." The reader is referred to Chapter 6 in this book (by Dr. M. Creak) for a current review of this area. This particular syndromic approach suggested that a schizophrenic disorder in childhood should be seriously considered if the majority of these nine criteria are fulfilled. The experiences of both Creak and her colleagues (and this writer) are contained in the following overview of these nine criteria:

1. Gross and sustained impairment of emotional relationship with people. This criterion is considered a primary sign of childhood psychosis by almost all workers in the field.
2. Apparent unawareness of his own personal identity to a degree inappropriate to his age. This is a very difficult clinical dimension to describe or delineate in a young child and hence is not universally accepted as a helpful criterion.
3. Gross and sustained pathological preoccupation with particular objects and certain characteristics of them, without regard to their accepted functions. This criterion is also felt to be a primary sign of childhood psychosis by almost all workers in the field.
4. Sustained resistance to change in the environment and a striving to maintain or restore sameness. Since the behavior subsumed under this criterion is often seen in the mentally retarded (Webster, 1963), in obsessive compulsive neuroses, and is also developmentally age-specific (for example, nursery school children need much structuring in this regard), it is not considered to be a specific sign of childhood psychosis.
5. Abnormal perceptual experience (in the absence of discernable organic abnormality) to sensory stimuli. Since so many psychotic children have little if any language, it is clinically difficult to substantiate this criterion. Also, children often have imaginary playmates. Therefore this is a borderline sign of psychosis.
6. Acute, excessive, and seemingly illogical anxiety as a frequent phenomenon. This is another borderline sign of childhood psychosis, since the clinician must rule out entities such as toxic disorders and others.
7. Speech either lost, never acquired, or showing failure to develop beyond a level appropriate to an earlier age. This is not specific enough as a criterion of psychosis, since it is frequently noted in childhood

aphasics and the mentally retarded. Perhaps "deviant" language would be more readily accepted by workers in the field.

8. Distortion in motility patterns. The specificity is not ample here, because entities such as choreoathetosis or musculorus deformans can easily parade as distorted motility, without psychosis being present.

9. A background of serious retardation in which islets of normal or exceptional intellectual function or skill may appear. This criterion is too frequently noted in many other disorders (among them childhood aphasia, Idiot Savant, "strong suits" in mentally retarded children, and artifacts or techniques of psychological testing) to be considered as specific for a psychotic reaction of childhood.

In their follow-up study concerning the responses of colleagues to the utility value of these nine points, Creak and her co-workers noted that criteria 1, 3, 5, and 6 were most commonly noted to suggest the presence of a schizophrenic syndrome in childhood.

Creak (1963) illustrated some of the basic problems encountered in applying these nine criteria to a schizophrenic syndrome of childhood by reviewing her experiences with a follow-up study of 100 cases of childhood psychosis. This is a significant paper, because she also underscores a major recurring problem: the differentiation of childhood psychosis from mental retardation (especially moderate and severe expressions of the syndrome of mental retardation). Since I shall also stress this particular diagnostic dimension, it may be prudent to note Creak's cautions (1963, p. 87):

Mental deficiency is the condition most readily confused with childhood psychosis, and indeed they have much in common. The psychotic child, while in the early withdrawn stage of his illness, is the most ineducable of any, and conversely, one meets among retarded patients odd skills, obsessional drives to no very obvious purpose, active withdrawal from social contacts, and many instances of bizarre behavior. The distinction where these are psychotic children, or examples of psychotic behavior in severely retarded children, is almost an academic one. Such children function at a grossly retarded level, even if it often seems that it is the emotional isolation that closes the doors of learning to them. These cases show that even with reasonable care and long-term oversight it is still possible to be in the dark as to the real diagnosis. Greater precision in diagnosis should be possible and the nine points were designated to help in this. We will always probably be faced with the problem "Is he mad because he is limited, or limited because he is mad?"—to put it crudely.

THE DIAGNOSIS OF A PSYCHOTIC REACTION IN CHILDHOOD

Phenomenological Aspects

Psychosis is not just a behavioral description; the clinician must assess the overall personality configuration. Many times the examiner has to almost put himself in the child's shoes (for example: What is his self-awareness system?). To illustrate the point: The *affect unavailability,* commonly observed in psychotic children, appears to be secondary to incongruent responses to a qualitative rather than a quantitative phenomenon; that is, it is *not affect instability* or *unaccessability.* Since it is a qualitative pheonomenon, the examiner must test his own responses to the child's reactions (for example: Does the child's laugh or smile seem incongruent as an emotional response?). Thus, we have noted that one of the major criteria for psychotic reactions of childhood is that the child consistently reacts inappropriately (or incongruently) to those stimuli and situations that ordinarily serve to integrate the personality.

The examiner must always attempt to ferret out the determinants of the observed behavior; otherwise he cannot tell about the self-system (the "I-Not I," or the "inside-outside" dimensions). To assess this self-system, the examiner must obtain a comprehensive past and current developmental and phenomenological overview of it. Accordingly, he must assess the child's integrative mechanisms for intake, integration, and output. For example, an *intake*-mechanism deficit can include the following: (1) There can be confused parental behavior, under which the child cannot trust the interpersonal environment and therefore can't develop stable (and satisfying) patterns to help him therein. These children seemingly do not experience pleasure often enough to trust the outside world (for example, childhood schizophrenia). (2) There can be special sensory defects such as a central language disorder (childhood aphasia), which make it hard for the child to tell the outside world from the inside world. These children obviously have a different world filtering into their central nervous system. In this particular instance, one notes fertile ground for both primary and secondary integrative deficits *and* a psychotic reaction of childhood. (3) In moderate and severe mental retardation in young children one frequently notes the problems of primary integrative disabilities. As

Benda (1952) pointed out, rather than regressing from reality, many of these children never had the keys to reality.

Such considerations become even more important when we consider children with multiple handicaps who have had a number of medical procedures (as frequently noted in the mentally retarded, and some children who are blind, deaf, or both). One notes that these children tend to be overly dependent on their parents, and in the initial interview session they may show a temporary regression (affect unaccessibility) that appears like psychosis unless one is aware of the past and recent clinical and personal histories.

Therefore, to say "psychosis," the examiner must spell out that it is based on observed reactions to different patterns of stimuli. The *quality* of the interactions of the psychotic child is what is important. These children appear to have a disturbed response to stimuli, and it suggests a "supra-reflex" level as to pain-pleasure and similar basic modalities of experience. At the same time, we have to ask what "raw data" are brought in and have to remember that affective responses are derivatives of raw receptive data (visceral) and that their appropriate elaborations depend on the intactness of the sensory organs and the central nervous system. Finley (1963) has reviewed this particular area with a degree of objectivity and neurological-developmental elaboration that is rarely noted in the psychiatric literature concerning possible intrinsic determinants of behavior in infancy and early childhood. These considerations are highly relevant to the previous underscoring of Piaget's findings that early personality development is highly dependent on the intactness of the primary sensory modalities (Piaget, 1952). Parenthetically, lack of such intactness in the primary sensory integrative systems is frequently noted in multi-handicapped and especially in mentally (both moderately and severely) retarded children who experience major emotional disturbances.

A Suggested Operational Diagnosis

One can summarize the previous comments concerning descriptive-diagnostic dimensions of a psychotic reaction in childhood, by defining it as a disorder in which there is a developmental failure (or dissolution) of the self-concept system that is consonant with the meaningful personal-social responses that ordinarily act to conserve both the identity and integration of the personality. Minimal criteria, in my opinion, are the following: *Affective unavailability,* which usually is present as refusal to interact. (For example, in the playroom setting one notes an inability to structure any interactive or reciprocal play with the child.) The psychotic child does not share his affect, nor does he react appropriately to the examiner's actions in the playroom situation. The clinical history strongly suggests a persistence of this type of relating as a reason for alienating the child from other personal-social relationships. The psychotic child shows a *major interest in inanimate objects,* the use of which is deviant from expected developmental expectations for the individual. (For example, there is lack of discrimination between these inanimate objects and animate objects, bizarreness of usage, and so forth.)

CLASSIFICATION: PROBLEMS AND GUIDELINES

In this section, I would like to discuss two major recurring diagnostic problems in classifying the psychotic reactions of childhood: general developmental language parameters and behavioral dimensions of young moderately and severely mentally retarded children with primitive behavior. Lastly, I shall offer a tentative diagnostic classification.

Developmental Language Parameters

The previously noted concepts of Piaget, that a certain level of sensory and cognitive development must occur before further more complex personality development can unfold, is well illustrated in the consideration of echolalia as a sign of childhood psychosis. Speech pathologists have noted that the early stage of language development (babbling) is cross-cultural in nature as to time of onset and type. However, the next developmental stage (echolalia) is not cross-cultural, and is a stage of language which is, so to speak, as far as the child can go without concomitant development of abstractive ability. It is this abstractive ability that is necessary for true formal language development to occur. Accordingly, in moderately retarded children one commonly notes echolalia as a sign of developmental delay, and not particularly as a sign of a psychotic reaction of childhood.

This dimension is extremely important in relationship to *both* general developmental delays and specific delays in the acquisition of language. Language is of crucial importance in the unfolding of the personality and the child's extended transactions with the external environment. Indeed, the very lack of further language development (beyond the echolalia stage) places such a child at a marked disadvantage for both initiating and continuing meaningful early interpersonal experiences. In this regard, I would agree with Rutter (1965), who stresses that language dysfunction appears to be one of the frequent crucial ingredients of severe behavioral disorders in early childhood. Indeed, it has been our experience that language dysfunctions are at the very crossroads of a number of major developmental problems of childhood. This relationship is schematically portrayed in Figure 5–1.

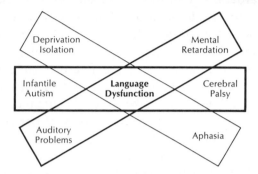

FIGURE 5–1 *Language Dysfunction: Relationships to Developmental Problems*

Brain-damaged children and children with cerebral-dysfunction syndromes (including the mentally retarded) are particularly prone to disorganization of personality from minimal stress. These children tend to have poorly integrated personalities in regard to impulse control and the limited settings in which they have the opportunity to understand and transact with the world around them. For example, their impaired integration is frequently noted in the assessment of figure-ground tests, in which such children report that the object (for example, an arrow) is literally jumping around. Their poorly stabilized internal system of reference (secondary to cerebral dysfunction) thus produces an excess need for them to have a very stable external support system. However, if such a child is in an "unstable" environment —either physically, emotionally, or both (for example, early institutional placement with associated deprivation features; elderly parents who are rather rigid; or families in which the child is looked after by his siblings whose interests are not focused on child care), the outside world can remain very fluid, and he will not be able to clearly define the external support system that he so desperately needs. Such considerations predicate that it would take minimal stress stemming from a relative lack of the extrinsic support system to initiate in such a child's personality a disorganization process that could reach a degree that would descriptively be termed a psychosis. Understandably, the assessment of the "real" etiology of a psychotic reaction in such children may quickly approach the hen-egg paradox.

Behavioral Dimensions of the Mentally Retarded

The studies on "early infantile autism" have stimulated a concerted review of *who* are the retarded, and the associated question of pseudo-mental retardation. Unfortunately, an "eyeball diagnosis" ("He looks retarded" or "He looks too bright to be retarded") is too often accomplished with young mentally retarded children, and a contemporary mythology has seemingly arisen concerning the "supposed" uniform behavioral parameters of the retarded child (hyperactivity, shortened attention span, impulsiveness, and so forth). These recurring professional postures persist because of inattention to the growing literature concerning the richness and variety of behavioral problems in the mentally retarded and disregard for the fact that *only* in anencephaly can the examiner be certain that the child is (or will be) mentally retarded. Rather than review similar pivotal issues, I would only comment that current psychiatric attention has unduly focused on the isolated symptom of "autism" as the basis for both the diagnostic reclassification and treatment of the severe emotional disturbances in early childhood. "Autism" has been studied (and debated) far out of proportion to both its frequency and inclusiveness. It has become a favorite of some training programs in child psychiatry the attitude being, "Tackle the big one!" and is most commonly viewed within the paradigm of "failure to thrive" syndromes rather than "failure to learn" syndromes such as mental retardation. Similarly, the autism and mutism so commonly seen in moderately and severely retarded children has been equated with the autism noted in emotionally disturbed young children who are not mentally retarded.

General Characteristics

Because of these and similar considerations, the personality characteristics of moderately and severely retarded children are too commonly viewed as "psychotic features" (or forerunners to them). Therefore, it may be timely to review some of the general characteristics of these mentally retarded children.

There is a high incidence of CNS dysfunction and complex motor, sensory and special sensory problems. This underscores the need for a thorough historical-medical overview of these children. For example, a history of "jackknife seizures" in the first year of life, followed by an asymptomatic seizure status later in childhood, is a very common history for infantile spasms (Paine and Cytryn, 1965). This clinical history can produce a child who has an intelligent facies, though he is most commonly moderately to severely retarded (and autistic!).

There are distinct delays in physical and personality development, usually from the start.

There are distinct delays in language development, and this frequently produces the clinical picture of the minimally verbal or mute child.

There are superimposed problems in motor integration which may mimic "bizarre" motor phenomena (for example, mild choreoathetosis or dystonia).

Behavioral Characteristics

As to behavioral characteristics of the moderately and severely mentally retarded, they frequently include the following aspects:

There are delayed personality development (Webster, 1963), as manifested by simplicity of the emotional life, a nonpsychotic type of autism with associated decreased flexibility of personality functioning, distinct problems in thinking (especially in regard to abstractive abilities in dealing with the concrete phenomena about them), and problems in emotional control which are usually clinically observed as affective and emotional lability.

There is also poorer development of social-adaptive mechanisms, with a resultant increase of the "at risk" status of the child for ongoing personality development.

We would also underscore that, since a high percentage of the moderately and severely retarded child population are seriously delayed in language development, the diagnosis of a concurrent emotional disturbance is commonly accomplished by means of a survey of available nonverbal behavior. Therefore, the diagnosis is often in the "eyes of the beholder," in his professional orientation, his choice of testing situations. Difficulties inherent in assessing the predominantly nonverbal behavioral indices in such children have prompted this writer and a colleague (Dr. Mary Haworth) to develop a standardized diagnostic play-interview technique (Haworth and Menolascino, 1968) for young children with primitive or disturbed behavioral profiles. We noted that psychotic mentally retarded children did *not* illustrate just primitive and immature behavioral patterns (as one would expect in the mental retardates without emotional disturbance who were progressing along the traditionally recognized delayed developmental pathways). Instead, these psychotic mentally retarded children displayed behavioral deviation from the expected developmental channels. The most commonly noted overall behavioral-play patterns represented withdrawal and disengagement, with inappropriateness of affect, deviantly inappropriate use of toys, minimal speech, and excessive manneristic behavior. The major behavioral characteristic of *affective unavailability* manifested as follows: (1) There was refusal to interact person to person, which took the form of passive withdrawal, walking away, or blandly ignoring the examiner's suggestions (for example, refusal to play ball and on telephones, staring off into space, assuming rigid poses, mouth movements and grimacing, licking or smelling objects, stereotyped gestures, or ritualistic finger movements or fingertapping). (2) Though some play patterns were noted in these psychotic mentally retarded children, those commonly noted in the retarded (for example, free play involved the exploration of isolated toy objects, rarely any combinative play), the psychotic retardates never engaged in any *interactive* play with the examiner at any time.

Another complicating factor, from the observation of the gross behavior itself, is the similarity of some of the behavioral pictures noted in the moderately and severely retarded children to the following: (1) the frontal lobe syndromes in adults (especially those that mimic the apathy of chronic schizophrenic reactions), (2) the initial stages of neurological degenerative diseases in childhood (this can also mimic schizophrenic disorganization), and (3) stereotyped behaviors and "programmed" autistic features such as rumination (Wright and Menolascino, 1966) in institutionalized moderately and severely retarded young children which can—on casual observation—lead one to consider a psychotic reaction of childhood.

In regard to these rather perplexing areas, we would stress that the moderately and severely retarded child is quite "at risk" as to ongoing personality functioning and tends to disorganize quickly (many times to minimal stress). At these particular times of disorganization, the child with a chronic brain syndrome and an associated severe behavioral reaction usually presents acute features of *primitive personality disorganization,* and one can say that he employs *primitive tactics* to deal with *primitive problems* (usually of motor control). In contrast, the child with a chronic brain syndrome and moderate (or severe) mental retardation who then develops a *functional* psychosis usually employs *primitive tactics* to handle rather *complex problems,* and here one notes *affect unavailability* and the lack of interaction (rather than problems of motor control as in the previously noted example). Thus one can differentiate in moderately and severely mentally retarded children the chronic brain syndrome with an associated severe behavioral reaction from the chronic brain syndrome with functional psychosis, and can arrive at the realization that both of these entities (unless one uses diagnostic caution) can mimic both each other and a primary functional psychosis of childhood.

A Tentative Classification

The heterogeneity of the etiologic and descriptive-behavioral spectrum in the psychoses of infancy and early childhood (in contrast to their usually implied homogeneity) suggests caution as to classification attempts. However, on the basis of the guidelines reviewed earlier in this chapter, I would like to suggest the following tentative classification of the psychotic reactions of infancy and childhood.

TABLE 5–3

Tentative Classification of Psychotic Reactions of Infancy and Childhood

A.	B.	C.
Developmental Arrest (primary or congenital). The child never had a functional ego. There is no concept of the self (there is an amorphic and formless personality —essentially no personality). Clinically, they reveal primarily self-generated activities with (1) little if any relationships with peers; (2) marked negativism (if pushed in an interpersonal setting one frequently notes negativism, withdrawal, out of contact [psychosis]); and (3) passive compliance to outside stimuli/demands.	*Deviational-Developmental* (e.g., "early infantile autism"). These patients never seem to develop a functionally complex ego early in life. This may be due to a *primary* integrative problem (e.g., minimal cerebral dysfunction, mental retardation, specific mid-brain deficits [Rimland, 1965]); or possible secondary integrative problems (e.g., it can be secondary to a negative intake process such as psychotoxic mothering, deprivation syndromes, combined sensory-general environmental input difficulties, etc.).	*Acquired (nonpsychotic) psychotic* (1) Regressive-dynamic: *Primary* (childhood schizophrenia). (2) *Secondary* (Propfschizophrenia). Organic Cerebral Insult/Dysfunction (e.g., infantile spasms syndrome and its residuals; traumatic etiologies, etc.). (3) Toxic psychoses (e.g., phenylketonuria). The toxic metabolic disorder literally disintegrates the personality relationship to reality—very similar to acute/chronic alcoholism in the adult.

If infantile autism is not a unitary syndrome, then some cherished notions concerning its etiology, description, and treatment must be reevaluated. This particular reevaluation epitomizes one of the major conceptual problems that presents a real dilemma to the psychiatrist in investigating both homogeneous and heterogeneous populations: the utilization of current nomenclatural systems that literally demand classification by etiology, whereas treatment-management techniques are based on behavioral and social constellation criteria. An extended discussion of this particular conceptual problem is reviewed in Part Five, Chapter 32, of this book.

INFANTILE AUTISM AND THE FAMILY

I have suggested that "infantile autism," in my opinion, is a most heterogeneous category of severe behavioral disturbances in childhood. Accordingly, no uniform (homogeneous) family "types" are noted or expected. I shall, therefore, keep my comments almost telegraphic in style and length.

It has been my experience that autistic children come from a variety of family backgrounds, and here the word "variety" encompasses socioeconomic classes, level of vocational attainments, ethnic and cultural dimensions, parental psychopathology and other variables. Clinicians have apparently had fixed attitudes and fadlike notions concerning the parents of these children. These have varied from "refrigerated parents," to "schizophrenogenic parents" (Bruner and Szurek, 1960), to specificity of types of psychosis and parental configurations (Goldfarb, 1963), to multifactorial etiologies (Sarvis and Garcia, 1961), to name but a few.

I have repeatedly been most impressed with the effects these particular children have on their families rather than vice versa. These experiences have repeatedly underscored the role such children can play in literally throwing the family "off balance" as an integral unit. Accordingly, it frequently becomes most difficult to differentiate the etiologic influences of family psychopathology from the effects *on* the family of having a chronically handicapped child in its midst. When this dimension is coupled with the apparently high incidence of emotional disturbances in our general adult population (see the Midtown Manhattan [1962], and Stirling County [1959] epidemiological studies), it does not become surprising that parents of such children are frequently described as "emotionally disturbed." The clinical challenge then becomes one of differentiating the primary role of family determinants in a given child's current disorder from reactive and similar dimensions.

As previously noted, my experiences with infantile autism are consistent with the viewpoint of multifactorial etiologies and hence a wide spectrum of family psychopathology and constellations. In other words, the heterogeneity of the clinical etiologies in such infants and children is seemingly matched by the heterogeneity of the associated families that accompany them for evaluation and treatment.

SUMMARY

Infantile autism was described and systematically discussed with regard to its possible relationship to associated disorders such as mental retardation, to the issues in clinical diagnosis it raises, and to the classification problems it poses. Finally, a tentative classification of the varieties of clinical disorders commonly subsumed under this rubric was presented.

Where are we in our current professional approaches to infantile autism? We have some knowledge of the etiologic beginnings, more knowledge of the descriptive aspects, some information as to intermediate types and developmental stages, and early suggestions of prognostic expectations. To fill in this currently impressionistic landscape of severe behavioral psychopathology in infancy and early childhood comprises a major future research challenge for child psychiatry.

―――

NOTES

1. This investigation was supported by United States Public Health Service Research Grants MH–08767 from the National Institute of Mental Health and HD–00370 from the National Institute of Child Health and Human Development, Washington, D.C.

2. This term is at times employed without regard to minimal diagnostic requirements such as marked disturbances of feeling, speech, perception, motility, ability to test reality, control of instinctual energies, or associated social isolation and withdrawal. The British working party's activities (Creak et al., 1961: Creak et al., 1964), in seeking further clarification of the concept of psychosis in childhood, emphasizing the different clinical problems here.

3. "Integrative capacities" is used here in its broadest sense, implying ego functions; physiological and neurological maturation; and intellectual and other dimensions of personality development.

REFERENCES

Alpert, A. A special therapeutic technique for certain developmental disorders in prelatency children. *Amer. J. Orthopsychiat.*, 1967, *27*, 256–270.

Anastasi, A., & Levee, R. F. Intellectual defect and musical talent: A case report. *Amer. J. Ment. Defic.*, 1960, *64*, 695–703.

Anthony, J. An experimental approach to the psychopathology of childhood autism. *Brit. J. Med. Psychol.*, 1958, *31*, 211–225.

Bellak, L. (Ed.). *Schizophrenia: A review of the syndrome.* New York: Logos Press, 1958.

Benda, C. *Developmental disorders of mentation and cerebral palsies.* New York: Grune & Stratton, 1952.

Bender, L. Autism in children with mental deficiency. *Amer. J. Ment. Defic.*, 1959, *63*, 81–86.

Bergman, P., & Escalona, S. K. Unusual sensitivities in very young children. *Psychoanal. Study Guide*, 1949, *3–4*, 333–352.

Bettelheim, B. *The empty fortress: Infantile autism and the birth of the self.* New York: The Free Press, 1967.

Bleuler, E. *Dementia praecox or the groups of schizophrenias*, trans. J. Zinkin. New York: International Universities Press, 1952, p. 63.

Bowlby, J. *Maternal care and mental health.* Geneva: World Health Organization, 1951.

Boyer, L. B. On maternal overstimulation and ego defects. *Psychoanal. Study Child*, 1956, *11*, 236–256.

Bruner, J. S. The cognitive consequence of early sensory deprivation. *Psychosom. Med.*, 1959, *21*, 89–95.

Bruner, J. S., & Szurek, S. A. Clinical childhood schizophrenia. In D. Jackson (Ed.), *The etiology of schizophrenia.* New York: Basic Books, 1960, pp. 389–446.

Creak, M. et al. Schizophrenic syndromes in childhood. *Develop. Med. & Child Neurol.*, 1961, *3*, 501–504.

————. Childhood psychosis: A review of 100 cases. *Brit. J. Psychiat.*, 1963, *109*, 84–89.

————. Childhood schizophrenia. *ACTA Paedopsychiatrica*, 1967, *34*, 365–370.

Despert, J. L., & Sherwin, A. C. Further examination of diagnostic criteria in schizophrenia illness and psychosis of infancy and early childhood. *Amer. J. Psychiat.*, 1958, *114*, 784–790.

Eaton, L., & Menolascino, F. J. Psychotic reactions of childhood: Experiences of a mental retardation pilot project. *J. Nerv. Ment. Dis.*, 1966, *143*, 55–67.

————. Psychotic reactions of childhood: A follow-up study. *Amer. J. Orthopsychiat.*, 1967, *37*, 521–529.

Ekstein, R., Bryant, K., & Freedman, S. W. Childhood schizophrenia and allied conditions. In L. Bellak and P. K. Benedect (Eds.), *Schizophrenia.* New York: Logos Press, 1959, pp. 555–693.

Finley, K. H. Behaviorial disorders and brain dysfunction. *Med. Clin. North America*, 1963, *17*, 1691–1710.

Goldfarb, W. Psychological privation in infancy and subsequent adjustment. *Amer. J. Orthopsychiat.*, 1943, *15*, 247–255.

————. *Childhood schizophrenia.* Cambridge, Mass.: Harvard University Press, 1963.

Goldstein, K. Abnormal mental conditions in infancy. *J. Nerv. Ment. Dis.*, 1959, *128*, 538–557.

Grunberg, F., & Pond, D. A. Conduct disorders in epileptic children. *J. Neurosurg. Psychiat.*, 1957, *20*, 65–68.

Harlow, H. Social capacity of primates. *Human Biol.*, 1959, *31*, 40–53.

Haworth, M., & Menolascino, F. J. Video tape observations of disturbed young children. *J. Clin. Psychol.*, 1967, *23*, 135–140.

————. Some aspects of psychotic behavior in young children. *Arch. Gen. Psych.*, 1968, *18*, 355–359.

Ingram, R. Chronic brain syndromes in childhood other than cerebral palsy, epilepsy, and mental defect. In W. Bax and R. MacLeith (Eds.), *Minimal cerebral dysfunction.* London: Heineman, 1963, pp. 10–17.

Ingram, T. T. S. Specific developmental disorders of speech in childhood. *Brain*, 1959, *82*, 450–467.

Kanner, L. Autistic disturbances of affective contact. *Nerv. Child*, 1943, *2*, 217–250.

————. Problems of nosology and psychodynamics of early infantile autism. *Amer. J. Orthopsychiat.*, 1949, *19*, 416–426.

————. To what extent is early infantile autism determined by constitutional inadequacies? *Proc. Assoc. Res. Nerv. Ment. Dis.*, 1954, *33*, 378–385.

————. The specificity of early infantile autism. *Z. Kinderpsychiat.*, 1958, *25*, 108–113.

————. Infantile autism and the schizophrenias. Presented at the Annual Meeting of the American Psychiatric Association, New York, 1965.

Lay, R. A. Q. Schizophrenia-like psychoses in young children. *J. Ment. Sci.,* 1938, *84,* 105–133.

Lanzkron, J. The concept of propf-schizophrenia and its prognosis. *Amer. J. Ment. Defic.,* 1957, *61.* 544–547.

Leighton, A. H. *My name is legion.* New York: Basic Books, 1959.

Lovaas, O. I., Freitag, G., & Kinder, M. I. Establishment of social reinforcements in two schizophrenic children on the basis of food. *J. Exper. Child Psychol.,* 1966, *4,* 109–125.

Mahler, M. S. On child psychosis and schizophrenia: Autistic and symbiotic infantile psychosis. *Psychoanal. Study Child,* 1952, *7,* 286–305.

Mahler, M. S., & Gosliner, B. J. On symbiotic child psychosis. *Psychoanal. Study Guide,* 1955, *10,* 195–212.

Menolascino, F. J. Autistic reactions in early childhood: Differential diagnostic considerations. *J. Child Psychol. & Psychiat.,* 1965, *6,* 203–218. (*a*)

———. Psychiatric aspects of mental retardation in children under eight. *Amer. J. Orthopsychiat.,* 1965, *35,* 852–861. (*b*)

———. The facade of mental retardation: Its challenge to child psychiatry. *Amer. J. Psychiat.,* 1966, *122,* 1227–1235.

Menolascino, F. J., & Eaton, L. Psychoses of childhood: A five-year follow-up study of experiences in a mental retardation clinic. *Amer. J. Ment. Defic.,* 1967, *72,* 370–380.

O'Gorman, G. *The nature of childhood autism.* London: Butterworths, 1967.

Paine, R. S., & Cytryn, L. Counseling parents of mentally retarded children. *Clin. Proc. Child. Hosp.,* 1965, *21,* 106–119.

Piaget, J. *The origin of intelligence in the child.* New York: International Universities Press, 1952.

———. *The construction of reality in the child.* New York: Basic Books, 1954.

Pollack, M. Brain damage, mental retardation and childhood schizophrenia. *Amer. J. Psychiat.,* 1958, *115,* 422–428.

Rank, B. Adaptation of the psychoanalytic technique for the treatment of young children with atypical development. *Amer. J. Orthopsychiat.,* 1949, *19,* 130–139.

———. Intensive study and treatment of preschool children who show marked personality deviations, or "atypical development," and their parents. In G. Caplan (Ed.), *Emotional problems of early childhood.* New York: Basic Books, 1955, pp. 491–501.

Reiser, D. Psychosis of infancy and early childhood, as manifested by children with atypical development. *New England J. Med.,* 1963, *269,* 790–798, 844–850.

Rimland, B. *Infantile autism.* New York: Appleton-Century-Crofts, 1964, pp. 17–22.

Rutter, M. The influence of organic and emotional factors on the origins, nature and outcome of childhood psychosis. *Develop. Med. Child Neurol.,* 1965, *7,* 518–528.

———. Children of sick parents: An environmental and psychiatric study. Oxford: Institute of Psychiatry Monograph, 1966, No. 16.

Sarvis, M. A. Psychiatric implications of temporal lobe damage. *Psychoanal. Study Child.,* 1960, *15,* 454–481.

Sarvis, M. A., & Garcia, B. Etiological variables in autism. *Psychiatry,* 1961, *24,* 307–317.

Schain, R. J., & Yannet, H. Infantile autism. *J. Pediat.,* 1960, *57,* 560–567.

Spitz, R. A., & Wolf, K. M. Anaclitic depression: An inquiry into the genesis of psychiatric conditions in early childhood. *Psychoanal. Study Child,* 1946, *2,* 313–342.

Srole, L. *Mental health in the metropolis.* New York: McGraw-Hill, 1962.

Szurek, S. A., & Berlin, I. N. Elements of psychotherapeutics with the schizophrenic child and his parents. *Psychiatry,* 1956, *19,* 1–9.

Tizard, J. Mental subnormality and child psychiatry. *J. Child Psychol. & Psychiat.,* 1966, *7,* 1–15.

Tredgold, R. F., & Soddy, K. *A textbook of mental deficiency* (9th ed.). Baltimore: Williams & Wilkins, 1956.

Webster, T. Problems of emotional development in young retarded children. *Amer. J. Psychiat.,* 1963, *120,* 34–43.

Weiland, I. H., & Rudnik, R. Considerations of the development and treatment of autistic childhood psychosis. *Psychoanal. Study Child,* 1961, *16,* 549–563.

Wenar, C. The reliability of developmental histories. *Psychosom. Med.,* 1963, *25,* 505–509.

West, R. Childhood aphasia. *Soc. Crippled Child. & Adults.* 1962, *16*, 31–42.

Wing, J. K. Epidemiology of early childhood autism. *Develop. Med. & Child Neurol.*, 1963, *5*, 646–647.

————. (Ed.). *Early childhood autism.* Oxford: Pergamon Press, 1966.

Wortis, J. Schizophrenia symptomatology in mentally retarded children. *Amer. J. Psychiat.*, 1958, *115*, 429–431.

Wright, M. M., & Menolascino, F. J. Nurturant nursing of mentally retarded ruminators. *Amer. J. Ment. Defic.*, 1966, *71*, 451–459.

: 6 :

Diagnostic and Treatment Variations in

Child Psychoses and Mental Retardation

Mildred Creak

INTRODUCTION

FEW people, once they have become familiar with both the concepts and the reality of autistic and psychotic children, can fail to wonder whether such children are, in fact, better seen as a variety of mentally retarded children. Wherein lies the justification for a separate category of "psychotic" children? Can the terminologies, differential diagnosis, and treatment-prognosis parameters commonly in use with autistic and psychotic children be clarified in relation to the concept of mental retardation in children? In this chapter, I shall attempt to review my past clinical experience and current reflections thereon.

TERMINOLOGY

Psychosis is commonly taken to mean a severe mental illness which, when it occurs, drastically alters the clinical condition of the child so affected. Mental retardation is usually accepted as referring to an inborn condition in which progressive development—in every aspect— fails to reach a normally accepted developmental level. At every point, and in every respect, the retarded child falls below the level normal for his chronological age. Clearly this may be somewhat modified by cultural factors and by intercurrent happenings. In contrast, the term "regression" is used in considering autistic and psychotic children, where a normal development fails to continue at the accepted rate, and where there is actual loss of skills previously gained. Yet there is much overlap between delayed development and regressive phenomena, both with regard to the causes and clinical description. For example, a highly intelligent child may regress in speech if, at an early stage of verbal development, he becomes severely deaf. Clinically, such a state of affairs should not be confused with an inborn retardation so severe that speech is never adequately developed. Yet a differential diagnosis between a congenital aphasia and the results of early deafness will sometimes pose an exceedingly difficult problem in differential diagnosis. The falling off in speech, or the failure to develop the ability to communicate verbally, is far harder to explain when it is seen as a pivotal point in a psychotic child, leading to confusion between the concepts of retardation and regression.

The term "early infantile autism" was used by Kanner (1943) as the title of his clinical description of a well-differentiated group of cases seen in early childhood where disturbances in speech and social contact, an "aloneness" in relation to his family and surroundings, a need to impose a rigid ritual or sameness in his behavior patterns and environment, and an attachment to objects rather than to people, coexisted in a child whose family Kanner observed were often of a coldly intellectual, even somewhat obsessional type. He regarded the condition as inborn or existing from a very early age (hence "infantile"), agreeing with other observers that even as babies these children failed to produce the usual anticipatory postural responses when picked up. He emphasized their normal appearance, the absence of stigmata, and that in certain achievements—notably their grace and skill in motor capacity—they were entirely different from those retarded children whose total development fails to achieve speech and the ability to communicate.

Wing (1966), commenting on Kanner's work and the problem of terminology, prefers "childhood autism" to cover all cases, since not all of them are manifest in the years of infancy, but eventually emerge as indistinguishable from the Kanner syndrome with an onset in the third or fourth years of life.

Bender (1959), Goldfarb (1961), and others use the term "childhood schizophrenia." Certainly the term "autism" was first used (by Bleuler) in connection with the solitary, self-immured quality manifest in adult schizophrenic patients. A degree of mental deterioration, or at least a diminishing capacity to function possibly due to disuse, is manifest in schizophrenics. Goldfarb's descriptions of clinical cases give a clear indication as to why this may apply to what is here called the "psychotic" manifestations seen in childhood; and why they might be associated not so much with a failure to retain capacity as a failure to achieve it. Certainly one would expect the impact of a schizophrenic illness to both threaten and distort the normal flow of development, when such impact happens in early childhood. Wing (1966) comments that these children are not like adult schizophrenics, do not develop the delusions, bizarre ideation, and hallucinatory experiences met with in the adult patient. He limits the term "schizophrenia" in children to those cases where an adult-type illness develops in childhood, leaving unexplored the problem of a common causation in the two conditions.

We are thus left with a clinical description of a group of children whose behavior and abilities render them unable to function normally within society. Development may be distorted almost from birth, and the net result may produce a degree of retardation which often appears to be secondary to their isolation in society and among their kind, and their inability to communicate and to both achieve and impart understanding. If the learning doors are blocked in this way, it may be exceedingly difficult to foster development in the normal social ways of children who live with their families. Nor can learning, in a more intellectual and tutorial sense, be imparted since nothing appears to be there at the receptive end. The clinical descriptions are clear and distinctive, whatever terminology is used, and we know and recognize the cases they refer to. Whether we can achieve a closer delineation of different varieties, suggested by the different terminologies used, will probably remain an open question, until a further step is taken in understanding how the condition is caused, and whether a uniform pathology exists. Bender (1959), perhaps more clearly than any of the other investigators, indicates the complexity of the overlap with some cases of mental retardation, when she distinguishes within her category of "childhood schizophrenia" a subgroup of "pseudo-defective" children. In her view, an all-round maturational lag is evident in every aspect of development.

What, then, are the characteristics of these psychotic children? Perhaps the outstanding feature is their total indifference to and disregard of their environment. They will focus attention on an object, held or twiddled in their own particular way, to the exclusion of unfamiliar objects offered to them. Whereas the crackle of a sweet wrapping which they know indicates a wanted object may evoke a response, a call or a loud noise, set to evoke response, will produce no reaction. A quality of unpredictability pertains, although those who know psychotic children can often be sure by many repetitions of what will alarm them. Such a child may be terrified of the vacuum cleaner, yet be perfectly competent at working the record player. While seemingly alert, they look past the investigator, avoiding contact or a direct glance. While their facial appearance is often beautiful, the features may be like those of a young child, and there is sometimes a marked degree of muscular hypotonia. They will climb and balance with the agility of a monkey, unscrew tops, and open doors, but the activity remains an end in itself rather than a means to an end and is often repeated monotonously. Frequently there is also an excess of bizarre and idiosyncratic activity such as tip-toe walking and twirling, tapping, or spinning objects. Many such children smell, mouth, or lick objects as soon as they take hold of them; their unexpected plunges and thrusts may cause damage, but they rarely fall or hurt themselves. Their appetites are unusual and often confined to a rigidly monotonous selection of foods. Water-play, sousing, and excessive drinking (for which no physiological reason can be found) are often prominent. Head banging and cot rocking may accompany their wakeful nights and, if interrupted, intractable screaming sometimes follows.

This type of behavior may evolve gradually from a rather quiet and passive infancy that was often regarded as normal at the time, but in retrospect showed even then a failure either to evoke or to respond to social contact and affective stimulation.

In other cases some event appears suddenly to deflect a hitherto more normal developmental pattern: in first-born children such an active withdrawal may seem to be fired off by the birth of a sibling.

This can be seen in contrast to "autistic" behavior in a child who appears to be primarily retarded. Here the slowness is shown from the start, often an unhealthily "good" (that is, quiet and inert) baby. Such children are slow to sit, are still slower to get on their feet, are timid and unwilling to try new skills—for the very good reason that the capacity to do so appears lacking, as is also the thrust of awakening interest and awareness. A need for long-continuing help with feeding and dressing, and slowness in recognizing games or bedtime stories suggest that when repetitive activities such as rocking begin, they do so as a simple pattern of perseveration, rather than as a protective monotony which, for the autistic child, appears to exclude unwanted demands.

Watching a retarded child develop makes one aware of a slower and simplified pattern, which in turn calls for a simplified form of social stimulation. Attempts to manipulate, to respond whether in speech or in action, are marked by hesitancy and a certain crude simplicity, that will only build up into a coherent response after a longer than usual period of trial and error. Learning of skills needs to be pushed home with infinite patience and care in selection. Such procedures do little to influence the inaccessible psychotic child, although in time they may succeed in getting around what is an active withdrawal rather than a failure in response which is derived from deficiency in resources in the true retardate.

ROLE OF LANGUAGE

Speech constitutes the human means of communication. Figuratively, it acts as a fertilizer of the thinking processes. We are aware of the extent to which language has to expand to meet the needs of deeper and more elaborate thought processes. We accept a certain literalness in the spoken expression of young children. An intelligent four-year-old, hearing her tired mother say, "Oh dear, my feet are not what they were," responded eagerly, "Oh—what were they?" An intelligent five-year-old carried in a dead bird to her mother and asked, "Who used to live in this?" which is a long way further on developmentally, but still with a very limited understanding of all the implications of the passage of time. Language in the retarded child develops slowly and tends to remain simple, even impoverished, and concrete in its expression. Concept formation, reflecting a delay in conceptual thinking, is only slowly developed. It will often need building up and amplifying with pictured images and acting-out experience.

The cessation of speech in the autistic child can be either abrupt, or it can be a gradual dying away of words and phrases learnt. In some, speech never develops; in others, who remain mute for long periods, a sudden appropriate sentence will be spoken, giving rise to the feeling parents often express with some irritation, that "he could speak if he would." Curious anomalies occur, such as children who can read before they speak, or spell before they can write. Skill with manipulating figures and spatial concepts may coexist with extremely limited speech and expressive powers. How far this predisposes to solitude and how far it arises from the extremely withdrawn social attitudes is often a matter of uncertainty. Almost certainly each has a tendency to increase the other. Thus, a most significant entry to the learning process remains closed, and even where speech is fluent it will often seem to belong to the repetitive habits rather than to subserve a need to be understood. Thus, thought processes remain undeveloped, abstract and sterile, without personal interchange enlightened by understanding.

For whatever basic reason, these psychotic children, besides being difficult to test reliably because of the lack of concern in cooperation, tend also to show a pretty widespread level of low ability. The concept of "islets of ability" will often lead to high, and totally unjustified, expectations. This is particularly true of those parents who, recognizing that this is not a problem of simple retardation, will comfort themselves that all is, or could be well, because of some odd and idiosyncratic capacity. A child seen after rejection by a class for severely retarded children because he was quite unable to cooperate, and apparently unable to learn, was seen at home correctly doing his "157 times table," the multiplication being fast and accurate. It required a deeper understanding to realize that this activity served no purpose and was of no practical use, even in a calculating world.

Recent work by Gillies (1965) suggests that the very oddness of these "islets of ability" may seem to imply a level of intelligence which is not borne out by careful testing. Making allowance for varying degrees of cooperation shown by the psychotic group, and matching them with a known mentally retarded group of children, showed the psychotic children to have greater variability and scatter, rather than a generally higher level of achievement. Nevertheless, the psychotics showed a more consistently higher performance level than vocabulary level although this was true of both groups, to some extent.

DIFFERENTIAL DIAGNOSIS

The fact remains that, in spite of much common ground with the mentally retarded, the psychotic child gives an impression of having a grossly disturbing process at work which disrupts behavior, stands in the way of normal human communication (affective response as well as verbal expression), and appears to prevent achievement of maturity. At one end of the scale are those who imply that emotional factors play a dominant role, and at the other end of the scale are those who believe an organic factor must be mainly responsible. In between come those clinicians who recognize autistic behavior in a variety of pathological conditions that operate during the early stages of a child's development process.

It is easy to see why the empty hours of an institutionalized retardate should be filled by rocking, banging, and other kinds of simple repetitive body play. What else lies within his range? It is easy to see why a deaf child's language may embody the same limitations as those seen in the psychotics, and how far his capacity to think, to adjust, and respond may be impaired by this very difficulty in conceptualization. One may guess that a similar blocking process may interfere in the case of the psychotic. In the absence of any definitive pathology, which requires a scrupulous search so the recognition may be clear, the interpretation and understanding of what has happened will inevitably vary with the style of the interpreter. In this connection, it is comforting to read accounts of such well understood diseases as typhoid and tuberculosis, written in the days before Jenner and Koch completed their definitive discoveries. Clinical observations were confirmed and fell into place only when this had happened. This has still to happen for psychotic children, and indeed for many mentally retarded children. However, one basis for differentiation may lie in the response to therapy, a point that will be discussed more fully elsewhere in this book.

TREATMENT CONSIDERATIONS

Used in its widest sense, the term "therapy" includes a range of procedures from drugs, physical methods of treatment, psychotherapy with specially organized education, counseling of parents, through to psychoanalysis. Whether or not organic factors are eventually laid bare, it seems clear that these children are so grossly deviant that in most of the cases therapeutic management is indicated, and in our present state of only partial understanding, the fact must be faced that in many of the cases, custodial care will be required. Since such care is likely to be found in an institution for the mentally retarded, and since it is also likely that some other distinguishing features will have become submerged in a general apathy and unresponsiveness by the time that this stage is reached, we may here be seeing one of the reasons for the way in which ultimately psychosis and retardation become merged and indistinguishable. Looking once again at the differential diagnosis, it is possible to distinguish certain patterns.

The date of onset of symptoms must influence the severity of the total effect. The child who withdraws before speech has ever been established stands a greater chance of failing to return to speaking even when the more blatant symptoms retreat, allowing a measure of "recovery."

Clinically, cases can be grouped in four ways:

1. One group from the onset appears to follow a slowly progressive downhill trend. Where in the course of this unusual features supervene, clearly the diagnosis is different. A clinical example follows.

A girl, an only child, became ill at the age of 5 years. Her upbringing had been disturbed by a severe physical illness in her mother. When she was 7 years old, the girl's behavior was so odd that she was regarded as a gross hysteric. Within a year she became progressively more withdrawn, silent, repeating some phrases, though at times meaningless. She displayed bizarre posturing and preoccupation with flicking and tapping certain objects. The illness progressed very slowly in a pattern similar to a hebephrenic psychosis. A one-sided extensor response, not present at the initial assessment, was noted when the girl was 14 years old, although no motor disability was then apparent. Later, occasional epileptic fits occurred and she became progressively physically handicapped, permitting of a diagnosis of Schilder's disease. This illness terminated fatally and was confirmed at autopsy in her 20th year.

Other degenerative diseases of the central nervous system, such as tuberous sclerosis, have been noted to produce, in the early stages, an autistic pattern of behavior. In some cases an end point is reached that amounts to quiet stagnation in institutional care without any evidence of organic disease.

2. Another group, including many cases of early infantile autism (Kanner's syndrome), become arrested at an early point in their development. They appear to withdraw progressively into themselves, only to have this process arrested, sometimes with and sometimes without the help of therapy. A slow and partial regeneration occurs and some learning patterns are resumed. The chaotic anxiety and the panic reactions of the early stages fade out, but they leave behind a somewhat odd, often rigid and limited personality. At this stage training can often result in satisfactory, if limited, achievement in both learning and creativity, but these children continue to seem odd and socially remote.

3. The final outcome is similar in a group in which progress seems to take over from an arrested development without noticeable regression in the early stages. These children's ultimate development remains limited.

4. Yet another group seems to show stagnation without any evidence of degeneration (deterioration). Speech is not lost but is limited, sometimes distorted into noncommunication, or at least is highly idiosyncratic. As time goes by, often with the help of skilled psychotherapy since these are accessible people on their own terms, some

sort of personality and ego-strength are built up with at least a compromise in regard to recognizing and accepting the reality of the social environment. Actual participation in the environment remains somewhat unpredictable, and ultimate success may well depend on innate endowment. "Emergence" is perhaps a better term than "recovery," and what emerges is often a person who protects himself against the full demands of a normal society.

In considering the question of diagnosis and prognosis by the results of therapy, it is of course important to observe and assess the child's environment. Parents may seek early institutionalization because of their own despair at trying to manage a psychotic child in the home environment with the inevitable impact this has on the family as a whole. Or they may have mistakenly believed that experts would succeed where they had failed. While inpatient care may be needed to pursue a full diagnostic investigation, hospitals and other residential units—geared to the needs of psychotic children—are few and far between. Requiring a high ratio of staff to patients, such units are costly to run; even with highly skilled intensive care, recovery of the patient is never certain. Still, the tendency to regard results as uniformly bad is no longer justified. At the same time, it is equally unrealistic to expect much from early hospitalization in a large unit. The work of Tizard (1964) has made clear for all time that however good the physical care, the large impersonal unit carries a high potential of impoverishing the child's social capacity particularly in the field of language.

SUMMARY

Throughout the preceding consideration of the as yet incompletely understood problem of autism runs an inevitable thread of indecision. Parents who have an autistic child wonder whether they should add further to their family. Physicians consulted on the care of these children may have seen few of them and may be at a loss to know what to prescribe. Cases referred to a child psychiatric clinic can only be taken on for intensive therapy in small numbers, and with uncertain results. Specialized residential units and special classes exist only in small numbers as yet, and they may seem not to justify their high cost by their results. Many persons may question the need to regard this problem as separate and different from mental retardation. Until ongoing research efforts give us further clues to the causation of both, we can do no more than continue trying to clarify the clinical picture.

———

REFERENCES

Bender, L. Diagnostic and therapeutic aspects of childhood schizophrenia. In P. Bowman & H. Martin (Eds.), *Mental retardation. Proceedings of the first international conference on mental retardation.* New York: Grune & Stratton, 1959, pp. 453–468.

Gillies, S. Some abilities of psychotic children and subnormal controls. *J. Ment. Defic.,* 1965, *9,* 89–101.

Goldfarb, W. *Childhood schizophrenia.* Cambridge, Mass.: Harvard University Press, 1961.

Kanner, L. Autistic disturbance in affective contact. *Nerv. Child,* 1943, *2,* 217–250.

Tizard, J. *Community services for the mentally handicapped.* London: Oxford University Press, 1964.

Wing, J. K. *Early childhood autism.* London: Pergamon Press, 1966.

: 7 :

The Life Course of Children with Autism
and Mental Retardation

Lauretta Bender

INTRODUCTION

TWO hundred children who were diagnosed as childhood schizophrenics on the children's ward of Bellevue Psychiatric Hospital between 1935 and 1950, when this author was in charge, have become subjects for a life-course study. From this pool of two hundred cases, fifty have been selected which fulfill the criteria of infantile autism as described by Kanner (1949). He spoke of an innate disturbance that is evident as early as the first and second year of life and is characterized by (1) an extreme autistic aloneness; (2) an obsessive desire for sameness in the environment, daily routine, and personal experiences; and (3) a language disturbance with mutism or noncommunicative language with echolalia, bizarre language, thought disturbances, and a failure to use first-person pronoun. He also described a poor object relationship except with nonhuman objects, and testing at a low level of intellectual functioning with some evidence of isolated areas of high cognitive ability.

These fifty children, besides their initial period of study and treatment at Bellevue Hospital, have been exposed to one or several subsequent follow-up studies (Bender et al., 1952, 1955, 1957; Bender 1959a, 1960, 1961a, 1963, 1964) and are again having their life courses reviewed to their present (1968) age of twenty-one to forty-two years.

It will be the purpose of this chapter to determine the current status and intervening history of each individual. This author knew each child when he or she was in Bellevue and again in the subsequent follow-up studies, as well as in this last one.[1] Thus the view is truly one of a life course and not one of a series of cross-sectional studies.

DEFINITIONS

I have previously defined childhood schizophrenia as a psychobiologic entity determined by an inherited predisposition, an early physiologic or organic crisis and a failure in adequate defense mechanisms (Bender, 1956). Schizophrenia persists for the lifetime of the individual, but exhibits different clinical, behavioral, and psychiatric features at different epochs in the individual's development and in relationship to compensating or decompensating defenses that can also be influenced by environmental factors. Thus we see the autistic and symbiotic features in infancy and early childhood, the psychosis of later childhood, and the pseudoneurotic (Hoch and Polatin, 1949) and the pseudopsychopathic (Bender, 1959a) features in adolescence. Many states of schizophrenia are not psychotic because of latency, remissions, adequate neurotic defenses, or in response to treatment.

I have also emphasized that the specific features of childhood schizophrenia are a developmental lag and an embryonic plasticity with a lack of differentiation of pattern formation and of boundaries in various areas of functioning; namely, in autonomic, motor, perceptive, cognitive, affective, and social behavior (Bender, 1966, 1968).

I have seen autism (Bender, 1959b) as a defense mechanism frequently occurring in young schizophrenic or brain-damaged or emotionally deprived children, who thereby withdraw to protect themselves from the disorganization and anxiety arising from the basic pathology. Menolascino (1965) has reported similar experiences.

In view of my definition, it will be necessary for me to seek out the evidence for features I have emphasized: the psychobiologic entity, the inherited predisposition, the physiological or organic crisis, the lifelong course, and the specific characteristic for each life epoch.

CASE MATERIAL

A cursory analysis of the case material suggested that the most variable factor is the organicity. Therefore I have divided this case material, with the variability of this factor in mind, into five groups:

I. Nine cases (18 per cent) in which an organic disorder has dominated the clinical picture from the beginning and progressively throughout life. Five of these individuals have died of causes related to their organic constitutional disorders.

II. Eight cases (16 per cent) in which both organic and schizophrenic features have coexisted throughout the life of the individual.

III. Eleven cases (22 per cent) in which organic disturbances during pregnancy, birth, or the first two years were recorded in individuals who consequently ran a life course of schizophrenia. The organic disorder is looked upon as the precipitating factor in relationship to the schizophrenic course.

IV. Ten cases (20 per cent) in which there is no recorded organic precipitating factor and the life course is one of schizophrenia.

V. Twelve cases (24 per cent) in which adults are making a social adjustment in the community.

To summarize, twelve individuals (24 per cent of the 50 sample cases) were (1968) adults between the ages of twenty-six and thirty-eight years of age, living outside of institutions; five (10 per cent) died between the ages of eighteen and forty years, and of the remaining thirty-three individuals (66 per cent), twenty-one to forty-two years old, are in institutions. The sample group comprised seven girls and forty-three boys.

The group's age range and mean age in years, in 1968, is shown in Table 7–1. It will be noted that the mean age is remarkably similar for all groups, except Group IV, which represents a life course of schizophrenia without known paranatal organicity suggestive of a precipitative factor. Here there were fewer of the older patients, which lowers the mean age to twenty-eight years as compared to the total mean age of thirty-one years.

These children were treated at Bellevue in the 1930's and 1940's,

TABLE 7–1

*Age Range and Mean Age in Years
of Grown Childhood Schizophrenics in 1968*

AGE	GROUP I PREDOMINANT ORGANICITY (9 CASES)	GROUP II ORGANICITY SCHIZ. (8 CASES)	GROUP III SCHIZ. WITH PARANATAL ORGANICITY (11 CASES)	GROUP IV SCHIZ. WITHOUT ORGANICITY (10 CASES)	GROUP V SCHIZ. WITH ADULT SOCIAL ADJUSTMENT (12 CASES)	TOTAL
Range	(died) 18–40 27–40 years years	21–42	25–40	23–33	26–38	18–42
Mean	32.5	31	32.5	28	32	31

before our knowledge of childhood schizophrenia was very complete. Consequently the early case histories have not always contained as much historical information as one would like and it has not always been possible to add to it later, when the individual becomes a chronic patient in an institution. In several instances the history has been enriched by reports of subsequently born siblings and their careers and by reports of other family members entering institutions for the mentally ill. In some instances subsequent information has denied family history of mental illness reported in the beginning. Therefore, the historical data concerning heredity, familial, and personal background, as well as that of the prenatal, paranatal, and early postnatal periods must be considered minimal.

The combined data from the original Bellevue records and the records from state institutions in New York and several neighboring states has been analyzed with regard to the following concerns for each of the five classifications of patients:

1. Cultural-religious, socioeconomic, and hereditary backgrounds.
2. Organic factors in pregnancy, the paranatal period, and early infancy.
3. Early developmental patterns, especially with regard to speech and the autistic features in early childhood.
4. The mid-childhood period, approximately between the ages of six to twelve years, with the presence of the schizophrenic disorder. It was during this period that most of the children were seen and treated on the children's ward of Bellevue Psychiatric Hospital and a diagnosis of schizophrenia was made. Some of the children were seen during their earlier childhood period, before the age of six.
5. The adolescent period, after the patients left Bellevue, with its variable pattern of home, school, and institutional experiences. During this

period there were a number of longitudinal and follow-up surveys made by a research team from Bellevue.[2] It was shown that the diagnosis of schizophrenia in 190 cases, eight to twelve years after the initial diagnosis, was confirmed in 66 per cent of the patients by the institution caring for them and in up to 89 per cent of the patients by the Bellevue research team (Bender et al., 1952; Bender, 1960).

6. The adult period, when visits and case studies in the state hospitals brought me in contact with many patients. During this time (after 1956), the extensive use of tranquilizing drugs and a liberalizing program of open wards with ground privileges, occupational therapy, recreation, television, frequent home visits, and trial periods at home, changed the pattern of many originally chronic backward patients; they became active patients responsive to treatment and some received a final discharge. Many others had frequent long periods at home that cannot be detailed in this report. Several follow-up studies have been derived from this period (Bender, 1960, 1961a, 1963, 1964).

DIFFERENTIATING FACTORS

Ethnic-Religious and Socioeconomic Backgrounds

The ethnic-religious origins (see Table 7–2) of these individuals might be expected to be representative of the city of New York during the 1930's and 1940's, when these children were first observed and treated under an unrestricted admission policy in a large, public, city hospital. But the actual classification is more limited. They have been classified as mid-European Jews, whose parents were the first or second generation immigrants from Poland, Russia, Austria, and Hungary; and as Western European Catholics, mostly of Italian and Irish stock. The Western European Protestants were for the most part not children of recent immigrants and came from English, Dutch, German and Scandinavian stock. There were two black children, one of Haitian parents and one of Panamanian parents from the Virgin Islands. There were no American Negroes or Puerto Ricans in this group. The mid-European Jews were predominant in the total series, representing 54 per cent, with Catholics and Protestants combined representing 22 per cent. This distribution was not the ethnic-cultural pattern of the total population from 1930 to 1950, nor is it the pattern in the 1960's.

It has been previously noted that a relatively high percentage of young schizophrenic children in the group are Jewish, and a minimal

TABLE 7-2
Ethnic-Religious Derivations

	GROUP I PREDOMINANT ORGANICITY (9 CASES)	GROUP II ORGANICITY AND SCHIZ. (8 CASES)	GROUP III SCHIZ. WITH PARANATAL ORGANICITY (11 CASES)	GROUP IV SCHIZ. WITHOUT ORGANICITY (10 CASES)	GROUP V SCHIZ. WITH ADULT SOCIAL ADJUSTMENT (12 CASES)	TOTAL	PER CENT
Mid-European Jews	3	3	8	6	7	27	54
West-European Catholics	2	2	1	3	3	11	22
West-European Protestants	3	3	1	1	2	10	20
Blacks	1		1			2	4
Total	9 (18%)	8 (16%)	11 (22%)	10 (20%)	12 (24%)	50	100

percent are American Negro children (Bender and Grugett, 1956). It is not believed that this indicates a different incidence of schizophrenia in these two ethnic groups, but rather that Jewish middle-class, usually professional, parents are more aware of deviations in child development and seek medical help sooner. What seems to be the low incidence of schizophrenia among Negroes may be a matter of failure at case finding.

The Jewish predominance does not hold for the two classifications with the most organic involvement, where there are six children of Jewish parentage as compared to eleven of non-Jewish parentage, or about one-third of the total. But for the two groups (III and IV) that represent, respectively, the predominance of schizophrenia over organicity, and Group V, which represents schizophrenia with adult social adjustment, there are twenty-one children of Jewish families as compared to twelve of non-Jewish families (see Table 7–2). The Jewish families thus represent about two-thirds of the total. This may be another expression of the same phenomenon.

Rimland (1964) discusses the high incidence of autistic children from Jewish parents, relating it to the high incidence of genius and intellectual eminence among Jews. At the same time, he quotes Fishberg (1911), Malzberg (1950), and Benda (1952), who have shown that Jews exceed their quota in terms of incidence of severe mental deficiency. Kanner (1954), as well as Cappon and Andrews (1957), also discussed the high incidence of Jews in their case material.

Fifteen, or 30 per cent, of the children studied had at least one parent occupied in one of the professions (Table 7–3). In three families, both parents were professionals. In spite of the high percentage of Jewish families, 60 per cent of the professional parents in the group were non-Jews. The professionals represented included college professors, teachers, physicians, engineers, and one lawyer. Three of the fathers were similar to the ones described by Kanner (1949). (See Table 7–4, "Kanner Syndrome Fathers.") Compared to the total child population in Bellevue in this period, the young schizophrenic children were represented by a much higher percentage of professional parents. This also appears to be due to the fact that these knowledgeable parents sought help for their deviate children at a time when Bellevue was one of the few places known to care for them.

Parents who were employed or had small businesses made up 40 per cent of the total (Table 7–3), probably for much the same reason as the professional parents. This group included medical technicians, accountants, bus drivers, patrolmen, shipping clerks, shoe factory workers, and a furrier.

TABLE 7–3

Social-Economic Background

	GROUP I PREDOMINANT ORGANICITY (9 CASES)	GROUP II ORGANICITY AND SCHIZ. (8 CASES)	GROUP III SCHIZ. WITH PARANATAL ORGANICITY (11 CASES)	GROUP IV SCHIZ. WITHOUT ORGANICITY (10 CASES)	GROUP V SCHIZ. WITH ADULT SOCIAL ADJUSTMENT (12 CASES)	TOTAL	PER CENT
Professional	3	4	2	2	4	15	30
Employed or small business owner	3	3	4	4	6	20	40
Marginal and dependent	3	1	5	4	2	15	30
Total	9	8	11	10	12	50	100

Heredity

In spite of the fact that our history for hereditary factors must be minimal, it is quite impressive (see Table 7–4). Where the term "psychotic" is used in that table, it means that the sibling(s) father, mother, or collateral relative was so diagnosed in a hospital or community agency from which records and confirmation of the diagnosis were obtained. These diagnoses mostly were dementia praecox or schizophrenia. "Deviate personality" refers to the seriously deviate, most of whom might well have been hospitalized; some were known to be patients in clinics or of private physicians, being treated for psychoneuroses, psychopathic personalities, or severe alcoholism. In one family the father and two uncles were symbiotically tied to their mother; they were unemployed, mute, and home-bound. The fourteen siblings of ten patients were all hospitalized schizophrenics, and eight siblings belonged to the pool of 200 schizophrenic children upon which this study draws.

The distribution of familial mental illness among the five classifications does not seem to follow a meaningful pattern. Perhaps this is so because of incomplete data. Each group had two, and Group I had three, families with a negative history. Yet Group I, which has the greatest predominance for organicity, reports two disturbed relatives for each of six families (Table 7–4). The difference among the groups, therefore, does not seem significant from the data available.

My earlier studies of heredity in childhood schizophrenia (Bender, 1963a) showed the following in regard to schizophrenic siblings: Of ninety schizophrenic children under seven years of age at Bellevue Hospital from 1935 to 1951, 15.5 per cent had schizophrenic siblings; of 100 schizophrenic children transferred from Bellevue to Letchworth Village as also retarded, between 1935 and 1957, 38 per cent had known retarded or mentally ill siblings. In the present study, 20 per cent had one or more schizophrenic siblings (Table 7–4).

Kallman and Roth (1956) studied the genetics of preadolescent schizophrenia in fifty twins and fifty singletons, with seventeen of the twin index cases monozygotic and thirty-five dizygotic. These investigators found that the schizophrenic rate of siblings was 12.2 per cent (compared to 14.3 per cent for adult schizophrenics).

Another significant genetic problem in schizophrenic children is the ratio of boys to girls. The incidence in boys is always higher than in girls before puberty, although this relationship is reversed after puberty (Kallman and Roth, 1956). In Bellevue between 1935 and 1951, 450 schizophrenic children between the ages of two to twelve years

TABLE 7–4
Heredity

	GROUP I PREDOMINANT ORGANICITY (9 CASES)	GROUP II ORGANICITY AND SCHIZ. (8 CASES)	GROUP III SCHIZ. WITH PARANATAL ORGANICITY (11 CASES)	GROUP IV SCHIZ. WITHOUT ORGANICITY (10 CASES)	GROUP V SCHIZ. WITH ADULT SOCIAL ADJUSTMENT (12 CASES)	TOTAL	PER CENT
Psychotic siblings	1	3	2 (1 with 2 sibs)	1 (4 sibs)	3	10 (14 sibs)	20
Psychotic mothers	4		1	2	2	9	18
Psychotic fathers	1			1	2	4	8
Psychotic collaterals	2	1	6		7	17	34
Deviate personalities	5	3	5	3		16	32
Kanner Syndrome fathers	1	1	1			3	6
Total	12	8	16	12	14	62	
Number mentally ill relatives per family	2.0	1.3	1.6	1.4	1.4	1.6	
Negative family history	3	2	2	2	2	11	22

were studied. The ratio of boys to girls was 2.7 (Bender, 1963*a*). This has been explained by the lessened capacity of the male to maturate smoothly (Falek, 1960), since a similar relationship has been noted in many other developmental deviations.

Pregnancies and Births

There is considerable pathology evident from pregnancy and birth histories (see Tables 7–5 and 7–6). Again the available histories must be minimal. Faretra and I (Bender and Faretra, 1962) studied 300 children with pregnancy and birth histories from a population different from these autistic schizophrenic children, but with similar diagnostic criteria. We attempted to compare children with schizophrenia and children with brain damage or organic factors with disturbed children who had neither problem. We found, however, the differences among the three groups were not great, and we concluded that approximately 66 per cent of all groups had a history of pregnancy or birth complications. In this study we made every effort to get as complete a history as possible.

In our schizophrenic children, 36 per cent of pregnancies (see Table 7–5) and 22 per cent of births (see Table 7–6) had a history of pathology. However, 32 (64 per cent) of the cases gave a history of either pregnancy or birth complication or congenital defects.

It is of some interest that whereas Group I, in which organicity was predominant in nine cases, had only two instances of pregnancy disorders, Group V, with twelve subjects who made a social adjustment as adults, had seven pathological pregnancies. The difference in pathology in Groups III and IV is a reflection of the choice of cases for each group: Group III represents a schizophrenic life course, with parental pathology seen as a precipitating factor, and Group IV includes ten cases without known paranatal pathology (see Table 7–5).

A good deal has been written about the birth ordinance of autistic, schizophrenic, and mentally defective children. Faretra and I (1962) found that more than two-thirds of the boys and one-half of the girls were first and second born. Rimland (1964) says categorically that infantile autism occurs primarily in the first born. He again sees an association between being the first born and high intelligence and superior achievement, but he again admits a relationship between the first birth and pregnancy pathology.

The present case material again shows a predominance of first born, twenty-seven of the fifty retarded children being first born (see

TABLE 7-5
Pregnancies

	GROUP I PREDOMINANT ORGANICITY (9 CASES)	GROUP II ORGANICITY AND SCHIZ. (8 CASES)	GROUP III SCHIZ. WITH PARANATAL ORGANICITY (11 CASES)	GROUP IV SCHIZ. WITHOUT ORGANICITY (10 CASES)	GROUP V SCHIZ. WITH ADULT SOCIAL ADJUSTMENT (12 CASES)	TOTAL
Stormy		1	1		1	3
Abortives			3		2	5
Bleeding		1	2		1	4
Nausea			1		1	2
Maternal illness		1[1]	1			2
Pathology, previous pregnancy	2[2]		1[3]		1[4]	4
Other			1[5]		1	2
Normal pregnancy	7	5	5	10	6	33

[1] Sinus infection with surgery.
[2] One had 2 miscarriages; and one had a stillborn-premature.
[3] 3 miscarriages.
[4] Tubal pregnancy.
[5] Twins.

T A B L E 7–6

Births

	GROUP I PREDOMINANT ORGANICITY (9 CASES)	GROUP II ORGANICITY AND SCHIZ. (8 CASES)	GROUP III SCHIZ. WITH PARANATAL ORGANICITY (11 CASES)	GROUP IV SCHIZ. WITHOUT ORGANICITY (10 CASES)	GROUP V SCHIZ. WITH ADULT SOCIAL ADJUSTMENT (12 CASES)	TOTAL
Premature	1	1	1		1	4
Postmature		1	1			2
Caesarian			1	1		2
Abnormal pre-sentation			2[1]			2
Other	1[2]		1[3]			2
Normal birth	7	6	6	9	11	39 (78%)

[1] 1 breech, 1 transverse.
[2] Cord around neck, with cyanosis.
[3] Instrument with injury.

Table 7–7). I have related this in part to the higher incidence of paranatal pathology in the first born.

In a previous study (Bender and Grugett, 1956) on some epidemiologic factors in young children with schizophrenia, it was found that, whereas twenty of thirty schizophrenic children were first born, only fifteen of thirty nonschizophrenic controls were first born.

Congenital Defects and Infantile Illnesses

Of the combined total of twenty-eight cases in the groups with organicity (I, II, and III), ten children had congenital defects (see Table 7–8).

My theory of childhood schizophrenia is based on the characteristic maturational lags and plastic or poorly differentiated and poorly patterned functioning that in the infant involve the autonomic nervous system and vasovegetative functions, including the general well-being of the infant—especially of his respiratory and gastrointestinal systems.

The impressive studies by Fish et al. (1966), have demonstrated the significant disorders in schizophrenic infants.

The history of these infants is not very impressive, due, I would like to assume, to the inadequacy of our early histories. In twenty-four cases, no history of infantile illness was obtained and it is assumed, perhaps incorrectly, that these individuals had a normal infancy (see Table 7–9). There were three sickly babies, seven instances of respiratory disorders, five cases of gastrointestinal disorders, and one child with skin disorders of the characteristic type. The respiratory illnesses ran the range from pneumonias, recurring bronchitis, and asthmatic attacks to recurring upper respiratory illnesses that were eventually ascribed to allergies. The gastrointestinal illnesses were colics and coeliac disorders, recognized by myself and others as frequent in autistic children (Bender, 1961b). A higher incidence of early infantile lack of well-being was reported by me in two other studies of young autistic schizophrenic children (Bender and Freedman, 1952; Bender, 1964).

Six of the children in the present study had convulsions during infancy, two each in Groups I, II, and III (Table 7–9). Eight children from Groups I and II developed convulsions in adolescence. Eleven (63 per cent) of seventeen children in the study, who had severe organic features throughout their lives, had convulsions (one of these during both infancy and adolescence). None of the subjects who were only schizophrenic and none of those who have made an adult social

TABLE 7-7

Birth Order

	GROUP I PREDOMINANT ORGANICITY (9 CASES)	GROUP II ORGANICITY AND SCHIZ. (8 CASES)	GROUP III SCHIZ. WITH PARANATAL ORGANICITY (11 CASES)	GROUP IV SCHIZ. WITHOUT ORGANICITY (10 CASES)	GROUP V SCHIZ. WITH ADULT SOCIAL ADJUSTMENT (12 CASES)	TOTAL
Only child	4	1	2	2	4	13 ⎫ 27 first born
1st born	2	1	4	4	3	14 ⎭
2nd born	1	4	3	2	3	13 ⎫ 23 subsequent born
3rd born or more	2	2	2	2	2	10 ⎭

TABLE 7-8

Congenital Defects

	GROUP I PREDOMINANT ORGANICITY (9 CASES)	GROUP II ORGANICITY AND SCHIZ. (8 CASES)	GROUP III SCHIZ. WITH PARANATAL ORGANICITY (11 CASES)	GROUP IV SCHIZ. WITHOUT ORGANICITY (10 CASES)	GROUP V SCHIZ. WITH ADULT SOCIAL ADJUSTMENT (12 CASES)	TOTAL
Microcephaly	1	2				3
Internal hydro- cephaly	1					1
Birth weight under 5 lb.	1	1				3
Other	1	2 [1]	1			3
Total	4	5	1	0	0	10

[1] 1-Lorraine-type dwarfism; 1-Acromegaly and other defects.

TABLE 7-9
Infantile Illnesses

	GROUP I PREDOMINANT ORGANICITY (9 CASES)	GROUP II ORGANICITY AND SCHIZ. (8 CASES)	GROUP III SCHIZ. WITH PARANATAL ORGANICITY (11 CASES)	GROUP IV SCHIZ. WITHOUT ORGANICITY (10 CASES)	GROUP V SCHIZ. WITH ADULT SOCIAL ADJUSTMENT (12 CASES)	TOTAL
Jaundice					1	1
Sickly baby	1	1	1			3
Ear trouble and mastoid			1	1	1	3
Respiratory	3		3		1	7
Gastrointestinal	1	1	1		2	5
Skin	1					1
Head injury	1			1		2
Calcium tetany	3			1		4
Childhood infections					1[1]	1
Infantile convulsions	2	2	2			6
Other			1[2]	1[3]		2
Normal infancy	3	4	2	7	8	24

[1] Whooping cough and measles.
[2] Circumcision at 18 months, followed by regression.
[3] Thyroid treatment for lethargy.

TABLE 7–10

Language Development and Usage at Age Five Years

	GROUP I PREDOMINANT ORGANICITY (9 CASES)	GROUP II ORGANICITY AND SCHIZ. (8 CASES)	GROUP III SCHIZ. WITH PARANATAL ORGANICITY (11 CASES)	GROUP IV SCHIZ. WITHOUT ORGANICITY (10 CASES)	GROUP V SCHIZ. WITH ADULT SOCIAL ADJUSTMENT (12 CASES)	TOTAL
Normal development and usage	1		2			3
Slow development and retarded usage	4	1		3		8
Slow development and schizophrenic usage		3	2		4	9
Normal development with regression and retarded usage	2	2	1			5
Normal development with regression and schizophrenic usage	1	2	2	5	5	15
Precocious development with schizophrenic language	1		3 [1]	2	2	8
Other			1 [1]		1 [2]	2

[1] Always remained mute except for occasional words, but developed superior ability to read and write within the symbiotic relationship to his mother, a school teacher.

[2] Always nearly mute, but understood what was said and made average score in WISC performance test at age 12 years.

adjustment (Groups IV and V, respectively) had convulsions, not even in reaction to phenothiazine medication.

Language Development and Usage to the Age of Five Years

Kanner, in his original series of cases of infantile autism, found that the capacity of the child at five years of age to use language communicatively proved to be a measure of their adjustment in school in adolescence (Eisenberg and Kanner, 1957). His description of the "irrelevant and metaphorical language" in these cases of early infantile autism is well known (Kanner, 1946).

In the present series of fifty cases, all but three had deviate development and usage of language at the age of five years. Eight had retarded language at the age of five years, and five more used language in a retarded fashion, although they had developed language normally before the age of five, but had regressed. Thirty-four children at the age of five years were using language in a schizophrenic and noncommunicative fashion. The most common pattern (fifteen children or 30 per cent) was reported as normal development of speech to the age of two to three-and-one-half years, followed by regression to a noncommunicative schizophrenic language by five years.

Many different forms of language disorder were presented, and often the language was variable from day to day or over months. It included mutism, either with full understanding or total inattention; failure to use the first pronoun; neologisms; mumbling; incoherent language often used egocentrically; explosive obscenities; private language; echolalia; and repetitive questions without waiting for an answer.

Precocities were represented by one child who was able to play classical music by ear at the age of one to two years; another child, who indicated his ability to distinguish between Beethoven's symphonies; and a third child, who spontaneously spelled and read street signs when he was between three and four years old. There appears to be no relationship between language development and usage at the age of five and the prognosis in adulthood in these fifty cases.

Intellectual Development and Deterioration

The fifty patients in the present study had repeated psychometric tests of their intelligence. Figures 7–1 through 7–5 illustrate the trends. They were derived from verbal scores on the WISC (Wechsler Intelligence Scale for Children), the Wechsler Bellevue Scale for Adults, or the Stanford-Binet Test. The solid lines are artifacts indicating the

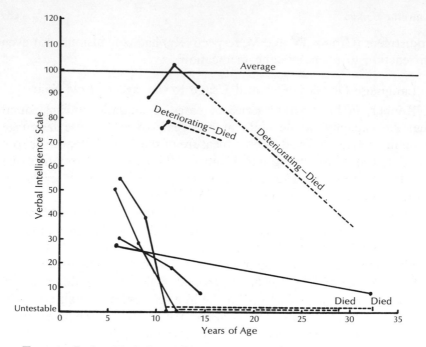

FIGURE 7–1 *Verbal Intelligence Scores for Group I Cases—*
Predominantly Organic

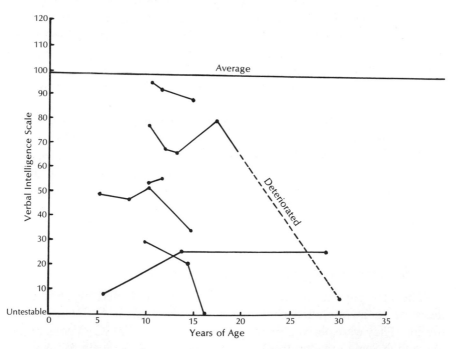

FIGURE 7–2 *Verbal Intelligence Scores for Group II Cases—*
Schizophrenic and Organic Features

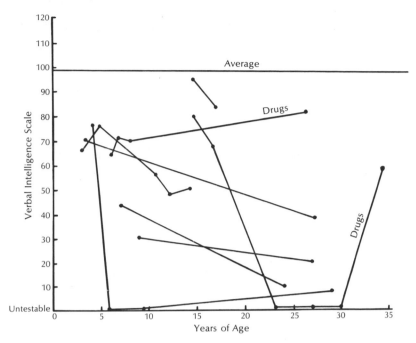

FIGURE 7–3 *Verbal Intelligence Scores for Group III Cases—Paranatal Organicity and Schizophrenia*

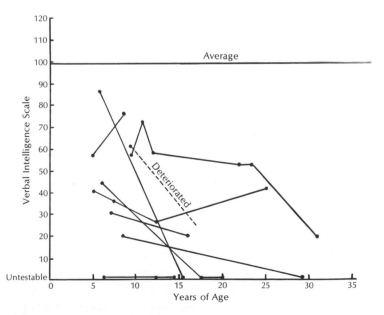

FIGURE 7–4 *Verbal Intelligence Scores for Group IV Cases—Schizophrenia without Organicity*

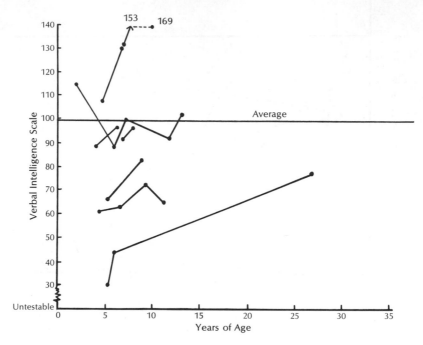

FIGURE 7–5   *Verbal Intelligence Scores for Group V Cases—*
Schizophrenia with Adult Social Adjustment

length of time between tests for the same individual and fail to show
the variations that probably occurred during that time. When a patient
is reported "untestable," this is recorded as zero in this scale.

Some general observations may be made at this point. With the exception of the group of patients who have made an adult social adjustment (Figure 7–5), the trend has been for the intelligence score to
drop, or for intelligence to deteriorate from childhood or early adolescence. There were two exceptions in Group III, where one patient became testable again and another one improved in connection with the
use of tranquilizers in the past ten years (see Figure 7–3). I have demonstrated this before (Bender, 1964). In general the intelligence
among the fifty subjects was low. Two or three individuals scored
above the defective level in childhood in each of the groups, and one
subject scored in the average range in Groups I, II, III. In Group IV,
none of the subjects attained the average range, and in Group V, five
of the twelve subjects were in the average range and one in the genius
range. Schizophrenic children who have developed normally into
early childhood rather than showing early autism tend to show a
more normal range of intelligence. Pollack (1967) has argued that,

since mental subnormality is the rule rather than the exception in children diagnosed as having "schizophrenia" or "infantile autism," the diagnosis is too broad and has nothing in common with adult schizophrenia and that the diagnosis of chronic brain syndrome should be used. Even if some autistic children prove to run a course of "chronic brain syndrome," which appears to be true of three or four of these fifty, we still have the typical adult schizophrenic course in all. It is clear, however, that a combination of certain organic features and schizophrenia from an early age on does interfere with intellectual development. More serious, however, is the intellectual deterioration that occurs in the presence of schizophrenia, with or without organicity (see Figure 7–4).

Another important observation is the variability of scores which emerges when several tests are performed in a short period. In such cases the curves are never smooth as would be expected for normal children of the age range of five to fifteen years. Wechsler and Jaros (1965) have shown that variability is the characteristic of schizophrenic patterns in children.

LIFE COURSE IN DIFFERENT GROUPS

Group I (Predominant Organicity)

There were nine patients in whom the life course seemed to be one of organic defect and deterioration. Five of these died, two in convulsive episodes at the respective ages of eighteen and thirty years, one of whom had strong schizophrenic features and family history, as well as infantile illnesses. The other had an uncertain family history of schizophrenia, early autistic features with internal hydrocephalus and a steady course of organic dilapidation. Three with no family history of schizophrenia were markedly dysplastic from birth; had a life history of organic disease; and died of cardiac failure, cardiac dysplasia, and inanition.

Two others—still living—showed early infantile illness as well as autistic behavior before the age of six years and failed to develop mentally; they settled into institutions for the retarded as low-grade defectives. One of them had a mentally ill mother, the other had a family history without mental illness.

One girl from a family without mental illness had as an adult a head circumference of eighteen and one-half inches and failed to develop speech beyond a few words, which she seemed to lose after a mastoidectomy at the age of two and one-half years. Her course was also that of a low-grade defective.

The ninth child had a schizophrenic mother and a schizophrenic sister who was also mildly retarded. His birth weight at full term was five pounds three ounces. He never developed beyond the two-year level and was epileptic from adolescence on. He and his schizophrenic older sister were observed and diagnosed together, but his sister was not autistic nor as defective as her brother and was able to return to her home.

To what extent did these nine children in Group I, who were grossly retarded throughout their lives, show autistic features in infancy and early childhood? History for mental illness was negative in three subjects' families. In two families the mother had been hospitalized with psychosis, in one of these families a sister was also schizophrenic. The two remaining families recorded one or both parents as grossly deviate and probably psychotic (see Table 7–4).

Three of the nine children in Group I were congenital deviates: one was a hydrocephalic, one had a small head, and the third was altogether too small. These children were all reported to develop normally until they reached one and one-half to two years, when speech did not develop or only a few words, which were soon lost. Regression and withdrawal were recorded in relation to a mastoidectomy at thirty months of age; birth of a sibling at thirty-four months of age; and mild upper respiratory diseases at twenty-two months of age. The hydrocephalic son of a Pulitzer Prize musician-father was a musical prodigy at the age of two years, playing Beethoven on the piano from ear, but lost this skill before he was three years. All of these defective children were mute, fearful of strange situations, of doctors, of dogs; they clung to familiar people, routine, and environment. None had any object relationship.

Three of these nine children in Group I developed, even precociously, to the age of one and one-half to two years, speaking in full sentences and having a good relationship to their parents. One parent was of the type described by Kanner. The children regressed after obscure illness starting in the early months, such as intestinal allergies, eczemas, colds or "flu" with high fever, or head injuries. The regression was severe by the age of three and one-half to four years. Diagnosis of Heller's disease and Schilder's disease was offered in two cases. The regression was accompanied by fright, panic states, wild running around in circles, wakeful nights, screaming, gradual withdrawal, and loss of interest in environment and object relationships. In two of these children the withdrawal and regression seemed to start before they were two years old and before the severest illnesses. They also showed a slight improvement after the severe regressive stage.

In intelligence (see Figure 7–1), three of the nine children in Group I were always untestable, four always tested in the defective range and deteriorated steadily, and two who scored in the normal range of intelligence deteriorated to the time of their deaths at the ages of eighteen and thirty years respectively.

The physiological treatment these patients received at Bellevue was metrasol convulsive treatment in five cases and electric convulsive treatment in three cases. One patient had no convulsive treatment. He developed convulsions in adolescence, as did two of those who received convulsive therapy. As a result of convulsive therapy, three of the patients were unaffected, but five improved in habit training and speech and were less disturbed in behavior. One was able to be cared for at home for two years during early adolescence before going to a state hospital. Three were treated with anticonvulsant medication in their final institutionalization. All received various tranquilizers during the last ten years of this study, with varying degrees of control in disturbed behavior.

Four of these individuals were transferred to state institutions for the retarded which comprised a hospital and school; four went to state hospitals; and one was in several institutions of both kinds and died in convulsion in a state hospital.

In three of these cases it is doubtful if the patients ever were schizophrenic, their whole development and life course being that of congenital defect and organic pathology. The other six, though dominantly organic, seemed also to have schizophrenia. The institutions in which most of Group I spent a major part of their lives agreed with this diagnostic opinion in four cases. In the other five cases, the diagnosis of psychosis with mental deficiency or psychosis with organic brain disease was offered.[3] This author agreed in three of these five cases. Seven of these original nine patients were seen once or oftener as adults in the institution caring for them either by this author or one of the Bellevue research team (1949–1952), and the diagnoses were reconfirmed.

One individual in Group I was dysplastic from birth. He had been born with the umbilical cord around his neck, and always showed autonomic-nervous-system and polyglandular disorders. He was an inert passive baby, who regressed after an illness when he was eighteen months and completely withdrew with negativism after the birth of a brother when he was two years old. He had spurts of maturation connected with organic disorders and psychotic phenomena, especially at puberty when he scored a verbal IQ of 93. From the age of nineteen years on he was considered a deteriorated hebephrenic until his death with cardiac aplasia. His family history was negative (Bender, 1964, p. 135).

The nine children in Group I were not lacking in autistic features in early childhood, although the organic factors seemed to dominate their lives from birth through many years in institutions, and to death in five instances.

Group II (Schizophrenia and Organic Disorders)

Included in this category are schizophrenia and severe organic features such as convulsive states (two in infancy and four starting at puberty); low-grade retardation throughout life, except for two boys (see Figure 7–2); and congenital defects including general immaturity, a mild microcephaly, a twin with prematurity, and dysplasia with several structural defects including acromegaly.

This group of eight patients differed from Group I, which were considered essentially organic (including those who died). The schizophrenic features in Group II seemed unquestionable and were so recognized in the final institution except for two who were in institutions for the retarded (see Note 3 at the end of this chapter.) One boy in this group was studied and reported on, with reproduced illustrations from his drawings, by J. Rapaport (1949) and also was represented by photographs in this writer's *Aggression, Hostility and Anxiety in Children* (Bender, 1952, pp. 162–170). This boy demonstrated the feature of introjected objects in schizophrenic children.

In two of these children, a negative family history for mental illness was claimed. Three had one schizophrenic sibling each who is included in this study (see Table 7–4). Four fathers in this group were professionals; three were employed or had a small business; and one was dependent on public welfare (see Table 7–3).

As child patients in Bellevue, two of the group had metrasol convulsive treatment and five had electric convulsive treatment. One, who later became a serious and dangerous epileptic, had no convulsive treatment. Two patients with metrasol convulsions showed dramatic improvement. All who received electric convulsions, except one girl, showed moderate improvement.

Two of the males who developed convulsions in adolescence, became dangerously disturbed as adults and at this writing are in facilities for the criminally insane. Five patients went to institutions for the retarded, where the schizophrenia was recognized in one case but not in the other four cases. All but one of these patients were seen and the diagnoses of schizophrenia as well as retardation were confirmed. One girl remains in a state hospital as a chronic simple schizophrenic; she is now twenty-one years old.

One boy in Group II with a strong family history of schizophrenia was autistic from infancy. He was evaluated and diagnosed as such in three other medical centers besides Bellevue. In early puberty he was given a diagnosis of pleuriglandular syndrome with Lorraine-type dwarfism. He had fever treatment for failure to grow. There was possible meningitis when he was eleven years old, followed by a more acute psychosis. He was then in Belleyue and had twenty-six metrasol shock treatments with a marked but brief remission, when his intelligence scored in the average range. This was followed by insulin-shock treatment during seven years of state hospitalization, when he was considered hebephrenic. Death came in the form of drowning when he was twenty-two years old and attempted to escape from an island hospital.

Group III (Schizophrenia Precipitated by Organic Factor)

A common pattern in childhood schizophrenia starting with autistic features in early childhood is the coincidence of organic factors paranatally and severe early infantile illness. The eleven children in Group III had organic factors that appeared to precipitate an autistic disturbance and schizophrenia, which continued as such throughout the life of the individual—apparently uncomplicated by further evidence of organic impairment.

All eleven children in Group III were boys. Six were first born, and a seventh was his mother's first full-term birth after miscarriage (see Table 7–7). There were seven cases of complications of pregnancy and birth, with the following records: A prolonged breech delivery; a pregnancy following three miscarriages, with spotting at six weeks and which was delivered at ten months by caesarian section; a seven-day labor terminated by instruments in which the infant was said to be injured; a pregnancy that bled at the third month and was associated with severe nausea; a stormy pregnancy in which abortives were used, terminating in a difficult birth by forceps from the transverse position; a pre-eclamptic condition in the mother at birth; and the attempted use of abortives in a pregnancy that had an excess of amniotic fluid (see Tables 7–5 and 7–6). Three of the infants resulting from these atypical pregnancies and births were also ill from birth with chronic

diarrhea and vomiting as well as chronic bronchitis and other recurring infections.

The remaining five infants had severe illnesses such as pneumonia
at two months; a head injury and croup with intubation before two
years; prematurity and calcium deficiency convulsions at nine months,
treated with x-ray to the thyroid; and intestinal allergies with vomiting
and diarrhea and failure in thriving from birth to the age of four
years. In one child, a circumcision at eighteen months was the point
of regression.

Two of the hereditary histories in Group III were negative for significant data (see Table 7–4). Three families had several members
hospitalized with schizophrenia. In the first, a paternal uncle, a maternal aunt, and a brother were hospitalized; the father had a breakdown
labeled "psychoneurosis"; and the mother and her sisters and their
mother had operable thyroid disease. In the second of these schizophrenic families a maternal uncle and two maternal cousins were hospital patients. In the third of these families, the maternal grandfather
and two aunts, as well as the father and his brother, were in institutions with various diagnoses of psychoses with psychopathic personality and paranoid schizophrenia. Incest was known to have occurred in
this family, and our patient probably was the result of incest between
his mother and her father.

Five of the families in Group III had conspicuous personality
deviants as members, but these were not hospitalized. For example, a tyrannical grandmother dominated a withdrawn, often mute,
unemployable father. Two of the father's brothers were like him.
They were said to have suffered "shell shock," although they were
never in the war. Another child was fathered by a "mean bombardier"
and a confused apathetic woman who abandoned the baby and whose
whereabouts became unknown.

Eight of the eleven families in Group III were of mid-European
Jewish background, the parents being immigrants (see Table 7–2).
This has been shown to have been characteristic of New York City's
minority class in the 1930's, when these children were studied.

One father in Group III was a college faculty member with the
characteristics described by Kanner for the fathers of the children he
recognized as having infantile autism. One father, a Haitian, was an
unsuccessful entertainer who abandoned his family. One father was
university trained in Europe in languages and worked as a shipping
clerk. Five of the families were marginal or dependent economically
(see Table 7–3).

Early maturation to the age of three years in one of the children in

Group III has been reported in the study "The First Three Years in the Maturation of Schizophrenic Children" (Bender and Freedman, 1952). He is called "Don." Photographs of him appear in *Aggression, Hostility and Anxiety* (Bender, 1953). He was described as an irritable, crying baby, who was rocking on his hands and knees at four months, would not allow his mother out of his sight, disliked crowds and strangers; he was shy. He sat up and stood up within one week at eight months, played best alone, but cried if taken to a strange place or if a stranger entered his home. At fifteen months he could walk alone and followed his mother everywhere. He was fearful of many things. Between eighteen and twenty-four months he was precocious in language development and was interested in books, pictures, nursery rhymes, and puzzles. Yet he was anxious and regressed in toilet training, was dependent on his mother, and ignored his baby brother and other children. When he was thirty months old he had lost his previous interests, played only with pots and pans in the kitchen, compulsively shutting all doors and turning light switches off and on, and pulling electric plugs. He was withdrawn, destructive, and obsessive-compulsive. At three years he was removed from nursery school on request. He was negativistic, wet and soiled, and masturbated compulsively. He had a fetish for a quilt. He had temper tantrums. He continued to be autistic, manneristic, and apathetic with severe anxiety. At four years he had electric convulsive treatment at Bellevue and was less dis, bed alone with his mother for a while, but he again regressed and was placed in an institution for retarded children. At the time of writing he was still there, twenty-six years old.

Five patients in Group III talked early, were precocious in their verbal development at three and four years of age, regressed rapidly without evident reason, and did not have communicative language at the age of five (see Table 7–10). They were admitted to Bellevue Hospital between the ages of four and eight years in a regressed, disturbed, anxious, compulsive state.

The other six in Group III developed speech slowly, had some communicative language at five years of age, and had IQ scores from 65 to 90 before they were admitted to Bellevue. Four of these children did not come to Bellevue until they were ten and eleven years of age with a puberty-type schizophrenic episode associated with definite obsessive compulsive features and paranoid ideation. Another came with mute catatonic episodes, but would communicate in writing.

Eight of the boys in Group III were treated with electric convulsive therapy and two with metrasol while they were in Bellevue. One was admitted to Bellevue before the convulsive therapies were available.

Before entering a state institution, four of the eleven had a period at home. Five who were regressed went to state schools for retarded children, and six went to the children's services of state hospitals. For the most part they have remained in the institutions to which they were originally sent, but they have had numerous home visits. Many other treatment methods have been employed including ECT, insulin, glandular therapies, and glutamic acid. Since 1956, all have had tranquilizing drugs. Two showed an improvement in their intelligence score with medication (see Figure 7–3).

In the state institutions to which the eleven children in Group III were sent, the diagnoses of schizophrenia held for all but two, who were in institutions for the retarded. I saw all these patients as adolescents or adults, most of them more than once, and retained my conviction that they were schizophrenic and several of them also mentally retarded.

I presented a complete case history of one of these boys in this group, "Melvin," in "The Origin and Evolution of the Gestalt Function: The Body Image and Delusional Thought in Schizophrenia" (Bender, 1963b). The article is also illustrated with reproductions of his drawings. I summarized his case by saying (p. 61):

Melvin was schizophrenic from earliest infancy. From the first he had primitive perceptual problems, the separation of the perceived object from the background, his own identity, separating his identity from mother, father, and brother (the latter was also mentally ill), problems in the construction of the body image, and the identity of the sexes. Through the years he tended to withdraw and disorganize increasingly until the advent of the drug therapies. The lag in maturation and plastic characteristics of all his functioning are clearly demonstrated in Melvin and interfered with his normal development.

Group IV (Schizophrenia without Organicity)

Ten children (four girls) were considered in a group because there was no history of any organic factor during pregnancy, birth, or early childhood that might have precipitated the development of early autism and schizophrenia which eventually completely crippled these individuals. The lack of such a history, of course, is not conclusive that some pathology might not have existed during pregnancy, birth, or early infancy, either unknown to the parents or not reported by them (see Tables 7–5, 7–6, and 7–7). The ethnic-religious and socioeconomic backgrounds as well as heredity were not significantly different from that of the other groups (see Tables 7–2, 7–3, and 7–4).

A family history of mental illness was denied in three families in Group IV. In another three families, a grandparent and an aunt or uncle were recognized as deviate personalities. One child had a hospitalized schizophrenic great-aunt. Two girls had a schizophrenic mother, one of whom was symbiotic with our patient. One girl belonged to a sibship of four, all of whom were schizophrenic in childhood and were studied at Bellevue, but this girl was autistic by the definition of this study (see Table 7–4).

Six of the ten children in Group IV came from a family of mid-European Jewish background; three families were Italian Catholic; and a family with four schizophrenic children had a father who was an alcoholic Dutch seaman (see Table 7–2). Of the parents, two fathers were professionals, one father was an independent businessman, one a taxi driver, and two were otherwise employed. Four families were marginal or dependent (see Table 7–3).

Three of these children were retarded in development, five boys developed normally until they were two to three years old and then regressed to schizophrenic language by the age of five. Two were precocious in development and interests until they were three and a half years old. They then regressed without known reasons. None had communicative speech at five years (see Table 7–10).

All ten of the children in Group IV had been seen at some other medical center or child guidance clinic before they were admitted to Bellevue between the ages of four to nine and nine to twelve years (mean seven years). At that time, three children could not be scored on a psychometric test, but the IQ of thc other seven ranged from 32 to 70, with a mean IQ of 52 (see Figure 7–4).

Three of these children had been seen by Leo Kanner. One was diagnosed as a case of Heller's disease, one as infantile autism, and one as schizophrenia. The downward course of intelligence by deterioration is shown in Figure 7–4 for all of these individuals except for one girl, A., who might have been able to leave the hospital had she had some home other than one with a symbiotic, near-psychotic mother.

Nine children in Group IV had electric convulsive treatment at Bellevue. One of these, R. L. was reported by Kanner and Eisenberg (1955, p. 238) to have deteriorated as a result of the therapy, although it does not appear that his subsequent clinical condition was different from that of other autistic children who have failed to respond with or without any form of treatment. One child, diagnosed a schizophrenic and treated with fifty insulin comas in another hospital, did not improve and was sent to Bellevue for long-term placement. One child had a year of histamine treatment (Sackler et al., 1952) after leaving Bellevue with some improvement in behavior. He was cared for in a private school for problem children until he was fifteen years old, when he was admitted to a state hospital.

Two girls, A. (already mentioned) and F. received intensive psychotherapy by Saul Gurevich (Bender and Gurevich, 1955), both while they were in Bellevue and for extended periods after leaving the hospital. A. had psychotherapy twice a week for a year and was placed in a treatment home while her mother was hospitalized for schizophrenia. When she was eight and a half years old, she was sent to a children's unit of a state hospital, where the diagnosis of childhood schizophrenia was confirmed. She has been in and out of the hospital often, but cannot remain out permanently both because of her autistic, dependent behavior and the schizophrenic state of her mother. A. was not only verbal; her most provocative symptom was her constant, obsessive questioning about her own identity, about time, and place, and especially about the texture of materials and objects.

F. was an isolated case of autism in an otherwise normal family. She was the first born and much loved. She never developed speech. She received daily therapy in Bellevue at the age of five years and twice a week for three years after leaving the hospital. Her habit training improved, but she did not acquire speech and remained withdrawn. At the age of ten years she went to an institution for retarded children for some months, then returned home for two years while receiving more psychotherapy. When she was fifteen, she was institutionalized as a chronic patient and is recognized as a case of retardation and schizophrenia.

One boy, at the age of ten years, had venous anastomosis or revascularization of the jugular vein, an operation performed with the hope that it would improve intelligence. This boy's behavior was less disturbed and he was more content, but his intelligence was not improved.

Altogether four of the ten children in Group IV were placed in state hospitals, where the diagnosis of schizophrenia was confirmed. The other six were placed in institutions for retarded children, where two were considered also schizophrenic. In the four who were considered only retarded, this author confirmed by repeated interviews the presence of schizophrenia as well as retardation.

Group V (Schizophrenia with Adult Social Adjustment)

Twelve men of the group of fifty are living in the community in some sort of social adjustment. These are men who are twenty-six to thirty-eight years of age (see Table 7–1). Seven come from a mid-European Jewish background; three were West-European Catholics, and two were Protestant (see Table 7–2).

Two of the families of men in Group V were on welfare. Another two are out-of-wedlock children of psychotic mothers and were raised in foster homes. Four fathers of patients were professional men or white-collar employees, and in two of these families the mother was similarly employed. The other six men had families at a marginal level of independence. In three of these, the father worked below capacity and education because of autistic preoccupation (see Table 7–3).

Of the twelve families in Group V, two denied a history of mental or personality disorders. In two families, personality deviations of a schizoid nature were recorded by agencies and psychiatrists who took care of the children. Several members of one family had private psychiatric care outside of institutions. Two fathers and two mothers were institutionalized psychotics, and four families had several institutionalized mentally ill grandparents, aunts, and uncles (see Table 7–4).

Three of the twelve socially adjusted men in Group V had siblings institutionalized for schizophrenia before puberty. Of the total in Group V, four boys were only children, and three were the first born of their mothers (see Table 7–7). Among the five later born children, one was the second of three, one the third of three, and one the fifth of six.

The pregnancy and birth data on the twelve men in Group V are given in Tables 7–5 and 7–6. Organic factors in pregnancy or paranatally were denied by four mothers. Two mothers reported taking abortives. A history of severe alcoholism was obtained from one mother from whom the infant was taken and placed in a foundling hospital. She had three more children who developed normally, but were also placed in the foundling hospital before she, herself, was sent to a mental hospital.

One mother in Group V was pregnant for the first time at the age of thirty-nine years and carried the infant three weeks overdue before labor was induced. The infant weighed ten pounds, eleven ounces. His head was marked by instruments, but he seemed normal the first year.

Three mothers in Group V had stormy pregnancies. The first had two abortions prior to being pregnant with our patient. She tried to abort this pregnancy also and bled in the second month and again in the last three weeks. The infant was jaundiced at birth. He had pneumonia at nine months of age and developed slowly. He walked at the age of seventeen months, at which time the sixth child of the family was born and our patient was placed in a nursery for a month. There he regressed and never recovered.

The second mother had an operation for a tubal pregnancy and had her remaining tube blown out to permit conception. She had a miscarriage and then conceived our patient. During the pregnancy, she vomited excessively. The infant developed autistically from the beginning.

The third mother who had a complicated pregnancy was an x-ray technician who was exposed to an erythematous dose of x-ray early in pregnancy and had an accidental electric shock two weeks before birth which stopped fetal movements for a week. The birth occurred at seven and a half months, and the infant appeared to be premature although he weighed seven pounds. He did not thrive, was colicky, and had coeliac disease until he was two years of age.

Thus, twelve autistic children in Group V who have graduated to social adjustment experienced a wide range of pathologies of pregnancy, birth, and early infancy comparable in every way to the four other groups of patients who have remained in institutions.

It may be significant that the history in the case of five of these twelve children contains the statement that the child was very much wanted and loved by the family who remained devoted throughout and made heroic efforts to have the boy home as soon as possible. This includes one foster child, who was born of a psychotic mother and at the age of one month was placed with foster parents with whom he still lives.

Autistic features appeared, sometimes in retrospect, according to histories given by the parents during the first two years of life and the features progressed until the children were admitted to the children's service of Bellevue Hospital between the ages of five and a half and ten and a half years (the mean age was eight and a half). All had had professional medical evaluation and shorter or longer periods of treatment in either a private office, a public clinic, or a residential treatment facility before referral to Bellevue.

Before the age of two years, some of those twelve boys were quiet, easy to care for but slow in developing, and generally remained immature with maturational lags in physiological functions. Others in the group of twelve from the beginning had eating and sleeping problems, were irritable, and showed poorly patterned or embryonic behavior. Still others were, in addition, withdrawn, not contacting parents, or were fearful. Two were precocious in walking and speech development. Four had an even and steady progression of maturational disturbances into a psychotic state after five years. The others showed early maturational disorders with a severe regression or an acute exacerbation of more disturbed behavior: in one boy at the age of nine months after pneumonia; in three boys at the age of two and a half years after a severe fright or fall; and in another two boys after a marked change in family pattern, and without other apparent cause. Three children became more disturbed at the age of three and a half to four years, one after he had measles and otitis media, another with the birth of a sibling, and the third with a change in foster homes.

The behavior in Group V after the age of two years was characterized by massive symptomatology in physiological areas: motility; withdrawal from sensory stimuli and social contact; a wide variety of language and speech disorders; outbursts of disturbed behavior against the physical and social environment; compulsiveness; demand for sameness in the environmental routine or superimposition of bizarre compulsive patterns on the environment; clinging, symbiotic behavior; demand for reciprocal behavior from the mother in some cases; precocities in language or structured play or drawings in some cases; and a short remission with more normal language and behavior in two cases. In all twelve patients there was an all-pervasive anxiety and distress.

It is significant for this group of children, who eventually attained some level of social living in the community, that they could all be evaluated on psychometric tests, and that their scores ranged from 61 to 106 per cent with the exception of one score of 39 per cent (the mean score was 74.5 per cent; see Figure 7–5). By Kanner's criteria all but one of these twelve children had developed speech before the age of five years (see Table 7–10). Four children had earlier lost it, but two of these regained speech before the age of five years. The child without useful language did have echolalia by the time he was five years old and could score at an average level in a performance test. This boy, C., with an IQ of 39 at the age of five and a half years, gradually increased his intelligence during adolescence until he reached a borderline level.

While in treatment at Bellevue, all of the twelve children in Group V took part in ward activities that included school, art, music, and puppet shows. Nine boys in the group had rather extensive psychotherapy. Eight of the twelve had electric convulsive treatment. Two had metrasol convulsive treatment, and one of these also had insulin-coma treatment. One child had no physiological therapy but extensive psychotherapy, speech training, and private tutoring until he was entered in a state hospital where he had electric convulsive treatment at the age of fifteen years. What follows are thumbnail descriptions of three of the boys who received convulsive treatment.

T. entered the ward at Bellevue in a panic, screaming that he was poisoned with bad medicine. He threw his head back into an opisthotonus posture, said his mind was being read. His motility was impulsive and whirling or immobile with mutism. He dominated the interview with the doctor with verbal precocities concerning time and space, and he dominated the children on the ward with his arrogant violence, kicking out, and spitting.

After electric convulsive treatment, there was a dramatic change in T. He became cooperative in all activities and clinging and dependent on adults. At the worst, he sat for hours, if undisturbed, reading in a corner, indifferent to the environment. His IQ on the Stanford-Binet Test rose from 106 to 153. He was able to return to his devoted foster home (he was the boy whose mother was hospitalized schizophrenic) for two years, when another episode of bizarre, narcissistic, manneristic psychosis necessitated transfer to a state hospital where the diagnosis of schizophrenia was confirmed. He quieted down in early puberty. He then displayed arrogance because of his intelligence, expressed an interest in science, occupied himself with reading, and engaged in some homosexual acting-out.

T. had many home visits with his foster parents. They attempted to keep him out of the hospital by the time he was 14 years old, but his seclusiveness made this impractical. However, at 17 he was able to stay out of the hospital and to obtain and keep a position as a shipping clerk while shopping among rehabilitation and psychotherapy centers and still living with his original foster parents. At the time of writing (1968) he was 31 years old.

C. came to Bellevue at the age of 5½ years—a beautiful, babyish, fragile child. He was anxious and disturbed, knocking toys together as his only play pattern and using people as objects. He had a peculiar rocking, weaving gait, walking on tiptoe in circles and flapping his hands in the air. He also had poor tissue tone, was pale, and had numerous upper respiratory illnesses that postponed all treatment programs several times. His speech was singsong, with a high-pitched metallic, ventriloquistic quality. The content of his speech and fantasy was limited and dealt with immediate reality objects. He had two courses of electric convulsive treatment within a year. As a result, he became much more robust and less babyish in physical appearance, but his mental picture did not change much.

While C. was with us, a younger brother of his was admitted as a severely defective, malnourished 3½-year-old. At birth the brother was so poorly developed and thrived so poorly and was so homely that the mother was ashamed and hid and neglected him. When he came to us, this younger boy functioned like a 4-month-old baby. But under our care he learned to walk within three months. At the age of 27 years, C.'s brother is a large, robust, acromegalic individual who weighs 200 pounds and has the mentality of a 3½-year-old. He has convulsions and is aggressively dangerous. During adolescence, he appeared bizarre and typically schizophrenic.

C. was transferred to a state school for retarded children. In the institution he was always considered a familial mental retardate. He was seen in follow-up studies twice by members of the Bellevue staff and a third time by the author. In these interviews he always appeared to be schizophrenic. When C. was 12½ years old, the Rorschach and TAT results were typically schizophrenic. At 19 years of age he was shy, manneristic, and aloof. He whirled on the longitudinal axis and said he believed he could fly if he tried, but the idea frightened him. He continued to benefit from the educational and work-training program of the training school. He learned to read and write and scored a full scale of 70 on the WISC, with a verbal score of 76 and a performance score of 67. In the end, he became a reliable worker and left the school of his own accord at the age of 27 years. He has lived in his parents' home for three years and has remained independent.

E. was 7 years old when he entered Bellevue. He had been precocious in kindergarten, being able to read and spell simple words spontaneously and being active in drawing. In the first grade he regressed to disturbed behavior, attacking other children whom he accused of teasing him and using obscene words and sexual gestures. He was in treatment in a child guidance clinic, which referred him to Bellevue.

At the time of admission to Bellevue, E. was anxious, restless, and inattentive. Play with toys revealed his preoccupations, but the structure of his play was disorganized and fragmented. He was preoccupied with hatred for his father: he made "little men" with clay and promptly destroyed them, saying, "the man died." He maintained that he had a little man inside him, littler than a baby, that can hardly talk; then he heard the voice in his head, directing him to bad behavior. Small bits of clay he called penises. He sucked them or crushed them between his fingers.

E. was disinterested in the activities and children on the ward, and was verbally abusive and obscene. In school he refused routine studies and occupied himself with crude drawings or remained inactive. As to his motility, he whirled on the longitudinal axis and had poor muscle tone and vascular motor lability, with the usual pallor changing readily to flushing.

His play therapy with a psychiatrist (biweekly) continued for many months after E. left Bellevue. He attended school and progressed satisfactorily, but he was a problem at home and with his peers, mostly because of his fears. He claimed he obeyed his father rather than his mother because his father had been a soldier in World War I and had killed Germans. He wanted to sleep with his father because he was afraid of kidnapers, but this ploy was rejected. He also was afraid of his mother's sharp knife. He played only with very small children.

At the age of 11 years he became very troublesome in school because of his conflicts with other children, the explosive obscenities he uttered, and his negativistic behavior with teachers. Both at home and at school he asked interminable questions about the eyes of people, why he was not a good ball player, and distance to places. He was returned to Bellevue.

In psychiatric interviews or therapeutic sessions he distracted the psychiatrist talking about baseball, or else refused to talk or play or draw. He had electric convulsive therapy when he was 11½ years old. At home he became unmanageable and in the streets was restless, picking fights and hitching rides without thought for danger. He was sent to a state hospital where the emphasis on his acting-out asocial behavior led to a diagnosis of "primary behavior problems," in spite of his manneristic behavior, compulsive questions, and inappropriate mood. His behavior improved and after seven months he was sent home. The discharge note read ". . . impression of childhood schizophrenia . . . offers little hope for continued adjustment."

While he was at home, E. made a follow-up visit to Bellevue at the age of 13 years, eighteen months after his electric convulsive treatment. His IQ on the Bellevue Wechsler Scale gave a composite of 97 (verbal 102, performance 92) in contrast to his pretreatment score of 93 on the Stanford-Binet Test. It was noted that his EEG had also improved, although there was a moderate dysrythmia for his age. Before the convulsive treatment there had been bursts of slow activity, with good underlying alpha activity for his age. He had leveled off his aggressive behavior, but was somewhat withdrawn and preoccupied with the same problems of identity, time, and space. He went to another state hospital at the age of 13½ years. He was noted to be anxious, manneristic, grimacing, whining, and empty. He was diagnosed a schizophrenic. About the time he was 17 years old, he developed paranoid ideation associated with instability. Later on, grandiose ideas seemed to help him feel more contented. He went home at the age of 17½ years under convalescent supervision, which was extended several times until he was 24 years old, because of his adjustment at home and his unwillingness to seek employment. He wanted to attend art school and hang around at home.

At the age of 24 years E. was returned to Bellevue because he molested a girl on the street. He was found to be dull and withdrawn, with some paranoid ideation and numerous somatic complaints. He was placed on tranquilizers and after a year was discharged to his father, although he was not considered employable. His adjustment continued at a dull, inactive, dependent level.

Five other members of the twelve in Group V, who eventually adjusted to the community, also had varied hospital careers. Three have been living at home since they were 18, 25, and 27 years of age respectively. They have been dependent on their families, have not been employed, and have continued to use tranquilizing drugs. One with a particularly stormy career involving a year of wandering about with an alcoholic father who committed suicide and a year in a hospital for the criminally insane because of his dangerously assaultive behavior, was released to the community at the age of 27, a known overt homosexual who had been trained as a beautician and thus supported himself for three years. The fourth left the hospital at 18, lived with his parents, has been employed steadily as a printer, and drives his own car. He voluntarily visits his former psychiatrists, revealing all his former manneristic habits and grimaces but maintaining an affable and friendly stance.

Three of the men in Group V never went to a state institution. Two were kept in the home by solicitous, almost symbiotic mothers, despite grossly psychotic, withdrawn, catatonic behavior. One of the three has continued in this state. His mother gives the excuse that his father died in a state hospital and she does not want her son to do the same. Another had a six-month period of treatment in a private sanitarium, which was followed by several years of a deteriorated schizophrenic state. Surprisingly, he suddenly remitted, obtained a civil service job as a park attendant by examination, and has been so employed for several years.

The third of the boys kept out of a state institution, the son of professional parents, has had his life carefully planned, with attendance at residential schools appropriate for each phase of his life. He is independently employed as a shipping clerk and has an active social life in a sheltered organization. Though his level of functioning is below his family's expectation, he has not grown to feel anything but contented with his lot.

SUMMARY

A pool was formed of 200 case files of individuals who, as children under the age of twelve years, were diagnosed childhood schizophrenics on the children's ward of Bellevue Psychiatric Hospital in the period from 1930 to 1950. Since then, these patients have been subjects of repeated follow-up studies in the state institutions to which they were transferred.

The fifty patients selected from this pool were chosen because they were autistic during early childhood. A study of their life courses was made from the accumulated data. The material was studied with regard to the following aspects:

1. Ethnic-religious, socioeconomic, and hereditary backgrounds.
2. Paranatal organic pathology.
3. The early developmental pattern with the autistic feature. Special consideration was given to development of communicable speech by the age of five years.
4. The intellectual level measured by verbal intelligence at intervals throughout the life span.
5. The childhood period roughly from four to twelve years, when the deviate behavior led to hospitalization at Bellevue and schizophrenia was diagnosed.
6. The adolescent period with various experiences at home, in the community, in schools, or in hospitals for the mentally ill, and institutions for the mentally retarded.
7. The adult period.

Six of the fifty have died, five in convulsive disorders or heart failure and a general physiological failure, and one drowned. Those surviving have reached the ages of twenty-one to forty-two years. Twelve are making a social adjustment in the community, mostly with dependance on a tolerant family, and thirty-three (66 per cent) are still chronic patients in institutions.

An effort was made to evaluate the treatment to which these patients had been exposed. Subsequent diagnosis from the institutions where each individual was treated was determined. In most cases, the author reexamined available patients.

Some of the important conclusions of this study are that children who are diagnosed as having schizophrenia, but whose presenting picture is autism, show a wide range of schizophrenic disorders in adulthood. A few (three individuals, or 6 per cent of this series), appeared not to be schizophrenic but organically defective and to run a life course of mental deficiency, with and without convulsions. Other subjects who were equally organically defective, and considered to be mental defectives in the institutions where they were cared for, appeared to this author to be also typically schizophrenic and to run a life course of mental deficiency and schizophrenia. Still others (22 per cent) of the series with histories of paranatal pathology developed schizophrenia in early childhood and ran a life course of schizophrenia. There was also an equivalent group (20 per cent) in whom there was no history or known evidence of paranatal pathology, which ran a similar course of schizophrenia. Of course, since histories are notoriously inadequate for paranatal pathology, this lack of evidence cannot be considered conclusive in these cases.

Twelve (24 per cent) of the patients in the series have made social adjustment in the community as adults. This varies from a complete psychotic dependency in a tolerant home to various degrees of independence; emotional, social, and financial. This group varied from the others by having a tolerant home; testing on psychometric procedures in the normal range and not deteriorating intellectually during the adolescent and adult periods; and responding to therapeutic efforts, especially the psychoactive drugs and socializing activities in the last ten years they were under study.

The young schizophrenic child with autism does not have a unique life pattern. In adulthood he presents any possible type of schizophrenia with any possible organic defect or disturbance.

NOTES

1. Because of my position as Consultant in Child Psychiatry for the New York State Department of Mental Hygiene, it has been possible for me to see those patients who were sent to hospitals for the mentally ill and schools for the retarded, and to have free access to their records. I have been appreciative of the warm cooperation given to me especially at Letchworth Village and at Central Islip, Kings Park, Middletown, and Rockland State Hospitals and at Wassaic and Willowbrook State Schools.

2. A 1949–1952 follow-up study was supported in part by a National Institute of Mental Health grant No. 171–C1. The research staff included A. M. Freedman, W. Ray Keeler, A. M. Magruder, R. Rabinovitch, S. Gurevich, and Mrs. A. E. Grugett, Jr.

3. In New York State a state hospital and school for the retarded will generally not recognize a diagnosis of schizophrenia since, by definition, this is a psychosis and these institutions accept and care for mentally retarded and not psychotic patients. However, they recognize in some extreme cases that mental deficiency and schizophrenia may exist in the same patient or that a mentally deficient patient may have some schizophrenic features.

REFERENCES

Benda, C. E. *Developmental disorders of mentation and cerebral palsies.* New York: Grune & Stratton, 1952.

Bender, L. *Aggression, hostility and anxiety in children.* Springfield, Ill.; Charles C Thomas, 1953.

———. Schizophrenia in childhood: Its recognition, description and treatment. *Amer. J. Orthopsychiat.,* 1956, *26,* 499–506.

———. The concept of pseudopsychopathic schizophrenia in adolescents. *Amer. J. Orthopsychiat.,* 1959, *29,* 491–512. (*a*)

———. Autism in children with mental deficiency. *Amer. J. Ment. Defic.,* 1959, *63,* 81–86. (*b*)

———. Diagnostic and therapeutic aspects of childhood schizophrenia. In P. W. Bowman (Ed.), *Mental retardation. Proceedings of the 1st International Medical Conference.* New York: Grune & Stratton, 1960, pp. 453–468.

————. Childhood schizophrenia and convulsive states. In J. Wortis (Ed.), *Recent advances in biological psychiatry*, Vol. 3. New York: Grune & Stratton, 1961, 96–103. (*a*)

————. Coeliac syndrome in schizophrenia. Letter to the Editor. *Psychiat. Quart.*, 1961, *35*, 586. (*b*)

————. Mental illness in childhood and heredity. *Eugen. Quart.*, 1963, *10*, 1–11. (*a*)

————. The origin and evolution of the gestalt function: The body image and delusional thought in schizophrenia. In J. Wortis (Ed.), *Recent advances in biological psychiatry*. New York: Plenum Press, 1963, p. 38. (*b*)

————. Twenty-five year view of therapeutic results. In P. Hoch & J. Zubin (Eds.), *Evaluation of psychiatric treatment*, New York: Grune & Stratton, 1964, p. 129.

————. The concept of plasticity in childhood schizophrenia. In P. Hoch & J. Zubin (Eds.), *Psychopathology of schizophrenia*. New York: Grune & Stratton, 1966, pp. 354–365.

————. Childhood schizophrenia: A review with critical evaluation by Clemens Benda, Stella Chess, Rudolf Ekstein, Seymour Friedman and Margaret Mahler. *Internat. J. Psychiat.*, 1968, *5*, 211–263.

Bender, L., & Faretra, G. Pregnancy and birth histories of children with psychiatric problems. Proceedings of the 3rd World Congress of Psychiatry, 1962, pp. 1329–1933.

Bender, L., & Freedman, A. M. A study of the first three years in the maturation of schizophrenic children. *Quart. J. Child Beh.*, 1952, *4*, 245–272.

————. When the childhood schizophrenic grows up. *Amer. J. Orthopsychiat.*, 1957, *27*, 553–565.

Bender, L., Freedman, A., Grugett, A. E. Jr., & Helme, W. Schizophrenia in childhood: A confirmation of the diagnosis. *Trans. Amer. Neurol. Assoc.*, 1952, *77*, 67–73.

Bender, L., & Grugett, A. E., Jr. A study of certain epidemiological problems in a group of children with childhood schizophrenia. *Amer. J. Orthopsychiat.*, 1956, *26*, 131–145.

Bender, L., & Gurevich, S. Results with psychotherapy with young schizophrenic children. *Amer. J. Orthopsychiat.* 1955, *25*, 162–170.

Cappon, D., & Andrews, E. Autism and schizophrenia in a child guidance clinic. *Canad. Psychiat. Assoc. J.*, 1957, *2*, 1–25.

Eisenberg, L., & Kanner, L. Early infantile autism, 1943–1955. *Amer. Psychiat. Assoc. Res. Rep.*, No. 1, 1957, pp. 55–67.

Falek, A. Review of T. Larsson & T. Sjogren's: A clinical and genetic population study. *Amer. J. Human Genet.*, 1960, *12*, 379–380.

Fish, B., Wile, R., Shapiro, T., & Halpern, F. The prediction of schizophrenia in infancy: A ten year follow-up. In P. Hoch & J. Zubin (Eds.), *Psychopathology of schizophrenia*. New York: Grune & Stratton, 1966.

Fishberg, M. *The Jews: A study of race and environment*. London: Walter Scott, 1911.

Hoch, P., & Polatin, J. Pseudoneurotic forms of schizophrenia. *Psychiat. Quart.*, 1949, *23*, 448.

Kallman, F. J., & Roth, P. Genetic aspects of preadolescent schizophrenia. *Amer. J. Psychiat.*, 1956, *112*, 599–606.

Kanner, L. Irrelevant and metaphorical language in early infantile autism. *Amer. J. Psychiat.*, 1946, *103*, 242–246.

————. Problems of nosology and psychodynamics of early infantile autism. *Amer. J. Orthopsychiat.*, 1949, *19*, 416–452.

————. To what extent is early infantile autism determined by constitutional inadequacies? *Proc. Assoc. Res. Nerv. & Ment. Dis.*, 1954, *33*, 378–385.

Kanner, L., & Eisenberg, L. Follow-up studies of autistic children. In P. Hoch & J. Zubin (Eds.), *Psychopathology of childhood*. New York: Grune & Stratton, 1955, pp. 227–239.

Malzberg, B. Sex differences in the prevalence of mental deficiency due to birth traumas. *Amer. J. Ment. Defic.*, 1950, *54*, 427–433.

Menolascino, F. J. Autistic reactions in early childhood: Differential diagnostic considerations. *J. Child Psychiat. & Psychol.*, 1965, *6*, 203–218.

Pollack, M. Mental subnormality and childhood schizophrenia. In J. Zubin & G. Jervis (Eds.), *Psychopathology of mental development,* New York: Grune & Stratton, 1967, pp. 460–471.

Rapaport, J. Phantasy objects in children. *Psychoanalyt. Rev.,* 1949, *3,* 316–322.

Rimland, B. *Infantile autism.* New York: Appleton-Century-Crofts, 1964.

Sackler, M. D., Sackler, R. R., LaBurt, H. A., Co Tui, & Sackler, A. M. A psychobiologic viewpoint on schizophrenias of childhood. *Nerv. Child,* 1952, *10,* 43–58.

Weschler, D., & Jaros, E. Schizophrenic patterns on the WISC. *J. Clin. Psychol.,* 1965, *3,* 288–291.

: 8 :

Down's Syndrome: Clinical and Psychiatric Findings in an Institutionalized Sample

Frank J. Menolascino

INTRODUCTION

DOWN'S Syndrome has for many years presented clinical and behavioral dimensions that have been of interest to a variety of workers in the field of mental retardation.[1] The high frequency and reported homogeneity of this particular subgrouping of the mentally retarded population present multiple challenges for clinical research. Formal diagnostic approaches had reached a point where these patients were considered to be a homogenous group among themselves, with differences being primarily the addition or absence of associated anomalies (for example, cardiac anomalies). This seems rather strange when one considers that this group was one of the first diagnostic entities to be separated from the previously amorphous population of the mentally retarded (Kanner, 1964). However, recent cytogenetic advances in Down's Syndrome, based on chromosomal findings, suggest the possibility of a number of subgroupings. These are likewise being extended to insights concerning possible clinical manifestations or metabolic findings in each of the delineated cytogenetic subgroupings (Baumeister and Williams, 1967).

The behavioral dimensions of Down's Syndrome have similarly been viewed traditionally as a homogeneous phenomenon and have culminated in the impression that these children represent the "Prince Charming" of the mentally retarded population. The "Prince Charming" behavioral stereotype comprises a cheerful disposition, amusing mimicry, and indiscriminate affection toward others (Domino et al., 1964). Similar to the clinical findings and descriptive reevaluation of traditional impressions, the behavioral parameters of these children have also been reassessed and a multiplicity of behavioral patterns and disturbances have been reported in contrast to the previously noted stereotypes (Beley and Lecuyer, 1960; Webster, 1963; Menolascino, 1965).

In this report we shall review the clinical-psychiatric findings in a randomly selected sample of ninety-five individuals with Down's Syndrome who are currently residing at an institution for the mentally retarded. Our initial research questions were the following two: What types and frequencies of psychiatric disturbances are noted in a randomly selected sample of institutionalized individuals with Down's Syndrome? What are the significant factors that correlate with the presence of a psychiatric disturbance in this sample?

SAMPLE

The study was conducted at a public residential facility for the mentally retarded. From a total of 263 individuals with Down's Syndrome, a sample of 95 was randomly selected. Each of the ninety-five subjects was studied retrospectively as to general information (family, medical, reasons for admission, and so forth). Physical and neurological examinations were carried out on each child and particular attention was focused on the frequency and type of cardinal stigmata in this particular syndrome.[2] A dermatoglyphic assessment of each of these individuals was obtained (finger and palm prints), employing the method of Walker (1957). A cytogenetic evaluation was arrived at on each,[3] and awake and asleep electroencephalograms were obtained.[4] Each patient was evaluated by means of an individual psychiatric interview, with a modified diagnostic play-interview technique for the children in the sample (Haworth and Menolascino, 1967). The interview of the adolescent and adult subjects assessed the current level of personality functioning and signs or symptoms of overt behavioral disturbance. Included in this assessment was a combined review of the recent behavioral adjustment of each individual and an overview of his previous clinical-psychiatric history—both before and since admission.

The nomenclature systems of both the American Association on Mental Deficiency (A.A.M.D.) and the American Psychiatric Association (A.P.A.) were used in this study. Necessary modifications pertinent to this particular group are in keeping with those reviewed in a previous study by this author (Menolascino, 1965).

RESULTS

For clarity, the results will be presented in two parts: medical-psychiatric findings and clinical-historical findings.

Medical-Psychiatric Findings

Diagnostic Stigmata

We elected to employ the diagnostic criteria of Oster (1953) as to the cardinal stigmata of Down's Syndrome, since there is some disagreement on the generally accepted minimal criteria of medical examinations in this disorder (Benda, 1960; Gibson and Frank, 1961; Gibson et al., 1964). Our overall medical diagnostic approach in this area has been previously reported (McIntire et al., 1965), so that only the results of the checklist of diagnostic stigmata [5] which accompanied the medical examinations of our ninety-five patients are presented in Table 8–1.

TABLE 8–1

Cardinal Stigmata Frequency and Cytogenetic Types

	CYTOGENETIC TYPE		
	TRISOMY 21	TRANSLOCATION	TRISOMY 21 MOSAIC
Number of patients	85	5	5
Mean frequency of stigmata	6.5	7.0	6.7
Standard deviation	1.4	1.6	1.62

Briefly, no distinct differences in the type or frequency of the diagnostic stigmata in each of the three cytogenetic subgroups were noted. Since the other medical-clinical findings will be reported in more detail in a forthcoming publication, the following overall review is within the context of the presence (or absence) of emotional disturbance:

1. The prevalence of associated congenital anomalies (beyond stigmata) in the total sample was quite high (43 per cent), though they were *not significantly* related to the presence or absence of emotional disturbance.
2. Similarly, the dermatoglyphic results (ATD angle, fingerprint patterns, etc.) did not differentiate either among the cytogenetic types or among the emotionally disturbed/not disturbed groups at statistically significant levels.
3. The prenatal, natal, and neonatal histories revealed a high percentage of "at risk" factors (41 per cent of the total sample), yet were not significantly related to the current psychiatric status.
4. The distribution of intellectual levels in this group revealed that 2.1 per cent were mildly retarded, 58.9 per cent were moderately retarded, and 35.8 per cent were severely or profoundly retarded. Three of the patients (3.2 per cent of the total sample) were untestable owing to the presence of overt psychotic features.

Electroencephalography

Turning now to the electroencephalographic (EEG) findings, we note that 130 EEG's were recorded and analyzed independently of any knowledge of clinical data. Twenty-five (26 per cent) of the patients yielded one or more abnormal EEG's as follows: mild diffuse slow activity, four; focal seizure activity, six; and 14/6-per-second positive spikes, three. EEG abnormality was maximal between thirty-six months and thirteen years of age. In that age range, 33 per cent of sixty-one EEG's were abnormal, all but one of which showed seizure activity. A total of 19 per cent of the thirty-one EEG's recorded at less than thirty-six months of age and only 15 per cent of the forty-eight EEG's of patients over fourteen years of age were abnormal.

No statistically significant differences (t-test) were found between groups of patients with normal and abnormal EEG's with respect to any of the following variables: sex, karyotypes, positive family, prenatal or birth history, cardiac or other associated anomalies, and neurological or psychiatric status.[6]

Of the twenty-five abnormal EEG's reported in our total sample, nine (36 per cent) were noted in patients who were emotionally disturbed. Though there is a suggested correlation here between emotional disturbances and associated EEG abnormalities, this relationship was not statistically significant when compared to those with abnormal EEG findings who were not emotionally disturbed.

Clinical-Historical Findings

Another part of this study focused on the possible determinates present in the clinical-personal histories of each patient in an effort to elucidate some of the current psychiatric problems noted. The collation of this information was plagued with the constant problems of assessing the validity of the available information (Wenar, 1963; Donoghue and Shakespeare, 1967). The validity of problems concerning pregnancy through the neonatal period was determined on the basis of the documentation obtained (hospital records, family physician's specific reports, and so forth) by personal review of all information by the author. Even so, we encountered major difficulty with such entities as "breathing difficulties at birth" (extent and time not stated); "difficulties during delivery" (no further data).

Important dimensions of the clinical-historical information on these patients are age distribution, both current and at the time of admission. Table 8–2 reveals that 95.8 per cent of the total sample was under twelve years of age at the time of admission.

TABLE 8–2

Age at Admission and at Current Examination

	UNDER 12 MONTHS	12.1–36.0 MONTHS	3.1–6.0 YEARS	6.1–12.0 YEARS	12.1–18.0 YEARS	18.1–24 YEARS	OVER 24 YEARS
Admission [1]	20	15	25	33	2	0	2
Current [2]	4	12	13	13	36	10	7

N = 95

Male 54
Female 41

[1] Mean age: total sample, 6.2 years; disturbed group, 8.2 years.
[2] Mean age: total sample, 14.2 years; disturbed group, 16.2 years.

From this table it can be determined that there is little difference in the distribution of age between the disturbed group and the nondisturbed group. Average length of confinement shows even less differentiation with 8.3 years being the mean for the total sample, as compared to 8.4 years for the emotionally disturbed group.

The prevalence of emotional disturbance in our sample and the types of disturbances found have more significance when viewed in connection with the reasons for admission as are shown on Table 8–3. All but five of the disturbed patients in the sample were noted to cluster in three categories: "Needs of Sibs" (four patients), "Family Psychopathology" (nine patients), and most markedly, "Overt Psychiatric Disturbance" (seventeen patients). Of the remaining five patients, only two were admitted for realistic family factors and medical needs; the other three came for special education. None of those admitted on professional advice showed psychiatric disturbance. Further analysis revealed a number of factors which apparently precipitated the psychiatric disturbance in the subgroup whose families were noted by marked psychopathology at the time of admission, though these children were not *overtly* disturbed at that time. This category displayed frequent instances of dysfunctional families with little investment in their children's developmental emotional needs, the crisis of divorce, psychosis in one or both of the parents, and the inability to accept the child's "differentness," which resulted in isolation of the child.

Of the thirty-three patients who were admitted because of distinct psychiatric disturbances, all had been referred for admission *as if* these behavioral factors were expected features of their underlying Down's Syndrome. In other words, the presence of overt psychiatric disturbance apparently did not seem to suggest to the referral source that psychiatric services were the primary need at the time. True, the psychiatric symptomatology could have been the "ticket" to institutionalization, as could well be in the case of the sixteen who were admitted because they displayed overt signs of disturbance at that time and who now express normal behavior (for their developmental age). However, this more forcibly suggests the outcome of the traditional professional diagnostic posture which seemingly uniformly viewed symptoms such as head banging, rumination, and frequent temper tantrums as "expected" behavior in the mentally retarded (Wright and Menolascino, 1966). Ironically, the incongruity of these abnormal behavioral dimensions and the common "Prince Charming" stereotype of the emotional placidity in patients with Down's Syndrome were also overlooked.

Perhaps the most striking correlation in our study is the relationship between the initial reasons for admission and the current psychiatric status of the emotionally disturbed individuals in the sample. As is evident in Table 8–3, fifty-six (58.9 per cent) of our total of ninety-five patients had been admitted to this institution under circumstances which made them "at risk" as to their future emotional adjustment. The findings in regard to the children who had been admitted

TABLE 8-3

Reasons for Admission and Frequency of Type of Psychiatric Disturbance on Current Examination

	CBS[1] WITH BEHAVIOR REACTION	CBS WITH PSYCHOTIC REACTION	ADJUSTMENT REACTION OF CHILDHOOD	PSYCHO-NEUROSES	PROPF-SCHIZO-PHRENIA[2]	PERSONALITY TRAIT DISTURBANCE
Realistic family factors (12)		1				
Needs of sibs (9)	2		1			1
Family psycho-pathology (14)	6		2	1		
Realistic (physical-medical) needs (3)	1					
Overt psychiatric disturbance (33)	8	3	3	1	2	
Iatrogenic (11)						
Need for special education (9)			2	1		
No reason given (4)						
Total 95	17 (49%)	4 (11%)	8 (22.9%)	3 (8.6%)	2 (5.7%)	1 (2.8%)

N = 35

[1] Chronic Brain Syndrome.
[2] Refers to a schizophrenic reaction engrafted upon a primary mental retardation (Lanzkron, 1957).

because of "Needs of Sibs," "Family Psychopathology," and "Overt Psychiatric Disturbance," suggest a number of possible interconnections as to their documented clinical course after admission. Many of these children had started on the pathway to institutional life with a history of marked parental and sibling rejection, conflicting experiences with identification and authority figures, and with little preparation for the event itself. Our previously noted finding that only thirty-five patients from a matrix of fifty-six "potential" candidates for psychiatric care were indeed in need of such services at the time of our study, suggests that twenty-one of these individuals may have obtained personal-emotional help after admission to this facility.

TYPES AND FREQUENCY OF PSYCHIATRIC DISTURBANCE

The particular types [7] of psychiatric disturbance noted in our sample will be briefly reviewed with reference to possible significant etiologic determinates. Before we proceed with this task, however, we should clarify a problem of terminology.

CBS with Behavioral Reaction

The seventeen subjects in this group presented a rather uniform psychiatric-interview picture of hyperactivity, impulsiveness, short attention span, and overall difficulties in the modulation of overt behavior. Though these symptoms are amenable to intervention by outpatient treatment, they have been one of the major reasons for seeking admission for these children. As a result, these children are denied both the outpatient care and highly structured interpersonal environment of either the family unit or a special education setting which such a patient so desperately needs. Rather, the children are admitted to an institutional environment that is devoid of any comprehensive psychiatric services and is poorly staffed, thereby precluding any close or continuing interpersonal relationships. It is not surprising that the majority of children in this group continued to display the behavioral difficulties that had been noted at the time of their admission.

CBS with Psychotic Reactions

These four closely allied patients displayed periods of either complete uncontrollability, loss of contact with the external environment, or both. Though the common psychiatric treatment approach is a period of intensive inpatient care, with or without psychotropic adjuncts, and a strong collateral allegiance with the family, these children were admitted to the institution and all have shown a documented continuation of their psychiatric symptoms. The psychotic reaction, superimposed on major intellectual-adaptive problems, prevents these children from engaging in special educational approaches owing to lack of behavioral control and propensities toward frequent personality disorganization. The latter also robs the patients of possible positive influences from their peer groups and the development of corrective identification models with the institutional staff.

Adjustment Reactions of Childhood

This group of eight never overcame the transition to the institutional setting. Unresolved grief reactions, extended bewilderment as to "Where are Mommy and Daddy—when are they coming?" and associated "unanswerable" questions pertaining to the reasons for severing the crucial family support system which had precipitated these adjustment reactions in five of this group. The remaining three displayed a continuation of the adjustment difficulties they had experienced in their initial home environments, and the entry into the new setting was followed by exacerbation, rather than alleviation, of their symptomatology.

Psychoneurotic Reactions

In this group of three, one with chronic psychoneurotic anxiety reaction and two with chronic psychoneurotic conversion reaction, all had displayed similar symptomatology in the primary home environment. The symptoms were viewed by the parents and the referral source as behavioral "stigmata" of the underlying Down's Syndrome as is illustrated in the following quotation: "Peculiar statements about being sick all the time—which is just another part of being Mongoloid." The misinterpretation of such overt psychiatric symptomatology as being part of the behavior syndrome of this disorder causes one to wonder about the diagnostic acumen of the referral source and his interest in these children and their families.

Propf-Schizophrenic Reactions

Propf-schizophrenic reactions (Lanzkron, 1957) were displayed in the current findings of two children who were described as passive, quiet, and fearful at the time of admission. This behavior persisted for ten months in one child and sixteen months in the other, at which time both slowly underwent marked behavioral withdrawal, displaying several signs of autism which is typical of this reaction (Menolascino, 1965; Rutter, 1956). After extensive medical reevaluation, the behavioral changes were attributed to "Unknown degenerative neurological changes" in one and "Her severe mental retardation status" in the other. The latter, however, had consistently placed high in the moderately retarded range on formal psychometric evaluation (Stanford-Binet). The problems of the "invisible schizophrenic" in facilities for the retarded are illustrated in these two children as well as the descriptive-etiologic considerations in their cases (Potter, 1933; Wortis, 1958).

Personality-Trait Disturbance

The one patient with a personality-trait disturbance (passive-aggressive type) was admitted to this institution at the age of eighteen years. Much of her past manipulative and obstinate tendencies had been viewed as related to her "inability to understand—otherwise I know she wouldn't be that way" (mother's statement). Instead of being given access to interventive psychiatric care before (or in place of!) institutionalization, this patient had been allowed to literally extend her psychopathology within the context of the new interpersonal arena— with associated increasingly self-defeating results for herself.

The types of psychiatric disturbances noted in our sample have been reviewed to illustrate that there is little differentiation from those which could well be managed on an outpatient basis, as they are amenable to current psychiatric techniques and methods. This raises the question why psychiatric resources were *not* made available to these patients prior to or after admission to the institutional setting. As Potter (1965) has so eloquently noted, some of the reasons are attributable to the negative attitudes of many psychiatrists toward the mentally retarded. Similarly, Chess (1966) recently commented on both the therapeutic amenability of most emotionally disturbed mentally retarded individuals, and the incongruous rejection of such treatment challenges.

CONSIDERATIONS NOTED IN
THE CURRENT SAMPLE

Frequently noted in our sample of children with chronic brain syndrome and associated behavioral reactions were the symptoms of hyperactivity and aggressiveness which are quite reminiscent of primitive levels of personality development such as the "terrible twos" of normal development. These were particularly noted in children who also appeared to be striving for attention. What is frequently described as "overaffectionateness" in patients with Down's Syndrome, on closer evaluation appears to suggest a coping device that attempts to fulfill the affect hunger of these individuals.

Our reported finding that thirty-five (36.9 per cent) of our total sample of 95 patients were emotionally disturbed clearly reveals that the presence of an emotional disturbance was a frequent finding in this randomly selected sample of institutionalized individuals with Down's Syndrome. Further, no significant correlations were obtained on a variety of clinical-laboratory–examination indices explored in our study.

In a previous psychiatric study of eighty-seven patients with Down's Syndrome, in an outpatient multidisciplinary team setting, this writer (Menolascino, 1965) noted that eleven patients (13 per cent) were emotionally disturbed. The findings from our current sample of institutionalized patients is quite similar as to the *types* of emotional disturbances noted and will be elaborated on in this discussion. However, the *frequency* of psychiatric disturbances reported in the current study was three times as great. Experiential dimensions pertaining to the reasons for admission to this facility (especially the emotional status of the family and the future patient at that time, with particular focus on the difficulties of personality adjustment the child was having in his everyday living-developmental situation) were highly correlated with the frequency of an emotional disturbance at the time of this study. Possible factors involved in this marked increase in frequency of psychiatric disturbances in the current sample will be reviewed. The incidence of clinical-medical findings (including EEG) was not significant in contrast to our previously reported outpatient study. These comparative features suggest that a variety of clinical, experiential, and temporal factors are probably operative in the psychiatric aspects of Down's Syndrome.

As an overall view, it can be said that emotional disturbance does exist at a rather alarming rate in this institutionalized sample of mongoloid individuals. It appears that there is a consistently "firm" professional opinion that these persons can most appropriately be managed by means of institutionalization even though, as noted by Webster (1963), mentally retarded children need considerable external stimulation and interpersonal structuring in their environment—or otherwise they will display a persistent "nonpsychotic" type of autism. This suggests an instrinsic vulnerability of these children with lowered adaptive abilities and their associated need for more investment from the meaningful persons in their immediate interpersonal and physical environments.

These considerations underscore the need for further psychiatric research in the area of mental retardation as exhibited in the wide diversity of clinical and psychiatric findings in our sample and in other groups of emotionally disturbed mentally retarded individuals (Wortis, 1956). This is particularly true when viewed in the context of the part these services will play in the evolving community health centers. Herein lies a great opportunity and challenge for the psychiatrist to aid emotionally disturbed retarded individuals (Menolascino, 1967) and actively practice principles of preventive psychiatry (Caplan, 1964).

SUMMARY

The clinical-psychiatric findings in a sample of institutionalized individuals with Down's Syndrome were presented and reviewed. The frequency of psychiatric disturbance noted in this sample was relatively high (37 per cent). No significant correlations were discovered on a variety of the clinical variables studied. These were physical, neurological, cytogenetic, and dermatoglyphic features; stigmata frequency; electroencephalographic features; and personal clinical-medical-historical antecedents. However, presence and type of emotional disturbance seemed highly related to both the reasons for admission and the patients' subsequent reactions to this event. The need for both inpatient and outpatient services for similar groups of retarded individuals is discussed within a treatment-management context that stresses both interventive and preventative dimensions of psychiatric involvement and action.

NOTES

1. This investigation was supported by research grant No. HD–00370 from the National Institute of Child Health and Human Development Project No. 405 from the Children's Bureau, Dept. of Health, Education, and Welfare, Washington, D.C.

2. The physical and neurological findings represent the consensus of the three separate physicians who examined each subject. The cardinal stigmata of Oster (1953) were employed as the basis for a stigmata checklist on each of these individuals.

3. These were accomplished and interpreted under the direction of Dr. James Eisen, Director of the Human Genetics Laboratory, Nebraska Psychiatric Institute at Omaha. It should be noted that since the initial selection had been a random one (employing a book of random numbers), the cytogenetic (and other tests) were accomplished thereafter.

4. These were administered and interpreted under the direction of Dr. Robert J. Ellingson, Director of Electroencephalographic Laboratories, Nebraska Psychiatric Institute at Omaha.

5. The reliability of the reported evaluation [medical, psychiatric, and stigmata checklist (Oster, 1953)] was assessed by comparing the independent judgments of three examiners (including the author) on twenty-five patients with Down's Syndrome (not included in the current sample) and on the first thirty-two patients evaluated in the current reported sample. Agreement was complete in all but seven of these two initial samples, and discussion between the three raters subsequently resolved these differences. Thereafter, all questionable findings or ratings were discussed by all three raters. It is concluded that the currently reported ratings and findings reflect a reasonably high degree of reliability.

6. It is interesting to note that 14/6-per-second positive spikes were noted in three patients: two who were emotionally disturbed and one who was not. This finding is in contrast to a recent report (Gibbs, et al., 1964) which suggests that the absence of this particular electroencephalographic finding in their sample of individuals with Down's Syndrome may contribute to their emotional quiescence.

7. At times the descriptive diagnostic terms are confusing. All mongoloids have an anatomic dysfunction designated as a chronic brain syndrome (CBS), for example, congenital brain anomaly as manifested by simplicity of neuroarchitectural structure, smaller cerebral and cerebellum weights, and so forth. The term "CBS with Behavioral Reaction" refers to the behavior symptom complex of the impaired cognition, impulse control, sensorium, and so forth. However, the term "Adjustment Reaction" when applied to mongoloid, *also* implies the underlying presence of the anatomic dysfunction of a chronic brain syndrome. Thus, one has to mix a "tissue impairment" diagnosis and a behavioral descriptive term.

REFERENCES

American Psychiatric Association. *Diagnostic and statistical manual of mental disorders*. Washington, D.C., 1952.

Baumeister, A. A., & Williams, J. Relationship of physical stigmata to intellectual functioning of mongolism. *Amer. J. Ment. Defic.*, 1967, *71*, 586–592.

Beley, A. P. L., & Lecuyer, R. Les enfants arrieres mongoliens. *Re. Neuropsychiat. Infant*, 1960, *8*, 37–51.

Benda, C. E. *The child with mongolism*. New York: Grune & Stratton, 1960.

Caplan, G. *Principles in preventative psychiatry*. New York: Basic Books, 1964.

Chess, Stella. Treatment of the emotional problems of the retarded child and of the family. In William A. Fraenkel (Ed.), *First Brooklyn Medical Conference on Mental Retardation.* New York: Association for the Help of Retarded Children, 1966, pp. 25–36.

Domino, G., Goldschmid, M., & Kaplan, M. Personality traits of institutionalized mongoloid girls. *Amer. J. Ment. Defic.,* 1964, *68,* 498–502.

Donoghue, E. C., & Shakespeare, R. A. The reliability of pediatric case history milestones. *J. Devel. Med. Child. Neurol.,* 1967, *9* (1), 64–69.

Ellingson, R. J., & Menolascino, F. J. Clinical-EEG correlations in mongoloids confirmed by karyotype. *EEG Clin. Neurophysiol,* 1969 (in press).

Ellingson, R. J., Menolascino, F. J., & Eisen, J. D. Clinical-EEG correlations in mongoloids confirmed by karyotype. *Amer. J. Ment. Defic.,* 1970 (in press).

Gibbs, E. L., Gibbs, F. A., & Hirsch, W. Rarity of 14- and 6-per-second positive spiking among mongoloids. *Neurology,* 1964, *14,* 581–587.

Gibson, D., & Frank, H. F. Dimensions of mongolism: I. Age limits for cardinal mongol stigmata. *Amer. J. Ment. Defic.,* 1961, *66,* 30–34.

Gibson, D., Pozsony, J., & Zarfas, D. E. Dimensions of mongolism: II. The interaction of clinical indices. *Amer. J. Ment. Defic.,* 1964, *68,* 503–510.

Haworth, M. & Menolascino, F. J. Video-tape observations of disturbed young children. *J. Clin. Psychol.,* 1967, *23,* 135–140.

Heber, R. A manual on terminology and classification in mental retardation. *Amer. J. Ment. Defic.,* 1959, *60,* 493–497.

Kanner, L. *A history of the care and study of the mentally retarded.* Springfield, Ill.: Charles C Thomas, 1964.

Lanzkron, J. The concept of propf-schizophrenia and its prognosis. *Amer. J. Ment. Defic.,* 1957, *61,* 544–547.

Levy, R. J. Effects of institutional versus boarding home care on a group of infants. *J. Personal.,* 1947, *15,* 233–241.

McIntire, M., Menolascino, F. J., & Wiley, J. Mongolism—some clinical aspects. *Amer. J. Ment. Defic.,* 1965, *69,* 794–800.

Menolascino, F. J. Psychiatric aspects of mongolism. *Amer. J. Ment. Defic.,* 1965, *5,* 653–660.

———. Mental retardation and comprehensive training in psychiatry. *Amer. J. Psychiat.,* 1967, *124,* 459–466.

———. Parents of the mentally retarded: An operational approach to diagnosis and management. *J. Amer. Acad. Child Psychiat.,* 1968, *7,* 589–602.

Oster, J. *Mongolism. A clinicogenealogical investigation comprising 526 mongols living on Iceland and neighboring islands in Denmark.* Copenhagen: Danish Science Press, 1953.

Potter, H. W. Schizophrenia in children. *Amer. J. Psychiat.,* 1933, *12,* 1253–1270.

———. The needs of mentally retarded children for child psychiatry services. *J. Amer. Acad. Child Psychiat.,* 1965, *3,* 352–374.

Rutter, M. The influence of organic and emotional factors on the origins, nature and outcome of childhood psychosis. *J. Devel. Med. & Child Neurol.,* 1965, *7,* 515–528.

Walker, N. R. The use of dermal configurations in the diagnosis of mongolism. *J. Pediat.,* 1957, *50,* 19–26.

Webster, T. E. Problems of emotional development in young retarded children. *Amer. J. Psychiat.,* 1963, *12,* 34–41.

Wenar, C. The reliability of developmental histories. *Psychosom. Med.,* 1963, *25,* 505–509.

Wortis, J. A note on the concept of the "Brain Injured Child." *Amer. J. Ment. Defic.,* 1956, *61,* 204–206.

———. Schizophrenic symptomatology in mentally retarded children. *Amer. J. Psychiat.,* 1958, *115,* 425–431.

Wright, M., & Menolascino, F. J. Nurturant nursing of mentally retarded ruminators. *Amer. J. Ment. Defic.,* 1966, *71,* 451–459.

Rumination, Mental Retardation, and Interventive Therapeutic Nursing

Margaret M. Wright and Frank J. Menolascino

INTRODUCTION

IN this report, we would like to discuss our experiences with the syndrome of rumination in four young mentally retarded children, to present our treatment approach to this syndrome, and to discuss both general and specific interventive therapeutic nursing programing for these children.[1] The role of the nursing profession in providing comprehensive care in response to this particular clinical challenge will be underscored.

The occurrence of rare syndromes in human beings is interesting to observe, rather easy to describe, but at all times difficult to interpret. The syndrome of rumination in children well illustrates these principles. Though initially described in the seventeenth century in adults, a number of reports have documented its occurrence in children during the past century (Cameron, 1925; Gaddini and Gaddini, 1957; Richmond and Eddy, 1957). Our recent experiences with the rumination syndrome in four institutionalized young mentally retarded children is contrary to reports that state that it is a rare phenomenon in mentally retarded children (Gaddini and Gaddini, 1957; Richmond and Eddy, 1957). Indeed, most reports on rumination in childhood tend to list the disorder as a psychosomatic entity occurring in relatively normal children who sustained emotional deprivation in early childhood secondary to failure of the individual mothering relationship. Thus our experiences with four mentally retarded children, all of whom had been institutionalized for varying periods, are contrary to recently reported findings of other workers in this area and also suggest that multiple dynamic factors are present and operative.

Rumination can be defined as the bringing up into the mouth of previously ingested food, generally requiring considerable efforts on the part of the child, and is accomplished by manipulation of the tongue and muscles of the throat, or by putting the fingers in the mouth. At times, the regurgitated food may be swallowed, but it is frequently allowed to drool from the mouth. It differs from ordinary regurgitation of food because it occurs only with obvious effort on the part of the child. Often, it is evident that the achievement of the rumination process may produce irritation and crying. The ability to ruminate tends to evolve over a period of time, and, in its earlier manifestations, rumination is often mistaken for vomiting and viewed as a possible symptom of gastrointestinal pathology. In many cases rumination is associated with behavioral disturbances such as autistic postures, excessive genital and fecal play, body rocking, head banging, and excessive thumb-finger sucking. Mortality rates in rumination have been reported as ranging from 25 to 50 per cent, and death has most commonly been attributed to prolonged malnutrition, dehydration, or a lowered resistance to intercurrent diseases (Kanner, 1957).

REVIEW OF THE LITERATURE

A review of the literature reveals only a limited number of publications on rumination, and most of them appear to be concerned with rumination in early infancy. One of the earliest reports by Cameron (1925) focused on constitutional factors. The more recent series of cases recorded by Gaddini and Gaddini (1957) and Richmond and Eddy (1957) have focused very strongly on the general factor of deprivation or the child's learning of new adaptive techniques for coping in the etiology of rumination. Richmond and Eddy (1957, p. 9) summarized one of the current interpretations of the syndrome of rumination as follows: "Inasmuch as the infant's communication with the outer world is largely through feeding and fondling, we may speculate that lack of comfort and gratification which ordinarily comes from without causes him to seek and re-create such gratification from within." They further state that, since much of the early experiences of the child with significant people in his environment centers around the gastrointestinal tract, this may be a phase specific crisis of early infancy. In this regard, Richmond and Eddy state (p. 10): "The gustatory, olfactory, tactile and kinesthetic senses play a large role in the early periods and are ones which are intensely tied into the feeding process. Traumatic events surrounding this process may lead to a variety of symptoms which may persist into adult life or to more severe symptoms such as rumination." Gaddini and Gaddini (1957) documented their observations of their series with filming of the process of the act of rumination, and in the supporting information on the mothers they noted significant disturbed mothering in the early history of the mother-child relationships. They write (p. 180): "We are dealing with babies who had some gratifying experiences, but not nearly enough to compensate for the frustration that they have suffered as a result of a profound alteration in the symbiotic relationship with the mother figure." Pertinent theoretical constructs that have added clarity to this particular mother-child interactional disturbance have been contributed by Benedek (1956), Spitz (1945), Greenacre (1958), and Louri (1955).

Among the other theories that have at one time or another been discussed as possibly causative of the syndrome of rumination, are: heredity, insufficient mastication in older children, aerophagy, finger sucking, boredom analogous to "cage sickness" in animals, and tension in the physical environment which prevents the feeding process from being a satisfying one (Kanner, 1957).

Since we plan to discuss our own treatment approach to these children with rumination syndromes, it may be appropriate to review some of the available literature as to treatment considerations here. Various methods of treatment have been explored which range from surgical approaches attempting to correct gastrointestinal dysfunction to skull trephining and—more recently—pharmacological agents such as hydrochloric acid, atropine, phcnobarbital, and carphenazine (Carter, 1961). Numerous mechanical devices have been periodically recommended, such as a "ruminating cap," which was applied to the skull and had strings which were tied tightly under the child's chin so that he could not move his jaws between feedings. Another mechanical device suggested was an inflated fish-bladder balloon, which was placed in the esophagus (with the aid of a stomach tube) after each meal to block the passage of food from the stomach in a retrograde fashion. Symptomatic treatments such as thickened feedings have also been reported. Experiential and environmental considerations, including manipulation of the physical environment, active physical intervention with the child such as more structured play activities, and added attention and affection have been reported. This latter trend was summarized by Kanner (1957) when he suggested a symptomatic treatment regime planned to help the child learn to trust those around him while simultaneously studying the child's symptoms so as to predict within limits when rumination would occur, and then try to structure the environment more appropriately at that time. Kanner also recommended frequent physical contacts with the child in an effort to provide a general background of satisfaction and stimulation for him. Other recent treatment reports have recommended a combined approach: an attempt to fulfill the child's deprivation features, and active psychotherapeutic intervention with the mother (with the possible need for substitute mothering figures at times).

Significantly, a review of the literature reveals no specific treatment recommendations for rumination when it occurs in young mentally retarded children. Accordingly, much of our own methods of treatment with our particular group of children had to be based on general principles of nursing and child management while incorporating some of the features of the previously reviewed treatment attempts.

METHOD OF STUDY

Four young children, all residents of institutions for the mentally retarded, were referred for consultative opinion, and our final impression was that their major current clinical problem was a rumination syndrome. A brief synopsis of their presenting problems is presented in Table 9–1.

Principles of Treatment

Our methods of nursing-treatment intervention in these children with persistent rumination syndrome were based on the following principles: (1) collaborative use of all nursing personnel and physical facilities as the enlargement of the child's interactive social and physical environments. This necessitates changes in such areas as food intake and type, the need for varying intensities of response to close interpersonal relationships, and the size and extent of social groups; (2) consistent and close relationships with the nursing personnel in an effort to allow the child to develop trust and meaningful relationships with the nursing personnel, and also seek substitute stimulation outside the self; (3) provision of external stimulating experiences that are closely scheduled with emphasis on both the need for substituted external experiences and the frequency and their duration. These scheduled external stimulating experiences were considered doubly important, since mentally retarded children generally seem less able to seek out external stimulation by themselves (Webster, 1963);

(4) modifications in the frequency and type of interactive experiences with ongoing developmental changes. This necessitated a flexible nursing-treatment approach geared to the child's changing activities and his increased availability to accept more complex structuring of his environment as he improved in any given area; (5) support of general developmental needs; regardless of the child's stage of therapeutic progress.

Phases of Treatment

Initial Phase

In practice, these treatment "ingredients" were preceded by a thorough diagnostic evaluation with a resultant therapeutic program prescription. Depending on a variety of factors (nature of the child's previous mothering, chronicity of the child's rumination, presence of physical problems that might limit motor mobilization, type and number of personnel interested and available, and others), the initial phase of our treatment approach to the retarded child with a rumination syndrome focused on the establishment of a relationship with the child. Tactile stimulation, verbalizations, continuity of nursing personnel, and neutral physical surroundings were stressed. Interestingly, it was observed that most of these children were noticeably frightened (with an associated prominent increase in their rumination) if too many treatment persons or a sharp increase in sensory input (for example, talking of children or adults nearby, action toys) was initially attempted. Rhythmic music (without words) was played at selected times during the day (especially at feeding times) and was noted to have an appreciably calming effect on these children. An associated problem of this initial phase of treatment was the anxiety levels of the treatment personnel; since the rumination itself tended to be repugnant as to odor and sight and the children's frequent postrumination smiling tended to precipitate feelings of anger and frustration in those immediately around them. Scheduled treatment seminars allowed for ventilation, acceptance, and correction of staff reactions in these areas.

Middle Phase

The middle phase of the treatment regimen concentrated on graduated exposure to new experiences as the child would allow and seemingly enjoyed them. Essentially, the dependent and trusting relationship established with the child in the initial phase of treatment was extended into helping him explore other adaptive techniques—

TABLE 9–1

General Aspects of the Rumination Syndrome in Four Institutionalized Mentally Retarded Children

CASE	SEX	AGE AT INSTITUTIONALIZATION	AGE AT OUR INITIAL EXAM.	ETIOLOGIC DIAGNOSIS [1]	CLINICAL HISTORY HIGHLIGHTS
1	M	5½	6	Prematurity; difficult to assess residuals of early gastrointestinal surgery and prolonged hospitalization for same (deprivation?); severe mental retardation	Feeding problem immediately after birth; surgical repair of tracheo-esophagol fistula at age 3 days, with stormy postoperative course necessitating 3 months of continuous hospital care at that time. Very slow developmental milestones with associated failure to thrive physically, frequent regurgitation, and uniform developmental delays. Initially noted to be happy and affectionate, despite multiple problems. Onset of rumination features prior to institutionalization with sharp increase in rumination shortly thereafter
2	M	5	10	Perinatal; severe mental retardation	Surgery for pyloric stenosis at age 3 weeks.[2] Slow development with minimal language evolution. Hyperkinetic behavioral picture ushered in his institutionalization. Autoerotic aspects of the rumination syndrome appear as part of an overall behavioral reaction in which the child attempted to obtain interpersonal distance

CASE	SEX	AGE AT INSTITUTIONALIZATION	AGE AT OUR INITIAL EXAM.	ETIOLOGIC DIAGNOSIS [1]	CLINICAL HISTORY HIGHLIGHTS
3	M	1½	7	Postnatal etiology—cause unknown; convulsive disorder; severe mental retardation	Deterioration of previous developmental attainments after onset of myoclonic seizures at age 11 months. Difficulty in feeding thereafter; initial poorly controlled seizure disturbance. Focus on feeding and seizure management had previously necessitated much professional involvement. Good seizure control had sharply decreased the amount of nursing attention the child then received
4	M	3	8½	Prenatal etiology—cause unknown; multiple congenital anomalies; moderate mental retardation	Multiple congenital anomalies. No previous feeding problems prior to institutionalization. Rumination as initial response to institutionalization with resolution of same with good aide-child relationship. Reassignment of a new aide ushered in recurrent rumination features

[1] Gaddini & Gaddini (1957) have commented on the possible role of early gastrointestinal disturbances as a factor in "choice of symptom" in later rumination syndromes. (May also apply to Case #1).

[2] Etiological considerations are consistent with those of the American Association on Mental Deficiency (Heber, 1959).

techniques ranging from his response to food intake to his increasing ability to enjoy and participate in social interactions. Our experiences in this middle phase of treatment tended to support the contention that a warm and dependent relationship with consistent adults is a necessary prerequisite to both the resolution of old habit patterns and initiation of the learning-to-learn posture in the child, regardless of whether the "subject matter" is the recovery from environmental deprivation or the child's learning of new adaptive techniques for coping with the outside world (Mowrer, 1960). It was fascinating to watch these children improve, from their initial looking at the nursing personnel's faces with fear, then with puzzlement, then fingering their facial features, allowing guided efforts during feeding (passive spoon feeding to assisted active spoon feeding to the lips, then unassisted to the lips, then autonomous feeding), and subsequent introductions into larger circles of children in a variety of activities. Thus this middle phase of treatment focused strongly on active intervention in the children's previous rumination and associated behavioral manifestations, while also initiating a series of self-help skills.

Final Phase

The final phase of treatment attempted to solidify the children's previous gains and maximize their developmental potentials. Self-help skills were stressed with focus on the children's ability to do for themselves and develop more effective methods of communicating their needs (physically and emotionally) by verbal and nonverbal methods. They became more comfortable in large group settings, their interpersonal interactions were flavored with much affective overtone, and they played with toys actively and purposefully (at their respective developmental levels). In association with quite obvious emotional and developmental improvements, these children *all* displayed dramatic gains in general physical well-being. Though the interruption of their rumination syndromes produced concomitant weight increases, we were more impressed by their increased affective availability and their developmental spurts in finger dexterity, general muscle tone, and increased range of motor abilities.

CASE HISTORIES

The following four case histories will attempt to show the direct application (and results) of our previously discussed treatment methods. The first case history to be presented is that of a child who was treated in a special clinical research unit for young mentally retarded children; the other three children illustrate the application of our treatment methods within the context of the child's original institutional placement.

Case 1

Personal history. A 6-year-old boy was seen in consultation at a home for the retarded because of marked feeding problems with associated persistent weight loss. The child's personal history revealed that he was the third child born to a 23-year-old mother. Pregnancy was normal—except that the child was born eight weeks before the expected date of confinement. The delivery was uneventful; the birth weight was 4 pounds. Umbilical and bilateral inguinal hernias were noted at birth. On the second day of life the child displayed regurgitation and marked feeding difficulties; clinical evaluation revealed a tracheo-esophageal fistula. Surgical repair of the fistula and hernias was accomplished on the third day of life. A stormy postoperative course, complicated by his prematurity status, eventuated in the child's remaining in the hospital until the age of 3 months. Upon returning home, he continued to have sporadic regurgitation difficulties. He achieved the normal developmental milestones extremely slowly throughout his early life, so that at the age of 3 years he weighed 23 pounds. Formal psychological examination suggested severe mental retardation, and an extensive medical evaluation eventuated in the impression of "chronic brain syndrome, cause unknown; mental retardation—severe." At this age the child was reportedly unable to sit, walk, or speak, although he did make sounds and "appeared happy and contented." (This may have been spurious, because his mother also described him as "never crying—very quiet–seems happy all by himself playing with his hands.") He had continued to have sporadic periods when eating, chewing, and swallowing seemed to bother him. At the age of 4 years, regurgitation became more frequent (ruminative features were described, but *not labeled* as such), and in view of the increasing feeding problem, the family conceded to institutionalization of their child at the age of 5½ years. Upon admission to the institution, his feeding problems became more marked; instead of sporadic periods of regurgitation, the child began to display persistent rumination phenomena. Feeding problems became of extreme concern to the staff at the institution and the child's general physical welfare prompted their seeking our consultation. The clinical picture was consistent with the diagnosis of a rumination syndrome and suggested a therapeutic program at our Clinical Research Unit.

On admission, the boy weighed 16½ pounds and was extremely emaciated and apathetic. He would accept a toy handed to him, but would hold it rather listlessly and would glance at the examiner with a dull and disinterested look. His jaws were in almost constant motion and teeth grinding was prominent. Lying in bed, he would wave his hands in the air in front of his eyes and look at them for prolonged periods. He frequently sucked his thumb, or the blanket, and masturbated quite regularly. He would begin to ruminate within five minutes after eating, often even before finishing his meal—moving his jaws and tongue or putting his fingers into his mouth to initiate the activity. He became tense when people were around him, and the rumination tended to increase in response to any noise or confusion in the immediate environment.

Treatment and outcome.   Elements of the previously reviewed general treatment principles were employed. Initially, the child was held for one and a half hours to two hours after each feeding and was provided emotional support and attention through cuddling, patting, stroking of his face and arms, holding him close while rocking, and talking or crooning to him softly. It was hoped that this would facilitate his engagement in an ongoing interpersonal relationship. At first the child was fed with the other children, but he became very distracted and disturbed with the noise and confusion surrounding the group feeding. Thus it was felt to be necessary to begin to offer him new experiences on a more graduated basis, and the decision was made to feed him alone in his room. Repetitiously rhythmic music was employed as another modality for soothing the child; a record player was placed in his room and was put on during the feeding and postfeeding periods. His rumination did not diminish appreciably until one month after admission, but during this initial period he displayed recognition of and interaction with the persons caring for him (for example, he began to reach out and touch the aide's face, hair, and mouth).

Interestingly, as he gradually began to ruminate less, the staff noticed he began to masturbate more frequently as if giving up one gratification led him to seek others. As he showed evidence of being able to tolerate more noise and other persons in the environment, it was decided to move him from his room for increasingly longer periods to the dayroom so that he would be with the other children. He was also taken outside, which he enjoyed very much. He was given an increasingly greater variety of toys to play with and handle, and soon he began to reach out frequently and touch other children who were playing around him.

During the fifth week of hospitalization, his rumination had stopped and he seemed to be progressing well in his feeding. He was then placed in a high chair for his meals and was taught to feed himself; he became able to do so with assistance although he much preferred to be fed. He progressed from pureed foods to solids, and eventually he was enjoying a regular diet including meats, vegetables, sandwiches, potato chips, cake, and cookies. His play became more active; he used more toys and seemed happy and content with much laughing and primitive sounds. He exhibited varied but appropriate emotional responses including disgust and anger when the nursing staff did something which displeased him. He enjoyed being held and would cuddle up closely to the person holding him. He began to assume a teasing kind of relationship with the staff (for example, he would pull the nurse's ear lobes and laugh, or playfully put his fingers in her mouth). He thoroughly enjoyed his tub bath and the period of bathing and getting ready for bed seemed a particularly happy time for him. During the last month of hospitalization, efforts were started at toilet training with some measures of success.

At the time of discharge (four and one-half months after admission) he weighed 31½ pounds, nearly double his admission weight. Psychological evaluation at this time (Stanford-Binet) revealed functioning in the upper portion of the severely retarded range. He had become a very friendly, winsome child who, with his sidewise glances, little grin, and happy playfulness, made one attracted to him immediately. He was an almost totally different child—both physically and emotionally—from the one he had been at the time of admission. Since his return to the home for the retarded, his improvement has persisted to the time of this report (one year).

Case 2

Personal history. We were asked to see a 10-year-old institutionalized boy in consultation because "He plays with his food off and on—doesn't do it all the time—but when he gets going on it he can do it for two or three months at a crack. Otherwise he's noisy, always tries to demand attention—which is awful hard to follow because he doesn't speak" (ward attendant). This boy's personal history revealed he was the second born child of a 28-year-old mother; the pregnancy was described as within normal limits. At the time of birth, the umbilical cord was noted to be wrapped twice around the neck, and the child had a rather stormy neonatal course with prominent anoxic difficulties. At the age of 3 weeks, he underwent surgery for correction of a pyloric stenosis disturbance; he tolerated the procedure without any known residuals. From then onward, he had no major medical illnesses, and the developmental timetable was entirely within normal limits except for extremely limited language development. He had only four words at the age of three years and developed only six more words in the next two years. His family history was negative for any hereditodegenerative diseases. His parents were warm and empathic individuals who had attempted to help their son in many ways, but his increasing hyperactivity, impulsiveness (with destructive overtones), and increasing problems in home management finally eventuated in the family's reluctant consent to institutionalize their son at the age of 5 years. Interestingly, except for the gastrointestinal difficulty immediately after birth, he had had no further difficulties in regard to digestive or nutritional aspects while in his home.

Shortly after admission to the home for the retarded, he was noted to begin to lose weight, became a management problem because of undifferentiated aggression, and it became increasingly more difficult to structure his educational or recreational activities because of his limited language. After the first six months of institutionalization, he began to have periods wherein he would "Chew his food, play with it, spit it up, keep some more in his mouth and play with it for hours" (nurse's notes). During these periods of rumination he would be relatively quiescent (except for infrequent periods of body rocking) and appeared very content from outward facial appearance. These periods of rumination would then be substituted (at four-to-six-month intervals) by similar lengths of time wherein he would become extremely boisterous with many primitive sounds, teeth grinding, and facial grimaces when people approached him. The degree of his motor restlessness would frequently necessitate psychotrophic medication and physical isolation. This alternating pattern of rumination-behavioral problems had continued for almost three years prior to our consultative contact. We were asked to examine him primarily because the last period of "feeding trouble" had lasted for seven months, with the child losing weight rapidly, and the question of surgical intervention had been considered. We were asked to see him on a consultative basis as to "helping us slow down his behavior [rumination and body rocking] so we can get him into better physical shape for exploratory surgery. We can't do any x-ray studies because he's so uncooperative. We'll have to do an exploratory, there must be something wrong with his duodenum or stomach" (ward physician).

On initial observation, the child was noted to be slowly and rhythmically chewing on obvious bits of food substance, and when seen at a distance he appeared quite pleased and relaxed. However, when one attempted to make verbal or nonverbal contact with the child, the rumination tended to decrease in frequency and he alternately would spit at the examiner and grind his teeth, or run to the corner of his room, when the rumination would become more marked. Nursing personnel stated they felt the child had "somehow sensed that we are planning surgery—we've given him so much attention lately—now he's not his usual happy self when he's chewing his cud—he seems to be a mixture of his ornery self and his happy cud-chewing self."

Treatment and outcome. A therapeutic program was planned with the nursing staff to increase stimulation, with particular reference to choosing personnel who could accept the child's rather primitive aggressive behavior and still try to make affective and tactile contact with him. After two rather stormy initial weeks in which he tested the limits quite actively

Margaret

(spitting at anyone in close range, grimacing when one tried to get physically closer, outbursts of physical aggression when one attempted to directly interact with him as to toys, play materials, etc.), he began to accept closer interpersonal interactions and a regular feeding schedule that focused on more involvement with the child in both emotional and physical dimensions. He slowly displayed fewer of the rather menacing distancing devices previously noted. Within two months, he had begun to gain weight consistently, rumination was no longer an obvious feature, and his behavior became more outgoing and predictable without aggressive propensities. Presently, though he tends to remain on the periphery of his ward group, he does interact to the best of his adaptive abilities. Rumination has not recurred in the last one year.

Case 3

Personal history. A 7-year-old boy was admitted to an institution for the retarded at the age of 1½ years because he was "spastic, profoundly retarded, and in a world all his own." This boy's personal history revealed that the child was the product of the third pregnancy in a 28-year-old mother; the pregnancy, birth and early neonatal development had been entirely within normal limits. At the age of 11 months the child had a series of myoclonic seizures and a rather rapid deterioration course, with loss of all previously attained developmental milestones, increasing spastic features, loss of speech, and stereotyped hand movements that were highly personalized. After his acute illness at 11 months of age, the parents had had increasing difficulty in feeding the child because of his frequent seizures and limited responsiveness to parental attempts at both feeding and emotional engagement. Because of the poorly controlled seizures, the developmental deterioration course, and the increasing medical bills the child was institutionalized. The feeding problems persisted after entry into the institution, and it appears that the nursing staff had attempted different feeding techniques and food supplements in an effort to keep the child's nutritional status adequate.

From the time he was 3½ years old, his seizures became less frequent, and shortly thereafter he began to display rumination features. Seemingly, as the child's seizures became medically controlled, the nursing staff's preoccupation with the "challenge" of his feeding problem diminished and, concomitantly with these changes, general attention from the nursing staff also dwindled. The child had slowly lost weight for the last year prior to our seeing him in consultation—and this was one of the children who had been "spotted" by a nurse who had attended one of our inservice training lectures on rumination.

Treatment and outcome. It is of interest that the child's problem of dwindling weight had been viewed as a cohesive part of his underlying medical problem, and the staff had seemingly reconciled itself to a slowly terminal prognostic course. We called this to the attention of the nursing staff, and raised the question as to the possible *increased* availability of the child because of the *diminished* seizure problem; the child's rumination phenomenon was interpreted as a possible response to decreased interpersonal stimuli in his environment. A total push program of nursing-care involvement with the child was outlined with more personalized feeding attention, increased interpersonal involvement, and reappraisal of the physical environmental stimuli. Within three weeks the rumination ceased, the boy became more alert, the autistic features receded, and he displayed an ability for interpersonal engagement which was beyond that previously described when he was a "feeding problem—but we get him to eat." It is interesting to speculate in this particular case whether the dire medical opinion in regard to the child's possible prognostic course had not indeed compromised the nurse's opinion and judgment of how much she should be involved with the child. Rather than considering this an error in nursing judgment, we wonder about the engagement and enthusiasm of the attending physician and about the role of his negative influence on the nursing members of the professional team.

Case 4

Personal history. An 8½-year-old boy was admitted to a home for the retarded at the age of 3 years. This boy's personal history revealed that he was the product of a normal pregnancy in a 31-year-old mother. At the time of birth, he was noted to have multiple congenital anomalies, as manifested by absence of the left eye, skull asymmetry, webbing of toes, and hypospadia. In early childhood his slow developmental course, only partial vision, and a psychologist's impression of moderate mental retardation had led the family physician to recommend institutionalization to the family. Living in a rural community with little hope for the availability of special educational facilities for the boy, the family reluctantly agreed to his institutionalization at the age of 3 years. He had not had any appetite or weight problems during his stay in his own home. Within a week after entering the institution, he was described as initially quite restless; next, a period of frequent crying and screaming followed. This persisted for the first two months of institutionalization. His parents considered taking him back home, but were reassured that, "He'll get over it, he'll learn to like us—he seems so retarded I don't think he really understands whether he's home or not." During his initial periods of emotional upset, his appetite pattern became rather irregular, but he did not lose weight. During the remainder of his first year of institutionalization he was commonly described in the nursing notes as "quiet, sad looking, likes to play around with his tongue and his food—but seems to eat enough to get along." However, during the following year distinct rumination features were described; he became a feeding problem and slowly began to lose weight. Interestingly, the ward personnel recognized and were empathic with the child's increasing adverse reactions to institutional life and appointed one of the older girl residents to be his exclusive "feeder" and helper. Within a month, his rumination ceased, he became more outgoing and demanding, enjoyed playing in the ward sand box and on the outdoor recreational equipment. We were asked to see him approximately three months after this period and the staff was quite concerned about the rapid return of his former pattern of "playing with his food," sadness, and rapidly declining weight. On examination, rumination was very much in evidence, the child's gaze was averted, and his behavior was very autistic with much psychomotor slowing. A review of the total clinical situation revealed that the child's daily "feeder and leader" had been placed in a vocational rehabilitation program three months previously, and the girl who replaced her had rather mechanically attempted to fulfill her duties to the child. We discussed the boy's problems with the child's new helper, and it became apparent that the child's cosmetic handicaps, low developmental level, and dependency-demandingness had all become rather repugnant to her. She bitterly complained about his "playing games with me with his food—if I get it down, he brings it back up; then he seems to have fun just chewing it in his mouth and looking at me with a funny look on his face—like he's laughing at me or something."

Treatment and outcome. In this particular instance, the exacerbation of the child's former rumination phenomenon appeared reactive to interpersonal environmental changes and the markedly altered relationships with his primary care giver. We were considering the replacement of the child's present care worker by another young lady (with attributes similar to the first child helper), when the child's mother became very interested in his recent feeding problems. In view of newly established outpatient community facilities for the moderately retarded in their home town, she asked to take the child home with her. We discussed with her the essence of the foregoing clinical information, reviewed his therapeutic needs, and supported her interest in and relationship with the child. On last report (six months after discharge) the child was doing very nicely at home and had no further appetite or feeding problems (including rumination).

DISCUSSION

The behavioral manifestations of young mentally retarded children have most frequently been described as developmentally delayed and in keeping with their general levels of endowment. Apparently, there has not been sufficient attention to the primitive behavioral manifestations of severely and moderately retarded young children, even though they are frequently encountered (Webster, 1963; Mowrer,

1960; Menolascino, 1965). In the past, symptomatic behavior or manifestations in mentally retarded children (such as head banging, autistic hand play, and so forth) were viewed as part of the underlying retardation process itself (Barr, 1904). However, as Collins (1965) has demonstrated, behavioral manifestations such as chronic head banging in severely retarded children are related to external environmental factors and can be modified or removed. Similar considerations have prompted our reevaluation of the manifestations and treatment of rumination in young mentally retarded children.

A review of our initial contact with each of the four children in this report underscores the nurse's need for a high index of suspicion so as to recognize the symptomatic nature of rumination and the collateral need for a specialized nursing regimen. The nature of the presenting complaints that we noted from the ward personnel, though they all revolved around the problem of food intake and concern about the children's nutritional status, had given little import to the rather prominent extenuating circumstances, both in the recent and remote past. It has been noted that two of the children reported herein were directly referred after an inservice training lecture on rumination. Thus, these two children could very easily have been "missed" by the ward personnel, with the children's eating habits being viewed as rather idiosyncratic in nature, but not particularly in need of therapeutic nursing intervention. Interestingly, two of the case histories reported suggest that there was information available to the administrative and nursing personnel *before* the onset of the rumination features that later prompted the consultation requests. Similar considerations underscore the nurse's role and possible contribution to the admission team's treatment programming for such children in facilities for the mentally retarded.

We are aware that service programs in mental retardation must be attuned to realistic personnel and time parameters to be feasible for large-scale application. We would submit that our previously outlined treatment methods are readily applicable to rumination syndromes in young mentally retarded children, since an excessive number of personnel, treatment time, or equipment was not necessary in our experience. What appeared essential to our treatment regimen were (1) alertness to and appreciation of the symptomatic manifestations of deprivation phenomena and their inimical effect on a child's development, (2) administrative flexibility and support permitting therapeutic nursing intervention, (3) modification of attitudes in the nursing personnel, (4) emphasis on providing the child with stimulating experiences to offset self-stimulatory activities, and (5) the need for ongoing collaborative efforts among all members of the therapeutic team. Accordingly, it would appear feasible to extend this treatment approach to more general programming of services for the large population of institutionalized young retarded children in order to positively alter or prevent symptoms of deprivation.

A closely allied challenge for therapeutic interventive nursing is the approach to children who are repulsive to their caretakers because of their physical anomalies or allied disorders. We frequently noted the circular pattern of repugnance leading to rejection of the child—with resultant isolation, deprivation, and finally rumination symptoms.

In closing, we would be remiss if we did not share some other possible implications of this report with our colleagues in public health nursing. The early prevention of similar problems in young children seemingly demands closer attention to those crises early in life which can so adversely affect a child's future developmental profile. In reviewing the four case histories presented in this report, the public health nurse may want to explore areas such as: How could these mothers and fathers have been helped in the initial crises of prematurity, the neonatal surgical interventions, the shock of the early diagnosis of mental retardation, or the persistent feeding difficulties? The public health nurse could have provided the mothers of these children much support and guidance in providing stimulating experiences within the home. Similarly, she can help support those mothers who care for children who give them little satisfaction or gratification in their mothering role. This interventive public health nursing service may prevent the frequently associated maternal feeling of inadequacy with its subsequent danger of maternal disengagement from the child. Thus, we need to be cognizant of and active in our role in the early detection and therapeutic intervention into those instances of the "at risk" childhood population so as to prevent those personal, social, and environmental experiences which can have such adverse psychosocial-developmental consequences. Research in nursing has already explored some of these problems, but much more needs to be done in this area as well as in many of the other nursing problems we commonly encounter in caring for retarded children.

SUMMARY

An interventive therapeutic nursing approach to the rumination syndrome in four young mentally retarded children was presented. Questions were raised as to the significance of the role of nursing in both the treatment and prevention of such symptoms. The closely allied nursing challenges of programing for close and consistent interpersonal relationships, intervening in or rechanneling self-stimulatory behavior, and ongoing attempts to provide nurse-child relationships that are conducive to maximizing the developmental potentials of mentally retarded children were underscored. Some preventative and other dimensions of nursing care for mentally retarded children which would warrant further research by institutional and public health nurses were noted.

NOTE

1. This investigation was supported by U.S. Public Health Service Research Grant HD–00370 and Project 405 from the U.S. Children's Bureau.

REFERENCES

Barr, M. W. *Mental defectives: Their history, treatment, and training.* Philadelphia: Blakiston's Son and Co., 1904.

Benedek, T. Toward the biology of the depressive constellation. *J. Amer. Psychoanal.,* 1956, *4,* 389–427.

Cameron, H. C. Some forms of habitual vomiting in infancy. *Brit. Med. J.,* 1925, *1,* 878–886.

Carter, C. H. Carphenazine in mental defectives: A specific antiemetic. *Arch. Pediat.,* 1961, *78,* 349–356.

Collins, D. T. Head banging. *Bull. Menninger Clinic,* 1965, *29,* 205–211.

Gaddini, R. O. B., & Gaddini, E. Rumination in infancy. In L. Jessner & E. Pauestadt (Eds.), *Dynamic psychopathology in childhood.* New York: Grune & Stratton, 1957, pp. 166–185.

Greenacre, P. Toward an understanding of a physical nucleus of some defense reactions. *Int. J. Psychoanal.,* 1958, *39,* 69–76.

Heber, R. A manual on terminology and classification in mental retardation. *Amer. J. Ment. Defic.,* Monogr. Suppl., 1959, p. 64.

Kanner, L. *Child psychiatry.* Springfield, Ill.: Charles C Thomas, 1957.

Louri, R. S. Experience with therapy of psychosomatic problems in infants. In P. H. Hoch, & J. Zubin (Eds.), *Psychopathology of childhood.* New York: Grune & Stratton, 1955, pp. 254–266.

Menolascino, F. J. Emotional disturbance and mental retardation. *Amer. J. Ment. Defic.*, 1965, *70*, 248–256.

Mowrer, O. H. *Learning theory and behavior.* New York: John Wiley & Sons, 1960.

Richmond, J. B., & Eddy, E. Rumination: A psychosomatic syndrome. *Psychiat. Res. Rep.*, 1957, *8*, 1–11.

Spitz, R. Hospitalism: An inquiry into the genesis of psychiatric conditions in early childhood. *Psychoanal. Study Child.*, 1945, *1*, 53–74.

Webster, T. E. Problems of emotional development in young retarded children. *Amer. J. Psychiat.*, 1963, *120*, 34–41.

PART TWO

===

Treatment Approaches

[A]

INDIVIDUAL
APPROACHES

: 10 :

Psychotherapy of the Mentally Retarded:
Values and Cautions

George Lott

PSYCHOTHERAPY, with due respect to its limitations and special indications, can be of assistance to the mentally retarded, especially those who are verbal and are aware of their handicaps. It is a mistake to assume that mental retardation, with its associated dimension of limited comprehension, is a firm barrier to the use of psychotherapy.

First, let us determine what we mean by "psychotherapy," a term that is too often used as a label to cover all the relationships between client and professional consultant of whatever persuasion or training.

WHAT IS PSYCHOTHERAPY?

Let us inspect a theologian's definition of psychotherapy as an illumination of how much depends upon the personality and training of the therapist. According to Close (1966),

Psychotherapy is a deliberate and intensive relationship between two persons whose goal is mutual forgiveness. The patient reveals himself to the therapist so that he may be forgiven for being the way he is—particularly for his arrogance, and the therapist offers forgiveness to the patient. Each brings a need to be forgiven and to forgive. If there is no felt need for this mutual forgiveness, then therapy has not really begun. But when a mutual forgiveness has been accomplished, the deeper purposes of therapy have been fulfilled.

The illuminating and intriguing manner in which Tarachow (1962) outlines an overall conceptualization of all psychotherapeutic techniques is more pertinent to our concerns in this chapter. He defines the difference between conventional counseling psychotherapy and psychoanalytic psychotherapy by reviewing the task or goals of treatment and defines psychotherapy and psychoanalysis as follows:

In psychotherapy real events are treated as reality, while in analysis they are treated as expressions of the patients' fantasies and as determined by the inevitable needs of his solutions of his unconscious conflicts. If the relationship between therapist and patient is taken as real, then both the therapist and patient turn their backs on the unconscious fantasies and anxieties. If the real relationship is set aside then both therapist and patient turn toward an understanding and working through of the unconscious fantasies.

Tarachow suggests three principles within whose limits any psychotherapeutic technique should be comprehensible. The first principle is to supply the infantile object in reality. This is the "unanalyzed transference." In analysis, the analyst rejects the patient as object and teaches the patient to reject the analyst as object. Under such conditions, problems are resolved by interpretation. In psychotherapy, the therapist and the patient retain each other as objects and varying areas of the patient's life remain uninterpreted. The two have entered each other's lives as real objects.

The second principle suggested by Tarachow is to supply displacements. These include maneuvers in which the therapist selects the more ego-syntonic aspects of a problem and interprets only them, leaving the more troublesome factors undisturbed. The author breaks down the area of displacement into three headings: displacements in the benign phobic sense; projection; and introjection.

Tarachow's third principle is that of supplying stability. In general this also acts in support of defensive structures. Stability may be supplied both by ego and superego support. For example, ego support can be given by reality discussions of real events and by participation in decisions. Education and information enlarge the powers of the ego and so strengthen it. Superego support is given by commands, prohibitions, and expressions of morals and moral values. Changes in the environment might also contribute to stability. Explicit verbal support has dangers. The most effective support is permitting oneself to be real to the patient in some implied or indirect way; such joining in the realities of the patient presents the fewest dangers.

Tarachow outlines the process of his psychotherapeutic approach as follows: (1) There must develop a relationship between the patient and the therapist, during which the problem is stated. Its onset and development is then followed by a picture of the patient's background and early development. (2) Soon there should be a talking out of aggressive, hostile, and probably guilt-tinged feelings, which are likely to be directed (projected on) at the therapist. (3) When released, these feelings must be worked through and ameliorated in the relationship with the therapist. Too many cases are opened up by well-meaning counsellors, only to be left like an open destructive sore without completion of the last step. This last is the *crucial* stage, and is an attribute of *real* therapy, which gets beyond the stage of support and leads to more mature emancipation with less vulnerability. There are some exceptions to the need for this particular stage. For instance, the second or release stage is usually followed by relief and a resumption of normal emotional development. Also, an adult's symptoms will occasionally clear up after a moving religious conversion.

Dr. E. James Anthony, in an address to the Sixth International Psychotherapy Congress held in London, 1964, stated his view of this matter as follows:

There are two phases in child psychotherapy, phase one and phase two, with all save the "relatively rare" patient getting what therapy he needs in the first phase. The kind of therapy offered in the usual guidance clinic was strictly phase one treatment, and apparently none the worse for that in most cases. Phase one is based on a symbiotic type of relationship, in which unconscious and preconscious elements are at a premium, regression is used in the service of gratification, transference is incoherent, and countertransference may be related to infantile frustrations in the areas of care, contact, and control. Phase two is founded on a working therapeutic alliance, in which analysis and working through take the place of "corrective experience" and catharsis. The therapeutic regression is incorporated into the analytic work, which is carried out on a secondary level with cognitive elements at the forefront. The transference neurosis is fully developed, and genital or erotic feelings may express themselves in countertransference.

Anthony noted that, given these descriptions of phases one and two, two main questions arise: Is it absolutely necessary for the child to move from phase one to phase two before his treatment could be regarded as completed, or could he safely be left to his own developmental resources after the "corrective experience"? Is the essential difference between child therapy and child analysis related to the shift from the first to the second phase? Anthony's answer to the first question was in the negative. He stated: "It is only in a relatively few cases that it is necessary to proceed into the second phase, and the selection of such cases is determined by the criteria of analyzability." His answer to the second question was, in his view, decidedly positive: "The tendency in child psychotherapy, as practiced in the usual child guidance center, is to remain within the confines of phase one." Most of the examples of case treatment given in the literature more nearly follow the phase one psychotherapeutic model.

The concept of reality therapy should be kept in mind to illustrate the wide divergence of psychotherapeutic models available for the mentally retarded. This is especially so if there is any chance to encourage motivation for joining the "success group." The need for psychotherapy is not a simple problem of illness, as it is compounded by an inadequate decision making process and by a lack of committed motivation for behavior change. All agree that symptoms are too often accompanied by a secondary utility or gain. For example, school phobias have many causes, but some authors believe in getting the youngster back into school promptly (Eisenberg, 1966) rather than calling such children sick and excusing them from adjustment effort and automatically acquiring a self-inflicted failing label. The choice is to go with others who care and try, rather than to hide alone. A basic need of all individuals is to be needed, to be considered worthy of others' attentions. Along with basic needs, Thorne (1948) notes that most individuals, before the fifth grade of elementary school, begin to segregate themselves into two classes: (1) the "success group," who continue in the mainstream of satisfaction, "usually college," and (2) the "failure group" (50 to 60 per cent), who continue to puzzle and think of themselves as failures. If their natural needs for recognition become pressing, they may seek "counterfeit successes" by prominent delinquent acts—certainly a prime example of wrong choices. Therapy then could consist of aid to make better choices of more responsible behavior, a success status with committed motivation, perhaps because someone (therapist or friend) "cares." Mulling over symptoms and causes may be helpful, and possibly necessary in some cases with guilt-drenched, misinterpreted, and possibly buried experiences.

REVIEW OF THE LITERATURE

As far back as the 1940's, Thorne (1941) reported that psychotherapy for the emotionally disturbed retardate, had been found both possible and profitable. Of sixty-eight children so treated, forty-five were improved, sixteen remained unchanged, and seven became worse. Heiser (1954) reported that fourteen children were given a median of thirty-four treatment hours. He found some improvement, especially in two who were able to return home, and concluded (p. 217) that, "as a result of the first year's work, we see no reasons for pessimism; on the other hand, we believe that it is not sensible to predict or expect drastic results from psychotherapy in an institutional setting with mentally handicapped children."

Weber (1953) felt that support from psychotherapy was possible in developing and integrating constructive potentials in borderline defective delinquents. Munday (1957) reported on her psychotherapeutic results with twenty-three institutionalized moderately retarded young adults who had both neurotic and associated behavior problems. She concluded that such individual psychotherapy was both feasible and justified. Denton (1959) treated twenty mentally retarded children (with a mean IQ of 60) by means of individual psychotherapy sessions (twenty-four therapeutic hours per case) with optimistic results. Freedom from the original symptoms (which had led to commitment) and an improved adjustment to institutional life occurred in one-third of the patient sample. Chase (1953) and Burton (1954) report the values of psychotherapy in an institutional setting for the mentally retarded. Friedman (1965) reported the successful rehabilitation of a mildly retarded delinquent boy, by means of an intensive eighteen-month program of individual psychotherapy. Crowley (1965) and Ogle (1963) found psychotherapy a significant treatment-management tool in helping the emotionally disturbed mentally retarded.

On the other hand, Albini and Dinitz (1965) reported that they had found no significant improvement in the behavior of the disturbed mentally retarded patients during or subsequent to therapy. They had treated thirty-six patients with a maximum of forty-eight half-hour sessions. The control group showed a much more positive change in attitude and behavior. No details are given of the contradictions that might have been revealed in failures.

In a review of psychotherapeutic techniques useful with the mentally retarded, Sternlicht (1964) listed twenty-seven references. He spoke of the prevalent fallacy that psychotherapy is not applicable to the mentally retarded.

In contrast, Rogers (1954) claimed that psychotherapy for the retarded was not relevant because it required insight, verbal communication, and other elements inherent in normal intelligence. Sternlicht (1966) seriously takes issue with the assumption by Rogers that, since insight is necessary for successful personality change, such change is therefore not possible for mental defectives who "lack insight." Sternlicht noted that warmth and accepting relationships were most effective. Because intelligence is a crude average of varying capacities, the individual patient's attributes have to be considered. Gestures, grimaces, and mannerisms are always present, regardless of the handicapping factors present in communication (Ruesch and Kees, 1956). Nonverbal communication techniques listed by Sternlicht (1966) included figure drawings (also reported by Freeman, 1936), finger painting (also reported by McDermott, 1954, when she wrote of the value of art therapy for the retarded), and music therapy (as outlined by Murphy, 1957, and Heimlich, 1960) as a means of expression, with use of percussion tapping, pointing, and musical rhythms. Sternlicht also listed dance therapy (also reported by Rosen, 1954) with its focus on muscular expression in ballet as a method for reducing tension and providing for emotional expressions of conflicts.

Relationship therapy as reviewed by Neham (1951) has been reported as being successful with disturbed retardates. Sternlicht (1965) called attention to Freud's listing the lack of an ego ideal (usually furnished by the therapist) as being a main source of poor psychotherapeutic results. Yet such ego-supportive therapy was reviewed favorably by Neham (1951), and he views relationship therapy as having greater success with mental retardates. Stevenson and Knight (1962) inquired about social reinforcement and the influence of the worker's sex in the effectiveness of such an ego-supportive type of therapy. These investigators emphasized social casework as probably being more appropriate for the active rehabilitation of the emotionally disturbed mentally retarded—especially when practical, and immediate goals were the focus. Sternlicht and Wanderer (1963) reviewed experimental literature demonstrating the dissipation of tension and hostility by way of substitutive activity for earlier frustrations. Simple cathartic relief for acting out provocations were noted to be helpful for such tensions.

Play therapy for the mentally retarded was viewed by Cewen (1962) as being relatively neglected. Munday (1957) reported a controlled experiment benefiting twenty-five severely retarded children. Leland and Smith (1962) provided suggestions for unstructured materials in play therapy for the emotionally disturbed retarded. Axline (1947) and Maisner (1950) reported equally successful results. Abel (1953) reported a positive psychotherapeutic intervention with destructive early adolescent retardates by means of psychodrama.

Group therapy with groups screened for balance can be constructive with an especially alert therapist who can constantly structure and revise individual goals (Astrachan, 1955).

Hood (1957) wrote of a brain-injured child who was successfully treated by means of drugs, psychotherapy, and—above all—"the affectionate care of trained therapists and teachers." Clarke and Clarke (1958) reviewed comprehensive remedial approaches for the mentally retarded, one of which was psychotherapy. Remedial education, vocational and social rehabilitation, speech therapy, and the need for a serious reevaluation of the learning ability of the severely retarded were also discussed by these authors as closely allied issues.

Woodward, et al. (1960) reported on their efforts in a psychiatrically oriented preschool nursery. They point out (p. 169) that in their sample of twenty-six patients, between the ages of twenty-three months to four and one-half years, there was "a high percentage of considerable improvement, reaching the point where some tested within normal range."

Bills (1964) observed: "Evidence has shown that relationships among people have influenced their intelligence. Therefore, successful psychotherapy could produce more intelligent types of behavior which would thus enable the client to become more intelligent." Another successful application of group psychotherapy with mental retardates was also described by Goodman and Rothman (1961).

Group therapy and group play provide the challenge of keeping to limits and observing routine rules. Relative control of impulsiveness, a major problem for the organically impaired, can also be learned in these therapeutic group situations. Further, mutual acceptance of handicaps occurs, and social contacts are better understood, as well as the dictum, "We all have limitations."

Rogers' (1954) original argument that "self-reliance is intrinsic in psychotherapy and this trait is often absent in the mentally retarded," seems to miss the mark. No "normal" is self-reliant, except in a relative sense. The world of the institutionalized retardate is protected and limited, and so is his self-reliance. The confines of the institution limit him until he can be placed in the community. The arguments for self-reliance bring to light another aspect of mental retardation which is often overlooked when one thinks of psychotherapy for the retarded. In treating the maladjustments of preadolescents, many therapists—and this is also the established practice of most psychiatric outpatient clinics—will not see the child until the parents have been seen in treatment for at least a few months. The reasons for this are three-fold: (1) The cause of the maladjustment is frequently traceable to some psychological abuse by the parent or both parents; (2) The soil at home must be made conducive to the growth of the child; and (3) The preadolescent child is totally dependent upon his parents for his necessities. Sternlicht (1965) speculates whether one should not approach psychotherapy with an emotionally disturbed retardate in the same manner as preliminary treatment of the preadolescent children since, in fact, he is as dependent as a child on ward personnel, on his doctor, or extramurally on his parents. Perhaps the first step in the program of psychotherapy with a disturbed retardate should start by counseling those upon whom he is dependent for care.

In this review of the literature there were no reported studies of negative results with psychotherapy for the mentally retarded. The intent of quoting so many references is not to emphasize psychotherapy as a great therapeutic achievement, but to counteract the usual impression that people with "backward minds" cannot be responsive to "talking or relationship" therapy. Psychotherapy is beginning to be more widely used in the management of the mentally retarded. A further search of the literature published between 1964 and 1968 by the author (with the aid of the Milton S. Hershey Reference Library) noted six articles on psychotherapy for the retarded plus three on group counseling. This reflects a minimal, but increasing interest in mental retardation over the last few years. Tarjan (1966) chose the title "Cinderella and the Prince" in describing this paucity of professional involvement and publication dealing with mental retardation, representing the Cinderella who was still patiently waiting for her prince. A similar article had been written by Potter (1965) under the title "Mental Retardation, the Cinderella of Psychiatry."[1]

SYMPTOM VARIATION AND
MULTIPLE CAUSATION

The mentally retarded are most frequently recognized by their slow development. They do not learn satisfactorily in the slowest sections of the school grades and often not even in special classes. They cannot keep up with the youngsters who are dull, intellectually mediocre, but not mentally retarded. Stabilization training can be given these children to give them maximal vocational skills, without the need for group management in special classes and in residential training schools (Perry, 1965). However, variations in the capacity for treatment, training, and education need wider recognition by the medical profession (Heiser, 1954). Because of these variations of symptoms and allied treatment dimensions, the autistic group is so specialized that their treatment is omitted in this discussion, as is drug treatment. These topics have been reserved for consideration elsewhere in this book.

Some of the diagnostic confusion in the field of mental retardation is partly explained by a lack of understanding that these children represent a composite group with many types (and subtypes) of intellectual defects, organic defects, emotional handicaps, chromosomal abberrations, and perhaps other deficiencies. Accordingly, one encounters both specific etiologics and instances of complex or multiple causation. Separate diagnosis can be made for the asocial, autistic, schizoid children; the grossly organically brain injured; and some children with genetic-enzymatic deficits. Each type has its own special problems requiring individual plans for treatment. As in all of medicine, accurate comprehensive diagnosis is very important as a preliminary to treatment intervention.

There are, however, many children who do not respond adequately to examination and testing, and hence present unclear diagnostic pictures (Graham and Rutter, 1968). An assessment of what is going on in the minds and attitudes of a retarded group member helps indicate his or her correctional needs. The first step is to establish the presence of a truly retarded state, as differentiated from a pseudo-mentally retarded personality involving a specific handicap (Lott, 1958).

One of the most essential steps in the comprehensive diagnostic evaluation of the child (and his parents) amounts to an assessment of the various developmental phases of personality development, their evenness and possible regressions, and of other influences blocking normal forward moves in the psychological make-up of the growing child. At least two groups in child psychiatry have made outstanding progress in this area: Levy and his associates, in the 1930's; and Anna Freud and her group, since the 1940's.

Levy (1940) used an approach that involved matching the character structure of the youngster with the phases of personality maturity. This encompassed a thorough evaluation of normal infantile narcissistic self-interest; affection for others; sibling and other rivalries; various identifications with loved or admired older people; insecurities; reactive negativisms; aggression, hostility, and guilt balance; and of other factors such as tolerance to frustration and an adequate or inadequate self-concept. Development was often observed to be very uneven, and intellectual abilities varied widely. Many personality developmental phases were noted to have lagged or become tinged with blocking failure, guilt, or rebellion. Levy and his associates noted that various mental mechanisms could be operating and that, while many chronic conflicts were totally internalized, others were largely reactive. Thus it was important to know which mechanisms, and in what combination, were present in any given child. These conditions lent themselves to simple nontechnical descriptions, which are so important for individual, group, or conference communications. With this particular approach, and a careful history and clinical observation, the clinician could gauge the degree of general emotional maturity, the tolerance to frustration, the quality of the attention span, and the ability to escape inhibiting overwhelming hostility and guilt. Similarly, one could spot the rivalries and jealousies that would have to be expressed and worked through, especially when involving the love (oedipal) relationships in the family. These were all conceived as variations of natural strivings toward personality growth and maturity.

In the early 1930's the psychoanalytic concepts of anal, oral, primary oedipal, latency, and adolescent stages were found useful concepts among professionals, but only tended to confuse the layman. Starting in the 1940's and on through the early 1960's, the general validity of these personality-development stages was attested to by psychoanalytic studies of the child (largely with play therapy by Anna Freud and her coworkers, 1955). In the 1940's, this group became active in the study of children's and family problems. They apparently independently rediscovered and outlined detailed personality mechanisms, building on the body of orthodox Freudian psychoanalytic theory. Thus child psychiatry has been enriched, even though evolving more difficult psychoanalytic terminology that is most confusing to the lay public.

In an effort to clarify developmental stages, Anna Freud (1965) proposed a helpful method for general diagnostic clarity in her "Diagnostic Profile," which stresses the vicissitudes of regression and fixation points. Previously she had summarized the development of the sexual-drive sequence of libidinal phases as oral, anal, phallic (oedipal), latency period, preadolescence and adolescent genitality—with overlapping that corresponds roughly with specific chronological ages. Ego mastery, with the concommitant unfolding of the superego, was noted to operate concurrently for both emotional maturity and social object relationships which reflect general developmental expectations.

In her assessment of normal or pathological development, Anna Freud infers from the presenting symptomology the position of any given child in the developmental scale with regard to drive, ego, and superego development and infers also the child's possible amenability to teaching, which could induce progression from the pleasure principle to the reality principle. The presenting symptomatology implies asking whether the child has reached personality and developmental levels adequate for age; whether and in what respects he has gone beyond or remained behind; whether regressions or arrests have intervened; and if so, to what depth or what level? She noted that disharmony among developmental lines becomes a pathogenic agent *only* if imbalance in personality attributes is excessive. For example, there may be a long history of complaints from home and school, with disturbances with self and others, and the child does not accept community standards or fit into community life. The resulting distortion of behavior is alarming, particularly in the areas of acting out of sexual and aggressive trends, profusion of organized fantasy life, and clever rationalization of delinquent attitudes. Such children are usually termed "borderline" or "prepsychotic." Descriptively these children may be classified as, "lacking in concentration, has a short attention span, and is inhibited."

Either of these two approaches to assessing personality maturity can be used as a classification of conflicts as (a) external (child and environment), (b) at cross purposes, (c) internalized (identification with external powers and after introjections of their authority in the superego), and (d) as being truly internal conflict clashes between the id and the ego. Such a diagnostic aid not only helps to assess the presence or absence of mental retardation, but also helps to grade the severity of pathological developmental deviation that is present and points to what management may be most effective. These two approaches out-line conceptual yet practical schemes of assessing normal development. This is then applied to pathology in childhood, which is assessed not in terms of severity of the presenting symptoms, but rather by focusing on the factors interfering with normal forward moves in both person-ality and general development. A similar schemata, with comparative cultural-anthropological dimensions was presented by Erikson (1950).

Similarly, differential diagnosis can also eventuate in an assessment of the positive personality and developmental attributes that are pres-ent. Such stabilizing factors include dimensions such as high tolerance for frustration, good sublimation potential, effective ways of dealing with anxiety, and a strong urge toward completion of development. In this regards, sublimation capacity is valued as a safeguard to mental health. Similarly, children who have active ego resources such as in-tellectual understanding and logical reasoning, changes in external cir-cumstances, or aggressive counter attack (that is, by mastery instead of retreat) have a better outlook for normal personality growth.

One of the most common confusing differential diagnostic pictures in mental retardation are the children with "reading disability" (or "Gross reading retardation"), reported to afflict 10 to 15 per cent of the general population. They may falsely be labeled "behavior prob-lems" or "mentally retarded." Other confusions involve congenital or other forms of deafness and obscure metabolic, neurological or endo-crinological syndromes. Usually a careful history and comprehensive physical examination can eliminate these possibilities. Vague histories of early high "fevers" or convulsive episodes are indicative of possible encephalitis. Some children have signs suggesting congenital abnor-malities (Alvarez, 1965), while others have indications of autistic crippling isolation (Werry, 1968; Kysar, 1968). All these children may have difficulties in learning or display behavioral indices that may be organic, emotional, or both in origin (Kysar, 1968).

Many retarded youngsters who either realize their limitations or re-spond nonadaptively to their adverse environmental support systems tend to develop a variety of emotional inhibitions and complexes (Lott, 1949). It is often impossible to determine the level of intellec-tual capacity on the basis of formal tests, and it becomes necessary to combine medical, psychophysiological, and neuropsychiatric evalua-tions with psychological examinations. Special interest in the preven-tion, differential diagnosis, care, and rehabilitation for the mentally-retarded has developed (Chess, 1962; Doris and Solnit, 1963; Schachter, 1962). A trial of investigative psychotherapy treatment has been extensively advocated in the last few years (Thorne, 1948;

Tarjan, 1966; Potter, 1965; Heiser, 1954; Sternlicht, 1965; Albini and Dinitz, 1965; Perry, 1965) in view of the growing tendency to keep higher performers within the community while training schools are assuming a greater responsibility for caring for the more disturbed retarded (Albini and Dinitz, 1965; Perry, 1965).

ILLUSTRATIVE CASES

The training school that is now the Institute for Mental Studies at Vineland, New Jersey, was founded in 1888. The training school operates a cottage program, an educational system for special training, and vocational recreational departments. Staff with psychiatric, psychological, and social work skills operate in every phase of the treatment program. Pilot studies at the training school from 1962 to 1964 led to some tentative conclusions concerning the utility of psychotherapy in emotionally disturbed mentally retarded patients (Lott, 1966). The following thumbnail sketches of the first six patients to be given psychotherapy illustrates both the advantages and disadvantages of this form of treatment. All of these patients were emotionally disturbed, but socially adequate adolescent slow learners. During treatment, undesirable acting out or abreactive incidents occurred in four of the six (Albini and Dinitz, 1965). While describing their parents, homes, or schools these patients briefly regressed to earlier childhood fears or misbehavior such as running away, stealing, shoplifting, insolence, and combativeness. It should perhaps be pointed out here that this kind of acting out during treatment may interfere with concurrent social and educational training.

Case 1. This 17-year-old boy had been in residence for six years. He was moderately retarded and had achieved the fourth grade scholastically. For a period of five weeks during psychotherapy he repeatedly took money from two affectionately disposed mother-substitutes: his vocational supervisor and his teacher.

These thefts continued until he recalled stealing his parent's pills and being punished; his father had repeatedly referred to him as a thief for some time thereafter. After a lull of two months, having described an ostensibly pleasant visit home, he started running away and did so repeatedly for six weeks thereafter.

Supportive psychotherapy had reached some depth-precipitating resumption of previous behavior from an earlier developmental phase.

Therapy was finally accompanied by a spurt in maturity growth, but the impaired emotional control remained.

Case 2. This adolescent 16-year-old orphan girl, who had been one and one-half years in a detention home before admission, had frequent temper tantrums. She was mildly retarded and had achieved a fifth-grade education scholastically. After two months of psychotherapy, her overwhelming resentments came to the fore as she described her home. She attacked her housemother on the smallest provocation, and she often struck out at other residents of the cottage. With support of the staff and six further months of supportive psychotherapy (with focus on alternate methods of handling her hostility), she became neater and performed better both socially and in class.

Caution in therapy when impulses are strong and defenses are weak is wise, but the successful result with this patient shows, nevertheless, that therapists may at times be too cautious and thus not persist in helping the patient to help herself.

Case 3. This 18-year-old girl, who had a brilliant brother, had had an episode of encephalitis in early childhood, followed by a persistent convulsive disorder. The convulsions were inadequately controlled by drugs until a neurosurgical procedure at the age of 12 years removed calcified local areas of the cortex. Psychological tests describe her as educable (IQ 55), but this was not considered representative. She had only achieved fifth grade scholastically. At the training school this girl constantly expressed a feeling that she "should" be pleasant and nice to others. She quoted her mother, housemother, and various teachers who had lectured, and indeed begged her to be congenial. While the patient appeared to accept these standards, she was constantly demanding and touchy with both peers and adults. She repeatedly disrupted cottage life, often refusing to go to classes, and she was occasionally aggressive if her demands were abruptly denied. At home the patient had been unmanageable because when her demands were not met, her parents were usually bullied into "giving in." A well-developed dutiful attitude toward authority was in conflict with her persistent childish emotional wants.

During seven months of biweekly hour-long interviews, progress could be observed in three stages. Free association brought out with great intensity rebellion and anger associated with being told to do anything (e.g., "I want to decide myself, and not have to be told"). This idea of self-determination was encouraged, although the cottage staff felt at first that this would be "spoiling" the patient more than ever. She was frequently heard repeating to herself, "I've got to make up my own mind." The staff finally realized that no one, either normal or handicapped, could be happy living dutifully at someone else's dictation, especially at eighteen years of age.

For a time the patient's behavior became even more difficult. However, in interviews, she gradually overdeveloped the feeling that she was being mistreated until even she could see the absurdity of her statement, "I won't do it unless it's my way." Still later, she would say, "I'll try to get my own way," and then smile apologetically. Meanwhile, those in charge did their best not to tell her how she could feel and behave, so that reinforcement of the inner conflict between the girl's feeling of duty to authority and her infantile egocentric desires might be avoided. The "getting my own way" theme gradually came to be seen by the patient as incongruent—an expression of the everdetermined wants of her childhood and quite unsuitable to her chronological age of 18 years and the attendant roles and needs thereof.

Here we see that psychotherapy of the retarded, as with normals, may involve more than overcoming secondary failure or other emotional problems which prevent success in adaptation. Skills in manipulating vulnerable parents or parent substitutes and self-love "wants" may also obscure the picture. As they grow older, these patients tend to have more than the usual difficulty in achieving self-mastery. Finding their own identity involves emancipation from detested dependency and achievement of some measure of a balanced self-determination. In such situations, psychotherapy may not only be supportive, but may also lead to greatly increased insight and emotional reeducation (Scott, 1964).

Case 4. This patient, a pleasant-appearing girl aged 18 years, was adjusting well after four years of residence. Her progress in classroom learning was limited. Her intellectual level was high borderline and she had managed to achieve a sixth-grade education. She was referred for psychotherapy because her conflicts with staff members tended to preclude her placement into a community job opportunity. The patient had good work habits but moped over the "mother," a foster mother who had a large family. This woman was suffering from a fatal disease. The patient's own parents had speech and hearing defects and were unable to manage well. In the past, each succeeding visit home on vacation was more trying. Ambivalent feelings toward her own mother made her more devoted to the foster mother, whose death revived in her a sense of abandonment. A new housemother alternately showered the patient with attention or became restrictive and punitive.

In the initial psychotherapeutic interviews, the patient tended to hold the therapist responsible for the new housemother's actions. The girl's disturbed state was aggravated by the crisis caused by her foster mother's death. It was suspected that the patient's oedipal rivalries with her mothers were having a delayed emergence, and this required sympathetic and adroit handling. She was quite concerned with "Getting my father back to my mother." The grief reaction finally passed and the patient became absorbed in the details surrounding her return to the community and living with some of her foster family. Finally, she revealed, "I feel guilty to my mother for teasing and being mean sometimes. I finally figured I can make it up to her by being good to my father. I figure my mother's (foster mother) spirit will be near where he is and that she will know." The four months' treatment reached a constructive point when the patient, after indirectly expressing more resentment to the therapist (father?), stated, "You tell me things. Then I have to put them down in my own mind." She added, "I have the right to be angry when I feel that way, but of course, I have to learn to control it."

Emotional storms arising from developmental and neurotic problems interfered here with the prompt community placement of a well-trained educable retardee. Psychotherapy enabled this patient to face an adjustment in the community as well as to her own feelings toward her handicapped true parents.

Case 5. This 22-year-old young man was seen once weekly for five months. Psychological evaluation had revealed high borderline ability with irregular gaps of ability—evidently of organic origin. He was attaining fifth-grade achievement.

There were wide variations in his intellectual and social-adaptive ability. A history of convulsions associated with measles encephalitis at the age of 20 months, delayed speech until the age of 6 years. Both ailments were suggestive of brain damage secondary to postnatal infection. The patient had much difficulty in integrating knowledge previously acquired. This educational handicap had extended from the very first grade, after which he was "carried" for about three years in a parochial school, followed by five years in a special education class for the retarded in a public school. A psychiatric examination had uncovered "no special personality disorders" at the age of 15 years. The defensive character disorder already mentioned evidently appeared soon afterwards.

His social relationships were fair, but he could not keep up with the group in a special technical high school course. He seemed to have developed an effective defense of "talking big" in a rather circumstantial and fragmented manner. Clarity of speech and self-expression were impeded by many hesitations and evasions. These features comprised his greatest handicap in making a good first impression.

In interviews the patient gradually went over his previous experiences in more detail, and an air of hopefulness began to replace his original chronic feeling of depression. During this time he was assisting the gymnasium teacher with three different groups of moderately retarded children. He described his activities with the children in order to develop their abilities. He could anticipate their "childish" actions, thus helping them to achieve a feeling of success, while simultaneously being able to empathize with their feelings of inferiority and failure. He slowly began to be drawn out of himself without egotism or childish fantasy, and appeared to become more realistic in his ongoing interpersonal relationships. He slowly began to compete on more equal terms. The patient's speech also gradually became a little clearer and he expressed the opinion that he was more capable than he had thought. "I finally came here and let you know me for what I am, and now I know that I've done the very best I can."

This young man appreciated the respect with which he had been treated and the opportunity to achieve relative successes. The treatment relationship contained elements of acceptance and mutual sympathetic feelings. There were beginnings of insight into his major problem: a tendency to "talk big" as a defense against his longstanding feelings of failure.

Case 6. This 19-year-old boy had been at two previous residential schools early in life: a military academy for four months at the age of 12 years, and a therapeutically oriented coeducational boarding school from 14 to 16 years of age.

At the age of 5 years the patient had a chronic mastoiditis, which healed after an operation. Thereafter, a considerable degree of tone deafness was noted. This complaint improved markedly with speech therapy and tutoring from the ages of 6 to 12. More correct sounds could then be substituted for the distorted ones he had heard and was using for language, but clear speech was very retarded until adolescence. The patient's original mildly retarded–borderline intelligence estimations finally yielded a minimal IQ of 106 and an eleventh-grade level of academic achievement. Thus, in spite of his at least average intellectual ability, he had repeated many grades and was considered a "slow learner."

His speech and hearing problems became complicated by a persistent obstinancy; this prompted his referral for psychiatric care. During four months of weekly psychotherapy, while undergoing vocational training, the patient was stimulated to reevaluate himself in the light of his history and to become more confident and less sensitive to criticism. His problem was to try to overcome the underlying rebellious negativism he had developed over the years. The first advance occurred when the patient was encouraged to dissipate these accumulated frustrations. One day he said, "When you're ordered to do something, you don't do it, but if you don't have to, you do it anyway. . . . I had a lazy attitude, but now I can do more. I'm not weak minded." When the patient left the Training School it was with the object not only of making up sufficient vocational high school credits to assure a certificate, but also of trying to obtain employment.

Occasionally, extreme passive-resistive conflict of this kind occurs and, in conjunction with normal adolescent negativism, it may reach a point where it interferes with learning. As we have seen, some children find themselves labeled retarded and yet have normal intelligence (Thorne, 1948; Doris and Solnit, 1963). Psychotherapy can be instrumental in rectifying this situation, as well as in bringing out hidden defects. Scott (1964) reported two cases of "pseudo-retarded" persons who were greatly aided by psychoanalytically oriented psychotherapy from neurotic blocks to learning. Similarly, Sarwer-Foner (1963, p. 306), published an account of intensive psychoanalytic psychotherapy of a brain-damaged "pseudo-retarded" fraternal twin who was "transformed from a drooling, confused, and awkward individual into a fairly coordinated young man over the course of seven years (from the ages of 16 to 23) of therapy."

However, as much as psychotherapy may be advocated, it has been pointed out that there are contraindications. For example, there are instances in which there is a high anticipation that the retardate might repeat previously shown severely difficult behavior. In these instances, the alternate utilization of indirect treatment, special training, and educational methods may play a larger part than psychotherapy in smoothing the way to a share of happiness for them.

Psychotherapy is an aid in the general treatment and training of the mentally retarded (Watkins, 1960). The impression that it is a holistic remedy can be avoided by exercising caution in making even implied promises of benefit. Long experience has certainly borne out the need for coordinated contacts with the parents (Beck, 1962; Philips, 1962). Our work has convinced us that psychotherapy plays a definite role in the management of these exceptional children or adults.

ECLECTIC APPROACHES

A recent investigation of the application of psychotherapy to the mentally retarded was a survey (Woody and Billy, 1966) of the opinions and practices on counseling and psychotherapy for the retarded from the Fellows of the Section on Psychology of the American Association on Mental Deficiency. These investigators noted (82.3 per cent responses to the survey) a pattern that indicated a primary acceptance of an eclectic approach (encompassing any technique deemed by the therapist to be appropriate for the particular client) to counseling and psychotherapy. "It appears therefore, that the professional subjects active in the field felt that the mentally retarded of dull normal (IQ 75–90) and educable (IQ 50–75) intelligence can benefit most from individual counseling and psychotherapy, as opposed to group therapy or a combination of individual and group procedures." The areas of benefit were noted to include institutional adaptation, motivation for learning, peer-group association, familial relationships, control of unacceptable behavior, resolution of conflicts with authority figures, return to the home and community, and personality modification and improving employability. Woody and Billy also noted that the provision for counseling and psychotherapy for mentally retarded persons was occasionally incompatible with the general philosophy of the residential-therapeutic setting. They suggested that more effort was necessary to orient persons in the allied professions, such as school and clinic administrators, to values of counseling and psychotherapy for the retarded.

While considering types of psychiatric treatment for the retarded, it would be a gross oversight to omit those methods with the usual supportive and personal relationships that are inherent in most psychotherapies. We refer to individual remedial reading, operant conditioning, psychodrama, and group therapy (Scott, 1964; Akins, 1967).

Another major type of therapeutic effort, often used concurrently with psychotherapy, are the stabilizing, tranquilizing, and stimulating drugs. This particular treatment aspect and topic is fully reviewed in the chapters in this book by Freeman, Lipman, and Kurlander and Colodny.

INFLUENCE OF THE ANXIETY OR THE PERSONALITY OF THE THERAPIST

In the evaluation of treatment progress when using psychotherapeutic techniques and methods, Schlicht and William (1968, p. 442), noted: "It seems to be an incredibly difficult and an anxiety provoking task . . . ," and, "the therapist really can't shake the notion that improvement is a matter of opinion; the therapist and patient should jointly make this decision. However, the focus of the evaluation should be in the total picture that may accompany specific behavioral change." When a person tries to change through the use of will power, there are generally undesirable side effects of increased self-consciousness and loss of spontaneity. Schlicht and William conclude that the patient has a choice between changing the behavior itself, or changing his perception of the behavior—particularly as it affects his self-concept. For example, if a shy person can understand the reasons for this shyness, he might explore the situations and begin to discover what it is like to behave without shyness and the new rewards that result. Rogers and Dyamond (1954) emphasize increasing self-acceptance, whereas Wolpe (1958) belongs to the category of therapists who focus more on changing the patients behavior through reciprocal inhibition. Undoubtedly there are, or should be, many choices of therapeutic approach available, taking into consideration the personality and special sore spots and prejudices in the therapist. In some instances there may be a drift toward a psychotherapeutic model in which events and ideas may turn out to be reflections of the client's (and therapist's) unconscious needs rather than of stark reality (Whitehouse, 1967). Accordingly, the therapist must have an awareness of his own personal tendencies in these areas.

In the psychotherapy of the retarded, feeling tones are usually perceived nonverbally. The danger is that the retarded patient may be unconsciously grossly underrated or overrated by the therapist, and then the therapeutic process becomes seriously handicapped.

SUMMARY

The retarded are just as human as normal people. They have the same varied emotional quirks, inhibitions, frustrations, guilt feelings, conflicts, and erroneous self-concepts as do others. Their intellect, however, is feebler, and their abilities are less adequate in correlating experiences and initiating original ideas. The need of the retarded to sublimate probably is just as great, if not greater, than that of the average person, and the retarded are probably more in need of defense mechanisms to smooth or complicate their path through life. When we add his frequently less effective powers of inhibition and tolerance of frustration, it becomes clear why the retardate may often need conflict-resolving psychotherapeutic measures.

Many retarded persons (especially the more capable ones) who have primary or secondary emotional problems (or scattered deficits attributable to brain injury) would benefit from the more formal types of psychotherapy. Those suffering from aphasia, deafness, and speech problems may only be functioning operationally as retarded and may need remedial education and supportive psychotherapy. Some retardates are not formally testable and trials of investigative treatment may be required before their diagnosis, prognosis, and degrees of training or educability can be determined. Improvement resulting from such psychotherapy may represent the difference between a return to the community and permanent institutionalization in a residential facility for the retarded.

Psychotherapy, both superficial and deep, often aided by the inhibitory control of psychoactive drugs, may help greatly in these purposes if the usual limitations of such forms of therapy are kept in mind. The overall treatment and training of most retarded persons, especially of those who are organically handicapped, needs a properly paced activity program that strongly focuses on personality development. Psychotherapy may aid in overcoming primary or secondary personality problems if these complicate the picture. The concomitant attention to early specific diagnosis and individually planned education or training can prevent further complications and promote personal happiness for these chronically handicapped individuals.

N O T E

1. Very helpful in this brief review of the literature was a computer printout furnished by the National Clearing House for Mental Health Information of the National Institute of Mental Health.

R E F E R E N C E S

Abel, T. M. Resistances and difficulties in psychotherapy of mental retardates. *J. Clin. Psychol.*, 1953, *9*, 107–109.

Akins, Keith. A psychotherapeutic approach to reading retardation. *Canad. Psychiat. Assoc. J.*, 1967, *12*, 497–503.

Albini, J. L., & Dinitz, S. Psychotherapy with disturbed and defective children: An evaluation of changes in behavior and attitudes. *Amer. J. Ment. Defic.*, 1965, *69*, 560.

Alvarez, W. C. Hereditary diseases (20) that can injure the brain of a newborn infant. *Mod. Med.*, 1965, *33*, 86.

Anthony, E. J. Child Psychotherapy. Address to the Sixth International Psychotherapy Congress. London, 1964.

Astrachan, M. Group psychotherapy with mentally retarded female adolescents and adults. *Amer. J. Ment. Defic.*, 1955, *60*, 152–156.

Axline, V. M. *Play therapy: the inner dynamics of childhood.* Boston: Houghton Mifflin Co., 1947.

Beck, H. L. Casework with parents of mentally retarded children. *Amer. J. Orthopsychiat.*, 1962, *32*, 870–877.

Bills, Robert F. Persons or processes. *Kansas Stud. Ed.*, 1966, *4*, 66–78.

Blackhurst, A. E. Sociodrama for adolescent mentally retarded. *Training Sch. Bull.*, 1966, *63* (3), 136–142.

Blatt, A. Group therapy with parents of severely retarded children. *Group Psychother.*, 1957, *10*, 133–140.

Bradley, C., & Bowen, M. School performance of children receiving amphetamine (Benzedrine) sulphate. *Amer. J. Orthopsychiat.*, 1940, *10*, 782–788.

Burton, A. Psychotherapy with the mentally retarded. *Amer. J. Ment. Defic.,* 1954, *58* (3), 486–489.

Cewen, E. L. *Psychotherapy and play techniques with the exceptional child and youth.* Englewood Cliffs, N.J.: Prentice-Hall, 1962.

Chase, M. E. The practical application of psychotherapy in an institution for the mentally deficient. *Amer. J. Ment. Defic.,* 1953, *58,* 337–341.

Chess, S. Psychiatric treatment of the mentally retarded child with behavior problems. *Amer. J. Orthopsychiat.,* 1962, *32,* 863.

Clarke, A. M., & Clarke, A. D. B. (Eds.). *Mental deficiency: The changing outlook.* Glencoe, Ill.: Free Press, 1958.

Close, Henry T. Psychotherapy. *Voices,* 1966, *2,* 1.

Crowley, Francis J. Psychotherapy of the mentally retarded. A survey and projective consideration. *Training Sch. Bull.,* 1965, *62,* 5–11.

Denton, L. R. Psychotherapy with mentally retarded children. *Bull. Maritime Psychol. Ass.,* 1959, *8,* 20–27.

Depalina, N. Group psychotherapy with high grade imbeciles and low grade morons. *Del. State Med. J.,* 1956, *28* (8), 200–203.

Doris, J., & Solnit, A. J. Treatment of children with brain damage and associated school problems. *J. Amer. Acad. Child Psychiat.,* 1963, *2,* 618–635.

Eisenberg, L. The management of the hyperkinetic child. *Devel. Med. Child Neurol.,* 1966, *8,* 593–598.

Erikson, E. *Childhood and society.* New York: Norton & Co., 1950.

Freeman, M. Drawing as a psychotherapeutic intermedium. *Amer. J. Ment. Defic.,* 1936, *41,* 182–187.

Friedman, E. Individual therapy with defective delinquents. *Amer. J. Psychiat.,* 1965, *121,* 1014–1020.

Freud, A. *Psychoanalytic treatment of children.* New York: International Universities Press, 1955.

————. *Normality and pathology in childhood-assessments of development.* New York: International Universities Press, 1965.

Goldberg, B. Children's psychiatric residential institute, London. *Canad. Psychiat. Assoc. J.,* 1962, *7,* 140–146.

Goldstein, E. A., & Eisenberg, L. Review of psychiatric progress. *Amer. J. Psychiat.,* 1965, *121,* 655–659.

Goodman, L., & Rothman, R. The development of a group counseling program in a clinic for retarded children. *Amer. J. Ment. Defic.,* 1961, *65,* 780–782.

Gorlo, L., Butler, A., Einig, K. G., & Smith, J. A. An appraisal of self attitudes and behavior following group psychotherapy with retarded young adults. *Amer. J. Ment. Defic.,* 1963, *67,* 893–898.

Graham, R., & Rutter, M. Reliability and validity of psychiatric assessment of the child. *Brit. J. Psychiat.,* 1968, *114,* 563–579.

Haworth, M. R. (Ed.). *Child psychotherapy.* New York: Basic Books, Inc., 1964.

Heimlich, E. P. Music as therapy with emotionally disturbed children. *Child Welf.,* 1960, *39,* 6–10.

Heiser, K. F. Psychotherapy in a residential school for mentally retarded children. *Training Sch. Bull.,* 1954, *50,* 211–218.

Hoffman, N. E. Therapeutic value of music and its treatment implications. *Forum,* 1966, *3* (1), 39–60.

Hood, O. E. *Your child or mine: The brain injured child and his hope.* New York: Harper Bros., 1957.

Joseph, H., & Heimlich, E. Therapeutic use of music with treatment resistant children. *Amer. J. Ment. Defic.,* 1959, *64*(1), 41–49.

Kysar, J. E. Two camps in child psychiatry: A report from a psychiatrist father of an autistic and retarded child. *Amer. J. Psychiat.,* 1968, *125* (1), 103–109.

Lavalli, A., & Levine, M. Social and guidance needs of mentally handicapped adolescents as revealed through sociodrama. *Amer. J. Ment. Defic.,* 1954, *58*(4), 544–552.

Leland, H., & Smith, D. Unstructured material in play therapy for emotionally disturbed, brain damaged, and mentally retarded children. *Amer. J. Ment. Defic.,* 1962, *66,* 621–624.

Levy, D. Seminar on child psychiatry. New York: Psychoanalytic Institute, 1940.

Lott, G. Mental defectives can become community assets. *Hygeia*, 1949, *7*, 548–549.

———. Story of human emotions. *Formal learning*. New York: Philosophical Library, 1958, p. 225.

———. Psychotherapy of the mentally retarded: Values and cautions. *J.A.M.A.*, 1966, *196*, 229–232.

McDermott, W. H. Art therapy for the severely handicapped. *Amer. J. Ment. Defic.*, 1954, *59*, 231–235.

Maisner, E. A. Contributions of play therapy techniques to total rehabilitative design in an institution for high grade mentally deficient and borderline children. *Amer. J. Ment. Defic.*, 1950, *55*, 235–250.

Munday, L. Therapy with physically and mentally handicapped children in a mental deficiency hospital. *J. Clin. Psychol.*, 1957, *13*, 3–9.

Murphy, M. M. Rhythmical responses of low grade and middle mental defectives to music therapy. *J. Clin. Psychol.*, 1957, *13*, 361–364.

Neham, S. Psychotherapy in relation to mental deficiency. *Amer. J. Ment. Defic.*, 1951, *55*, 557–572.

Ogle, W. A. Psychotherapeutic treatment in mental deficiency: Report of a case. *Canad. Psychiat. Assoc. J.*, 1963, *8*, 307–315.

Perry, S. E. Middle class and mental retardation in America. *Psychiatry*, 1965, *28*, 107–118.

Philips, I. The application of psychiatric clinic services for the retarded child and his family. *J. Acad. Child Psychiat.*, 1962, *1*, 297–313.

Potter, H. W. Mental retardation, the cinderella of psychiatry. *Psychiat. Quart.*, 1965, *39*, 537–549.

Rogers, C. R. *Client-oriented therapy*. Boston: Houghton Mifflin Co., 1951.

Rogers, C. R., & Dyamond, R. F. *Psychotherapy and personality change*. Chicago: University of Chicago Press, 1954.

Rosen, E. Dance as therapy for mentally ill. *Teachers Coll. Rec.*, 1954, *55*, 215–222.

Ruesch, J., & Kees, W. *Nonverbal communication*. Los Angeles: University of California Press, 1956.

Sarwer-Foner, G. J. Intensive psychoanalytic psychotherapy of a brain damaged pseudo-mental defective fraternal twin. *Canad. Psychiat. Assoc. J.*, 1963, *8*, 296–307.

Schacter, F. F., Meyer, L. R., & Loomis, E. A. et al. Childhood schizophrenia and mental retardation: Differential diagnosis after one year of psychotherapy. *Amer. J. Orthopsychiat.*, 1962, *32*, 584–595.

Schlicht, J., & William, J. The anxieties of the psychotherapist. *Ment. Hyg.*, 1968, *52* (3), 439–444.

Scott, W. C. M. Psychotherapy of mental defectives. *Canad. Psychiat. Assoc. J.*, 1964, *8*, 293–295.

Sternlicht, M. Establishing an initial relationship in group psychotherapy with delinquent male retarded adolescents. *Amer. J. Ment. Defic.*, 1964, *69*, 39–41.

———. Psychotherapy techniques useful with mentally retarded: A review and critique. *Psychiat. Quart.*, 1965, *39*, 84–90.

———. Psychotherapeutic procedure with the retarded. In E. Nurmad (Ed.), *International review of research in mental retardation*, Vol. 10, No. 2. New York: Academic Press, 1966, 279–354.

Sternlicht, M., & Wanderer, Z. W. Group psychotherapy with mental defectives. *Amer. J. Psychother.*, 1963, *67*, 214–220.

Stevenson, H. W., & Knight, R. M. Social reinforcement with normal and retarded children as a function of pre-training sex. *Amer. J. Ment. Defic.*, 1962, *66*, 866–871.

Stubblebine, J. Group psychotherapy with epileptic mentally deficient adults. *Amer. J. Ment. Defic.*, 1957, *61*, 725–730.

Tarachow, S. Interpretation and reality in psychotherapy. *Internat. J. Psychoanal.*, 1962, *43*, 377–387.

Tarjan, G. Cinderella and the prince: Mental retardation and community psychiatry. *Amer. J. Psychiat.*, 1966, *122*, 1057–1059.

Tarvis, E. Some notes on group psychotherapy for severe mental defectives:

Reasons for attempt and evaluating patients responses. *Del. State Med. J.,* 1961, *33* (10), 301–307.

Thorne, D. C., & Dolan, K. M. The role of counseling in a placement program for mentally retarded families. *J. Clin. Psychol. Monogr. Suppl.,* 1953, *9,* 1–8.

Thorne, F. C. Psychotherapy in relation to mental deficiency. *Amer. J. Ment. Defic.,* 1941, *45,* 135–141.

———. Counseling and psychotherapy with mental defectives. *Amer. J. Ment. Defic.,* 1948, *52,* 263–271.

Watkins, J. G. *General psychotherapy: Outline and studies guide.* Springfield, Ill.: Charles C Thomas, 1960, p. 196.

Weber, H. Borderline defective delinquent. *British J. Delinq.,* 1953, *3,* 173–184.

Werry, J. S. Empirical analysis of the minimal brain dysfunction syndrome. *Arch. Gen. Psychiat.,* 1968, *19* (1), 9–16.

Whitehouse, F. A. Concept of therapy: A review of some essentials (individual therapy programs multifaceted). *Rehabil. Lit.,* 1967, *28* (8), 238–247.

Wilcox, G. T., & Guthrie, G. M. Changes in adjustments of institutionalized female defectives: Following group psychotherapy. *J. Clin. Psychol.,* 1957, *13,* 9–13.

Wolpe, J. *Psychotherapy by reciprocal inhibition.* Palo Alto, Calif.: Stanford University Press, 1958.

Woodward, K. F., Brown, D., & Bird, D. Psychiatric study of mentally retarded preschool children. *Arch. Gen. Psychiat.,* 1960, *2,* 156–170.

Woodward, K., Jaffe, N., & Brown, D. Psychiatric program for very young retarded children. *Amer. J. Dis. Childhood,* 1964, *108* (3), 221–229.

Woody, R. H., & Billy, J. H. Counseling and psychotherapy for the mentally retarded: Survey of opinions and practices. *Ment. Retard.,* 1966, *4,* 120–123.

: 11 :

Use of Behavior Therapy with

the Mentally Retarded

William I. Gardner

INTRODUCTION

SOME of the most exciting work in the application of behavior principles to treatment of developmental and behavior problems has been that involving the mentally retarded. Recent results of the application of the behavior modification techniques described in the clinical and research literature provide illustration of behavior change of a range, degree, and rate which most psychiatric, psychological, and educational personnel had not thought possible owing to the limitations imposed by the term "mental retardation." The techniques and related behavior principles discussed in this chapter have had, and will continue to have, a great impact on the general area of psychological aspects of mental retardation. In fact, it is felt by some that this impact will be as great as that of any other single contribution since the introduction of mental testing in the early decades of this century. It has been demonstrated that at least a significant degree of the behavioral limitations of the retarded may well reside in an inappropriate or limited learning environment, rather than being an unalterable manifestation of the individual's retardation. Severely and profoundly involved retardates who for years were beyond help or hope have, as a result of treatment programs using the systematic application of behavior-modification procedures, developed language, motor, perceptual, cognitive, affective and social skills that have rendered them more independent and more able to experience a meaningful personal and social existence. Additionally, other less disabled retardates exhibiting an array of maladaptive behavior patterns have responded favorably to behavior modification efforts. Experiences of behavior therapists who work with mentally retarded children between preschool and eighteen years of age will be described in this chapter. While a comprehensive review of reported studies will not be attempted, examples will be provided of the range of problems treated, the methods used, and the results obtained.

A brief presentation of the assumptions and behavior principles that lend direction to the treatment procedures followed in dealing with a variety of problem behaviors will provide a perspective for the discussion to follow. Reference should be made to Eysenck (1960), Kalish (1965), Ullman and Krasner (1965), and Wolpe (1958) for more extensive descriptions of the nature of behavior therapy, as well as to recent works by Bijou and Sloane (1966), Bucher and Lovaas (1968), Gelfand and Hartmann (1968), and Leff (1968) for comprehensive reviews of the use of behavior therapy with a range of childhood disorders. Although the following discussion will focus on those problems which are typically viewed as clinical (for example, treatment of a self-destructive child [Tate and Baroff, 1966], or treatment of an emotionally disturbed child with an inappropriate psychophysiological reaction [Wolf et al., 1965]), illustrations of the treatment of developmental and educational deficits (for example, teaching eating skills to the profoundly retarded [Gorton and Hollis, 1965], or remediation of academic difficulties [Birnbrauer et al., 1965]) are included to demonstrate the basic and essential similarity among the behavior-changing procedures employed regardless of the nature of the problem treated.

BASIC CONCEPTS

Behavior modification [1] is a term that applies to a number of different treatment techniques which have the goal of altering human behavior in a beneficial manner. These techniques are based on concepts of various learning theories and on behavior principles and experimental data concerning stimulus-response relationships. In short, as Ullman and Krasner (1965, p. 1) have suggested, "The basis of behavior modification is a body of experimental work dealing with the relationship between changes in the environment and changes in the subjects' responses." The learning concepts that provide the basis for most of the behavior-modification work with the mentally retarded are those derived from the operant conditioning model of Skinner. In addition, concepts from other reinforcement learning theories and from the work by Pavlov and Hull on classic conditioning have provided direction to some of the techniques used.

In the behavior-modification model, behaviors typically described as inadequate, inappropriate, neurotic, maladaptive, or pathological are viewed simply as learned behaviors. As Ullman and Krasner (1965, p. 20) have suggested, "the development and maintenance of a maladaptive behavior is not different from the development and maintenance of any other behavior. There is not discontinuity between desirable and undesirable modes of adjustment or between 'healthy' and 'sick' behavior." The behavior therapist looks to learning concepts to help him answer the questions "How can inappropriate behaviors be weakened or eliminated?" and "How can new forms of behavior be developed?"

The focus of treatment is the overt behavior that is creating difficulty or concern for those responsible for the child. Explanation of psychological problems is not in terms of internal events. Rather, stated simply, the causes of the behavior are viewed as those environmental events which are effective in influencing the occurrence or nonoccurrence of the behavior. The problem behavior is not viewed as being symptomatic of some more basic or central underlying difficulty, and as problem behaviors are modified suitably, treatment is terminated. This approach is in sharp contrast to the general psychodynamic model that views the treatment goal as that of modifying the basic internal pathology that is assumed to be causing the symptomatic problem behavior. In reference to this point, Skinner (1953, p. 373) observed: "Where, in the Freudian scheme, behavior is merely the symptom of a neurosis, in the present formulation it is the direct object of inquiry." Similarly, Eysenck (1960, p. 3) has stated: "Learning theory does not postulate any such unconscious causes, but regards neurotic symptoms as simple learned habits; there is no neurosis underlying the symptom, but merely the symptom itself. Get rid of the symptom and you have eliminated the neurosis."

Such a view places the major cause of inadequate behavior in the environment rather than on factors within the child, as for example, his "emotional disturbance," his "low motivation," or his "inadequate personality." It also removes from consideration such devastating explanations of behavior as "he can behave appropriately when he *wants* to," or "he can dress himself when he's in the *mood* to do so." The implicit assumption is that the child behaves as he wishes or wants to, and that it is the child's fault that more appropriate behavior does not occur. Such pseudoexplanations remove the responsibility for the undesirable or inconsistent behavior from the environment and place it within the child. Meyerson et al. (1967, p. 215) have suggested that this kind of approach "not only places an overwhelming, needless, and often unfulfillable responsibility on the client to be the architect of his own rehabilitation, but also neglects two other basic variables that can be manipulated for the client's benefit: his environment and, as a result of the manipulation of his environment, his behavior."

Although diagnostic activity in the traditional sense is not pursued in developing a treatment program, the therapist does engage in what might be termed a behavioral analysis (Kanfer and Saslow, 1965). The behavior therapist initially seeks a specification of the problem behavior. What behavioral deficits or excesses are creating difficulty or concern in what environmental situations? Emphasis is on rendering this description as precise and quantitative as possible. To illustrate this point: It is not sufficient to indicate that the child is schizophrenic or emotionally disturbed. For example, Lovaas (1967, p. 110), in his behavior-therapy approach to childhood schizophrenia raises the possibility that schizophrenia does not constitute a psychological variable in a functional sense and suggests that "instead of addressing treatment to the hypothetical condition, 'schizophrenia,' one could concentrate treatment on some of the behavioral deviations covered by that term. . . . This kind of approach leads to the attempted modification of functionally identifiable behaviors in such areas as verbal, intellectual, and interpersonal behaviors." It is even necessary to translate more circumscribed behavior descriptions such as "aggressiveness," "cries easily," "hyperactivity," and "socially isolated" into terms of specific behavioral reactions and to describe the frequency of occurrence under specific environmental conditions.

Only after the problem behaviors have been pinpointed is the behavior therapist in a suitable position to develop treatment goals and to decide upon the treatment techniques to be used. In delineating treatment goals, emphasis is on precise quantitative specification whenever possible. Goals such as "motivate him more," "decrease his disturbance," "strengthen his ego," and "increase his sociability" are much too general. These are translated into specific frequency behaviors in specific situations. "Motivate him more" becomes, for example, "increase the frequency of his initiating classroom work behavior without teacher intervention." In summary, the behavior therapist identifies those behaviors which should be developed, strengthened, eliminated, or altered. The treatment goals are then stated in behavioral terms: What environmental events must be changed (added, eliminated, or rearranged) to strengthen present behaviors or to develop new behaviors, to alter the factors that control present behaviors, to insure the continuation of present behaviors under new conditions, or to decrease or eliminate the occurrence of behaviors under certain circumstances or under all conditions?

In the behavioral analysis, the therapist seeks to identify those environmental events which have the effects of increasing or decreasing the occurrence of behavior when presented contingent upon that behavior. These reinforcing events will vary considerably from child to child and even—from time to time—for any given child. Although social reinforcement in the form of praise, approval, smiles, or attention is effective with some, studies have found nonsocial reinforcers such as food, toys, trinkets, or access to preferred activities to be more effective with other retarded children (for example, Bijou et al., 1966; Birnbrauer and Lawler, 1964). In addition, the behavioral effects of aversive or punishment consequences vary considerably when used with the retarded, as Striefel's work (1967) with a time-out from positive reinforcement procedure has demonstrated. Bijou (1966) has suggested that many of the behavioral limitations present in the retarded are due to the inconsistent, inappropriate, or infrequent nature of the reinforcements provided by the environment. That is, many retardates are unable to exhibit certain behaviors because these behaviors have not been followed by appropriate, frequent, and consistent consequences. Such a supposition emphasizes the necessity for identifying a range of stimulus events that are potential reinforcers for the retardate being treated by behavior therapy. This task can pose some real problems as suggested by Watson's discussion (1967) of the considerable variability among the more severely retarded in the effectiveness of reinforcing events.

The diagnostic goal stated in behavioral terms may be viewed as the specification of the conditions under which certain behaviors can be obtained. In some cases, an unsuccessful behavior-modification program may have diagnostic implications in that it will reveal the conditions under which a behavior cannot be obtained. Further, the deficit responsible for this may become evident. As there are no projective, psychometric, or interview procedures available which have suitable powers for reliably predicting these conditions, it frequently becomes necessary to "try out" the initial stages of a program of behavior change prior to reaching a decision concerning the acceptability or rejection of a client for treatment or for reaching other major decisions concerning the conditions needed for suitable behavior change.

Kerr et al. (1965, p. 369) provide an example of the use of a limited behavior-therapy program to demonstrate that a severely retarded girl could profit from further rehabilitation efforts and to establish the conditions under which the desired behaviors could develop. In a matter of a few hours of contact with a three-year-old, mute, cerebral palsied, epileptic, emotionally disturbed, severely retarded child, the therapists followed a program based on the principles of reinforcement and "altered her mute, antisocial behavior in the direction of spontaneous vocalizations under the control of adult vocal stimuli and a first approximation to true echoic behavior."

In a related study (Baer et al., 1967), three severely retarded children ranging in age from nine to twelve years who lacked both initiative and verbal behaviors responded favorably to a behavior-modification program. These children developed both reinforced and generalized initiative behaviors. The results provided important information to the treatment personnel, as the conditions under which learning could take place were empirically identified.

In some cases that manifest striking deviations in behavior development, the range of reinforcing events may be too limited to expect suitable progress in the development of new behaviors. One basic abnormality may be viewed as a distortion in stimulus functions. That is, certain social events such as a smile, adult attention, closeness, approval, affection, and the like may have no reinforcing effect. In such cases, the range of reinforcing events available in the natural or even in a carefully designed treatment environment may be quite limited. The initial treatment program may be designed to alter stimulus functions so that previously neutral stimuli acquire reinforcing properties.

These new reinforcing events become quite valuable in the subsequent program of remediation of the deficit behaviors. Lovaas (1967), in his work with schizophrenic children, not only has demonstrated the value of altering stimulus functions, but also has emphasized the differences in treatment operations between this procedure and those concerned with the remediation of deficit behaviors, for example, speech or social interaction. In other cases, it may be necessary to attach aversive components to certain stimuli so as to provide for environmental control of certain inappropriate behaviors. Watson (1967) illustrates this strategy in his report of a procedure used in attaching a behavior control function to certain verbal stimuli.

As the focus is on modifying behavior that will be more suitable in the natural environments of the child, treatment frequently is conducted in the setting in which the problem occurs. Patterson et al. (1965), for example, chose the classroom as the location for treatment of hyperactivity in a mentally retarded boy with an impaired central nervous system to insure greater generalization of treatment effects. Additionally, the natural environment is chosen as the place of treatment because of the availability of both caretaker personnel and a wide range of possible reinforcing conditions. Wiesen and Watson (1967) used peers to reinforce social interaction in an isolated mentally retarded boy. Teacher personnel implemented the plan for treatment of a number of behavioral and psychophysiological reactions of a mentally retarded girl (Wolf et al., 1965).

In using a general functional analysis of behavior methodology, the behavior-therapy approach offers the therapist a specific means of evaluating the effectiveness of the treatment procedures (Baer et al., 1968; Gelfand & Hartmann, 1968). In the initial behavioral analysis when the behavior problem is being specified, the therapist obtains a reliable record of the frequency of occurrence of the behavior. These data serve as the base line against which behavior changes that may accompany treatment can be evaluated. If no effect is noted within a reasonable period, the treatment variables can be changed and further systematic observations can be obtained under a new treatment regimen. The therapist does not have to wait for an extended period before deciding if treatment has its effect, as is the case in many other therapeutic practices.

In summary, the focus of behavior modification is on the relationship between the child's behavior and environmental consequences. The goal is to change aspects of the current life situation which control the occurrence of inappropriate behaviors or which impede the development and maintenance of more appropriate ways of responding. The emphasis is not on the child's deficiencies, but rather on the development of behaviors that are more suitable to the behavioral requirement of the environment in which the child resides. In practice the treatment techniques seek to modify the relationship between the behavior and those stimulus events which control the behavior— either those discriminative stimuli which mark the time or place in which the behavior will result in suitable reinforcers, or those reinforcing stimulus events which maintain or increase the rate of occurrence of the behavior. By altering the stimulus events, the behavior is altered in its rate or frequency of occurrence, or in the conditions necessary for its occurrence or continuation. In short, as Ullman and Krasner (1965, p. 29) put it, "all behavior modification boils down to procedures utilizing systematic environmental contingencies to alter the subject's response to stimuli."

APPLICATION TO THE RETARDED

As suggested initially, the use of various behavior modification procedures has resulted in some most significant changes in the behavioral characteristics of individuals functioning within the retarded range. Evaluation of these reports emphasizes the particular applicability of these treatment procedures to the retarded, as no particular characteristics such as speech or a certain level of cognitive development are necessary for treatment effects. Every retardate, even the most profoundly involved, is a possible client for behavior therapy, as the Fuller (1949) and the Rice and McDaniel (1966) studies with "vegetative" patients have demonstrated. Additionally, there is ample illustration in published reports, as suggested previously, that various behavior-modification procedures can be applied by caretaker personnel in the setting in which the retardate resides. This is of especial significance in view of the limited number of trained psychiatric personnel who are presently available to provide service to the mentally retarded.

The following sections will describe the application of behavior-modification procedures to developmental, behavioral, and educational problems presented by children and adolescents who range in level of functioning from mild to profound mental retardation. Treatment goals were directed toward both reduction or elimination of inappropriate behavior patterns and development or strengthening of more appropriate ways of behaving. Although there are no essential differences in the procedures and related learning concepts used, the cases reported are described under the three major headings of clinical, developmental, and educational problems. As a brief chapter presentation does not permit a comprehensive exposition of the behavior therapy techniques available to those working with the mentally retarded, an effort is made to include examples of a wide range of applications. This sampling should offset the seemingly isolated and circumscribed focus of some of the individual studies described. It should also be noted that the application of behavior therapy to a range of problems presented by the retarded is of recent origin. Many of the studies reported represent pioneer efforts which merely suggest possible procedures and related results.

Clinical Problems

A significant emphasis in most of the clinical studies and reports which describe behavior-therapy techniques with the retarded has been that of eliminating or reducing in frequency or severity specific inappropriate behavior patterns. In addition, most of this work has involved the more severely retarded. The studies described below illustrate three general techniques for the elimination of undesirable behavior. First is that of extinction, which involves the removal of those contingent stimulus events which are reinforcing the behavior. The report of Wolf et al. (1965) illustrates the successful use of this procedure. Owing to the practical difficulties involved in using an extinction procedure in numerous instances, various techniques having punishment or aversive components have been used, especially in work with the more chronic behavior problems presented by the severely involved. Finally, the therapist can choose to develop behavior patterns that are incompatible to or which compete with and replace the inappropriate behavior patterns. Patterson et al. (1965), for example, illustrate this general technique in reinforcing a variety of attending responses that successfully competed with hyperactivity. In other instances, the aversive components associated with certain environmental events can be extinguished by a combination of repeated graded presentations of the conditioned aversive stimuli and the concurrent reinforcement of more appropriate behaviors in the presence of the feared event. Blackwood (1962) illustrates this approach in his work with a retarded child who exhibited a fear of walking down steps. All studies using extinction and punishment procedures to eliminate excessively occurring inappropriate behavior patterns reported the concurrent reinforcement of appropriate ways of behaving. It is frequently reported that these new ways of responding add considerably to the reduction and eventual elimination of the punished behaviors.

Extinction Procedures

Wolf et al. (1965) provide one of the first examples of the successful use of behavior modification in work with a clinical problem presented by a mentally retarded child. This nine-year-old girl, diagnosed as suffering from mental retardation, cerebral palsy, aphasia, hyperirritability, and brain damage, resided in an institution for the mentally retarded and was enrolled in a school program which met three hours daily. After a few weeks in class, the child began to vomit occasionally. This rate increased until within three months vomiting became practically a daily class occurrence. Drug therapy was of no value in reducing this rate. Noting that the child frequently was returned to her dormitory following a vomiting episode, the therapists hypothesized that such consequences were reinforcing and thus maintaining the vomiting behavior. The major modification procedure followed in eliminating this behavior was based on the learning principle of extinction. As noted earlier, this principle suggests that behavior will decrease in strength upon the removal of those stimulus consequences which maintain it. The treatment consisted of keeping the child in the classroom throughout the class period and of attempting to shape desirable behaviors by providing tangible and social reinforcers contingent upon the occurrence of such appropriate responses. Under such a program, vomiting behavior declined to a zero level over a period of thirty class days. Other behaviors that occurred with virtually every vomiting episode—screaming, clothes tearing, and destruction of property—also declined to a zero level along with the vomiting. It was noted that productive classroom behavior and responsiveness to the teacher's requests improved markedly.

In order to determine if the elimination of the vomiting and related tantrum behaviors was due to the extinction operations imposed, the original consequences were reinstated. After the occurrence of the vomiting behavior in the classroom for the first time in a number of weeks, the child was immediately returned to the dormitory. Vomiting gradually increased until it occurred in over one-third of the class sessions over a three-month period. The extinction procedure was reinstated with the result that the vomiting episodes were again virtually eliminated. This reversal or replication procedure demonstrated that the vomiting behavior was operant in nature and could be controlled in its occurrence by providing or removing the reinforcing consequences.

This treatment report also provides illustration of other characteristics of behavior-therapy programs. For example, the behavior was not assumed to be a symptom of some internal psychological disturbance. Further, it was not deemed necessary to delve into the history of this behavior to identify factors associated with its development, even though the child had been vomiting in the dormitory since being admitted to the institution. This illustrates the position that the reinforcement that led to the behavior's initial development need not be the same as the current reinforcement. Nor is it assumed that the reinforcement that maintains maladaptive behavior in one setting is necessarily the same reinforcement that maintains it in another. Additionally, behaviors other than those chosen as the focus of treatment may show change in a desirable manner. The temper tantrums in this case abated, although this behavior was not given specific and systematic attention. Numerous other studies in the literature on behavior modification report the same results. Finally, a behavior-therapy program not only seeks to eliminate maladaptive behavior, in this case vomiting episodes in the classroom, but attempts to provide more suitable behavior as a replacement. Had vomiting behavior been eliminated without replacing it with "increased productive classroom behavior," the treatment program would have been only partially fulfilled.

Although valuable for the elimination of behavior in numerous cases, serious limitations in the application of an extinction procedure are encountered when working with the retarded. As has been suggested by Hamilton et al. (1967), analyzing and controlling the reinforcing contingencies—especially of complex behavior and behavior of long standing—may be a most difficult undertaking. First, it is difficult to identify the reinforcing events and to control them once identified. Even with the severely retarded it must be concluded that for a large class of behaviors the complete elimination of reinforcement is impossible. Secondly, as noted by Lovaas et al. (1965), in the early phase of extinction there may be an actual increase in the rate of behavior prior to a decremental effect. This was noted in study by Wolf et al. (1965) as the number of vomiting episodes reached a high of twenty-one in one day during initial extinction prior to its elimination and a high of twenty-nine during the second extinction period. This characteristic renders this procedure highly undesirable in those instances in which the behavior is either highly disruptive or of potential danger to the client or others. In such cases, there is need for a treatment procedure that would result in a relatively immediate reduction in the frequency or intensity of the problem behavior. Furthermore, as most behaviors have developed under and are maintained by a partial reinforcement schedule, a strategy of behavior elimination based solely on extinction operations promises to be a slow undertaking. This was noted by Birnbrauer et al. (1965, p. 360) in attemping to eliminate behavior problems of groups of retarded boys in a classroom setting by an extinction procedure, that is, by ignoring instances of inappropriate behavior. After some experience, a punishment procedure was added "since extinction is often difficult to implement effectively in a classroom . . ."

Bucher and Lovaas (1968) used an extinction procedure with a seven-year-old severely retarded boy who, because of a high-rate self-injurious behaviors, was kept in complete restraints twenty-four hours a day. After eight days of being released from restraints for one and one-half hours daily, the behavior was gradually reduced to near extinction level by removal of a presumed source of reinforcement. However, during this extinction process the child hit himself in excess of 10,000 times. In another case of severe self-destructive behavior in a sixteen-year-old retarded girl with psychotic features, Bucher and Lovaas (1968, p. 91) reported that "because of the extreme severity of her self-injurious behavior . . . it is impossible to place such a child on extinction. Marilyn could have inflicted serious self-injury or even killed herself during an extinction run."

Watson's observation (1967, p. 13) is also quite pertinent:

When a child is engaged in acts that are physically damaging, such as breaking windows with his head, arms, or hands, beating his head against the wall, stabbing himself or others with a safety pin, or throwing another child down with great force, the cottage staff cannot wait for the effects of extinction to gradually end or eliminate the behavior. Someone might be injured severely before the effects of extinction could eliminate the behavior in question.

It is evident from these observations that considerable difficulty is frequently encountered in the use of an extinction procedure in a field situation, especially with cases of extreme behavior deviation. In these instances, extinction at times is a highly inefficient and thus impractical procedure. Obviously more humane behavior-treatment procedures must be applied.

Certain characteristics of the more severely involved mentally retarded further emphasize the need for using every useful treatment approach that is available. Limited language and general cognitive skills, a rather primitive social motivation system, and a restricted range of stimulus events that are controlling or reinforcing—all of these aspects render extinction and behavior-shaping treatment attempts with this group quite difficult. In addition, for a large number of severely and profoundly retarded, a disproportionate amount of their total behavior is of a sort that creates considerable management problems. It is not unusual to find in this group such behaviors as dangerous self-mutilation; rectal digging; feces smearing and eating; violent and unpredictable temper outbursts; physical attacks on peers and attendants; chronic and high-rate repetitive movements; disruptive screaming and crying; and destruction of windows, clothing, furnishings and the like.

Punishment Procedures

Some treatment procedures that have gained recent consideration in work with the severely retarded are those having punishment or aversive components. Many of the reports describing experience with punishment have been products of relatively new clinical research programs aimed at creating a more effective total rehabilitation environment for the retarded; few have been products of systematic experience in clinical treatment programs. This is not surprising, as most clinical treatment personnel categorically reject the use of punishment procedures as a legitimate approach to behavior change. Punishment procedures are typically viewed as inhumane, deplorable, unethical, and nonprofessional. This attitude is perhaps understandable in relation to the mentally retarded in residential settings, as various punishment techniques all too frequently have been applied as punitive measures instead of being used as treatment techniques in a deliberate, systematic fashion. In addition, it is assumed by many that the decelerating effects of punishment are temporary, and that punishment produces undesirable side effects, including disruptive emotional states and disruption of social relationships. It even appears that these attitudes and extrapolations from animal research have greatly restricted the clinical use of punishment with the retarded. For example, a recent review chapter (Spradlin and Girardeau, 1966) on the moderately and severely retarded reports no studies in this area. In general it appears that punishment is frequently rejected as a treatment procedure, not on the basis of an objective evaluation of scientific data, but rather on the basis of ethical, philosophic, and social-political considerations.

Punishment procedures that have been used with the retarded can be grouped into two classes on the basis of the operations followed.

The first class includes those procedures which result in the *presentation* of certain stimulus conditions that follow a response that is to be eliminated. These would include (1) primary aversive stimuli, for example, electric shock (Tate and Baroff, 1966), (2) physical restraint, for example, strapping to chair or bed (Hamilton et al., 1967), placing in restraining jackets (Giles and Wolf, 1966), and (3) conditioned aversive stimuli, for example, "No" paired previously with removal of food and physical restraint (Henriksen and Doughty, 1967). The second class includes those procedures which result in the *removal* of certain stimulus conditions that follow the behavior to be eliminated. Various procedures of time-out from positive reinforcement, for example, placement in an isolation room after inappropriate behavior (Wiesen and Watson, 1967), illustrate this class of procedures. On occasion the time-out is used in combination with a response-cost procedure (Weiner, 1962); for example, the subject is isolated and in addition loses certain tangible positive reinforcers that are available to him (Hamilton and Allen, 1967).

In most of the studies to be described, regardless of the specific punishment procedures used, the children not only had alternative response possibilities available in the punishment situation, but in addition were provided positive reinforcement for more suitable alternative behaviors. Azrin and Holz (1966) emphasize that such an alternative response situation results in maximum suppression by a given intensity of punishment. Resulting behavior change should be viewed as a result of the combined treatment strategies.

Primary Aversive Stimulation

The presentation of primary aversive-stimulus conditions contingent upon inappropriate behavior has been used in a number of behavior-modification programs in an attempt to eliminate a variety of self-destructive, aggressive, and disruptive behaviors. In a recent report, Bucher and Lovaas (1968) described the application of electric shock in suppressing the high rate of self-destructive reponses of three retarded subjects with psychoticlike behavior. All had long histories of self-injurious behavior (SIB), all were hospitalized, and all were kept in constant restraints. In all cases the self-destructive behaviors were suppressed immediately and virtually eliminated after a series of response-contingent electric shocks usually delivered by a hand-held indoctorium and distributed over a small number of sessions.

Risley (1968) used shock to control dangerous climbing behavior in a six-year-old hyperactive brain-damaged girl described as asocial, with no speech or imitative behaviors. Repetitive head twisting was eliminated by a procedure of shouting at and shaking the child. Previous withdrawal of attention, isolation for ten-minute time-out periods contingent upon the climbing behavior, and reinforcement of incompatible behaviors all proved noninfluential. As the behavior was dangerous to the child and destructive to the home, and as the child's aggressive behavior toward her younger brother was causing parental concern, it was felt that an effective control procedure having immediate effects was needed.

Shock was applied by a hand-held inductorium to the child's leg contingent upon climbing behavior. Climbing behavior, which was occurring at the rate of one climb every ten minutes, was eliminated in a laboratory room after six contingent applications of the shock over eight sessions. No climbing occurred in the therapist's presence during the subsequent twelve sessions, but it did reappear in the following session. No shock was administered during the subsequent eleven sessions, with climbing occurring an average of 4.9 times per hour. As Risley (1968, p. 29) emphasized, "Clearly, the effects of the shock punishment were reversible (not permanent)." A single response-contingent shock again eliminated the response, with no further climbing occurring during the next fifty-nine sessions.

The procedure was applied in the home, where the inappropriate climbing was at an average rate of twenty-nine times daily. The rate was reduced to two per day within four days of response-contingent shock, with a zero rate obtained within a few additional days. Aggressive behavior against the younger brother resulted in shock. Within three weeks this behavior rate was reduced to zero and was not reported to occur during the subsequent seventy days of follow-up. The repetitive head-rolling behaviors were virtually eliminated within ten sessions of response-contingent shouting ("stop that") and vigorous shaking.

In evaluating the question of possible negative side effects associated with the use of a punishment procedure, Risley (p. 33) concluded: "The most significant side effect was the fact that eliminating climbing and autistic rocking with punishment facilitated the acquisition of new desirable behaviors." Both frequency of eye contact with the therapist and rate of imitation behavior were increased. Risley suggests the possibility that stereotyped behaviors of deviant children are "functionally incompatible" with the development of new socially desirable behaviors. In the case reported, socially appropriate behaviors were established as stereotyped behaviors were eliminated.

Tate and Baroff (1966) described the successful use of response-contingent electric shock in work with a nine-year-old blind boy residing in a state institution for the mentally retarded. The boy engaged in various SIB's including head banging, face slapping, punching his face and head with his fist, hitting his shoulder with his chin, and kicking himself. He was reported to enjoy bodily contact with others. The child spent most of his time restrained in bed. Electric shock was used in this case on the assumption that such aversive consequences would result in rapid deceleration of the SIB. This was deemed essential as the risk was present that further SIB would completely destroy the retina of his right eye in which some light-dark vision was present. An earlier treatment procedure consisting of brief termination of physical contact with an adult produced dramatic results, but was replaced by the primary aversive stimulation procedure. This time-out procedure will be described in the following section.

Shock was delivered to the lower leg contingent upon SIB. Previous base line rate of SIB was approximately two per minute. After response-contingent shock a rapid deceleration effect was noted, with only twenty SIB's of light intensity observed during a five and one-half hour period (average of 0.06 responses per minute) on the first day after shock. On the second day, there were only fifteen SIB's during the entire day (rate of 0.03 per minute). During subsequent days, the subject spent nine hours daily out of bed. He was observed for 167 days after the beginning of shock, with no SIB's observed during the last twenty days of treatment.

After initiating use of electric shock, these writers observed that no deleterious emotional or social interaction effects were evident. On the contrary, punishment frequently resulted in a more alert, cooperative, smiling and relaxed child. Bucher and Lovaas (1968) and Luckey et al. (1968) reported highly similar reactions of decrease in whining, fussing, and crying and an increase in alertness, affection, and general social responsiveness in their similar treatment of retarded and autistic children. In all cases, these new behaviors were provided ample reinforcement by the therapists and other caretaker personnel having contact with the child.

Time-Out Procedures

Wiesen and Watson (1967) describe the behavior treatment of an institutionalized severely retarded six-year-old boy who exhibited excessive attention-getting behavior. This behavior, directed toward adults, was described as "almost unbearable" and consisted of constant grabbing, pulling, hitting, untying shoelaces, and the like. It was further noted that this boy totally ignored other children. Unlike a psychodynamic model, which would view the behaviors as, for example, a symptom of "emotional disturbance" or of an "excessive need for affection," the behaviors were hypothesized to be maintained by the adult attention such behaviors brought. Wiesen and Watson (p. 50) hypothesized that the excessive rate (over six responses per minute during the base-rate observations) was being maintained by "an inadvertently established partial reinforcement schedule carried out unwittingly by harried attendant counselors who periodically reinforced Paul with prolonged attention."

Elimination of this highly disruptive behavior and development of peer social interaction were identified as the treatment goals. One element of the treatment procedure, that of removing the child from the presence of the reinforcing adults immediately after inappropriate attention-seeking behavior, is based on the suggestion from experimental and treatment studies that time-out from positive reinforcement functions as an aversive event and thus decreases the strength of the preceding behavior (see Ferster and Appel, 1961; Wolf et al. 1964). A time-out procedure consisting of removal of the boy from all possible social reinforcement and placing him outdoors for five-minute periods were made contingent upon excessive attention-seeking behavior. Concurrent tangible reinforcement was made contingent upon appropriate interaction with peers. An interesting aspect of this procedure consisted of the manner in which reinforcement was provided this behavior. Over the twenty-one day treatment program, peers presented the tangible reinforcement to the boy whenever he interacted with them. These peers in turn were reinforced by the attendant counselors. Removal of clothing and soiling behaviors which were observed to occur during the isolation or time-out period resulted in an extension of the aversive-consequence condition. Additionally, report Wiesen and Watson (1967, p. 51) following soiling "no bathing was permitted until five minutes had elapsed and water temperature was maintained at below room temperature."

This treatment program produced a rapid decrease in the rate of attention-seeking behavior. Although the child was removed a large number of times during the first few days of the program (over forty times during the first day), this decreased rapidly. The investigators (p. 52) note that "Soiling, which had occurred as often as nine times per day before conditioning, had been extinguished with only nine episodes of spontaneous recovery." Rate of social interaction behaviors were reported to become a "major response."

Hamilton et al. (1967) describe the use of a combination of time-out from positive reinforcement and physical restraint in a program designed to eliminate a range of destructive and aggressive behaviors exhibited by severely retarded residents. After inappropriate behaviors the retardate was restrained in a padded chair in an isolated area for periods ranging from thirty to sixty minutes. Head and back banging, which occurred literally thousands of times daily in one resident, was dramatically eliminated after initiation of treatment and remained at a zero level during a nine-month follow-up period. Positive changes in social behavior were reported to follow the elimination of this stereotyped behavior. A variety of aggressive and destructive behaviors were either eliminated or drastically reduced in frequency of occurrence in a group of other residents using the same procedure.

The treatment plan used with one resident illustrates the value of application of response-contingent punishment over the use of the same negative conditions in an unsystematic manner. Owing to a number of bothersome behaviors, including the habit of breaking windows with her head, an adolescent was restrained to her bed for extended periods prior to initiation of treatment. She averaged one broken window daily during the short periods when she was released for eating, bathing, toileting, and exercising. After initiation of the program, whenever she broke a window, the girl was immediately restrained to her bed for two-hour periods, with no attention provided beyond that essential for medical treatment of cuts for the broken glass. Within a week this behavior had dropped to a minimal frequency. During the next seven weeks she broke only eleven windows, after which the behavior did not reoccur during an eleven-month follow-up period. Once prolonged restraint and window breaking had been eliminated, two other classes of behavior—body slamming and clothes tearing—were selected for deceleration programming. The occurrence of either behavior resulted in immediate bed restraint. After a few weeks the behavior virtually dropped out and remained so over an extended follow-up period.

One of the criticisms of a treatment program that deals with specific behavior difficulties is that the basic psychological problem causing the symptomatic behavior is being avoided. The appearance of other equally undesirable behaviors in the form of symptom substitution is expected. Addressing themselves to this question, these investigators (Hamilton et al., 1967, p. 586) reported that "there has not been one observed case of negative symptom substitution or any other undesirable side effect. On the contrary, residents whose unacceptable behaviors were suppressed as a result of the punishment procedure were judged by the ward personnel to be more socially outgoing, happier, and better adjusted in the ward setting."

Henriksen and Doughty (1967), in a program to eliminate in young profoundly retarded boys undesirable mealtime behaviors consisting of rapid eating, eating with hands, stealing food, hitting others at table, and throwing trays on the floor, interrupted the misbehaviors and held the child's arms down in his lap. Secondary aversive cues of verbal disapproval were developed by pairing these cues with movement restraint. Proper eating habits were encouraged by various social reinforcement procedures.

Peterson and Peterson (1967), in a program designed to eliminate the SIB of a severely retarded eight-year-old, successfully used time-out from primary (food) and secondary (brief termination of social interaction) reinforcement. An additional punishment procedure of requiring the child to walk across the room and sit in a chair was included. These procedures functioned as mild forms of punishment and facilitated the reduction of the inappropriate behaviors.

As suggested in an earlier section, Tate and Baroff (1966) used a brief time-out from physical contact in an effort to eliminate undesirable SIB in a nine-year-old blind boy. Previous observations of this subject strongly indicated that physical contact with people was reinforcing to him and that being alone, especially when he was standing or walking, was aversive. A three-second time-out period from physical contact immediately followed each occurrence of a self-injurious response. In addition, during the time-out period the therapist ceased conversation with the subject. A median average rate of 6.6 responses per minute was obtained for five control days prior to the initiation of the time-out procedure. This average declined sharply with the initiation of the time-out procedure to an average of 0.1 responses per minute. The results of this study indicate that the relatively simple procedure of immediate brief withdrawal of physical contact produces a dramatic reduction in the frequency of chronic self-injurious behavior. The usual extinction procedure of ignoring the behavior was not effective in reducing its frequency of occurrence.

Development of Incompatible Behaviors

The studies of Patterson et al. (1965) and Patterson (1965) illustrate the procedure of developing behaviors that are physically incompatible with the maladaptive ways of behaving. This work also demonstrates the possibility of modifying hyperactivity of a neurologically impaired child by means of a behavior-treatment procedure. These and similar results support the assumptions, as suggested by Lindsley (1964), that even though a class of behavior is highly correlated with organic factors, the behaviors may be modifiable by environmental conditions. The Patterson et al. (1965) study involved the conditioning of attending behavior in a brain-injured hyperactive ten-year-old mildly retarded boy. Although the "hyperactivity" was present in a child who demonstrated obvious CNS impairment, the behavior was viewed as potentially responsive to treatment procedures based on learning concepts. The child was described as having a short attention span, being aggressive to younger children, and being very hyperactive. This disruptive, nonattending hyperactivity was defined more precisely in terms of seven different response categories, and quantitative measures of the frequency of occurrence of these behaviors in the classroom were taken. Treatment procedure consisted initially of the immediate reinforcement of brief intervals of attending behavior. After improvement, reinforcement was provided on a variable interval schedule. To insure the cooperation of the other children in the classroom, the tangible reinforcers the boy earned were shared with his classmates. There was a significant reduction in the nonattending behavior in comparison to that shown by a control subject. Thus, the hyperactivity was reduced by developing responses that were incompatible with this behavior pattern.

Developmental Problems

Experience with the retarded has demonstrated that the systematic use of reinforcement procedures can facilitate the development of a variety of skills of eating (Gorton and Hollis, 1965; Spradlin, 1964; Blackwood, 1962; Bensberg et al., 1965), dressing (Roos, 1965; Minge and Ball, 1967), toileting (Hundziak et al., 1965; Giles and Wolf, 1966; Watson, 1967), grooming (Gorton and Hollis, 1965; Girardeau and Spradlin, 1964; Bensberg et al., 1965), socialization (Bensberg et al., 1965; Wiesen and Watson, 1967; Gorton and Hollis, 1965; Girardeau and Spradlin, 1964), locomotion (Meyerson et al., 1967) and language (Sloane et al., 1968; MacAulay, 1968; Kerr et al., 1965). As suggested earlier, even the young and more severely retarded are suitable subjects for this type of treatment, as little prerequisite language or specific cognitive or "understanding" skills are assumed essential for adequate progress. Bensberg (1965) provides an excellent description of the principles and techniques of training a variety of self-help skills to the young retarded child. Simply stated, these developmental skills have been facilitated by a behavior-shaping or successive-approximation technique. Complex behaviors such as self-feeding or self-dressing are organized into a series of small discrete units. Reinforcement is provided for behaviors that approximate each segment, with progressively more complex behavior being brought under the control of the reinforcement procedure. A wide variety of food, trinket, activity, and social reinforcers have been used in these behavior-development programs, with an empirical attitude being maintained by the therapist as to the type of reinforcing event that should be used. For the interested reader, Spradlin and Girardeau (1966) and Watson (1967) provide a review of the types of reinforcers that have proven most successful. Typically, the desired behavior is initially reinforced immediately upon its occurrence. Reinforcement is presented in large quantities, as the behavior is being established and then gradually reduced in magnitude and frequency. In some instances (for example, Giles and Wolf, 1966), positive reinforcement is used in conjunction with punishment procedures. The clinical experiences reflected in these references would suggest that even the more profoundly retarded can be taught a number of basic self-care skills. Again, with sound empirical support, a behavior-therapy approach would place the blame for the presence of poor self-care skills not in the "mental retardation" of the retarded, but in the poor environment that is under the control of the family or the professional staff of the residential facility.

Educational Problems

The extensive work at Ranier School in conjunction with the University of Washington provides excellent examples of the use of a variety of behavior modification-procedures for influencing the academic, motivational, and social behavior of the mentally retarded in a classroom group setting. Both the mildly retarded child (Bijou et al., 1966; Birnbrauer et al., 1965; Birnbrauer et al., 1965) and the trainable child (Birnbrauer and Lawler, 1964) have responded favorably to such programs. Bijou et al. (1966) describe the classroom program used to develop a motivational system for strengthening academic and appropriate social behaviors. Initially, teacher approval that was bestowed on desirable classroom behaviors was ineffective in strengthening these classes of behavior. After the introduction of a token reinforcement system, higher rates of effective study and cooperation behaviors became evident. Various "study habits" including such behaviors as sitting quietly, paying attention to and complying with instructions, and working productively for sustained periods were strengthened and a range of disruptive behaviors was eliminated. Techniques involving frequent token and social reinforcement for appropriate social and study behaviors, and those utilizing extinction and punishment (time-out from positive reinforcement) operations were used by the teaching personnel. The results of these behavior-modification procedures, along with the use of programmed materials, can best be depicted by describing the study behaviors developed in one of the retardates. It should be noted that initially the children were poorly motivated for academic achievement. Bijou et al. (1966, p. 512) report:

Instead of being given his assignment by the teacher he obtained his own "work folder," set his own watch, and entered the date and starting time on his daily record sheet. He chose his first task, completed it, and went on to the next. Starting and finishing times were entered for each item. When all the work was completed he called a teacher and together they checked his work. Marks (token reinforcement) were given at this time.

These authors provide an excellent discussion of the basic principles that guided the development of the procedures and materials used. Specific techniques for the development of the motivation system, prerequisite academic behaviors, and programmed instructional materials are provided and should be consulted by those interested in developing a behavior-modification program for use with the mildly retarded in a classroom environment.

Birnbrauer and Lawler (1964) discuss the use of operant learning principles in development of classroom skills for the more severely retarded child. Thirty-seven children with IQ scores below 40 were able to achieve rather well in a few months after reinforcement of approximations to desirable social and study behavior by having inappropriate and incorrect behaviors ignored and by receiving punishment for dangerous behavior patterns. A case report of a moderately retarded child with severe behavior problems illustrates the value of the techniques in development of behaviors such as working cooperatively with peers in a small group, waiting one's turn for individual instruction, responding to several verbal requests, control of aggressive and self-destructive outbursts, and the like. At the beginning of the program, this child was described as aggressive, destructive, extremely hyperactive, and with behavior that was uncontrollable and violent.

These reports and the clinical experiences of numerous others working with the retarded child in an educational setting provide suitable support for the usefulness of various behavior-modification procedures. As noted earlier, there is undeniable evidence that, under an appropriate "designed environment," the retarded can learn to behave in a mature and productive manner "in spite of his mental retardation."

CONCLUSIONS

The recent development of behavior-modification techniques has opened a new and exciting chapter in the area of psychological treatment of the mentally retarded. The studies reviewed in the present chapter, although reflecting a rather limited application both in terms of the range of problems treated and the techniques used, do offer results that provide enthusiasm to those who for so long had few viable concepts of behavior change offering some specific treatment direction and had even fewer successful treatment techniques available for dealing with many of the severe and chronic problems presented by the retarded. Psychiatric, psychological, child development, and educational personnel can no longer categorically dismiss the mentally retarded as being unsuitable for therapeutic intervention. A learning approach to behavior change has produced some dramatic results.

At the same time, the early exploratory nature of the behavior-therapy approaches renders it necessary to maintain a strict experimental attitude concerning the use of these procedures. Considerable laboratory and clinical research must be completed prior to a general use of the behavior-modification approach. The experimental background from which behavior modification procedures have evolved does provide the methodological base for continued development and evaluation. A major danger, however, lies in the unqualified application of procedures by personnel working on the practical level who neither have the theoretical knowledge nor the experimental skills to evaluate the influence of their therapeutic attempts. As Bachrach and Quigley (1966, p. 510) have suggested,

. . . we must be sure that there are scientists (research personnel) to provide the necessary thinking through and analysis of the techniques used by applied personnel. It is undoubtedly true that the field of behavior therapy, with its worthy social goals, its theoretical simplicity (deceptive though it may be), and its empirical success (under certain circumstances), will attract many psychotechnicians. It is, therefore, a field in danger of being ruined by amateurs.

NOTE

1. Although some writers use the term "behavior modification" in a broad sense to refer to many types of behavior change, including educational programs, and reserve the term "behavior therapy" specifically for those behavior-changing procedures which are used in dealing with clinical problems, this writer follows the practice of Ullman and Krasner (1965), Reyna (1965), and Bachrach and Quigley (1966) in using "behavior modification" and "behavior therapy" as interchangeable terms.

REFERENCES

Azrin, N. H., & Holtz, W. C. Punishment. In W. K. Honig (Ed.), *Operant behavior: Areas of research and application.* New York: Appleton-Century-Crofts, 1966, pp. 380–447.

Bachrach, A. J., & Quigley, W. A. Direct methods of treatment. In I. A. Berg and L. A. Pennington (Eds.), *An introduction to clinical psychology* (3rd ed.). New York: Ronald Press, 1966, pp. 482–560.

Baer, D. M., Peterson, R. F., & Sherman, J. A. The development of imitation by reinforcing behavioral similarity to a model. *J. Exper. Anal. Beh.,* 1967, *10,* 405–416.

————, Wolf, M. M., & Risley, T. R. Some current dimensions of applied behavior analysis. *J. Appl. Beh. Anal.,* 1968, *1,* 91–97.

Bensberg, G. J. *Teaching the mentally retarded.* Atlanta, Ga.: Southern Regional Education Board, 1965.

————, Colwell, C. N., & Cassel, R. H. Teaching the profoundly retarded self-help activities by behavior shaping techniques. *Amer. J. Ment. Defic.,* 1965, *69,* 674–679.

Bijou, S. W. A functional analysis of retarded behavior. In N. R. Ellis (Ed.), *International review of research in mental retardation,* Vol. I. New York: Academic Press, 1966, pp. 1–20.

————, Birnbrauer, J. S., Kidder, J. D., & Tague, C. Programmed instruction as an approach to teaching of reading, writing, and arithmetic to retarded children. *Psychol. Rec.,* 1966, *16,* 505–522.

————, & Sloan, H. N. Therapeutic techniques with children. In I. A. Berg and L. A. Pennington (eds.), *An introduction to clinical psychology* (3rd ed.). New York: Ronald Press, 1966, pp. 652–684.

Birnbrauer, J. S., Bijou, S. W., Wolf, M. M., & Kidder, J. D. Programmed instruction in the classroom. In L. P. Ullman and L. Krasner (Eds.), *Case studies in behavior modification.* New York: Holt, Rinehart, & Winston, 1965, pp. 358–363.

Birnbrauer, J. S., & Lawler, J. Token reinforcement for learning. *Ment. Retard.,* 1964, *2,* 275–279.

Birnbrauer, J. S., Wolf, M. M., Kidder, J. D., & Tague, C. Classroom behavior of retarded pupils with token reinforcement. *J. Exper. Child Psychol.,* 1965, *2,* 219–235.

Blackwood, R. O. Operant conditioning as a method of training the mentally retarded. Unpublished doctoral dissertation, Ohio State University, Columbus, Ohio, 1962.

Bucher, B., and Lovaas, O. I. Use of aversive stimulation in behavior modification. In N. R. Jones (Ed.). *Miami symposium on the prediction of behavior, 1967: Aversive stimulation.* Coral Gables, Fla.: University of Miami Press, 1968, pp. 77–145.

Eysenck, H. J. (Ed.). *Behavior therapy and the neuroses.* New York: Pergamon Press, 1960.

Ferster, C. B., and Appel, J. B. Punishment of S$^{\Delta}$ responding in match to sample by time-out from positive reinforcement, *J. Exper. Anal. Beh.*, 1961, *4*, 45–56.

Fuller, P. R. Operant conditioning of a vegetative human organism. *Amer. J. Psychol.*, 1949, *62*, 587–590.

Gelfand, D. M., & Hartmann, D. P. Behavior therapy with children: A review and evaluation of research methodology. *Psychol. Bull.*, 1968, *69*, 204–215.

Giles, D. K., & Wolf, M. M. Toilet training institutionalized, severe retardates: An application of operant behavior modification techniques. *Amer. J. Ment. Defic.*, 1966, *70*, 766–780.

Girardeau, F. L., & Spradlin, J. E. Token rewards in a cottage program. *Ment. Retard.*, 1964, *2*, 345–352.

Gorton, C. E., & Hollis, J. H. Redesigning a cottage unit for better programming and research for the severely retarded. *Ment. Retard.*, 1965, *3*, 16–21.

Hamilton, J., & Allen P. Ward programming for severely retarded institutionalized residents. *Ment. Retard.*, 1967, *5*, 22–24.

―――, Stephens, L., & Allen, P. Controlling aggressive and destructive behavior in severely retarded institutionalized residents. *Amer. J. Ment. Defic.*, 1967, *71*, 852–856.

Henriksen, K., & Doughty, R. Decelerating undesirable mealtime behavior in a group of profoundly retarded boys. *Amer. J. Ment. Defic.*, 1967, *72*, 40–44.

Hundziak, M., Maurer, R. A., & Watson, L. S. Operant conditioning and toilet training of severely mentally retarded boys. *Amer. J. Ment. Defic.*, 1965, *70*, 120–128.

Kalish, H. I. Behavior therapy. In B. B. Wolman (Ed.), *Handbook of clinical psychology*. New York: McGraw-Hill, 1965, pp. 1230–1253.

Kanfer, F., & Saslow, G. Behavioral analysis: An alternative to diagnostic classification. *Arch. Gen. Psychiat.*, 1965, *12*, 529–538.

Kerr, N., Meyerson, L., & Michael, J. A procedure for shaping vocalizations in a mute child. In L. P. Ullman and L. Krasner (Eds.), *Case studies in behavior modification*. New York: Holt, Rinehart & Winston, 1965, pp. 366–370.

Leff, R. Behavior modification and the psychoses of childhood: A review. *Psychol. Bull.*, 1968, *69*, 396–409.

Lindsley, O. R. Direct measurement and prosthesis of retarded behavior. *J. Educ.*, 1964, *147*, 62–81.

Lovaas, O. I. A behavior therapy approach to treatment of childhood schizophrenia. In J. Hill (Ed.), *Symposia on child development*, Vol. I. Minneapolis, Minn.: University of Minnesota Press, 1967, pp. 108–159.

Lovaas, O. I., Freitag, G., Gold, V. J., & Kassorla, I. C. Experimental studies in childhood schizophrenia: Analysis of self-destructive behavior. *J. Exper. Child Psychol.*, 1965, *2*, 67–84.

Luckey, R. E., Watson, C. M., & Musick, J. K. Aversive conditioning as a means of inhibiting vomiting and rumination. *Amer. J. Ment. Defic.*, 1968, *73*, 139–142.

MacAulay, B. D. A program for teaching speech and beginning reading to nonverbal retardates. In H. N. Sloane, Jr. and Barbara D. MacAulay (Eds.), *Operant procedures and remedial speech and language training*. Boston: Houghton Mifflin, 1968, pp. 102–124.

Meyerson, L., Kerr, N., & Michael, J. L. Behavior modification in rehabilitation. In S. W. Bijou and D. M. Baer (Eds.), *Child development: Readings in experimental analysis*. New York: Appleton-Century-Crofts, 1967, pp. 214–239.

Minge, M. R., & Ball, T. S. Teaching of self-help skills to profoundly retarded patients. *Amer. J. Ment. Defic.*, 1967, *71*, 34–68.

Patterson, G. R. An application of conditioning techniques to the control of a hyperactive child. In L. P. Ullman and L. Krasner (Eds.), *Case studies in behavior modification*. New York: Holt, Rinehart & Winston, 1965, pp. 370–375.

Patterson, G. R., Jones, R., Whittier, J., & Wright, M. A. A behavior modification technique for the hyperactive child. *Beh. Res. & Ther.*, 1965, *2*, 217–226.

Peterson, R. F., & Peterson, L. R. Mark and his blanket: A study of self-destructive behavior in a retarded boy. Presented at meeting of the Society for Research in Child Development, New York, 1967.

Reyna, L. J. Conditioning therapies, learning theory, and research. In J. Wolpe, A.

Salter and L. J. Reyna (Eds.), *The conditioning therapies*. New York: Holt, Rinehart & Winston, 1965, pp. 169–180.

Rice, H. K., & McDaniel, M. W. Operant behavior in vegetative patients. *Psychol. Rec.*, 1966, *16*, pp. 279–281.

Risley, T. The effects and side effects of punishing the autistic behaviors of a deviant child. *J. Appl. Beh. Anal.*, 1968, *1*, 21–34.

Roos, P. Development of an intensive habit-training unit at Austin State School. *Ment. Retard.*, 1965, *3*, 12–15.

Skinner, B. F. *Science and human behavior*. New York: Macmillan, 1953.

Sloane, H. N., Jr., Johnston, M. J., & Harris, F. R. Remedial procedures for teaching verbal behavior to speech defective young children. In H. N. Sloane, Jr., & Barbara D. MacAulay (Eds.), *Operant procedures and remedial speech and language training*. Boston: Houghton Mifflin, 1968, pp. 77–101.

Spradlin, J. The Premack hypothesis and self-feeding by profoundly retarded children: A case report. Working Paper No. 79, Parsons Research Center, University of Kansas, Parsons, Kan., 1964.

Spradlin, J. E., & Girardeau, F. L. The behavior of moderately and severely retarded persons. In N. R. Ellis (Ed.), *International review of research in mental retardation,* Vol. I. New York: Academic Press, 1966, pp. 257–298.

Striefel, S. Isolation as a behavioral management procedure with retarded children. Working Paper No. 156, Parsons Research Project, University of Kansas, Parsons, Kan., 1967.

Tate, B. G., & Baroff, G. S. Aversive control of self-injurious behavior in a psychotic boy. *Beh. Res. & Ther.*, 1966, *4*, 281–287.

Ullman, L. P., & Krasner, L. (Eds.), *Case studies in behavior modification*. New York: Holt, Rinehart & Winston, 1965.

Watson, L. S., Jr. Application of operant conditioning techniques to institutionalized severely and profoundly retarded children. *Ment. Retard. Abstr.*, 1967, *4*, 1–18.

Weiner, H. Some effects of response cost upon human operant behavior. *J. Exper. Anal. Beh.*, 1962, *5*, 201–208.

Wiesen, A. E., & Watson, E. Elimination of attention seeking behavior in a retarded child. *Amer. J. Ment. Defic.*, 1967, *72*, 50–52.

Wolf, M. M., Birnbrauer, J. S., Williams, L., & Lawler, J. A note on apparent extinction of the vomiting behavior of a retarded child. In L. P. Ullman and L. Krasner (Eds.), *Case studies in behavior modification*. New York: Holt, Rinehart & Winston, 1965, pp. 364–366.

Wolf, M. M., Risley, L., & Mees, H. Application of operant conditioning procedures to the behavior problems of an autistic child. *Beh. Res. & Ther.*, 1964, *1*, 305–312.

Wolpe, J. *Psychotherapy by reciprocal inhibition*. Stanford, Calif.: Stanford University Press, 1958.

: 12 :

Early Psychiatric Intervention for Young Mentally Retarded Children

Katharine F. Woodward, Norma Jaffe, and Dorothy Brown

INTRODUCTION

THE very young child with retarded functioning who does not fit clearly into any of the well-defined organic categories continues to be terra incognita. Parents become alarmed when they find that their child does not develop as other children do. In their search for help they often receive conflicting opinions or inadequate guidance. The fact is, there are very few existing resources for this kind of child. There are even fewer resources that attempt to explore such a child's intellectual potential before making a final judgment. A start is now being made in accumulating knowledge and techniques of therapy both for children and for their parents in this situation.

The authors have previously reported on a three-year psychiatric program for preschool children with retarded functioning, some of whom were helped to achieve performance within normal limits. From this study emerged our assumption that psychogenic factors can play an important role in causing the inhibition of mental development and that a comprehensive treatment plan, aimed at overcoming the effect of these psychogenic factors, might help these children to an improved intellectual functioning.

Since that time we have had the opportunity to study and work with many more children, and of an even younger age, and to involve their parents in a more intensive therapeutic process.

The conclusions reached have supported our earlier convinction that the exploration of possible psychogenic aspects affecting each case must be considered an important treatment approach with these children.

Relatively little material has been published regarding psychogenic factors in retarded functioning. Bornstein (1930) and Chidester and Menninger (1936) have given detailed accounts of psychoanalytic therapy in older children. Rappaport (1961) has told us about a two-year treatment period of a brain-damaged child with severe hearing loss. Kaplan et al. (1948) report therapy with a boy of borderline intelligence who offered a mixed picture of cerebral damage and superimposed neurotic disturbance. Axline (1949) and Heiser (1954) report cases where the measurable quotient has risen to the normal range after therapy.

It appears to be fairly well established from the literature that children who function at a retarded level may be helped by various programs to improved or even normal functioning.

Kirk (1958) instituted an educational program for retarded children between three and six years of age. There were two groups, one in an institutional setting and one in the community with matched control groups. He found that the children who had the special program made greater gains than those in the control groups, as measured by the Stanford-Binet, Kuhman, and Vineland tests. Fifty per cent of the children with demonstrable organic lesions and 79 per cent of the "nonorganic" cases showed accelerated growth in response to the special program.

Skeels and Dye (1939) reported that fourteen of fifteen children, functioning at a retarded level in an orphanage, showed a mean rise in measurable IQ of 27.5 points when they were transferred to a school where they received extra attention from a group of older girls and attendants. Heath (1941–1942), Garfield and Affleck (1960), and Martz (1945) have reported cases whose functioning rose to the normal level after several years in institutions. Cobb and Wilber (1959) have reported greatly improved functioning in young children when transferred from institutions to foster homes.

Tizard (1960) selected sixteen severely retarded children in an institution and gave them a specialized program, with separate quarters and much individual attention. In two years, there was a rise in the verbal mental age averaging fourteen months compared to only six months in a group of matched controls who had no special program. Barsch (1962), Strazzula (1956), Jubenville (1962), and Sloan (1952) have reported gains in severely retarded young children after they were placed in special programs or day care centers.

DESCRIPTION OF THE PRESENT PROGRAM

In the early study, the group was fixed as to number of children and length of time of attendance. Since then it was found that more flexibility is advantageous, and we now regard the first three months in the program as a "clinical trial." After the diagnostic study has been completed, the child who is under study has individual or group sessions with a teacher and a social worker, perhaps both, and the parents have interviews with the social worker. The purpose of this trial is to confirm our diagnostic impression and form prognostic judgments. If, at the end of this period, it is our considered opinion that the child and his family cannot profit by a longer period in the program, the parents are helped to find other resources. Frequent, almost daily communications among staff members of the different disciplines, in addition to the regular weekly staff conference, is vital to our program. Written reports are regularly submitted by each member of the team.

The therapeutic team consists of a psychiatrist, a psychologist, a social worker, and teachers. We operate as part of a well-equipped general hospital and are able to include in our diagnostic evaluation pediatric, neurological, speech and hearing examinations, and any other studies which are indicated. We depend much on the speech therapist who, in the role of consultant, gives the teachers advice on techniques of speech stimulation. In cases that make good progress, speech often develops without special help. We have found speech therapy particularly valuable when some organic factor is interfering with the development of speech.

As soon as the preliminary examination is completed, the children are placed in the group that best fits their needs at the time of referral. The groups are kept small; maximum size is six children with two teachers. The teachers work with the children in a framework as much like that of a normal nursery school as possible. Within this setting of constant routine, they try to stimulate creative play, expression of emotion, interest in outer reality, and—above all—communication.

An important and perhaps unique feature of our program is the use of the teachers in individual sessions. These sessions are regarded by us as the initial stage of psychotherapy. The teacher's major aim here is not to teach, but to encourage the use of various types of play equipment. Resistances to forming a good working relationship with an adult are often worked through in these sessions. Some children are not ready for group participation until they have had these individual sessions for a period of time.

We review grouping arrangements frequently so as to be able to change this plan for any particular child when necessary. The child is placed in a particular group on the basis of his social need and capability rather than on the basis of diagnostic category or age. Work with parents is a crucial part of the program. Mothers are seen once a week, regularly, for casework treatment. Individual or group therapy (or both) is available for the fathers. We have learned that, with some insistence on our part, many more fathers have been willing to participate.

THE FAMILIES

The families who have come to us so far have a wide variety of racial, ethnic, and religious backgrounds. None have been from the extremely underprivileged group, and only a few are of marginal economic status. Intellectually, all fall at least within thc average range of intelligence, and a large percentage have higher than average intelligence and have been able to complete their college education and go on to professional careers. All the families showed severe marital stresses, but the majority had remained intact; one-parent families proved to be very much the exception. Most of the families had other children with personality problems, but in no instance with impairment of their intellectual functioning.

As a group the parents appeared to be unusual in their efforts to find help for their retarded children and in their willingness to follow a program at a considerable sacrifice of time, energy, and money. They came from all over the metropolitan area and even from outlying suburbs, and yet it is noteworthy how regular their attendance has been. In previous papers it was suggested that possibly this effort was in part stimulated by guilt feelings about unconscious rejection of the child. Yet, it also means that the children in the group were not rejected or neglected without appreciable conflict.

Casework interviews with the parents revealed deeply fixed emotional disturbances not necessarily related to the birth of the retarded child, although seriously aggravated by this. This had not been apparent upon initial contact. Among the mothers, we became aware of marked immaturity, strong hostile dependent ties to their own mothers, and depression as predominant features of their disturbed functioning. Fathers also showed markedly infantile reactions and either related on a sibling level to their children or remained withdrawn and remote from the family. In many instances the deviant child was singled out for infantilization, sometimes on the basis of the sex of the child or ordinal position. This seemed especially striking in view of the fact that other siblings were handled differently. We had the distinct impression, however, that these parents did not show any more pathology or resistance to the therapeutic process than parents of child patients in a psychiatric clinic.

CATEGORIES OF CASES STUDIED

The categories of cases we studied are (1) neurotic patterns, (2) neurotic patterns with schizoid or autistic features, (3) possible psychosis, with marked negativism as the most prominent feature, and (4) minimal or debatable brain damage.[1] (A group of children with clearly defined autism, although given treatment by us for variable periods, was excluded from the study for reasons explained in a note at the end of this chapter.)

Of the sixty-one children whom we treated and evaluated, forty-one were studied and followed up intensively and form the basis of our presentation. At the time they came to us, these children ranged in age from fifteen months to five years. At the beginning there were an additional nine children who were supposed to be studied and followed up, but they were withdrawn after an attendance of from only two to six months. In this group of nine, the parents in all instances save one, resisted exploring the possibility of their emotional involvement and preferred to seek programs where the diagnosis of organicity was made. Most of these parents appeared to feel greatly relieved when they could find someone who would pronounce their child organically damaged. All the children were behind their respective age groups in at least two of the following five areas: motor development, speech development, toilet training, self-care, and use of materials and equipment. Retarded functioning was the only basis for selection.

In the group that showed no demonstrable organicity, all the children gave evidence of emotional disturbance of varying degrees. Although no two children were entirely similar and there was, in fact, considerable variation, in general they fell into four categories: (1) neurotic patterns; (2) neurotic patterns with schizoid or autistic features; (3) possible psychosis, with the most prominent symptoms being marked negativism; and (4) minimal or questionable brain damage.

In the evaluating the progress of each child, all members of the team came to agreement through the study of the combined observations. In this present study, "good" progress indicates that these children are testing in the normal range, are able to attend schools for normal children, and are without severe problems of adjustment. "Fair" progress indicates that these children are still functioning below the normal range, but that their use of their abilities has improved and that they are without serious problems of adjustment. At preacademic levels, most of them can attend a normal group but when they are ready for academic work they require special classes. Neurotic traits will be diminished although present to a sufficient degree to interfere with optimum functioning. "Slight" progress indicates minor degrees of improved functioning and lessening of neurotic traits. "No progress" speaks for itself.

Neurotic Patterns

Recognizing that it is not possible to make a clear-cut diagnosis at this age level, we are placing into the category of neurotic patterns those children in whom neurotic traits predominate, such as feeding and sleeping problems, fears, phobias, separation anxiety, obsessive phenomena, and habit disturbances. Most of these sixteen children showed negativism in varying degrees, but not as severely as those to be described in category 3, and depressive features were common. The progress of this group was as follows: Cases, sixteen; good progress, six; fair progress, seven; slight progress, three; no progress, none. The history of the boy which follows illustrates the group of children with neurotic patterns:

Group A.

An only child of college-educated parents, was referred two weeks before his second birthday because of generally retarded development. Delivery had occurred three weeks after it was expected. Forceps were used because of slowing contractions. The baby's birth weight was 9 pounds, 14 ounces. Physicians believe he took feedings poorly during the first five days of his life because of excessive mucus. He had an operation for torticollis at the age of 5 months, after which he had to wear a leather collar for several weeks. For the first two days of wearing it, he cried excessively. At the age of 9 months he had a herniorrhaphy that was uneventful.

The boy's motor development was delayed. At the time of referral he was not yet walking alone, although he was crawling actively and walking with support. His speech was limited to three words, which he had recently acquired. Toilet training had not been attempted. His neurotic traits were minimal. He had resisted solid food until 9 months of age. While without specific fears, he was described as "overcautious." He seemed anxious when held, clutching and clinging to the adult. At the age of 18 months he had a high fever for twenty-four hours during which eye-rolling was noticed.

When first seen, he appeared to be functioning at a level slightly under 1 year. He was an attractive child who was friendly and responsive and crawled around actively and said "Hiya" to everyone he saw. He showed little interest in toys and equipment. He cooperated reasonably well on the psychological test and achieved an IQ of 55 on the Cattell Infant Intelligence Scale.

The boy responded very well to the program. He walked alone at 2½ years, and his gross motor coordination became reasonably good. His speech developed rapidly; he was using four- and five-word sentences at the end of a year. Toilet training was achieved during this period. After nine months in the program, at the age of 3 years and 2 months, he achieved an IQ of 90 on the Stanford-Binet Test. He is 10½ years at the time of writing. He was able to attend normal nursery, kindergarten, and first grade classes. Since the second grade he has been in a special public school class. His academic achievement has been uneven. He reads on grade level, but has lagged behind in mathematics and other abstract work. He has had problems of social adjustment for which psychotherapy has been given.

In this case, the favorable results probably were due largely to the casework with the mother. Both parents had regarded themselves as without serious personal problems at the time of referral, and both were reluctant at first to come for interviews. The mother in particular felt she was well read in child development. In her interviews she made it belligerently clear that she believed in rigid and repressive techniques for rearing children. She expressed disappointment in her expectations for her husband and child, and anger that she could not make them conform to her standards. It soon came to light that the marriage relationship was exceedingly poor. She nagged, scolded, and criticized, and her husband responded with massive negativism.

The marital relationship improved considerably during the casework contact. The mother's attitude toward her son also softened, which resulted in a much better handling of him and more realistic expectations of him. The most interesting aspect of the casework contact, however, was discovering this mother's unconscious need to see her child as brain-damaged and retarded. She was very much disturbed when the second psychological test indicating normal intelligence was reported to her and had difficulty accepting these results. Later she was able to see that her attitudes toward the child had tended to hold back his growth; examples were her reluctance to wean him, to give him table food, to encourage activity, to toilet train him.

Group B.

These six children did not show the severe withdrawal typical of the autistic child. They were able to relate to adults and other children, although in an immature way. Initially, some of the children showed some degree of posturing, some mildly bizarre mannerisms, and some degree of echolalia. As they grew older and became able to verbalize, they had difficulty in reality testing, although not to a severe degree. They tended to remain relatively narcissistic and to be much slower than the average child in understanding the feelings and rights of others. The progress of the group was as follows: Cases, six; good progress, four; fair progress, two; slight progress, none; no progress, none. The case history of the boy which follows is one example of the group of children who have neurotic patterns with schizoid or autistic features.

A boy was referred at the age of 2½ years because of slow development in all areas. Pregnancy and delivery had been uneventful. His feeding history proceeded routinely except that he was rather slow taking bottles at the beginning and refused to eat anything but pureed foods. He was described as an infant who was not very responsive to people, but interested in objects. Because of delayed motor development, he was admitted to the children's ward of another hospital at the age of 18 months. Here all examinations were negative but the prognosis seemed poor. His parents elected to send him away, and he spent the next six months in a foster placement. During this period he became more responsive and made a few oral noises. Much encouraged, the parents took him home where, soon after this, he began to say a few words, became toilet trained without difficulty, and improved in motor coordination. He had a wide variety of bizarre mannerisms from time to time, but these disappeared during his stay in the foster home. Rocking had occurred when he was about 1 year old, but had stopped in the foster home. There had been some transient fears. He still clung to his bottle.

The parents were an intelligent couple, both college graduates. The father was quite successful in his business and was not aware of personality problems. The mother had always tended to worry excessively. Despite her cooperation in all practical aspects of our program for her son, she remained unable to work on her role in his development and kept herself free of any emotional involvement in her casework. A 6-year-old sibling was reported to be bright and without problems. The patient, at 2½ years, was an attractive, well-developed child whose gross coordination was somewhat awkward. He clutched his bottle constantly and would not separate from his mother. He was able to relate to the examiner and to enter into some play with her.

On the Cattell Infant Scale he cooperated enough to achieve a quotient of 74, with a mental age of 16 months. Pediatric and neurological examinations including skull X-ray and EEG were entirely negative. He had had very little illness.

This boy had individual sessions three times weekly with the teacher for a six-month period. His first three months of sessions consisted of a vigorous unremitting attempt on his part to control both mother and teacher. After the separation from the mother was effected, he relaxed, became more friendly with the teacher, began to enjoy the resources of the playroom, and improved greatly in speech. He made good progress and has adjusted well to normal groups since. He has just completed fifth grade in public school, and reports from the home and the school have been very favorable. He had four years of psychotherapy, which terminated when he was 9½ years old.

Psychological tests were given him at intervals. The results are seen in Table 12–1.

TABLE 12–1

AGE	TESTS	IQ
2½	Cattell	74
3	Stanford-Binet (LM)	81
4	Stanford-Binet (L)	80
5	Stanford-Binet (L)	115
	(WISC Performance Scale)	89

Group C.

There were 6 children who presented a picture which thus far has not been described in the literature and which we presume is psychotic, although this was not apparent in the early stages of the study. The first observations indicated that they were children who could definitely relate to adults and other children although in an infantile way. In all six patients, depressive phases were noticed early and frequently. In these two respects they differ from the typical autistic child who tends not to relate to people, but mostly to objects, and who is withdrawn rather than depressed. Early in the contact the marked negativism became apparent. These children seemed incapable of reacting to anything but in an "opposite" way. This has been so persistent that they have been able to learn little or nothing while in our program. Speech was markedly delayed, and only two of the six children used a few single words although they seemed able to understand what was said to them. Motor function was almost normal. Children like these, in our experience, have remained uneducable and untrainable in spite of the fact that they have good motor abilities and some capacity for object relationships. The negativism tends to take a passive form and is usually not recognized except by experienced observers. The history of a girl which follows is illustrative of this negativistic group.

A girl was referred at the age of 3 years. Her history revealed that pregnancy and delivery were uneventful. Her early development appeared normal. She smiled early, sat alone when she was 7 months, stood with support when she was 11 months, and said a few words when she was 1 year old. At the age of 14 months she had a severe attack of laryngitis during which she could not make any oral sounds. After she recovered, she did not say any words until she was over 2 years of age. At the time of referral, she had been heard to say about ten words, although she did not use them consistently. She walked alone at the age of 17 months. Toilet training was attempted when she was 1 year old, without any response; her mother discontinued her efforts after a few months. When the child was 2½ years old, she began to lead her mother to the toilet and became continent. She had few fears. At the age of 2 she had a prolonged screaming spell when left with a sitter whom she knew. She waked crying each night for several months after this episode. She was still taking bottles at the time of referral, although she could drink from a cup. Her health had always been unusually good. Her parents were an intelligent, educated couple. The father had a good job but was less ambitious and aggressive than the mother. The mother was aware of her preference for older children over infants. She stated that she had been pleased when the child, as an infant, had been content to sit for long periods in front of the TV set.

The girl at 3 years of age was a pretty child, at first rather passive and inactive. Her facial expression was somewhat vacant, except when something caught her interest and there would be a transient smile. She seemed aware of the examiner and did not show typical autistic withdrawal. The psychologist found her entirely untestable at the time of referral and throughout the contact. Pediatric and neurological examinations were negative on several occasions, as well as the skull X-ray and EEG.

The child was in our group program for three years. She had individual psychotherapy during the second and third years. She early appeared to be a responsive child with ability to become strongly attached to an adult in an infantile way. Her language usage progressed very little during the four years of our work with her, although she occasionally used single words appropriately. For a year we tried speech therapy, but she proved quite resistant. She showed marked negativism from the beginning. Her reactions were so regularly negative that one could almost estimate her abilities from them. She always put her shoes on the wrong foot; she always began looking at a book upside-down, starting with the last page; she always held the scissors by the blades and tried to cut with the handles. She made little progress during the program. With much individual attention and much patience, it was possible to get her to do some of the table activities, but there would be little carry-over for the next occasion.

Psychotherapy was likewise quite unsuccessful. She developed a strong attachment to the therapist, so much so that she would become withdrawn and depressed if, on her visits to the group, the therapist paid attention to any other child. In therapy sessions her major interest was to try to get the therapist to participate with her in infantile activities, or to do something that would make the therapist look ridiculous. Her mother showed a good deal of resistance to her own therapy. She kept her appointments as a rule, but made very little real progress. The father avoided participation. Both parents have been unwilling to bring her back for follow-up visits.

Group D.

In this group are thirteen cases with minimal or questionable brain damage; it is a very heterogeneous group. These cases will be reviewed by their etiologic aspects and illustrated by eleven brief histories.

Premature Birth

Case 1. This girl had a positive EEG, which showed some rhythmic sharp wave activity over the left tempero-occipital areas which was frequently absent on the right. There was very slow development until the child was 2½ years old. She gained rapidly in our program. The measurable IQ was 84 at the end of one year. For a time she attended a normal kindergarten. She was very shy and socially immature, and the school transferred her to a class for the brain damaged where the children have normal intelligence. Psychotherapy is planned for the coming year because she still has personality problems.

Case 2. This boy had had convulsions at long intervals with negative neurological findings and a negative EEG. He had many neurotic traits and conduct disturbances. He showed some progress when he was in the program, but has regressed since he was removed. Casework with his parents was relatively unsuccessful as they were unusually immature and openly rejected the child. He was finally placed in a state institution, where he has remained.

Case 3. This boy showed negative neurological findings and an EEG within normal limits. He had a severe hearing loss. He did well in the program, which included speech therapy. At the time of writing he is attending a small private school for normal children and is continuing speech therapy.

Case 4. This boy had repeated severe respiratory infections during early life. His development was markedly delayed in all areas. His neurological examination was negative. His EEG throughout the tracing showed intermittent paroxysmal bursts of irregular sharp waves and slow waves from all head regions. In addition, there were prolonged runs of rhythmic square-top waves of high voltage at about two per second from the occipital area bilaterally. The EEG showed a marked bilateral abnormality with definite paroxysmal features of the type seen in convulsive seizures arising from deep midline structures. He showed no progress in the program. Toward the end of his period here, the pediatricians suspected progressive muscular dystrophy. The parents refused to have a special test done to establish or rule out this condition. He was later transferred to a state institution, where he died of pneumonia.

Difficult Delivery

Case 5. This boy is very small for his age and poorly nourished. He had shown delayed bone age. Otherwise the physical findings were negative. His EEG showed some diffuse abnormality over the tempero-occipital areas bilaterally. After six months in the program, his measurable quotient rose from the high moron level to a borderline level (IQ 77). Psychotherapy was given in the hope that his functioning might be further improved. At the time of writing he is in a special residential school.

Brain Injury Due to Accident

Case 6. This girl was without positive neurological findings. Her EEG showed random and occasionally rhythmic slow waves of low-to-moderate voltage over all head regions. There was a diffuse slow-wave activity. She had a sensory aphasia. She responded well to the program combined with speech therapy. A psychological test indicated that she had a potential within normal limits. At the time of writing she is in a class for "neurologically damaged" children making moderately good progress. Psychotherapy seemed strongly indicated because of excessive anxiety, but this could not be worked out because of the distance factor.

Spotting During the Pregnancy

Case 7. This boy showed generally retarded development and some movements of the arms and legs that appeared slightly spastic. His measurable IQ at the time of the intake study was 65 on the Stanford-Binet Test. Since he has many fears, especially of doctors, examinations tended to be unsatisfactory. Brain damage was suspected, but never proved neurologically. His general adjustment has improved; he is no longer fearful and speaks better. Tests showed a dull normal range of general intelligence. At the time of writing he is in a special residential school, where he is making moderately good progress.

Possible Cerebral Palsy

Case 8. This girl had no presenting abnormality at birth, but showed markedly delayed motor development. The diagnosis of cerebral palsy was considered, but never was clearly established by the special outpatient clinic. Her EEG was within normal limits except for some intermittent random high-voltage waves from the occipital areas bilaterally. These were considered to be of questionable clinical significance. Her response to the program was favorable. Her measurable IQ rose from 59 to 82. She attended a health class in public school for four years. At the time of writing she is doing very well in a small residential school for mildly retarded children. In this case, a prolonged period of psychotherapy contributed to her improved adjustment.

Case 9. This girl had brain damage probably due to paranatal factors. There was a history of early convulsions. This child made rather slight gains in our program. She is now attending a school for brain injured children near her home. In this case, the family proved rigid and inflexible and resisted following recommendations.

Case 10. This boy has symptoms suggesting the Charcot-Marie-Tooth Syndrome, with hearing loss and poor coordination. The syndrome does not ordinarily cause mental retardation, but in this case there was some question of this because of delayed speech development. There was also a history of bleeding during middle pregnancy. The child has responded well to a program that included group therapy, speech therapy, and regular sessions with a teacher-therapist. At the time of writing he is adjusting well in a normal kindergarten and is continuing speech and teacher therapy.

Case 11. This girl has multiple congenital defects including a cleft palate. She also was premature. A pediatric neurologist considered her to have a mixed picture of organic defect and emotional problems. She responded well to individual sessions with a teacher-therapist and made gains in speech and social relationships. In this case, open rejection of the child by the parents made planning difficult.

Progress of the group as a whole was as follows: Cases, thirteen; good progress, two; fair progress, six; slight progress, one; no progress, four.

At the time of writing, there are nine children (aged three to about six years) who have completed one school year in the program. Of these nine, seven show "neurotic patterns," one has mild organicity, and one shows a "neurotic pattern with schizoid features." All have shown substantial gains in expressive communication, motor skills, self-care, and social relations. The psychologist finds that at least three of the children show evidence of normal potential. The child who has made the least progress has an especially difficult home situation. All these children have had individual teacher sessions as well as group sessions, and all but two had speech therapy. We plan to continue these children in the program for at least another school year.

COMMENTS

Exclusive of the clearly defined autistic group,[2] there were sixty-one children who have been in our program for varying periods of time, forty-one of which have been studied intensively. Twenty-eight of these had no demonstrable organic basis for their retarded functioning and thirteen had minimal or questionable neurological findings. In most cases the psychologist did not offer a numerical IQ at the time of initial testing, feeling that at the age level and in the presence of emotional problems, test results were not accurate. The psychologist participated in the selection of the cases and agreed that all forty-one showed retarded functioning.

At the end of their participation in the program, it was considered that twelve of the children had made good progress, sixteen fair progress, six slight progress, and seven no progress. Of the seven children who showed no progress, six were in the group classified as possible psychosis with extreme negativism. Our statistics lead us to the conclusion that the most favorable cases for this program are from the categories here classified as "neurotic patterns" and "neurotic patterns with schizoid or autistic features." Of the twenty-two children in these two categories, ten showed good progress and nine showed fair progress. Our group of children with slight or questionable neurological findings is still too small to permit us to form any conclusive opinions. However, the results are sufficiently encouraging for us to plan to continue with them in the program.

There are two prevalent attitudes on the part of many practicing child psychiatrists in the New York City area [3] with which we differ strongly:

1. There is the attitude that a psychiatric diagnosis must be made in terms of either organicity or nonorganicity. Those holding this view seem unable to conceive of a mixed picture. Our experience would suggest that a mixed picture is common. To us it is irrational to say that a child with brain damage can have only one form of pathology, and that this explains everything. Why cannot a child have mild brain damage and a psychoneurosis?

2. There is the attitude that a child who has any evidence of brain damage at all, even a positive EEG without other evidence of CNS involvement, should not be offered psychotherapy. This attitude exists in spite of the known fact that children with brain damage may have normal intelligence. In our experience the results of therapy are always in proportion to the amount of psychopathology. There are some severely disturbed children who respond poorly to a psychotherapeutic program also among those who have no evidence of organic lesions. We believe that the decision whether a child should have psychotherapy depends on the estimate of his ability to profit by it, regardless of the presence or absence of organic pathology.

We are in agreement with Goldberg and Max (1962) who, in their report on studies of a large number of retarded children, write: "From the overall survey of the group, it appears that, in any one child, either organic or psychological factors may be of relatively greater importance. Failure to take both into consideration leads to faulty diagnosis and incomplete treatment." Webster (1963), in his studies of 159 cases of retarded children three to six years old, concluded that mental retardation is a clinical development syndrome that regularly includes an impairment in emotional as well as intellectual development.

We are usually unable to predict from the picture presented at the time of referral how the child will respond. We have found that if a child makes some gains early in response to the program, the chances are that he will continue to gain. Because of this, it has become our policy to consider our first three or four months as an observation period in which we clarify our diagnostic impression and form a prognostic opinion.

In the earlier years of our program, we found that when the children were ready for other programs in the community, they sometimes did less well than we had anticipated. The change to a large group in a public school or a smaller group in a private school seemed to be too drastic. In recent years, this situation has been helped by the formation of several private schools, which are primarily set up for children of normal intelligence with learning problems. New York State will provide a stipend to make attendance in such schools possible even for families of marginal income, if the public schools in the area do not have classes that will meet the child's needs. These private schools have proved to be invaluable in bridging the gap between our very individualized program and the average public school or private-school class. Eventually, we hope to enlarge our program so as to take care of the "gap" ourselves.

It will be noted that we have avoided the terms "brain damage" and "brain dysfunction," which have been discussed so often in the recent literature. We use the term "retarded functioning" rather than "dysfunction," because the latter term has come to be associated with organicity. Our experience with these very young children tends to place us among the "purists" (as classified by Clements, 1962), who believe that brain dysfunction can only be inferred when physiological, biochemical, or structural alterations of the brain are demonstrated.

The symptoms listed by Birch (1964) as suggesting brain damage in children of school age are disordered behavior, short attention span, emotional lability, social incompetence, defective work habits, impulsiveness and meddlesomeness, and specific learning disorders. Some of these symptoms have been observed in our preschool population. Since these symptoms tend to disappear when the psychiatric program is successful, it has been our inclination to regard them as psychogenic. Some psychologists have questioned the validity of psychological tests in establishing the diagnosis of organicity, especially in very young children and in the absence of neurological findings (Kessler, 1968; Graham and Berman, 1961; Beck, 1961; Koppitz, 1962; and Herbert, 1964). These authors emphasize the need for further study by all the disciplines, as do Birch (1964) and Work (1966).

We have not found it helpful to use the term "brain damage" in dealing with parents unless we are very certain of the diagnosis. As indicated earlier, some parents are eager to find their children "brain damaged" rather than to face their own emotional involvement. It is our experience that many physicians, psychologists, social workers, teachers, and speech therapists use this term too freely, without sufficient evidence of its validity in a given case.

SUMMARY

We described a psychiatrically oriented nursery program for preschool children with retarded functioning, the majority of whom showed no demonstrable organic damage or minimal or questionable damage. Until fairly recently, this population has been given little attention, especially of a psychiatric nature. Yet we have found that many of these children can profit from a program suited to their needs. A high percentage of those in our program showed considerably improved functioning. Some reached the point where they tested within the normal range. It is our opinion these gains are due in part to the active participation of the parents, a requirement we made in each case.

We conclude that retarded functioning without demonstrable organic basis in the very early years need not be regarded with pessimism. Our explorations have led us to the conviction that psychogenic factors frequently play a major role in the developmental lag. Therefore, treatment of both the child and his family in this crucial early stage can mean the difference for the child between life as a functioning member of society or an existence within the walls of an institution.

NOTES

1. It was our original purpose to exclude children of this category from the project since they have been extensively treated elsewhere. However, having had so many such referrals, we included some of these children in our program when no other facilities could be found for them. Most of these children were transferred to other agencies as soon as suitable resources were located. It interested us that in the referrals to a retarded children's program, there was included such a large proportion of autistic children.

2. A recent follow-up letter was sent to the parents of the autistic children who had been in the program, and forty-six responded. They reported: good progress, five; fair progress, twelve; slight progress, thirteen; and no progress, sixteen.

3. We have had no experience in any other area.

REFERENCES

Axline, V. Mental deficiency: Symptom or disease. *J. Consult. Psychol.,* 1949, *13*(5), 313–319.

Barsch, R. H. The subtrainable child: A community program. *Amer. J. Ment. Defic.,* 1962, *67,* 33–40.

Beck, H. S. Detecting psychological symptoms of brain injury. *Except. Child,* 1961, *27,* 57–62.

Birch, H. G. *Brain damage in children, the biological and social aspects.* Philadelphia: William & Wilkins, 1964.

Bornstein, B. On the psychogenesis of pseudodebility. *Internat. Zeitschr. f. Psychoanal.,* 1930, *16,* 378–384.

Chidester, L., & Menninger, K. A. The application of psychoanalytic methods to the study of mental retardation. *Amer. J. Orthopsychiat.,* 1936, *6,* 616–621.

Clements, S. D. Minimal brain dysfunction in children. Washington, D.C.: U.S. Department of Health, Education, and Welfare, 1962, NINDB Monograph No. 3.

Cobb, D., & Wilber, R. C. Explorations in family care placement for retarded children. *Amer. J. Ment. Defic.,* 1959, *63*(6), 1089–1092.

Garfield, S. L., & Affleck, D. C. A study of individuals committed to state home for the retarded who were later released as not mentally defective. *Amer. J. Ment. Defic.,* 1960, *64,* 907–915.

Goldberg, B., & Max, P. Postnatal psychological causes of mental retardation. *Canad. Med. Assoc. J.,* 1962, *87,* 507–510.

Graham, F. K., & Berman, P. W. Current status of behavior tests for brain damage in infants and preschool children. *Amer. J. Orthopsychiat.,* 1961, *31,* 713–718.

Heath, S. R. Making up for lost time. *Training Schl. Bull.,* 1941–1942, *38,* 1–5.

Heiser, K. T. Psychotherapy in a residential school for mentally retarded children. *Training Schl. Bull.,* 1954, *50,* 211–216.

Herbert, M. The concept and testing of brain damage in children: A review. *J. Child Psychol. & Psychiat.,* 1964, *5,* 197–201.

Jubenville, C. P. A state program of day care for severely retarded. *Amer. J. Ment. Defic.,* 1962, *66,* 829–837.

Kaplan, S., Abbott, J. A., & Waldfogel, S. Clinic on psychosomatic problems: Feeblemindedness or pseudoretardation? *Amer. J. Med.,* 1948, *5,* 891–896.

Kessler, J. W. Why either . . . or . . . ? *Clin. Psychologist,* 1968, *21*(3), 22–26.

Kirk, S. A. Early education of the mentally retarded: An experimental study. Urbana, Ill., University of Illinois Press, 1958.

Koppitz, E. M. Diagnosing brain damage in young children with the Bender Gestalt test. *J. Consult. Psychol.,* 1962, *26,* 541–549.

Martz, E. W. A phenomenal spurt of mental development in a young child. *Psychiat. Quart.,* 1945, *19,* 52–57.

Rapaport, S. R. Behavior disorder and ego development in a brain injured child. *Psychoanal. Study Child,* 1961, *16,* 423–435.

Skeels, H. M., & Dye, H. B. A. A study of the effects of differential stimulation on mentally retarded children. *Proceedings of the American Association of Mental Deficiency,* 1939, pp. 114–119.

Sloan, W. Preschool class at Lincoln state school and colony. *Amer. J. Ment. Defic.,* 1952, *56,* 755–759.

Strazzula, M. Nursery school training for retarded children. *Amer. J. Ment. Defic.,* 1956, *61*(1), 141–149.

Tizard, J. The residential care of mentally handicapped children. London conference of the scientific aspects of mental deficiency. *Brit. Med. J.,* 1960, pp. 1041–1046, 5178.

Webster, T. G. Problems of emotional development in young retarded children. *Amer. J. Psychiat.,* 1963, *120,* 37–43.

Woodward, K. F., Siegel, M. G., & Eustis, M. J. Psychiatric study of mentally retarded children of preschool age: Report on 1st and 2nd years of a 3-year project. *Amer. J. Orthopsychiat.,* 1958, *28,* 376–380.

Woodward, K. F., Brown, D., & Bird, D. Psychiatric study of mentally retarded preschool children: Report four years after initiation of project, with emphasis on psychiatric and teaching approach. *Arch. Gen. Psychiat.,* 1960, *2,* 156–170.

Woodward, K. F., & Siegel, M. G. Psychiatric study of mentally retarded children of preschool age: Preliminary report. *Pediatrics,* 1957, *19,* 119–124.

Work, H. H., & Haldane, J. E. Cerebral dysfunction in children: A review. *Amer. J. Dis. Child.,* 1966, *111,* 571–572.

[B]

PSYCHOPHARMACOLOG- ICAL APPROACHES AND ISSUES

: 13 :

Psychopharmacology and the Retarded Child

Roger D. Freeman

INTRODUCTION

THE retarded have received fluctuating attention over the years, varying from extreme pessimism and neglect to extreme optimism (Kanner, 1964).[1] We are still on an upswing of optimism ("the retarded *can*
be helped") provided (in part) by governmental support, success of
psychoactive drugs in treating psychiatric patients, and publicity
about possible enhancement of learning and memory by pills (Spencer, 1966).

The behavior problems of retarded persons have been a major
problem for the families and communities in which they live and for
the institutions and schools which train (or contain) them. Lack of adequate staff in state institutions makes the management of psychiatric
disorders difficult; the promise of chemical "tranquilization" (if not
enhanced learning) is naturally received with enthusiasm. Apart from

such justifiable uses, the prescription of a drug may serve less rational purposes: it may get the physician "off the hook" temporarily and it has multiple (sometimes magical) connotations to children, parents, and staff which may be of demonstrable significance in affecting results (Rosenthal, 1967).

The physician who wishes to use the psychoactive drugs is on the horns of a dilemma: the claims made in promotional material are optimistic, yet reading the fine print on adverse reactions could lead to therapeutic nihilism. Pilot studies are almost uniformly favorable, yet many of these drugs are banned or disappear from the market within a few years.

This chapter is divided into two parts. The first summarizes and attempts to assess past studies and methodology; the second is a concise status report on current usage. Every effort has been made to include important studies, even on drugs not available commercially in the United States, but no claim of completeness is made, particularly for the foreign literature.

As will be seen, the variety of adverse drug effects is large and continually expanding with increased use. The reader should *not* depend solely upon information contained in this chapter, which will of necessity be somewhat out of date by the time of publication. The physician's responsibility is clearly to be aware of such effects through reading package inserts and relevant scientific literature.

It would also be wise for the reader to keep in mind Leon Eisenberg's statement (1964): "The first law of psychopharmacology might be formulated to state: the certainty with which convictions are held tends to vary inversely with the depth of the knowledge on which they are based."

AN OVERVIEW OF THE PAST THIRTY YEARS

General Methodological Considerations

A few problems commonly neglected in drug studies will be concisely presented. No extensive coverage of this subject is necessary here because its comprehensive treatment is reviewed in other chapters of this book. Reference may also be made to Nash (1960), Liberman (1961), Cole (1962), Davis (1965), and Zubin and Katz (1966). The book by Fisher (1959) contains several chapters of interest for those working with children.

In any scientific study of the effects of an independent variable (that is, the drug) upon one or more dependent variables (for example, activity level, destructiveness, or other aspects of behavior), the phenomena to be studied (criteria of change) must be specified, a population of subjects (sample) defined, and valid and reliable test instruments chosen for measurement.

When the phenomena to be studied involve personality (feelings, motivations, enduring patterns of behavior), the criteria for measurement are usually imprecise and often subjective. Environmental circumstances are also likely to be a major influence. Laboratory or test situations may be a poor basis for generalization to more natural settings. Recently Zrull and others (1966) showed that different sources of information may disagree with each other about a child's behavior. They suggested that perhaps school and parent observations are more valid indices than clinical measures. Interest is increasing in carrying out observations of the child in his natural setting (Freeman, 1967), including actual measurement of defined behaviors in the classroom (Werry and Quay, 1968). In the past, many drug studies have not adequately described the setting in which the investigation was carried out (Liberman, 1961).

Criteria of change often involve value judgments. The doctor may regard increased aggressive behavior in an inhibited patient as an improvement, although ward staff or parents are likely to find it troublesome and a cause for complaint. Is better adaptation to the peculiar environment of a state hospital to be regarded as a sign of health or as a manifestation of pathology (Paredes et al., 1961)? There is also controversy over whether global, target-symptom (Hesbacher et al., 1968), or a combination of measures (Lipman et al., 1965) are most useful as criteria of change.

The characteristics of the sample are of basic significance. If the size is too small, individual variability may obscure true drug effects. Overall and others (1967) indicated that forty to sixty patients must be included in each group, and that the use of two raters instead of one only reduced the size of the sample needed by 15 to 20 per cent. Conflicting results in different studies may often be accounted for on the basis of sample differences. Particularly in institutional populations, there has been a regrettable tendency to include groups that are grossly heterogeneous in age, length of stay, and types of symptoms or diagnosis.

Multiple influences, many of which cannot easily be experimentally controlled, are at work in drug studies. Some of these are summarized in Table 13–1, which is modified from DiMascio and Klerman (1960).

TABLE 13–1

Factors Influencing Drug Studies

Drug Factors
1. Is the patient taking the drug? (Hare & Willcox, 1967; Maddock, 1967).
2. Route of administration.
3. Dosage: single, multiple; standard, individualized; short- or long-acting form (Cole, 1962; Ostow, 1965); different dose ranges may give *qualitatively* different results (for example, depressant or stimulant) (Chessick & McFarland, 1963).
4. Interaction with drugs previously or concurrently administered (Batterman & Lower, 1968; Berry & Turner, 1968); sequence of drug and placebo.
5. Individual metabolic differences may affect timing of peak action.
6. Duration of study and "washout" period between drugs.
7. Interactions with diet (Asatoor et al., 1963; Resnick, 1965).

Nondrug Factors in the Subject
1. Severity of symptoms, level of anxiety, degree of stress in experimental situation (Beecher, 1960; DiMascio & Barrett, 1965).
2. Constitutional, physiologic, ethnic-cultural, social, and personality factors.
3. Expectations and fantasies may enhance or obscure pharmacologic effect (Knobel, 1960; Fisher, 1962; Dinnerstein, Lowenthal, & Blitz, 1966).
4. Previous experiences with drugs.
5. Relationship between subject and experimenter.
6. Motivation of subject; preparation (or lack of it) for treatment.
7. Clinic patients may be "atypically unresponsive" (Cole, 1962).
8. Practice effects of testing.

Factors in Investigator and Staff
1. Attitudes and expectations which may influence observations (Rosenthal, 1967); if separate rating sheets are not used, seeing previous ratings may bias current ones (Jacobsen, 1965).
2. Attitudes and expectations communicated· to subjects (Uhlenhuth et al., 1959; Haefner et al., 1960; Nash, 1962; Ostow, 1965).
3. Expectations of staff dealing with the patient (or parents if child is at home).
4. Investigator and staff can often guess who is on drug, and who on placebo.
5. Physician's attitude toward "blind" research and use of placebos may be negative (Rickels, 1963).
6. Improper choice of rating scales or statistical methods of analysis.
7. Failure to specify uncontrolled conditions which might have influenced results.

The literature on placebo effects is large and conflicting but of considerable interest. Good general reviews are those of Kurland (1960), Boatman and Berlin (1962), and Liberman (1962). Suggestibility is not the only factor involved, contrary to many opinions, at least in adults (Hornsby et al., 1967). The incidence of placebo effects has been estimated at from 30 to 35 per cent in the studies reviewed by Beecher (1955). Toxic reactions (including extrapyramidal symptoms) may occur (Wolf and Pinsky, 1954). Correlations with personality types and diagnostic categories are unfortunately not well established, so that predicting such reactions in advance is not possible (Wolf et al., 1957). In most studies, a perfectly matched placebo (color, size, taste, and side-effects) is an impossibility. Lewis (1966) has even described a situation in which the active principle in a placebo confounded the phenomena being tested. For several years it has been recognized that separate, individual coding of placebo and drug is needed rather than labeling "Tablet A" and "Tablet B," for example. In the latter situation, side-effects developing in some patients on the drug may break the code for all (Cole, 1962).

Placebo effects are probably most effective when the patient is under stress (that is, "needs" them the most), as pointed out by Beecher (1960). Studies that report no placebo effect are regarded with skepticism by many. Although these problems and others make the use of placebos complex, omission of such usage invalidates many studies. It is common, for example, to read that because the patients had been unresponsive to other drugs given previously, this was considered sufficient to eliminate the need for placebos. It is also considered good practice, where possible, to have a "no-treatment" group which receives neither drug nor placebo.

Double-blind studies are one method, now commonly used, of controlling for the placebo effect and investigator bias. The subjects are "blind" in that they supposedly do not know when (or whether) they are receiving an active drug or a placebo; the investigator and staff are also "blind" in this regard, a third party holding the code until the study is completed. The techniques used in such studies were reviewed by Cass and Frederik (1965).

Unfortunately, there are many limitations in such a design: bias is not completely excluded (patients and staff may guess who is on drug or placebo); attitudes are altered; and small, heterogeneous groups cannot be effectively studied (Hoffer, 1967). Ethical questions have also been raised from time to time (Hoffer, 1967). Guy and others (1967) have suggested an "independent assessment team" as an alternative to the double-blind method. A "triple-blind" technique has also been employed, in which the additional degree of "blindness" refers to the staff's ignorance of the design of the study.

When matched groups are used, matching must be done on all of those variables known to influence the phenomena under study. This should include pre-drug ratings of mean symptom intensity (not just the presence of symptoms) since response to a drug may be correlated with severity of symptoms (Wolpert et al., 1968). Assignment to treated and untreated groups, after matching, should be random.

Perhaps the majority of drug studies are inadequate in design, significantly reducing the applicability and validity of results. More serious, however, is the lack of awareness of many investigators that their work does have such limitations. It is encouraging that this situation is changing, and that journals are upgrading their standards for acceptance. The favorable, uncontrolled pilot study with no reported side-effects is almost extinct.

Finally, it should be remembered that many studies which choose patients who are extreme on some variable will be invalid because of the so-called regression effect (that is, subsequently the mean of the observations would tend to be less extreme anyway), and that positive reports are more likely to be submitted for publication, somewhat biasing the literature.

Special Methodological Considerations with the Retarded Child

In order to demonstrate significant effects, natural variability in the population studied must be reduced or controlled as far as possible. Heterogeneity of a sample means increased variability and reduced power of statistical methods to demonstrate a true drug effect. Since there is no completely satisfactory scheme for classifying the retarded, this limitation is important.

Differentiation among the many labeled groups with developmental problems is frequently difficult. Young children may be categorized as autistic, psychotic, aphasic, brain-damaged, cerebral-palsied, deaf, blind, retarded, suffering from developmental lags, or multiply handicapped. Different professional workers may apply different labels to a child at any one time, utilizing imprecise criteria, and providing the parents with different prognoses and recommendations for management which, in themselves, may alter the child's subsequent development. Even in the same clinic, the category may change from year to year. Not infrequently the firm diagnosis of mental deficiency is the outcome of years of waiting or of therapeutic efforts [that is, it is applied to those children who do not improve or show some area(s) of age-appropriate functioning]. Even in cases with the stigmata of multiple congenital anomalies, assumptions about associated mental deficiency are sometimes too casually made (Koch et al., 1965). Paralleling the controversy in psychiatry over the medical or disease model in mental illness, there is much disagreement over the medical or defect model in mental retardation (Baumeister, 1967; Zigler, 1967).

Under these circumstances, drug research runs into formidable obstacles. In those individuals whose retardation is due to neurological factors (and there is disagreement about the size of this group), the response to drugs may be partly dependent upon which areas or functions of the central nervous system are altered or intact. There seems to be no good reason to assume that such alterations are of only one type, or that their effects are invariant with increasing age.

In the investigation of children in institutions (a group easier to study than out-patients) one must ask what characteristics of the child and his family led to his residence in that particular institution because admission requirements differ from place to place. Furthermore, it has been well established that institutions are not equally likely to produce secondary ("back-ward") syndromes of behavior. Attention given to relatively neglected patients may produce nonspecific effects. Patients from different categories, after long residence in an institution, may appear defective.

Baumeister (1967) has suggested that matching needs to be done not only for chronological and mental ages, but also for school experience, reinforcement history, comprehension of instructions, motor impairment, and other factors. There are few studies which actually have done this.

The prevalence and types of mental disorders in the retarded are other issues. Since criteria for psychiatric disorder are rather vague, this is not surprising. Craft (1959a) reviewed the literature and reported figures of 16 to 44 per cent psychiatric disorder among defectives. He showed that very different percentages could be arrived at using different criteria. Philips (1967) studied 227 retarded children and their families and concluded that most of the children could be termed "emotionally disturbed," but that this was not due to limited intelligence but to delayed, distorted personality development and interpersonal relationships with significant people in childhood. He felt that the kinds of psychopathology were not different in the retarded.

In summary, attempts to demonstrate group drug effects upon retarded children are beset with many complex difficulties, but the nature of the caretaking problems warrants such efforts.

DRUG STUDIES

General Introduction, Terminology, Classification

There have been a number of reviews of drug therapy in the neuropsychiatric disorders of childhood, the most helpful of the recent crop being those of Freed (1962), Grant (1962), Rosenblum (1962), Eveloff (1966), Fish (1968), and Kraft (1968). Attempts to modify the behavior and learning ability of retarded children have been reviewed by Kugelmass (1956, 1959), Craft (1959b), LaVeck and Buckley (1961), and Louttit (1965). A selected, annotated bibliography of drug therapy with the retarded has been prepared by Jones (1966), but it suffers from several errors. Freeman (1966) has surveyed drug effects on learning.

There is no completely satisfactory system for the classification of psychoactive drugs, though many have been proposed (Berger, 1960). There are also differences in terminology, which are particularly obvious when comparing North American and European literature. Table 13-2 summarizes some of the overlapping terms used. Part of

TABLE 13–2
Terminology of Psychoactive Drugs

Hypnotic. Used to induce sleep; in smaller doses may sedate.

Sedative. Agent which produces reduction in tension and excitation short of sleep, but with some impairment of intellectual functions. Many drugs have both hypnotic and sedative effects, depending upon dosage (for example, barbiturates).

Analeptic. A stimulant which counteracts narcosis, as in drug overdosage (for example caffeine, pentylenetetrazol, picrotoxin).

Psycholeptic. Term used infrequently in the United States, which includes drugs depressing mental activity (for example, hypnotics, sedatives, some tranquilizers).

Phrenotropic. Having an action upon the psyche or mental processes, rather than on psychomotor activity (sometimes used as equivalent to psycholeptic).

Neuroleptic. Having an action upon psychomotor excitation with production of neurological syndromes which were originally thought to be necessary to desired effect; now used interchangeably in the United States for "major tranquilizer" or "antipsychotic."

Tranquilizer. Used to include neuroleptics (*major;* antipsychotic) and *minor* or antianxiety agents. European usage sometimes distinguishes some of them from neuroleptics because of lack of neurological syndromes (minor agents).

Ataractic (ataraxic). "Ataraxy" means absence of anxiety or confusion; often used interchangeably with major, or major and minor, tranquilizers.

Psychic energizer. This term is approximately equivalent to *antidepressant, mood elevator,* and *thymoleptic.*

Stimulant. Increases activity of CNS; includes amphetamines and analeptics; some classifications include the antidepressants, others do not.

the difficulty stems from the purposes of classification: Should the basis be chemical structure, even though the mechanism of action is not known and different drugs may have almost identical effects? Or should it be mode of action, pharmacological effects in animal studies, or target symptoms which are presumably affected? Further complications ensue from the fact that several drugs belong to more than one chemical group. For the purposes of this review, a combination of approaches has been chosen, for which no special advantage is claimed.

Side-effects (adverse effects) of most of the psychoactive drugs are fairly common and of such variety that no complete or final description can be attempted. Major effects are discussed or listed with the drug description. Table 13–4 in the section Discussion and Conclusions contains a concise compilation, but recourse to the latest information and package insert is mandatory for anyone contemplating using a drug with which he is not familiar. Drugs listed under "others" are so designated because no significant studies could be found in the literature. Some of the more unusual drugs were classified with the assistance of the very helpful book by Usdin and Efron (1967).

In general, efforts to modify the behavior of retarded children with drugs began long ago with sedatives and hypnotics, proceeded to stimulants and anticonvulsants in the late 1930's, antihistamines by the end of World War II, minor tranquilizers in the early 1950's, and then passed on largely to the major tranquilizers in the mid-1950's.

The Major Tranquilizers

These drugs are also known as "antipsychotic" agents, though their use is certainly not limited to psychotic states. Although the groups differ pharmacologically, they have rather similar adverse effects. The reasons for this are not fully understood.

PHENOTHIAZINES

Since 1952 the phenothiazines have become one of the most frequently prescribed groups of drugs in the United States; new compounds are constantly being synthesized. Their site of action is presumably subcortical; that is, they probably act upon those structures which involve emotion rather than upon the cortex. Desired effects can therefore be obtained without impairment of consciousness, although the mechanisms of action are not well understood. They possess no great tendency to cause psychic or physical dependence.

Metabolism and Dosage. It is said that the more severely disturbed the patient, the higher the dosage of major tranquilizers he can tolerate without serious adverse effects (Kinross-Wright, 1967). It is not known why a person may respond favorably to one and not another drug of the same group. The rate of metabolic degradation and excretion of these drugs is significant in planning sequential studies and in considering experimental variables. Recently there have been several reports of prolonged excretion with marked variability in rate of degradation (Kinross-Wright, 1967; Curry and Marshall, 1968). Cowen and Martin (1968) reported that cortisone increases the rate of chlorpromazine excretion and that some elderly patients excrete the drug for as long as one to one and one-half years after ceasing medication. Differences in stress might affect blood levels through corticosteroid production and become a relevant variable. The significance of these findings in work with children is not clear. Long-acting and depot preparations seem to have little value (except perhaps in uncooperative patients on hospital leave who do not take prescribed medication).

Personality Type and Drug Responsiveness. Many attempts have been made to find correlations without much success. Some of the reasons for this disappointment are discussed by Zubin and Katz (1966). However, one clinical observation has been confirmed by Heninger and others (1965). Persons whose defenses center around psychomotor activity and "acting-out" behavior may feel the actions of these drugs as ego-threatening, whereas introspective, intellectualizing patients do not. Paradoxical reactions may be partly explicable on this basis.

Side-effects. The most common of these are due to the anticholinergic action of the phenothiazines: dry mouth, constipation, urinary retention, blurred vision, and so on. The remarkable list of adverse effects is constantly being expanded. Kinross-Wright's statement (1967, p. 463) seems apt: "It is conceivable that there does exist an adverse reaction which has not been attributed to the phenothiazines, but one doubts it. . . ." He attributed this variety to diverse pharmacological actions, widespread use, long duration of treatment with high doses, and perhaps certain psychophysiological quirks in persons taking them.

Most serious reactions are either dose-related responses due to effects upon the central or autonomic nervous systems, or idiosyncratic (allergic) responses. Only some of the more important and interesting effects can be noted here.

Extrapyramidal reactions were formerly thought to be necessary for therapeutic efficacy (the origin of the term "neuroleptic"), but there is much doubt about this now (Hollister, 1964; Chien and Di-Mascio, 1967; Kinross-Wright, 1967). There is disagreement as to whether children are more or less susceptible than adults (Hollister, 1964; Corless and Buchanan, 1965; Fish, 1968). Hollister (1964) stated that women are more susceptible than men. Encephalitis and meningitis can sometimes present similar pictures. Malitz and Hoch (1966) reported that extrapyramidal symptoms (EPS) are more common with the aliphatic (chlorpromazine-like) subgroup; others have indicated that the piperazine subgroup is more often the cause.

The EPS may be divided into *Parkinson-like symptoms* and *dyskinetic symptoms*. The Parkinsonian symptoms include tremors, cogwheel rigidity, shuffling gait, pill-rolling movements, excessive salivation, and masklike faces; incidence is reported (Hollister, 1964) to be between 15 and 45 per cent, increasing with age and occurring more commonly with the aliphatic subgroup. Dyskinetic symptoms may include sweating, pallor, abnormal movements of face, neck, and tongue, mandibular tics, difficulty in speech and swallowing, torticollis, oculogyric crises, and hyperextension of the neck and trunk (Hollister, 1964). The incidence is reported to be 2 to 3 per cent. Another type of reaction described in adults is *akathisia,* which involves inner restlessness and an inability to keep still. These manifestations may be managed with the antiparkinsonian drugs.

In adults, there is controversy over dyskinetic effects which appear late (even after the drug has been stopped) and may be irreversible (Kline, 1968; Crane, 1968). In children, such cases must be quite rare but have been described by Dabbous and Bergman (1966) and Angle and McIntyre (1968). Oculogyric crisis after a small single dose of perphenazine was reported by Kozinn and Wiener (1960). Corless and Buchanan (1965), in a tentative study, suggested that their three children who developed transient signs of an upper motor-neuron lesion might have been predisposed by dehydration. (Hyperthermia can result from these drugs, and heat seems to potentiate some of their adverse effects.) A neurological syndrome commonly encountered by Gupta and Lovejoy (1967) consisted of opisthotonus, torticollis, dystonia, rigidity, and hyperreflexia. They pointed out the need for a high index of suspicion because not infrequently the child, parents, and even physician may have forgotten that a phenothiazine was given. The symptoms may be episodic and partly controlled by conscious effort. Most frequently implicated were prochlorperazine and chlorpromazine; intravenous diphenhydramine (Benadryl) was said to be the best antidote.

Although the phenothiazines are often said to be contraindicated in patients with convulsive disorders, there seems to be little good support for this warning. In fact, although brain-damaged subjects may have a slight excess of seizures while taking the drugs (Logothetis, 1967), improvement in frequency of convulsive episodes has also been reported, at least with thioridazine (Baldwin and Kenny, 1966; Kamm and Mandel, 1967) and prochlorperazine (Carter, 1959).

Phenothiazines are the leading cause of drug-induced *blood dyscrasias* in the United States. The incidence is reported by Hollister (1964) to be one in 3,000 to 4,000 patients under long-term therapy. Periodic blood counts unfortunately offer little protection because the onset is usually sudden. Fever, weakness, sore throat, and other systemic signs should alert the physician.

Skin reactions include photosensitization, rashes, and a peculiar purplish discoloration (Greiner and Berry, 1964; Gombas and Yarden, 1967), which seem to be dose-related.

Jaundice usually occurs early in treatment and is almost always reversible (cholestatic rather than hepatocellular). It appears in less than 1 per cent of patients and only very rarely with thioridazine (Barancik et al., 1967).

Eye changes may include retinitis pigmentosa with thioridazine (Hagopian et al., 1966) and corneal and lenticular opacities (Greiner and Berry, 1964; Geiger and Lesser, 1967; Satanove and McIntosh, 1967). Reversibility is questionable; occurrence is more common than skin lesions (Kinross-Wright, 1967) and is dose-related. Most cases show no visual impairment despite the lesions.

Adrenergic blocking (sympatholytic) effect may result in hypotension, especially with chlorpromazine, promazine, thioridazine, and triflupromazine. Great caution should be used by starting parenteral administration with a low dose.

Electrocardiographic changes are sometimes noted (especially with thioridazine in high doses), and very rarely sudden death may occur, presumably due to cardiovascular effects (Leestma and Koenig, 1968).

(In the following descriptions, drugs 1 to 3 are aliphatic or dimethylaminopropyl derivatives; drugs 4 to 13 are piperazines; 14 and 15 are piperidines; 16 and 17 are in a miscellaneous category.)

1. *Chlorpromazine* (Thorazine, Largactil). The first major drug of this group, chlorpromazine, was preceded by phenothiazine itself (an antihelminthic) and methylene blue. It has yet to be clearly surpassed,

and is often used as a standard against which other major tranquilizers are compared (Peppel and Joynes, 1963).

Bair and Herold (1955) used chlorpromazine with the ten worst management problems in a training school and employed a matched control group. Their very enthusiastic conclusions were that 90 per cent of the drug-treated group improved in behavior without side-effects; they found that attention span was increased and tested IQ rose an average of 10.4 in the experimental subjects, as compared with only 2.5 for the controls. The size of the sample, however, was very small, and according to Rosenblum (1962) the test instrument chosen was not adequately standardized for this type of study.

Rettig (1955) performed an uncontrolled experiment and reported improvement in twenty-three out of twenty-seven highly disturbed patients who had failed to make progress on other drugs or management. Esen and Durling (1956) employed a small group (with an even smaller control group) and concluded that the drug was helpful in improving learning in hyperactive retarded boys. MacColl (1956) used no controls but felt that the 74 per cent improvement could be attributed to the drug. Of a very large group of retardates, about 70 per cent improved in an uncontrolled investigation by Tarjan and others (1957). Ison (1957) gave a standard dose to sixty-two retardates, ages eight to forty-eight, of above 40 IQ, and reported no changes in IQ after one month on the drug. A matched control group was used, but it is hard to see why changes should appear on psychological testing in so short a time.

A group of reports during 1957 all compared chlorpromazine with reserpine in severely disturbed, institutionalized retardates and found considerable benefit with both but no significant advantage of one over the other. No controls were used (Horenstein, 1957; Johnston and Martin, 1957; Sprogis et al., 1957; Wolfson, 1957). A double-blind study of forty retarded patients, ages eight to forty, with a control group matched for age, sex, weight, ward, mental age, etiology, and type of management problem was reported by Adamson and others (1958). Placebo effects in some groups ran as high as 70 per cent, but the drug-treated groups improved somewhat more, though there were no changes in intellectual functioning. Rudy and others (1958) used partial controls and found that twenty-two of twenty-five patients improved in behavior.

Control of hyperactivity in children of normal intelligence is said to be possible with chlorpromazine. Freed and Peifer (1956b) reported beneficial effects in hyperactive children and felt the drug "facilitated the learning process" and increased emotional control. The setting was a child psychiatric out-patient clinic, and no controls were used. Other studies with hyperactive children include Werry and others (1966) and Weiss and others (in press). These studies showed a reduction in hyperactivity but no benefit on cognitive functions. The latter investigation produced several other interesting findings: psychiatrists were able to guess, prior to breaking the code, 100 per cent of those children receiving the drug; this was thought to be due to the relatively high incidence of side-effects. Chlorpromazine was more reliable than dextroamphetamine in reducing hyperactivity, but the latter tended to improve cognitive functioning and had fewer side-effects.

Freed and others (1959) reported that retarded readers did better with the drug and remedial instruction than with drug alone or with instruction plus placebo; this seems to contradict the findings of Weiss and others (in press), although differences in the populations studied may help account for the discrepancy. A deficiency of the Freed and others (1959) investigation was the high rate of drop-outs (twenty-seven of seventy).

Several investigators have reported on use of the drug with children suffering from psychoses, neurotic reactions, and behavior disorders. Freedman and others (1955) found it more effective than placebo with hyperactive schizophrenic children. All of a small group of severely disturbed, acting-out boys were reported to improve more than a control group by Gatski (1955). Miksztal (1956) used chlorpromazine in an uncontrolled study of mixed neuropsychiatric disorders. Sixty-five to eighty-one per cent of seventy-four children showed moderate to marked improvement, depending upon diagnostic category. Other positive results with groups of mixed etiology were described by Freed and Peifer (1956*a*) and Hunt and others (1956). Negative results, with impairment in attention span, in paired-associate learning, and on the Porteus Maze Test were reported by Garfield and others (1962) and Helper and others (1963) in uncontrolled studies.

In conclusion, chlorpromazine has been used in a wide variety of conditions and seems to have a beneficial effect upon children (retarded or of normal IQ) who are highly disturbed, particularly if psychomotor overactivity is present. Adverse effects are varied and not uncommon, but in usual doses are rarely sufficient to require termination of treatment. High doses can directly impair learning and performance (Hartlage, 1965). Its usefulness in learning disabilities remains unsettled, probably depending partly upon whether excessive anxiety is impairing concentration.

2. *Promazine* (Sparine). This drug is not quite as potent as chlorpromazine and seems to have no advantage over it (Fish, 1968). Some

investigators report a higher incidence of seizures than with other phenothiazines (Kinross-Wright, 1967). Favorable uncontrolled reports with the disturbed retarded were published by Esen and Durling (1957), Benda (1958), Rudy and others (1958), and Bergin and Bergin (1958). A combination with meprobamate (Prozine) was used in a controlled study by LaVeck and Buckley (1961) of fifty-four disturbed, retarded children with spastic cerebral palsy. No statistically significant effects were demonstrated, and some drowsiness was encountered. Prozine was also used in an uncontrolled study by Faretra and Gozun (1964), who considered it definitely superior to the phenothiazines alone in both organic and nonorganic behavior disorders. The children were said to show more interest in learning.

Schulman and Clarinda (1964) measured the effect of promazine alone on the diurnal activity level of six hyperactive, retarded boys at four dosage levels, using an actometer to avoid bias in quantitative assessment. (The actometer is a modification of a self-winding wristwatch, worn on the wrist and ankle of the dominant side and read periodically to measure total activity.) In an attempt to diminish any placebo response, the staff were told that no effect might result from the drug and that placebo was being used half the time. No placebo effect was demonstrated, and no change in activity level occurred with the drug. Conceivably a true drug effect may have been masked by this "antiplacebo" method.

3. *Triflupromazine* (Vesprin). This drug was introduced in 1957 and reported to improve the behavior of disturbed adult retardates in an uncontrolled study by Himwich and others (1960). Shaw and others (1963) did a controlled, partially double-blind comparison of triflupromazine with trifluoperazine (Stelazine), thioridazine (Mellaril), and fluphenazine (Prolixin, Permitil). They reported no significant differences among the drugs. Sixty-eight per cent of the total group of severely emotionally disturbed children in a residential setting improved significantly. Triflupromazine had a higher incidence of troublesome side-effects than the other drugs, however.

Other aliphatic phenothiazines: Acetylpromazine (acetopromazine, Acepromazine); promethazine (Phenergan) is used as an antihistamine and in anesthesiology.

4. *Prochlorperazine* (Compazine, Stemetil; introduced in 1956). Despite early positive reports with disturbed retarded children (Bowman and Blumberg, 1958; Carter, 1959; Craft, 1959b; Mitchell et al., 1959; and Pilkington, 1959), Rosenblum and others (1960) found that a placebo group improved more than either an untreated group

or the prochlorperazine-treated group, and that the last had the least improvement.

In a well-controlled study, Cytryn and others (1960) found pro-chlorperazine no more helpful than placebo in behavior disorders seen in an out-patient clinic.

No investigations with retarded children utilizing adequate designs were found in the literature. The evidence in favor of this drug's usefulness is therefore slim.

5. *Perphenazine* (Trilafon; introduced in 1957). Perphenazine has a higher incidence of side-effects than many other phenothiazines. No significant difference from the placebo-treated group was found with a group of delinquent boys studied by Molling and others (1962). Both groups improved, but the placebo group maintained its gains *better* than the drug group.

A well-controlled study of neurotic and hyperactive children by Ei-senberg and others (1961) found brief psychotherapy alone as effective as the drug in changing behavior.

Jaquith and others (1967) reported their analysis of the rate of readmission among former mental hospital patients (about 9 per cent of whom were diagnosed as retarded) and concluded that the drug reduced duration of hospital stay and the risk of rehospitalization.

No studies of the retarded were found in the literature; the drug seems to have no benefit over chlorpromazine, trifluoperazine, or thioridazine.

6. *Thiopropazate* (Dartal; introduced in 1957). Laird and Hope (1959) reported favorably upon the use of this drug with hospitalized schizophrenic patients. Despite the use of placebo, the study was limited by a small sample. The results were not dramatic, and the drug, although available, is not described in the *Physicians' Desk Reference* (PDR).

7. *Trifluoperazine* (Stelazine; introduced in 1958). Although the phenothiazines are generally recommended for agitation, trifluopera-zine has been reported to have an "activating" effect upon withdrawn, apathetic patients, a group usually less responsive to the major tran-quilizers (Fish, 1960*b;* Himwich et al., 1960). Beaudry and Gibson (1960) described a normalization process in which severely disturbed retarded children with both withdrawn and hyperactive behavior lost their extreme symptoms.

Freed (1961) observed excellent improvement in fifteen of twenty-three child psychiatric out-patients who had failed to respond to other drugs, but no controls were used. Most of the children developed adverse reactions, but no seizures occurred, even in those with abnormal EEG's. Freed and Frignito (1961) felt trifluoperazine was useful in the management of autistic and psychotic children.

Hunter and Stephenson (1963) did a controlled study in which the nursing staff was encouraged to believe in the effectiveness of the placebos, which were given fictitious names. It was concluded that both chlorpromazine and trifluoperazine helped severely subnormal children regardless of age or etiology. Fine (1964) and Rosewell (1964), in uncontrolled studies, both reported that about one-third of their retarded patients improved.

Silberstein and others (1965) were able to keep eight out of ten psychotic children from being institutionalized with this drug, but no controls were used. A controlled study of twenty-two retarded autistic children, ages two through six, was reported by Fish and others (1966). Only the most severely impaired, nonverbal children improved, the verbal children tending to deteriorate. They suggested, as have others, that control and treatment groups must be matched for severity of illness.

In summary, too little work has been done to confirm the impression that trifluoperazine is more effective than other phenothiazines in treating the withdrawn, apathetic patient. Side-effects are probably somewhat more likely than with chlorpromazine or thioridazine.

8. *Fluphenazine* (Prolixin, Permitil; introduced in 1959). On a milligram-per-milligram comparison, fluphenazine is perhaps one hundred times as potent as chlorpromazine (Fish, 1968). Niswander and Karacan (1959) reported that the drug was effective but had a high incidence of side-effects. LaVeck and others (1960) found no statistically significant improvement in a small controlled study with hyperactive, aggressive, destructive, retarded children. A positive response was reported by Waites and Keele (1963) in an uncontrolled study of children and young adults with similar problems.

The potency of fluphenazine seems to offer no clear-cut advantage because the adverse effects are at least as common as with chlorpromazine and the drug has been less adequately studied in retarded populations.

9. *Acetophenazine* (Tindal; introduced in 1961). McLaughlin and others (1962) reported positive results in an uncontrolled study of out-patient children with emotional problems; no adverse effects were noted. In 1963, the A.M.A. Council on Drugs stated that the value of acetophenazine was "not established." Darling (1963) found it helpful in 72 per cent of child and adolescent ambulatory schizophrenics, with few side-effects except lethargy. McLaughlin and others (1964),

in a follow-up study on their earlier work, reported that hyperactivity was reduced and the great majority of children improved but no controls were employed. Finally, Madsen (1965) described the successful treatment of a seventeen-year-old autistic, retarded boy who had been resistant to chlorpromazine and chlorprothixene therapy.

No studies of sufficient numbers of retarded, disturbed children are available to assess the value of acetophenazine, which seems to have no advantage over the better-known phenothiazines.

10. *Carphenazine* (Proketazine; introduced in 1963). Carter (1961) used this drug in the management of 110 institutionalized, retarded vomiters. He found it to be exceptionally effective as an antiemetic, with additional benefits in modifying behavior, but no controls were utilized. No increase in frequency of seizures, or of extrapyramidal side-effects (EPS) were noted. However, the A.M.A. Council on Drugs (1963) stated that the EPS and somnolence were fairly common, especially in higher dosages. It was felt by the Council that the drug was useful in the treatment of schizophrenia.

In 1963, Peppel and Joynes found carphenazine to be superior to chlorpromazine with schizophrenic adults. However, it has not replaced chlorpromazine or the other better-known phenothiazines, and its use in the retarded child has not been adequately explored.

11. *Dixyrazine* (dixirazine; Esucos, Metronal; not available in the United States). The structure of this drug is a combination of promazine and hydroxyzine. A double-blind crossover study by Lindholm (1967) yielded favorable results in reduction of hyperactivity and anxiety in retarded patients, without significant adverse effects.

12. *Butaperazine* (butyrylperazine; Repoise, Randolectil; not available in the United States).[2] Rajotte and others (1965) studied the effect of this drug (used in France and West Germany) on forty chronic adult schizophrenics with a double-blind design. It was found to be comparable to prochlorperazine. No reports of its use with retarded children were encountered.

13. *Oxypertine* (not available in the United States). Two controlled studies indicated that it is not an effective drug, at least for adults (Robinson and others, 1965; Hunt, 1967). (It can also be classified as a butyrophenone.)

Other piperazines: Thioproperazine (Majeptil); methophenazine.

14. *Mepazine* (Pacatal; introduced in 1957). Gillie (1957) felt that this drug was of limited value in a controlled study of low-grade retardates, but the sample was small. Ten of the twenty-three patients treated by Rudy and others (1958) showed improvement. Side-effects

are now felt to render this drug less useful than others, and it is not recommended by Fish (1968).

15. *Thioridazine* (Mellaril; introduced in 1959). This drug has fewer side-effects than many of the aliphatic and piperazine subgroups and has been extensively studied (Hollister, 1964; Barancik et al., 1967).

All the available studies with retarded children are favorable: LeVann (1961), Oettinger and Simonds (1961), Badham and others (1963), Allen and others (1963), Abbott and others (1965), Leger (1966), Baldwin and Kenny (1966), Kamm and Mandel (1967), Pregelj and Barkauskas (1967), and Alexandris and Lundell (1968). These studies differ in the adequacy of their experimental controls but add up to an impressive recommendation.

Kamm (1965) and Leger (1966) both commented on reduction in disturbing sexual behavior in older patients, though no generally applicable results are available. For other neuropsychiatric disorders, positive studies include the following: Freed and others (1959) and Freed (1962) in uncontrolled trials with behavior and learning disorders in children of normal IQ; Alderton and Hoddinott (1964) in reducing aggressive, hyperactive behavior in severely disturbed children in a residential setting; and Lucas (1964) in Gilles de la Tourette's Syndrome. Sprague, Barnes, and Werry (unpublished manuscript), however, found that normal-IQ, learning-disability children suffered a decrement in performance as compared with methylphenidate, which enhanced performance and reduced hyperactivity.

Davis and others (1969) performed an investigation of the effect of thioridazine upon stereotyped behavior in nine severely retarded adolescent males who acted as their own controls. Confidence in the results is increased by the sophisticated methodology employed. The drug was found to significantly decrease stereotypy without affecting other behavior, as compared with placebo, no-drug, and methylphenidate conditions. Findings were felt to be consistent with the interpretation of stereotyped behavior as a consequence, rather than a cause, of states of arousal.

Mellinger and others (1965) found that thioridazine accumulates within three or four days, so that administration on a once-a-day basis should be adequate; long-acting preparations would seem to have no advantage.

With the exception of having no palatable liquid form, thioridiazine seems to be exceptionally safe for use with retarded children, and the literature is uniformly positive in its reports. The presence of a convulsive disorder is no contraindication to its use.

16. *Piperacetazine* (Quide; not available in the United States). This drug was reported to be beneficial in an uncontrolled pilot study of twenty-six chronic schizophrenic adults by Kirkham and Kinross-Wright (1964). No other investigations were found.

17. *Propericiazine* (pericyazine; Neuleptil, Neulactil; not available in the United States). Wartel (1966) and Daneel (1967) reported positive results in uncontrolled studies with retardates. A recent comparison with chlorpromazine by Weir and others (1968) failed to discuss results or indicate dosages, so that conclusions cannot be drawn.

Summary. There are no adequate comparative studies of the many phenothiazines in children. Hanlon and others (1965) investigated the comparative effectiveness of eight of these drugs. They found promazine and mepazine to be significantly less effective than chlorpromazine, thioridazine, perphenazine, fluphenazine, prochlorperazine, triflupromazine, trifluoperazine, and thiopropazate, all of which seemed approximately equivalent in patients over age eighteen.

The reputed activating effect of the piperazine subgroup (already mentioned under trifluoperazine) has not been well established in children. The usefulness of chlorpromazine and thioridazine in reducing psychomotor excitement and disorganized, psychotic behavior seems to be firmly based in numerous controlled studies. However, since individuals vary so much, a trial of another major tranquilizer may be indicated when one of these fails to produce the desired results.

Few new phenothiazines have appeared in recent years, perhaps because of discouragement in efforts to surpass chlorpromazine. Only time will tell whether anything dramatically new remains to be discovered among the derivatives of these drugs. In the meantime, there is still much work to be done in improving comparability of studies through selecting samples that are relatively homogeneous and of adequate size.

RAUWOLFIA ALKALOIDS (FOR EXAMPLE, RESERPINE)

This group of drugs has been used, in crude form, for many centuries in India for the treatment of mental illness. The name derives from the botanist Rauwolf in whose honor the root was named (Klotz, 1959). Since their introduction for psychiatric use around 1954, these drugs went through a period of wide usage but were rather quickly replaced by the phenothiazine drugs because of unpredictability of response and dangerous side-effects (Lucas, 1966; Fish, 1968). The derivatives still have a place in the treatment of hypertension and may still be used in psychiatry either where other drugs have failed or where cost is an important consideration (they are less expensive than phenothiazines). No improvement in tested intelligence has been reported in studies with the retarded. Because of their very limited usefulness, selected studies are listed in Table 13–3 rather than in the text.

TABLE 13–3

Studies with Reserpine in Disturbed Retarded Children

RESULTS POSITIVE		RESULTS NEGATIVE	
CONTROLLED STUDIES	UNCONTROLLED STUDIES	CONTROLLED STUDIES	UNCONTROLLED STUDIES
Timberlake et al. (1957)	Lehman et al. (1957)	Rosenblum et al. (1958)	
Adamson et al. (1958)	Pallister & Stevens (1957)	Kirk & Bauer (1956)	
Fischer (1956)	Horenstein (1957)		
	Johnston & Martin (1957)		
	Sprogis et al. (1957)		
	Wolfson (1957)		

THIOXANTHENES

This group of drugs is related to the phenothiazines. Despite occasional descriptions as "minor tranquilizers," their pharmacologic effects clearly place them in the major tranquilizer category. Used since the beginning of the 1960's in Europe, only two of these drugs have been introduced into the United States. Side-effects and contraindications are generally the same as for the phenothiazines, although some have claimed that the incidence of adverse reactions is lower.

Chlorprothixene (Taractan). This drug was the first of the thioxanthenes. Pilkington (1961) compared it to chlordiazepoxide in the behavior disorders of retarded children, but the group was small (twenty-one) and no controls were utilized. Oettinger (1962) reported that its effects were comparable to thioridazine in an uncontrolled study of habit, conduct, and neurotic disturbances. McCray and others (1963) used it on a long-term basis with adolescents and adults (including the retarded) and obtained good to excellent results in 52 per cent (uncontrolled study). Dietze (1963) reported a case of a thirteen-year-old retarded boy who had a typical dyskinetic reaction. In 1966, Harman and Winn compared it favorably with chlorpromazine in severely disturbed children, yet close examination of their data seems to indicate no significant benefit for either drug over placebo at the dosages used.

Thiothixene (Navane). This drug has been introduced only recently. Wolpert and others (1966) reported a favorable response among drug-resistant children with autistic features, but no controls were used in the small series. Hackett and others (1968) stated that thiothixene was especially useful in highly anxious, depressed patients; Filotto and others (1968) used it with good results in adult manic states. Wolpert and others (1968), however, found it slightly inferior to thioridazine in a controlled study of adult chronic schizophrenics.

Clopenthixol (Sordinol; not available in the United States). This drug has the same side-chain as perphenazine. Wolpert and others (1967) published an initial positive report on adult schizophrenia. Kordas and others (1968) compared it favorably with chlorpromazine in a similar group. Dehnel and his colleagues (1968) found more frequent and severe side-effects than with perphenazine in a controlled comparison, and no greater efficacy in their adult patients could be demonstrated. In adults, therefore, it seems to have no advantage over the older drugs. No studies on its use with children were found in the literature.

Summary. Only chlorprothixene has been used in a number of studies performed on children. It seems about as effective as chlorpromazine and related drugs but has no clear advantages. None of these drugs have been adequately tested in use with disturbed retarded children.

THE BUTYROPHENONES

These major tranquilizers are unrelated to the phenothiazines. They have been used since the early 1960's outside the United States, but the first, haloperidol, was only released here in 1967. Side-effects are similar to the phenothiazines, including EPS at relatively low dosage levels in adults. Central nervous system depressants may be potentiated, but anticonvulsants probably are not. EPS can usually be adequately controlled with antiparkinson agents.

Haloperidol (Haldol; introduced in 1967). In 1962, Jensen reported that this drug had a marked to moderate beneficial effect in 67 per cent of psychotic mental defectives, with rapid onset of action (uncontrolled study). Court and Cameron (1963) stated that the drug was actively antipsychotic and not merely sedative in their ten cases of manic or schizophrenic excitement. Gerle (1963) reported on three years' experience. He concluded that the drug was helpful in hyperactive retardates at a maintenance dose level of 1 to 2 mg per day (uncontrolled study).

Renard and others (1965) described twenty-five children and adolescents who received the drug in a school for maladjusted children, many of whom had IQ's in the mildly retarded range. Results were good to very good in sixteen cases. However, other drugs were given concurrently, confounding the effect of haloperidol. This was justified by the claim that the dose could be kept lower with the combination. Antiparkinson drugs were given routinely, rather than waiting for side-effects to develop. One very important feature of these drugs is mentioned: a tasteless, odorless concentrate is available, which permits easy administration in food or drink.

Another uncontrolled study was reported by Berthiaume, and his colleagues (1966). Thirty-six of the eighty-nine cases were retarded, and of these the best results occurred with the mildly defective without obvious brain damage. No increase in seizures was noted among epileptics. Side-effects occurred in 27 per cent of the patients but were usually readily controlled.

Jacobs (1966) found haloperidol most useful in states of psychomotor agitation, aggression, and self-mutilation, as well as excessive masturbation. Out of sixty-five children who received the drug, only two developed EPS, and there were no other major adverse effects in this uncontrolled study.

Crane (1967) reviewed the drug's usage and side-effects. Earlier reports of significant improvement in Gilles de la Tourette's Syndrome (multiple tics and coprolalia) were confirmed by Lucas (1967) and Connell and others (1967). The latter group found it to be superior to diazepam. [This author's own experience and a recent paper by Shapiro and Shapiro (1968) agree with the peculiar specificity of haloperidol for this rare and little-understood condition.]

LeVann (1968a) performed an uncontrolled study and reported that of one hundred patients 86 per cent improved, although in the retarded group only 37 per cent changed in a favorable direction that was rated "marked" or "moderate."

Recently three controlled studies have become available. Barker and Fraser (1968) studied seventeen children with different diagnoses. Side-effects were minimal, and the results of drug treatment were clearly superior to placebo. Burk and Menolascino (1968) performed a double-blind investigation of disturbed retarded children and adolescents. A two-week "drying-out" period (without drugs) was followed by administration of haloperidol to twenty-six patients and placebo to twenty-four control subjects, using a flexible dosage schedule. Nineteen per cent showed marked improvement, with some favorable change occurring in 81 per cent of the drug-treated group and in 25 per cent of the placebo-treated group. EPS appeared in three children but responded to dosage reduction.

LeVann (1968b) compared the drug with chlorpromazine in a double-blind study that omitted placebo and utilized a flexible dosage schedule. Global and target-symptom changes were rated, but the rating scale was not well operationalized (defined), which may somewhat limit the validity of the conclusions. Only three of seventy-eight patients receiving haloperidol developed EPS. The conclusion was that haloperidol was superior to chlorpromazine in controlling impulsive, hostile, aggressive behavior in institutionalized retardates. Incidence of side-effects was not significantly different from chlorpromazine.

The A.M.A. Council on Drugs (1968) concluded that haloperidol is a useful drug in treating the hyperactivity of psychotic patients. Approval for use with patients under age twelve may be forthcoming shortly but currently remains under investigation.

Trifluperidol (Triperidol; not available in the United States). This drug is often thought to be two separate drugs because of confusion about the trade and generic names. Gallant and colleagues (1963) found it to be superior to chlorpromazine in a double-blind study of chronic adult schizophrenics, as did Pratt and others (1964) with acute schizophrenics. Hollister and co-workers (1965) were enthusiastic in describing trifluperidol as the most effective drug they had ever used with paranoid patients, but no controls were used. Finally, LeVann (1968c) treated fifty children with mixed neuropsychiatric disorders in an uncontrolled study. Ten of fourteen psychotic retarded children were said to improve. No controlled study with retarded children was found in the literature.

Benperidol (benzperidol, Frenactil; not available in the United States). This drug was studied by Pellet and others (1967) in seventeen children, eight of whom were retarded; six of the eight children improved in this uncontrolled clinical trial. There were few cases of EPS. Schmidt and Daudet (1968) also described an uncontrolled clinical trial consisting of mostly retarded children, the majority of whom improved. "Side-effects subsided after the initial period. No controlled studies with children were encountered."

Summary. Haloperidol seems to be an effective drug for use with the disturbed retarded child, and especially in Gilles de la Tourette's Syndrome (where most children have normal intelligence). One controlled study which has some methodological flaws suggests it is at least as good as chlorpromazine. Drowsiness and EPS are the most common side-effects; apparently other more serious adverse effects are rare. Trifluperidol and benperidol seem to be similar in action and side-effects. Preparation as an odorless, colorless, tasteless concentrate makes administration simple for suspicious patients. No other major tranquilizer has this advantage. However, available data are insufficient for formulating a final conclusion about this group in comparison with other "neuroleptics."

MISCELLANEOUS MAJOR TRANQUILIZERS

Prothipendyl (Tolnate; not available in the United States). This drug is related to the phenothiazines. McKenzie and Roswell-Harris (1966) described it as a very helpful drug in the management of acute and chronic problems of adolescent and adult retardates. Toxicity was reported to be low.

Molindone. This drug is an oxygenated indole derivative distantly related to reserpine. In a pilot study of schizophrenics, Sugerman and Herrmann (1967) found it useful, with side-effects similar to the other major tranquilizers. No studies with the retarded were found.

The Minor Tranquilizers

DIPHENYLMETHANE DERIVATIVES

Diphenhydramine (Benadryl). This drug was introduced as an effective antihistamine around 1946. It is one of the oldest and safest of the psychoactive drugs and is also used as an antispasmodic, in motion sickness, and in the dramatic reversal of the dystonic syndrome caused by the major tranquilizers.

Effron and Freedman (1953) reported that it was especially useful in highly anxious children (uncontrolled study). Freedman and colleagues (1955) utilized a placebo control and found the drug superior to chlorpromazine, reserpine, and mephenesin in "primary" behavior disorders. In his review of the literature, Freedman (1958) concluded that it was also useful in controlling impulsive behavior. Fish (1960*b*, 1961) reported greatest benefits with anxious, immature younger children, with little effect after age ten. The latter conclusion has often been cited since then and is still asserted (Fish, 1968); however, no data from an adequate study have been published to support this observation and no sex differences, which might be expected, have been specified.

No well-designed study has determined the clinical effectiveness of diphenhydramine in promoting behavioral change in the disturbed retarded child. Its usage would appear to be relatively safe, side-effects consisting mainly of drowsiness, dizziness, dryness of the mouth, and (rarely) overexcitation. Drowsiness usually subsides after a few days of continued medication.

Captodiame (captodiamine; Suvren, Covatin). This drug is represented in the literature by two favorable studies: its use with forty brain-damaged children (Low and Myers, 1958), and Castner and

Noble's (1959) report that it helped stabilize agitation or depression in 75 per cent of their adult patients without side-effects. Although both trade preparations are still available, neither is described in the 1968 *Physician's Desk Reference*, probably indicating little use. No full evaluation of its effectiveness with the retarded has been made.

Azacyclonol (Frenquel). This drug has enjoyed some popularity as an antihallucinatory agent, but the claim for this effect has not stood the test of time. Wright (1958) tried it in an uncontrolled study of eight chronic schizophrenic retarded adults; most improved. Rudy and others (1958) found it inferior to the phenothiazines and reserpine in use with chronically disturbed retarded children and adults; placebo controls were utilized. In their review of azacyclonol, Paredes and co-workers (1961) concluded that it had been a disappointment.

Hydroxyzine (Atarax, Vistaril). This drug has been extensively employed in pediatric practice since 1956. It was reported to reduce hyperactivity, tension, and "psychosomatic symptoms" in disturbed retarded children in a residential school (Segal and Tansley, 1957). Placebo was used, and behavior ratings were made by teachers. Craft (1957) utilized hydroxyzine in a double-blind design with severely retarded children and adults who were described as hyperactive and difficult to manage. He found no significant differences in activity level, aggression, or social behavior in comparing drug and placebo conditions. Fish (1960*b*) reported that the drug was less effective than diphenhydramine (uncontrolled studies). Litchfield (1960) treated forty-one neurotic children and reported benefit in 93 per cent with few side-effects (also an uncontrolled study).

Other uncontrolled reports claiming positive results in a wide variety of disturbances are those of Dougan (1962) and Giannini (1964). Although the latter investigation employed so-called "control" subjects, they were given neither drug nor placebo, there was no "blindness" in the design, and therefore the term "controlled study" is a misnomer. Piuck (1963) reported no great benefit in an uncontrolled investigation of twenty-six emotionally disturbed out-patients.

The discrepancies reported may be due, in part, to variations in subjects, study designs, dosage levels, and durations of administration. There seems to be no definitive recent study to indicate usefulness with the disturbed child who is retarded.

Other diphenylmethane derivatives: Benzquinamide (Quantril); buclizine (Softran).

Summary. Side-effects with this group of drugs are unusual and rarely dangerous, but the effectiveness is also not very pronounced. Few good studies have been done. At present, diphenhydramine (Benadryl) seems worth trying in anxious nonpsychotic patients. Hydroxyzine is probably less potent but may also be worth trying if other drugs fail.

SUBSTITUTED DIOL DERIVATIVES

Mephenesin (Tolserol). This drug was introduced after its muscle-relaxant properties were demonstrated in 1947. In partially controlled studies of behavior disorders (Freedman and others, 1955) and brain damage (Freedman and others, 1955), improvements were reported, but interest in the drug waned because of its short duration of action, undesirable side-effects, and the appearance of the related drug meprobamate a few years later.

Meprobamate (Miltown, Equanil, Trelmar, plus many combinations with other drugs; introduced 1953). "Miltown" has become almost a household word. Although thought at first to be an ideal, nonaddicting tranquilizer, it was later found that true withdrawal reactions occur after prolonged use at high doses, occasionally with seizures. It is not useful in the psychoses.

With adults, Uhlenhuth and others (1959) found that the effectiveness of meprobamate depended partly upon the expectations of the prescribing physician. Positive reports include the following: Kraft and others (1959) in reading disability; Katz (1958) in reducing tension in cerebral palsied children; Kugelmass (1956) in the behavior disorders of the retarded; Litchfield (1957) with the prepsychotic or borderline child; Freedman (1958) with behavior disorders; Bender and Faretra (1961) with hyperactive, brain-damaged children; and Freed and Frignito (1961) with mixed behavior disorders. Unfortunately, most of these studies are methodologically inadequate.

A double-blind design demonstrated no benefit of the drug with low-grade, hyperactive, destructive retardates (Craft, 1958). Heaton-Ward and Jancar (1958) and Rudy and others (1958) also reported negative results. In a well-controlled study, Cytryn and co-workers (1960) compared it with placebo and found no benefit in children's behavior disorders.

Although widely used in treating neurotic adults, the effectiveness of meprobamate has been equivocal and it has no clearly established place in the management of the disturbed retarded child.

Tybamate (Solacen, Tybatran; introduced in 1965). This drug is a close relative of meprobamate; early assessment was reported by the A.M.A. Council on Drugs (1965). An uncontrolled study (Barsa and Saunders, 1963) reported it to be effective in reducing tension and anxiety in chronically psychotic adults and adolescents, some of whom were retarded. Assessment was complicated, however, by concurrent administration of antipsychotic agents. No studies have appeared on its use with retarded children, and it is not recommended for use with children under age six.

Phenaglycodol (Ultran; introduced in 1957). This drug is a weak muscle relaxant related to mephenesin and meprobamate (A.M.A. Council on Drugs, 1957). Its effectiveness is in doubt, and Zukin and Arnold (1959), in a controlled study with anxious adults, found it less useful than meprobamate, though better than placebo. Although still available, it is not described in the 1968 *Physician's Desk Reference*. No studies with retarded children were found.

THE BENZODIAZEPINES

Originally noted as having a "taming effect" upon wild animals, these drugs have also been found to possess anticonvulsant properties and have been widely used for neurotic disorders and (in combination with antispasmodics) in gastrointestinal psychosomatic conditions.

Side-effects include drowsiness, fatigue, ataxia, jaundice (rare), and paradoxical states of excitation.

Chlordiazepoxide (Librium). LaVeck and Buckley (1961) could demonstrate no reduction in seizures and found an increase in undesirable behavior (including hyperactivity) in a double-blind study with placebo of twenty-eight retarded children. Krakowski (1963), on the other hand, felt it was helpful in managing emotionally disturbed children, including the retarded; sixty-six per cent of children and adolescents improved, but no controls were employed. A recent study of adults (Gardos and others, 1968) reported that anxiety was effectively reduced in highly anxious patients but was *increased* in "low-anxious" patients, whose hostility was also exacerbated. They suggest that where it is preferable for the patient to express hostility, chlordiazepoxide would be better than oxazepam (see below), which reduced anxiety without increasing hostility. The implications of these findings for children are not clear.

Diazepam (Valium; introduced in 1963). This drug has been used with great success (intravenously) in controlling status epilepticus and with some apparent benefit in cerebral palsy and dystonic states. Its use in the psychiatric disorders of children is endorsed by some but felt to be of no value by others (Zrull et al., 1964). Galambos (1965) found it effective, with few side-effects, in long-term use with adult retardates with psychotic or less severe symptoms. It has never been fully assessed as to its usefulness with retarded children.

Oxazepam (Serax; introduced in 1965). This drug was reported by the A.M.A. Council on Drugs (1966) to be as effective as the others of this group in relieving anxiety in neurotic adults. No work with retarded children was found in the literature.

Nitrazepam (Mogadon; not available in the United States). This drug has been used (with mixed enthusiasm) as an anticonvulsant. One study of epileptics (Hagberg, 1968) reported that some children were calmer and easier to manage, but no large-scale testing has appeared.

Ro 5–4556. Closely related to diazepam, this drug is still for experimental use only. In an uncontrolled study of disturbed retarded children, Ucer (1968) reported that each of twenty-five patients improved to some extent; hyperactivity, anxiety, and interpersonal relations seemed to be benefited.

Summary. The use of the benzodiazepines in anxiety states unassociated with psychosis probably deserves a trial, although no adequate studies support any claim for efficacy in retarded children.

MISCELLANEOUS

No significant studies were found for the following drugs: benactyzine (Suavitil; in combination with meprobamate as Deprol), ectylurea (Levanil, Nostyn), and emylcamate (Striatran).

Sedatives and Hypnotics

Prior to the introduction of the barbiturates (barbital, 1903; phenobarbital, 1912), alcohol and the bromides (1857), chloral hydrate (1869), and paraldehyde (1882) were used. With the possible exception of alcohol and the bromides, all of these continue to have a place in formal medical management, although it may seem that recent additions to the field have overshadowed them.

Classification is not entirely satisfactory. Presumably their action is more at the cortical level than is the case with the tranquilizers. They are therefore of value in producing mild impairment of consciousness (sedation), sleep, and in the control of severely agitated or manic behavior.

The minor tranquilizers are used for mild anxiety states, though their superiority to the older sedatives has never been proven. The barbiturates are believed to aggravate behavioral difficulties in young hyperactive (especially nonepileptic) patients (Lourie, 1964; Eisenberg, 1966; Werry, 1968a; Fish, 1968), although the evidence for this is rather weak. The nonbarbiturate sedatives were introduced, for the most part, between 1956 and 1960, and include methyprylon (Noludar), glutethimide (Doriden), chlormezanone (Trancopal), oxanamide

(Quiactin), ethchlorvynol (Placidyl), acetylcarbromal (Paxarel), and others.

No adequate studies on the use of these compounds with retarded children were found in the literature; Fish (1968) stated that the hypnotic agents are not useful in the prepubertal child.

Stimulants

The drugs described here are not all chemical relatives; some authors combine this group with the so-called antidepressants, but the latter are presumed to have specific effects upon depressive states without producing generalized psychomotor stimulation. Although tried in states of depression, the stimulants have not proven effective in their management, at least partly because of the "let down" which follows mood elevation.

THE AMPHETAMINES

The amphetamines [amphetamine (Benzedrine), dextroamphetamine (Dexedrine), and methamphetamine (Desoxyn, Methedrine)] have been used since 1937 and are closely related to ephedrine, sharing its adrenergic effects. Amphetamine (Benzedrine) is the racemic mixture of the two optical isomers dextroamphetamine and levoamphetamine. The latter has much less direct stimulant effect upon the central nervous system and is used as an anorexiant in obesity. It will not be further described here. There seems to be no reason to expect that amphetamine would be superior, therefore, to dextroamphetamine, although purely on clinical grounds Laufer (1968) has found that some hyperactive children respond differentially to one or the other drug forms. Methamphetamine has central actions which are so similar to dextroamphetamine that it will be considered identical for purposes of the review. No studies on its use with children were found in the literature, although Kosman and Unna (1968) suggested that chronic administration of methamphetamine led to different results than with the other drugs of this group.

The amphetamines are potent sympathomimetic amines with respect to stimulation of the central nervous system. Dextroamphetamine is three to four times as potent as levoamphetamine, and one and one-half to two times more potent than the racemic mixture (amphetamine) (Goodman and Gilman, 1965, p. 500). Unlike other analeptics, the amphetamines do not cause seizures and are even used in the treatment of some of the convulsive disorders.

Some children have a seemingly paradoxical reaction to these drugs, being inhibited or quieted rather than stimulated, as seen with adults. Very occasionally extreme inhibition, superficially resembling catatonia, may be observed; tearfulness is also a common early reaction. Differential stimulation of subcortical inhibitory centers is usually given as the best hypothesis to account for the amphetamines' inhibitory effect.

Beneficial results were first reported by Bradley (1937) in an uncontrolled study of children with mixed disorders attending a residential treatment center; school performance seemed to improve. The earliest controlled study found in the literature of psychoactive drug use with children was performed by Molitch and Sullivan (1937), who gave fifty children, ages ten to seventeen, a standard single dose of amphetamine one and one-half hours before a standardized achievement test. These children were court-committed juvenile delinquents who varied in IQ. A control group of forty-six children received a placebo. Those who did not improve their scores were retested later, having been given twice the original dose. It was concluded that significant improvement in performance did occur, more with the older and higher-IQ children. This result is interesting because it contradicts the general impression that younger children do better.

Subsequent positive, uncontrolled reports include the following: Bradley and Bowen (1940); Bradley and Green (1940); Moskowitz (1941); Bender and Cottington (1942); Bradley (1950, 1957); Laufer and Denhoff (1957); Laufer and others (1957); Fish (1960b, 1961); and Solomons (1965).

Bender and Cottington (1942) and Freedman (1958) reported that no improvement could be anticipated in psychotic patients or in the psychopathic disorders.

Cutler and co-workers (1940) found no change in IQ or behavior in a controlled study of retarded children. Morris and others (1955) performed a controlled but not completely double-blind investigation of fifty adolescent and adult retardates, using a battery of intelligence and memory tests, as well as learning tasks. They concluded that the drug does not increase IQ, learning, performance speed, attention, or memory in retardates. Weiss and Laties (1962) reviewed learning and performance studies in adults and observed that although the amphetamines tended to influence motor performance and reaction time favorably, they created no significant improvement in intellectual performance unless normal functioning was impaired by fatigue or boredom.

Superiority over placebo was shown in delinquent institutionalized boys by Eisenberg and colleagues (1963). Burks (1964) performed a study with forty-three behavior-problem children, ten of whom had normal EEG's. He postulated that the normal EEG group improved more because of amphetamine's supposed effect upon diencephalic dysfunction (which would not show on the EEG), whereas the thirty-three children with abnormal EEG's had cortical and subcortical dysfunctions which would be less responsive to this drug. (There are several methodological short-comings in this study.) Burks' conclusions relate to the 1957 report of Laufer and others in "hyperkinetic impulse disorder" children. They felt a useful distinction between organic and nonorganic hyperkinetic children could be demonstrated by means of a photo-Metrazol test which activates the EEG pattern; amphetamines were said to raise the photo-Metrazol threshold. A diencephalic dysfunction was hypothesized as the cause of the hyperactivity and distractibility in these children, which appeared to improve gradually with maturation. This test has been cited many times, and the data seem convincing, but apparently no replication has been undertaken.

Zrull and co-workers (1964) compared dextroamphetamine favorably with diazepam and placebo in retarded, brain-damaged, and borderline psychotic children. The "slowing-down" inhibiting effect upon hyperkinetic children, mentioned earlier, was not confirmed in a triple-blind study of retarded children by McConnell and others (1964). (This study was unusual in that direct measurement of activity level was undertaken by means of a ballistographic chair.)

Eisenberg and colleagues (1965) compared the response of hyperkinetic and neurotic groups of children to brief psychotherapy and stimulant drugs, using placebo control and two objective tests. The hyperkinetic children did significantly better with stimulants, and the neurotics with psychotherapy. A further controlled study from Eisenberg's group (Conners et al., 1967) utilized a double-blind crossover design with a standardized dose of dextroamphetamine in fifty-two children with learning problems. IQ did not change, but classroom behavior improved, and this was thought to reflect increase in "assertiveness and drive."

A retrospective study of thirty-one "organic" and "nonorganic" hyperkinetic children by Conrad and Insel (1967) led to conclusions that emotional factors interfere with drug action, organic factors are primary in positive response, and organic children with good parent-child relationships respond best. No control group was employed.

In a preliminary study with institutionalized retardates, Sprague and others (1967) found a reduction in activity level and latency of responses. However, they were aware of a defect which made clear-cut interpretations of results difficult: the drug sequence was not counter-balanced (no "crossover"). Weiss and co-workers (in press) performed a double-blind uncrossed study of dextroamphetamine and placebo on a group of thirty-eight hyperactive children of normal intelligence. The drug was found to be superior to the placebo in reducing hyperactivity and improving the goal-directedness of behavior. In comparison with chlorpromazine, it was less reliable in reducing hyperactivity, but when it worked, its effects were more dramatic. Cognitive changes were not statistically significant, but there was a definite trend in a positive direction, whereas chlorpromazine was indistinguishable from placebo. (This report is also notable for its complete and interesting discussion of some of the research problems encountered in similar studies.)

A dissent from the previously described positive studies is reported by Alexandris and Lundell (1968) who found it inferior to thioridazine and only slightly better than placebo in hyperactive retarded children.

Side-effects. The side-effects encountered in the use of the amphetamines are likely to be due to exaggeration of intended effects or central nervous system stimulation: irritability, anorexia, insomnia, and so on. Recently Mattson and Calverley (1968) reported tic-like dyskinetic syndromes in children treated with dextroamphetamine, which resembled those seen with the major tranquilizers. These reactions were probably idiosyncratic and not dose-related.

Summary. Although amphetamines have been used for over thirty years, adequate studies have only begun to appear recently. The amphetamines seem to facilitate reduction in excess activity, better organization of behavior, and possibly assertiveness in children with poorly integrated behavior who are not psychotic. Studies specifically with the retarded are few, and in any case drug effects are likely to be rather weak as compared with psychological and educational variables (Werry and Sprague, in press). Use with psychotic children should probably be avoided. Administration should be on a morning and noon basis to avoid insomnia.

In children who are responsive, the age at which inhibition is replaced by psychomotor stimulation has not been accurately determined and must be individually monitored. The claims for miraculous benefits in the majority of hyperactive children have certainly been grossly exaggerated and may be based upon nondrug effects (McDermott, 1965). Predictive criteria are still unclear.

DEANOL

Deanol acetamidobenzoate (Deaner) is related to the amphetamines but lacks their adrenergic effects. It is presumed by some to be a precursor of acetylcholine. Increased attention span and accelerated mental processes were reported in uncontrolled investigations by Oettinger (1958) in brain-damaged children and Mebane (1960) in delinquents. Controlled studies, however, generally showed no benefit for this drug over placebo (Clausen et al., 1960; Bell and Zubek, 1961; LaVeck and Buckley, 1961; Kugel and Alexander, 1963). In fact, Bell and Zubek found that both deanol and dextroamphetamine were inferior to placebo with adults. Geller (1960) was the only investigator who reported positive effects in a controlled study, but there was so little placebo effect that Eveloff (1966) suggested that some bias might have been communicated to the subjects or they may have distinguished the drug from placebo because of side-effects. Not one child improved on placebo—a most unusual finding.

The recent publicity with regard to direct effects of drugs on learning led to at least one extravagant claim about deanol as reported by David (1966): "Already here—a drug to improve reading ability in 15 weeks . . . a remarkable study of 22 children (who) have normal intelligence but had been diagnosed by special tests as poor readers . . . major improvements in reading ability were noted in all 22 subjects."

Despite this statement for popular consumption, the majority of studies do not support the efficacy of this drug in improving either learning or behavior in children.

METHYLPHENIDATE

Methyphenidate (Ritalin; introduced in 1956) lacks the marked adrenergic effects of the amphetamines. A partially controlled study by Levy and co-workers (1957) demonstrated that it had some usefulness in alleviating the drowsiness caused by other psychotropic drugs in disturbed, retarded children.

Zimmerman and Burgemeister (1958) compared methylphenidate favorably with reserpine in a group of unresponsive, depressed children and adults with severe behavior disorders, some of whom were retarded. Reaction time was reduced without an increase in tested IQ; no placebo was employed. Reserpine was found to be superior to methylphenidate with hyperactive, irritable, aggressive patients.

Impulsivity of hyperkinetic, brain-damaged children was reported to be diminished, and a stimulating effect upon "cortical maturation and integration" was postulated in four papers describing uncontrolled studies (Lytton and Knobel, 1958; Knobel et al., 1959; Knobel and Lytton, 1959; and Knobel, 1962).

Conners and Eisenberg (1963) performed a relatively brief, double-blind study employing methylphenidate with hyperactive, emotionally disturbed children in a residential setting, some of whom were retarded. They concluded that the drug caused some decrease in impulsivity and improved performance on several learning tasks (especially with children of lower IQ), but the differences were small and further research was recommended. In a later paper (Conners et al., 1964) the authors speculated that some of the children in the 1963 investigation might have become aware that they were receiving the drug rather than the placebo because of side-effects.

Lourie (1964), agreeing with Laufer and others (1957), felt that this drug or the amphetamines could provide diagnostic clues to the etiology of hyperactivity in children, though no data were presented to support this view.

Other studies showed a favorable response of hyperactive, nonneurotic children (Eisenberg et al., 1965), increased verbal productivity in children with cerebral dysfunction (Creager and VanRiper, 1967), and conduct disorder children of normal intelligence (Werry, 1968a).

Sprague and colleagues (unpublished manuscript) recently demonstrated an increase in desirable behavior conducive to learning with this drug, as compared to thioridazine. The children involved were in a class for learning disabilities, and many would be categorized as suffering from "minimal cerebral dysfunction"; intelligence was in the normal range. Impulsivity, hyperactivity, and motor restlessness were all improved, as was attention span.

Side-effects of methylphenidate are insomnia, occasional anorexia and excitation; these may be reduced by omitting a late-afternoon dose.

No adequate studies have compared the relative efficacy of methylphenidate and the amphetamines in retarded children. Until such information is available, indications would seem to be similar for both. The preponderance of data favors the usefulness of methylphenidate in the overactive child who has difficulty in appropriately inhibiting his behavior.

PIPRADROL

Pipradrol (Meretran) is related to methylphenidate and to the diphenylmethane minor tranquilizer azacyclonol (Frenquel). In a preliminary, uncontrolled study by Oettinger (1955) it was not as effective as amphetamine in children's behavior disorders. Klingman (1962) reviewed clinical experience in tics and convulsive disorders but presented no data. Although still available, it is not described in the 1968 *Physician's Desk Reference* and seems to have no advantage over better-known and -evaluated stimulants.

PENTYLENETETRAZOL

Pentylenetetrazol (Metrazol) is an analeptic agent used also as a stimulant in geriatrics and as an activating drug in electroencephalography (Laufer et al., 1957). McGaugh (1968) has reported plans to test it on retarded children because of indications from animal experiments that it reduces task-learning time. No data are currently available.

MAGNESIUM PEMOLINE

Magnesium pemoline (Cylert) is not currently released for general use. It has been claimed that it improves memory in the senile and in animals, but its effects upon the learning process have more recently been attributed to enhancement of performance (as with the amphetamines and methylphenidate) rather than to stimulation of RNA metabolism (Gelfand et al., 1968; Yuwiler et al., 1968). No studies with the retarded were found in the literature, though it is likely that such work is being undertaken currently.

Antidepressants

Gardner (1967) has reviewed studies on frequency of depression in the retarded. He felt that the incidence was often underrated. Any investigation in this field is complicated, however, by the assumptions regarding "depressive equivalents" or "masked depressions," the self-limited nature, multiple etiologies, and lack of analogous conditions which could be employed in animal experiments.

Use of drugs alleged to have specific antidepressant activity dates from about 1957. However, the first suggestive observations were made in 1952 when patients with tuberculosis who were receiving iproniazid improved in mood. Other compounds were developed, some of which were used with institutionalized retardates, but all have potentially dangerous adverse effects. More of these drugs have been withdrawn from the market than has been true with the phenothiazines. Some of this group exhibit tranquilizing as well as antidepressant effects. Possible danger in aggravating latent psychoses is still controversial.

Reports of well-designed studies in children are few. In 1965 three papers appeared challenging the specific usefulness of these drugs in childhood and adult depression. Friend stated that the monoamine oxidase inhibitors (MAOI) were less effective than the iminodibenzyl (tricyclic) group. Hollister (1965) and Hollister and Overall (1965) asserted that there is no specific class of antidepressants; they reported that thioridazine and other phenothiazines were as good as imipramine, except with endogenous psychotic depressions.

Onset of desired action seems to be delayed, requiring from several days to several weeks, making conclusions about drug effect versus spontaneous remission difficult to establish. Excellent general reviews are those of Cole (1964) and Malitz (1966).

The stimulants were tried in depressive states but were not found to be effective. Malitz states (1964, p. 479):

Because of lack of sustained action, secondary slump, development of tolerance, possibility of habituation, and distressing side effects, the amphetamines do not provide an answer to the need for an effective and acceptable antidepressant. They still have a place, however, in the treatment of very mild depressions, and as an interim measure when used with those of the newer antidepressants that have delayed action.

MONOAMINE OXIDASE INHIBITORS (PHENYLHYDRAZINE GROUP)

Monoamine oxidase inhibition is a convenient way to classify these drugs and those in the nonphenylhydrazine group, but this activity may be unrelated to the clinical effects observed. Serious side-effects of a hypertensive nature may occur with alcohol, cheese (Asatoor et al., 1963), chianti, many foods also rich in tyramine, and from interaction with the sympathomimetic amines (such as amphetamine or others in cold preparations and patent medicines).

Iproniazid (Marsilid). This drug was the first of the antidepressant group. Although still used in other countries, it produced such severe adverse effects (including death) that it has been banned in the United States.

Isocarboxazid (Marplan; introduced in 1959). This drug was developed as a replacement for iproniazid. No adequate studies report its effectiveness in a retarded population. An uncontrolled favorable report was made by Carter (1960) based on work with 116 institutionalized retarded patients of all ages over a period of many months. Side-effects were not serious, except for increase in seizures in five cases.

However, adverse effects do require very careful medical supervision, difficult to implement outside an institution. Some of these reactions include hypotension, excitation, and cardiac dysrhythmias, as well as occasional blood, skin, gastrointestinal, genitourinary, and central nervous system abnormalities.

Phenelzine (Nardil; introduced in 1959). This drug was reported to be the best of the antidepressants available at that time (Thal, 1959) and has side-effects similar to isocarboxazid (Furst, 1959). Jaundice has been encountered, and convulsive disorders may be aggravated. Soblen and Saunders (1961) found the drug useful in an uncontrolled study of severely disturbed adolescents. Frommer (1967) assessed phenelzine as superior to both placebo and phenobarbital when combined with chlordiazepoxide in a double-blind trial with thirty-two children with depressive disorders.

No adequate studies with retarded children were found in the literature.

Nialamide (Niamid; introduced in 1959). This drug was reported to be helpful in retardates in uncontrolled studies by Davies (1961) and Millon and others (1965). Krupanidhi and others (1964) achieved positive results in a controlled investigation of ninety-two young disturbed retarded children in India. Other studies have produced conflicting results. Heaton-Ward (1962) obtained negative results in a controlled study of Down's Syndrome (mongolism).

Side-effects are not as serious as some of the drugs previously described, but efficacy is in question. It is listed, but not described, in the 1968 *Physician's Desk Reference*.

Pheniprazine (Catron). This drug was discontinued because of severe toxicity. The uncontrolled Soblen and Saunders study (1961) found it to be useful with disturbed adolescents.

Mebanazine (Actomol; not available in the United States). This drug has been used with adults. Gilmour (1965) reported on positive results in an uncontrolled study, but Barker and others (1965) found it to be no better than placebo when controls were utilized. No studies with the retarded were found.

Summary. This group of MAOI is represented now mainly by isocarboxazid and phenelzine. No studies with the retarded clearly justify their use in the face of potentially serious side-effects and the (at least) equal effectiveness of the iminodibenzyl group (see below).

MONOAMINE OXIDASE INHIBITORS (NONPHENYLHDRAZINE GROUP)

Etryptamine (Monase). This drug has been discontinued because of adverse effects and unproved efficacy.

Tranylcypromine (Parnate; introduced in 1961). This drug has had a checkered course since its synthesis in 1948. Initial reports were favorable, suggesting rapid onset of desired effects. It was combined with trifluoperazine for agitated depressions and marketed in Canada and Great Britain as Parstelin; this combination was never marketed in the United States. In 1964, tranylcypromine was withdrawn at the insistence of the Food and Drug Administration because of severe hypertensive crises. A protest resulted in reintroduction later that same year under more stringent regulations (A.M.A. Council on Drugs, 1964). Several controlled and uncontrolled studies with adult depressive patients demonstrated superiority over placebo but not over other drugs. Atkinson and Ditman (1965) have reviewed the reports up to 1964, as well as the pharmacology and toxicology of tranylcypromine.

No studies with retarded children were found in the literature. Efficacy is not established, and prescribing restrictions are stringent. Its use in children is not indicated except under carefully supervised residential conditions.

Pargyline (Eutonyl). Marketed as an antihypertensive, this drug is not yet approved as an antidepressant. It is unclear whether it possesses any advantages over other drugs (Oltman and Friedman, 1963). No studies with the retarded were found. In addition, potentially serious side-effects and potentiation of many other agents will probably limit its use if it is approved.

IMINODIBENZYL (TRICYCLIC) GROUP

Also known as dibenzazepines, these drugs should not be combined with the MAOI because of reports of serious reactions; they may also be dangerous with the benzodiazepines (page 321). They are structurally related to the phenothiazines. One possible side-effect which may cause increasing concern is the prolongation of A-V conduction time.

Imipramine (Tofranil). The first of this group, this drug was introduced around 1959. Like chlorpromazine in the phenothiazine group, this drug is the agent of reference for comparative studies of the antidepressants. Onset of action is from several days to several weeks, and there seems to be no sudden "lift" or "slump" as with the stimulants. Thousands of reports are now available on use with all age groups (Malitz, 1966). Most controlled studies demonstrate superiority over placebo in treating depressive illness.

Bender and Faretra (1961) were of the opinion that imipramine and the MAOI helped withdrawn autistic children. Pilkington (1962) selected the worst of the available disturbed retarded children and adults for an uncontrolled investigation. He divided the patients into two groups: "affective" (cyclothymic), and "nonaffective" (schizophrenic traits or undifferentiated behavior disturbances). About half of the first group improved markedly, but almost all of the second group deteriorated.

Rapoport (1965), in an uncontrolled study, indicated that 80.5 per cent of forty-one children and adolescents with behavior and learning problems improved.

Side-effects are not uncommon but are less serious than with the MAOI.

Amitriptyline (Elavil; introduced in 1961). This drug is a close relative of imipramine. Much has been written about the benefits, indications, and side-effects of this drug and others of this series, but nothing conclusive can be stated at present. Side-effects are mainly atropine-like, with rare hypotension, excitement, or convulsions.

In 1965, Krakowski reported that 72 per cent of fifty hyperkinetic children responded well in a double-blind design; only a few of these were retarded.

Lucas, and others (1965) concluded that amitriptyline was useful in managing severely disturbed in-patient children who were not retarded. The number of subjects (ten) was perhaps too small to lead to firm conclusions, despite the double-blind design with placebo.

Krakowski (1966) performed an uncontrolled investigation of psychosomatic disorders in children and reported that the drug was useful. Finally, Kraft and co-workers (1966) studied 123 children with behavioral disorders, finding that four of the five with retardation improved in an uncontrolled design. Studies with enuresis are covered in the section on special problems.

Nortriptyline (Aventyl; introduced in 1965). This drug was given a favorable rating by Splitter and Kaufman (1966) when combined with psychotherapy in underachieving adolescents, and by Kurtis (1966) with autistic children, both in uncontrolled studies.

Carter (1966), in a small-sample controlled investigation, found it at least as effective as chlorpromazine or a barbiturate in controlling severely disturbed behavior in institutionalized retardates.

Protriptyline (Vivactil; introduced in 1968). This drug was found by Williams (1968) to be equal in effectiveness and more rapid in onset when compared with amitriptyline in a double-blind trial with thirty-seven depressed adults. No adequate evaluation of its potential usefulness with the retarded has appeared.

Desipramine (desmethyl-imipramine; Pertofrane, Norpramin). Thought to be a metabolite of imipramine, it was hoped that this drug would have more rapid onset of effect. However, this was not borne out in practice. A study by Edwards (1965) showed it to be less effective than imipramine and to have no shorter onset of action. Its use with the retarded has not been established.

Opipramol (Ensidon; not available in the United States). The structure of this drug relates it to perphenazine. Effects have not been superior to others of this group (Splitter, 1963; Malitz, 1966).

Trimipramine (Surmontil; not available in the United States). This drug has been used in Europe and is closely related to imipramine. It was reported by Salzmann (1965) to be superior to the latter in a small comparison study with adults; use with the retarded has apparently not been reported.

Summary. Imipramine has not been replaced by any clearly superior compound of its class. These drugs are thought to have specific antidepressant effects, but they have been tried with a wide range of disordered behavior which cannot be subsumed under depression. The iminodibenzyl group is safer than the monoamine oxidase inhibitors, but a final place in the management of the disturbed retarded child is not yet taken, with the possible exception of the treatment of enuresis (see the section on special problems).

Anticonvulsants

Since the introduction of phenobarbital in 1912 and diphenylhydantoin in 1938, the management of convulsive disorders by means of drugs has received greater impetus. (Prior to these agents, the bromides were used to treat grand mal epilepsy.) However, there is little adequate data to evaluate the beneficial or harmful effects of these and other anticonvulsants in behavior disorders of the retarded child.

Some believe these drugs are useful in treating children who have episodic behavior disorders without seizures but associated with abnormal EEG's (Walker and Kirkpatrick, 1947; Jonas, 1965, 1967; Turner, 1967). However, others have reported such applications to be of no value (Pasamanick, 1951; Klein and Greenberg, 1967; Fish, 1968). This controversy has been exacerbated by claims in the popular press (*Life Magazine,* 1967) and subsequent criticism (Livingston, 1968).

Side-effects of anticonvulsants may be serious, including blood dyscrasias, renal changes, and personality alterations to the point of toxic psychosis.

In a partially controlled study, Guey and colleagues (1967) reported that ethosuximide (Zarontin) lowered tested IQ, produced slowness and perseveration, impaired memory, and tended to bring about deleterious psychic effects in retarded and nonretarded epileptic children. Wapner and others (1962) studied phenobarbital in a more adequately designed investigation and found no significant effect of the drug upon learning in either direction.

When a child with a convulsive disorder is having his alertness impaired by frequent seizures, is apprehensive that another one may occur, or is developing secondary emotional problems because of parental protection or social ostracism, there is little doubt that anticonvulsant treatment may have a significant ameliorative effect. Teachers who are aware of the sedative action of the barbiturates may falsely conclude that inattention in an epileptic child is due solely to the drug, which probably is only rarely the case. Children with poorly controlled seizures, however, may have to take high doses of several drugs, and may suffer impairment in coordination, alertness, and other aspects of learning.

In summary, these drugs have little place in the management of nonconvulsive behavior disorders, except in very carefully selected instances. In retarded children with a convulsive disorder, the anticonvulsants often have a basic role in ameliorating the multiple manifestations of the condition. In most of these cases, no gross change in learning or behavior is to be expected. Adequate research data are not yet available to assess the effects of most of these drugs on learning and behavior in children with different types of epilepsy. Some anticonvulsants may also be found to possess psychotropic effects independent of their anticonvulsant properties.

Compounds Part of Normal Metabolic Processes

HORMONES

Thyroid hormones. These preparations are necessary for children with hypothyroidism (cretinism) but must be begun as early in life as possible (Collipp et al., 1965). Despite early reports of benefit from hormone therapy of euthyroid retarded and psychotic children (Sherwin et al., 1958), such treatment seems to have no rational basis today, although it is widely employed as a form of quack or fringe method for all sorts of medical complaints, including Down's Syndrome.

Chorionic gonadotrophin. Gonadal immaturity was also thought to be a possible factor in retardation, and a group of thirty-two boys with "somatic immaturity" were treated with chorionic gonadotrophin by Berman and others (1959), who reported a slight gain in IQ and readiness to learn. However, Reiss and colleagues (1966) found no such effect with the same type of preparation and anabolic steroids.

Thus, no benefit seems to accrue from hormonal therapy except in early childhood in cases of hormonal deficiency.

VITAMINS

Like the hormones, there seems to be no good evidence to indicate usefulness of vitamins except in cases of deficiency. Houze and others (1964) reported some improvement in the behavior of twenty retarded boys (who had failed to improve on other drugs) from the administration of alpha-tocopherol (vitamin E). No controls were used, and no changes were noted in tested IQ.

5-HYDROXYTRYPTOPHAN

This compound is a precursor of serotonin (5-hydroxytryptamine) which has some role in brain metabolism. Bazelon (1968) found that infants with trisomy 21 Down's Syndrome (mongolism) have 20 to 50 per cent of the normal blood level of 5-hydroxytryptamine after six months of age. Elevation of these reduced levels with oral administration of the precursor was reported to improve hypotonia, tongue protrusion, and activity level. The fourteen treated patients had significantly higher scores on the Bayley Infant Scales and achieved motor milestones at earlier ages than usual for these children. However, double-blind and long-term studies are as yet unavailable to confirm these findings. Down's Syndrome has for many years been a fertile area for disappointed hopes after initial enthusiasm.

GLUTAMIC ACID

Glutamic acid (GA) and its salts and metabolites have been highly controversial since their introduction as anticonvulsants in 1943. (It was reported that children given GA for petit mal epilepsy improved in learning and behavior.) GA is a nonessential amino acid (that is, it can be produced by the body from its precursors) which has a role in cerebral metabolism.

Generally favorable reviews on the use of GA in improving the intelligence of retardates were published by Gadson (1951), Kugelmass (1959), and Zimmerman and Burgemeister (1959), but Lombard and others (1955), in a controlled study, reported no such benefit.

Astin and Ross (1960) reviewed a large number of previous investigations and concluded that most positive reports were based on uncontrolled studies, whereas the preponderance of controlled studies showed negative results. A more exhaustive review by Vogel and co-workers (1965) challenged this conclusion. They state:

A considerable amount of evidence indicates a role for glutamic acid in cognitive functioning. The sheer weight of this evidence is surprising; indeed, there is more sound experimental confirmation of the positive effects of glutamic acid than appears to exist for most of the psychotropic drugs now in common therapeutic use.

Positive studies with GA tended to use varying dosage schedules, administer the free form rather than the salt, employ out-patient populations, and utilize clinical as well as psychometric assessments. A further very important point made by Vogel and others is that repeated psychometric testing without opportunity to utilize hypothetically improved abilities is meaningless. Prior to the review by Vogel and others, GA had passed out of usage. One subsequent positive report on a small number of patients has been made by Babcock and Drake (1967), and it remains to be seen whether further definitive clinical work will finally settle the issue of GA's usefulness.

GAMMA-HYDROXYBUTYRIC ACID

GABA was described by Logue and Bessman (1968) as a new drug which helps induce natural sleep. No studies on its use were found in the literature.

Miscellaneous Drugs

LSD-25

Lysergic acid diethylamide has been very much in the news because of its abuse and reports that it possibly causes chromosomal damage. It has been used with autistic children with encouraging results (Bender et al., 1966; Simmons et al., 1966). No studies with the retarded were found in the literature.

LITHIUM SALTS

Lithium has been used in other countries since 1949, but only recently has it gained a place in the treatment of the affective psychoses (especially mania) in the United States. No specific reports on use with the retarded were encountered.

ALLOPURINOL

The rare Lesch-Nyhan Syndrome includes mental retardation, hyperuricemia, and peculiar self-destructive behavior (such as lip-biting). Newcombe and co-workers (1966) reported successful treatment of a four-year-old boy, but in older children there seems to be little, if any, response to uricosuric agents.

SICCACELL THERAPY

In this treatment, dried embryonic cells from the brains of animals are injected into retarded subjects, with the theoretical (but highly dubious) notion that the cells will migrate to the brain and there stimulate growth and function. Other organs have been utilized to "treat" many other conditions, and the treatment is widely regarded as an expensive form of quackery. Black and others (1966) performed a double-blind study of this method but not surprisingly were unable to demonstrate any benefit in retarded children.

BOVINE BRAIN HYDRATE

This treatment is somewhat similar to Siccacell therapy but does not use whole cells. Rather, some special lipid or amino-acid content is assumed which will be helpful when administered over a long period of time. Six pairs of monozygous twins were used (with co-twin control) in a two-year investigation by Inouye and co-workers (1966). Four of the individuals treated with the preparation were reported to improve, and two became worse, but the study had many defects: the preparation was not pure brain hydrate but included L-glutamic acid, vitamins B_1, B_2, B_6, C, and chondroitin sulphate; there was no crossover to control for the order effect, which was probably important since three of the four who improved, continued to improve while receiving placebo for a year; changes were noted in hemoglobin in those receiving the preparation, which may have been a confounding factor if those receiving placebo were somewhat anemic, and so on. The authors were encouraged but stated that there was no proof the results were not due to chance.

NEOSTIGMINE (PROSTIGMINE)

Louttit (1965) mentions negative results in trials with this parasympathomimetic agent.

CELASTRUS PANICULATA SEEDS

These seeds have been used in the Orient to stimulate learning and memory, but according to Louttit (1965) two well-controlled studies were unable to demonstrate any benefit.

BENZCHLORPROPAMIDE (BECLAMIDE, NYDRANE, POSEDRINE, HIBICON)

Benzchlorpropamide is a drug which does not fit clearly into any of the categories used in this review, although it has anticonvulsant properties. It is not available in the United States. Price and Spencer (1967) reported a double-blind study in which nineteen of twenty-two severely retarded patients with difficult behavior improved significantly. Epileptics did better than nonepileptics.

CYPENAMINE (2-PHENYLCYCLOPENTYLAMINE HCl)

This drug is listed as an "energizer." Kurland and others (1967) tried it with ten retarded children in an uncontrolled pilot study. They reported improvement without significant side-effects, but no other studies were found in the literature.

Special Problems: Stuttering and Enuresis

Kent (1963) reviewed the studies to that date dealing with stuttering in the retarded, including the trials of reserpine, meprobamate, chlorpromazine, and hydroxyzine. No clear-cut benefit was apparent, either with or without speech therapy. Subsequently, however, improvement in fourteen of twenty-eight children receiving amphetamine was reported by Fish and Bowling (1965) in an uncontrolled study. Eight of the fourteen who did not improve received some benefit from use of trifluoperazine. Most were maintaining their improvement at follow-up after six months. The susceptibility of stuttering to nonspecific effects, however, makes it impossible to draw any conclusions regarding the efficacy of drug therapy at this time.

Enuresis is a very common problem in childhood, and its relief makes the management of patients living at home or in a residential setting much easier. Improvement has been reported with a large variety of drugs (as well as training methods).

Dinello and Champelli (1968) reviewed the use of imipramine for enuresis and found that all of twenty-three uncontrolled studies produced positive results, while six of seventeen controlled studies did not. A study specifically with the retarded by Fisher and others (1963) failed to demonstrate benefits. However, a paper by Alderton (1967) asserted that the timing of drug administration is crucial: early administration is needed for enuresis occurring during the early hours of sleep, later medication for the later pattern. He felt that neglect of this variable might account for some of the conflicting evidence.

Poussaint and co-workers (1966) found amitriptyline better than placebo (72 per cent cured or improved) in children of normal IQ. Poussaint and Ditman (1965) tried protriptyline in an uncontrolled study and found it was effective for the enuresis but side-effects were worse than with imipramine or amitriptyline. Smith and Gonzalez (1967) used placebo with nortriptyline and reported that the drug was efficacious in retarded, institutionalized boys.

Enuresis has multiple causes. It cannot be expected, therefore, that any one treatment will be successful with the great majority of cases; delineation of more homogeneous groups according to etiology will probably be necessary before it is possible to make a more conclusive assessment of the usefulness of psychoactive drugs.

DISCUSSION AND CONCLUSIONS

Drugs Combinations

No attempt has been made in the preceding review to describe or evaluate the many drug combinations available in the United States and abroad. One of the best justifications for the avoidance of this onerous task has been provided by H. Freeman (1967) who exhaustively reviewed studies purporting to show the therapeutic value of combinations of psychoactive drugs. These fell into the categories of two major tranquilizers, a major and a minor tranquilizer, two antidepressants, an antidepressant and a major tranquilizer, and an antidepressant and a minor tranquilizer. With the possible exception of the combination of amitriptyline and perphenazine for use with schizophrenics with depressive features, no advantage was clearly demonstrable.

Where more than one drug is necessary, flexible ratios are advisable, which are made difficult by drug combinations in fixed proportions.

Critique of Methodology

During the approximately thirty years covered by this review, there has been marked improvement in research methodology, awareness of nondrug effects, and the quality of experimental controls utilized in psychopharmacological studies with the retarded. This positive trend is offset, however, by concurrent advances in methodology with which surprisingly few investigations have kept pace. Table 13–4, adapted from the excellent critique of child psychopharmacologic research edited by Sprague and Werry (1968), enumerates some of the many areas in which old and more recent studies have failed.

With full recognition of the limitations of double-blind and other types of controlled studies, there can be little question that some method of dealing with variability and bias must be utilized if we are to have any confidence in the conclusions of drug investigations. Fur-

TABLE 13–4

Common Flaws in Experimental Designs

1. Failure to utilize placebo and "blind" procedures.
2. Failure to test for "blindness" by having investigators guess who is on placebo, and who is on drug.
3. Tests may be needed to be sure patients are actually taking drug.
4. Duration of treatment may be unequal across subjects, or insufficient.
5. Failure to select sample or analyze data so as to control for possible developmental (age) differences in reactions to drugs.
6. Dosage is often fixed regardless of age or weight, or flexible, which may break the code by identifying subjects with side-effects. Several fixed levels according to body weight may be best plan.
7. Failure to choose (and specify) reasonable time between drug administration and assessment.
8. Failure to control for variations in behavior at different times of the day, and for sequence (order) effects.
9. Inappropriate sample size and matching, including on symptom severity as opposed to mere presence.
10. Failure to randomly assign subjects to conditions after matching.
11. Practice effects of repeated testing on the same or similar instruments are often not "partialled out" (taken into statistical account).
12. Rating scales are frequently nonoperationalized, unreliable, invalid, or not provided in the report. Testing of raters for consistent bias is needed.
13. Failure to utilize (and report) appropriate statistical techniques.
14. Confounding of results by the regression effect (not taking into account the selection of a sample because of its extremeness on a variable).
15. Global assessments alone, without target symptoms, are often employed.
16. Other drugs or forms of therapy may be applied concurrently.

SOURCE: Adapted from Sprague & Werry (1968).

ther efforts must be made to specify the circumstances under which the studies are carried out and to try to include observations in meaningful settings, such as the classroom or home. It would also be helpful if future investigators learned from the shortcomings of previous studies or consulted with experts in methodology and study design.

Again it should be reiterated that lack of proven benefit from a drug study does *not* mean the agent is inert or useless. The sample used may be inappropriate, the patients may be "atypically unresponsive," nondrug factors may obscure desired effects, dosage may be insufficient, or the assessment instruments may be insensitive to the changes which are to be measured.

Useful Drugs

Fish (1968) has pointed out that young children tend to respond to inner distress with irritability and psychomotor activity. As a consequence, overactive behavior is a "final common pathway" for many different factors, making differential diagnosis difficult. Ascribing hyperactivity to any one cause makes little sense (Werry, 1968*b*). Nevertheless, drugs which suppress psychomotor activity are likely to be very helpful in child psychiatry.

The drugs which have been clinically sifted and seem unquestionably useful are relatively few in number. The major tranquilizers have the greatest interest from this standpoint and have achieved moderate success. There is some evidence that they may slightly depress learning ability, but this limitation must be balanced against the potential benefits from relief of symptoms which are inhibiting the same learning process. The stimulants probably play a definite role in improving attention, reducing distractibility, and promoting goal-directed behavior in nonpsychotic hyperactive or brain-damaged children. There is suggestive evidence for slight enhancement, or at least no decrement, in behavior conducive to learning. These possible benefits are better supported by adequate studies than was the case only three years ago. The minor tranquilizers, anticonvulsants, antidepressants, and sedatives have a much more limited use.

It must be remembered that drugs provide, as yet, nothing which is absent from the individual's behavioral repertoire: they merely stimulate or inhibit functions already present. Training and rehabilitative efforts are required to take full advantage of the benefits conferred by psychopharmacological agents.

Biochemical Approaches to the Learning Process

Recent optimism regarding biochemical alterations in the hypothetical learning or memory processes seems premature. Results are conflicting. It is hard to imagine that direct enhancement of learning and memory will be possible for the majority of the retarded without similar utility for individuals with normal intelligence since most of the retarded have no specific defect. The implications of such general upgrading of intellectual functions are unclear but would undoubtedly have the most far-reaching consequences.

There is somewhat better reason for hope that the study of differential drug responses may lead to an understanding of central nervous system processes which may benefit those children in whom cerebral dysfunction is a significant factor in disturbed behavior and intellectual retardation.

Long-Term Effects on Child Development

Concern has been expressed over the eventual effect of prolonged psychoactive medication on the course of a child's development since the drugs may interfere with anxiety as a "signal" or with other emotional responses. Experiments with animals are inconclusive. Meier and Huff (1962) reported decrements in learning and performance of adult rats which had been given reserpine and deanol before maturity. No such effect was evident in studies on puppies by Fuller and others (1960) and by Fuller (1962). Unfortunately, no adequate assessment of this issue is available to guide those working with children. However, since drug effects are rarely, if ever, complete in suppressing emotions, apprehensions about the possible harmful consequences of an anxiety-free early development are probably unfounded.

Comparison of the Retarded and the Nonretarded

There is little good evidence to support intellectual ability or level as a major variable in the efficacy of the psychoactive drugs. This may be related to the presence of all psychiatric diagnostic categories among the disturbed retarded. Just as certain principles of psychotherapy, family management, behavior therapy, and common sense can be applied to both groups, so the effects of drugs at our present level of knowledge support the similarities rather than the differences between the retarded and other individuals.

Role of Drugs in a Total Treatment Plan

There is general agreement that drugs should not be used as the sole treatment modality but rather as part of a more comprehensive program which takes into account the assets, liabilities, and feelings of the child, parents, and staff. Such a plan attempts to develop new skills and build self-esteem through realistic success experiences. However, until society pays more attention to its neglected citizens, we may expect to see drugs used as substitutes for the more adequate programs of which they should be but one important component.

SUMMARY OF CURRENT USAGE

Some of the complex issues in drug evaluation were discussed at the beginning of this chapter. The paucity of solid data should be painfully apparent. Of what practical value is this rather academic information to the clinician who must decide which drug (if any) to use? What precautions should be taken? Which drugs are best to try in which types of problems? Some of these questions will be considered in this section. For convenience, Table 13–5 summarizes drug preparations, dosages, and common side-effects. Average initial dosages are indicated: the range may be great, and maintenance levels must be individually determined.

Several issues that are well known in work with adults are quite unsettled in child psychopharmacology, where no constant baseline is available. Are certain classes of drugs likely to worsen behavior? For example, the phenothiazines (perhaps with the exception of the piperazine subgroup) are felt by some to be contraindicated in depression. Antidepressants occasionally activate "latent" psychoses in adult depressed patients. These warnings do not seem to apply to children, at least. They have also been questioned in adults. Are adverse effects more likely in children than adults? Some authors report higher, others lower incidences. This may depend upon the drug, the age group, the diagnosis, and the side-effect under consideration. No general statements can be made. Are the minor tranquilizers superior to the older and less expensive mild sedatives? No clear superiority, at least in younger children, has been demonstrated.

Fish (1960a, 1968) has attempted to establish differential criteria for drug use in child psychiatry. She felt that diagnostic categories, by themselves, are useless, but presented some evidence that level of anxiety, activity level, and reduced intelligence had some effect. (It is hard to see why the last should be significant, unless it is because of associated organic dysfunction.) Because of methodological limitations, her conclusions must be accepted with caution: (1) schizophrenic, retarded, hypoactive children became drowsy with amphetamine and were depressed by low doses of chlorpromazine and diphenhydramine, although trifluoperazine (Stelazine) had a more stimulating effect; (2) hyperactive, retarded, schizophrenic children responded more favorably to chlorpromazine and diphenhydramine, but the latter was not effective against severe anxiety, decreasing only the hyperactivity; (3) less retarded children did better with diphenhydramine, although this drug's effectiveness almost disappeared by age ten; (4) chlorpromazine was effective over the entire spectrum of clinical disturbances; (5) amphetamine was helpful in neurotic children with behavior disorders who were better organized. [This last conclusion seems to contradict the findings of Eisenberg and others (1965), who found it ineffective for such children.]

In her recent report, Fish (1968) stated that drugs are only useful in aggressive behavior associated with affective or motor outbursts; negativistic children without these accompaniments may have little

TABLE 13–5

Drug Preparations, Dosage, and Side-Effects [9]

		MAJOR TRANQUILIZERS	
DRUG NAME	**AVAILABLE FORMS**	**DOSAGE**	**SIDE-EFFECTS AND COMMENTS**
Chlorpromazine (Thorazine)	Tabs (10, 25, 50, 100, 200) SR (30, 75, 150, 200, 300) Syrup (10/5cc) Conc (30/cc, 100/cc) Inj Supp	10–20 3–4x/day initially	Drows.; const.; jaundice; hypotension; photosensitivity; EPS; skin pigmentation; ocular changes; dry mouth; nasal stuffiness. CI with CNS depressants, epinephrine (norepinephrine or phenylephrine should be used to counteract hypotension), MAOI; caution with other psychotropic drugs and subcortical brain damage
Thioridazine (Mellaril)	Tabs (10, 25, 50, 100, 200) Conc (30/cc)	10 2–3x/day initially	As above: jaundice & EPS less common; retinitis pigmentosa with high doses for prolonged periods; weight gain
Trifluoperazine (Stelazine)	Tabs (1, 2, 5, 10) Conc (10/cc) Inj	1 1–2x/day initially	Side-effects similar to chlorpromazine; possibly more "activating"; EPS relatively common
Promazine (Sparine)	Tabs (10, 25, 50, 100, 200) Syrup (10/5 cc) Conc (30/cc) Inj	10–25 3–4x/day	Skin and ocular changes rarer, but felt to be less potent
Triflupromazine (Vesprin)	Tabs (10, 25, 50) Susp (50/5 cc) Inj	10 3x/day initially, up to 50 3x/day	Similar to others
Prochlorperazine (Compazine)	Tabs (5, 10, 25) SR (10, 15, 30, 75) Syrup (5/5 cc) Conc (10/cc) Inj Supp	2.5 2–3x/day initially	High incidence of EPS; less potentiating effect with CNS depressants
Fluphenazine (Prolixin, Permitil)	Tabs (1, 2.5, 5) El (0.5/cc) Inj	1 1–2x/day up to max. 3.5/dose	May increase conv. seizures; no photosensitivity or eye changes; long-acting; less sedative than chlorpromazine
Perphenazine (Trilafon)	Tabs (2, 4, 8, 16) SR (8) Syrup (2/5 cc) Supp Inj	2 2–4x/day initially	Potent antiemetic, may mask organic disease; may increase seizures; urinary frequency
Carphenazine (Proketazine)	Tabs (12.5, 25, 50) Conc (50/cc)	Not well established; lowest dose initially	Similar to others of this group, but shorter-acting; CI in severe agitation and anxiety in nonpsychotic pts.
Acetophenazine (Tindal)	Tabs (20)	No dose given for children in PDR	A milder drug, less useful in severe states of agitation; blood and liver changes rare

TABLE 13–5 (continued)

DRUG NAME	AVAILABLE FORMS	DOSAGE	SIDE-EFFECTS AND COMMENTS
Chlorprothixene (Taractan)	Tabs (10, 25, 50, 100) Conc (100/5 cc) Inj (over age 12)	10–25 3–4x/ day over age 6	Drows.; aggravation of seizures occ.; CNS drug potentiation; all other phenothiazine side-effects possible
Thiothixene (Navane)	Caps (1, 2, 5, 10)	1–2 3–4x/ day initially	Not yet recommended for children under 12; may aggravate seizures; phenothiazine-like side-effects possible
Haloperidol (Haldol)	Tabs (0.5, 1, 2) Conc (2/cc)	0.5–1.0 2–3x/day over age 12	Potentiates CNS depressants; EPS; drows.; possibly other effects like phenothiazines; conc. is odorless, tasteless
Reserpine (Serpasil)	Tabs (0.1, 0.25, 1, 2) El (0.2 & 1/4 cc) Inj	Not recommended	Potentially serious adverse effects are many; use as last resort
		MINOR TRANQUILIZERS	
Diphenhydramine (Benadryl)	Caps (25, 50) SR (50) El (10/4 cc) Inj	10–25 3–4x/ day, or 1/lb. body wt/day	Drows.; dizziness; dry mouth; occ. excitement; overdose may cause seizures; given i.v. for EPS (25–50 mgm.); may be used as night sedative in older pts.
Hydroxyzine (Vistaril, Atarax)	Caps (10, 25, 50, 100) Susp (25/5 cc) Syrup (10/5 cc) Inj	25 2–4x/day	Drows.; rare involuntary movements; some antiemetic, antihistaminic and antispasmodic effects; injection should not be in arm
Meprobamate (Miltown, Equanil)	Tabs (200, 400) SR (200, 400) Susp (200/5 cc)	100–200 2–3x/day initially	Drows.; rare allergic reactions: rash, purpura, edema, fever; rare blood dyscrasias
Tybamate (Solacen, Tybatran)	Caps (125, 250, 350)	125–350 3x/day	Drows.; dizziness, nausea, insomnia; rare rash or excitement; not approved under age six
Chlordiazepoxide (Librium)	Caps (5, 10, 25) Tabs (5, 10, 25) Inj	5–10 2–4x/ day	Drows., ataxia, confusion; rare EPS, skin, blood reactions, or overexcitation; not recommended under age six; withdrawal reactions
Diazepam (Valium)	Tabs (2, 5, 10) Inj	1–2.5 3–4x/ day	Drows., ataxia, fatigue, hyper-excited states, rare blood dyscrasia; CI in psychosis; anticonv. activity useful
Oxazepam (Serax)	Caps (10, 15, 30)	Not well established, 10 2–3x/day	Similar to diazepam; CI in psychoses; withdrawal reactions; not approved under age 6

TABLE 13–5 (*continued*)

DRUG NAME	AVAILABLE FORMS	DOSAGE	SIDE-EFFECTS AND COMMENTS
		SEDATIVES AND HYPNOTICS	
Chloral hydrate (Noctec, Dormal, Felsules, Kessodrate)	Caps (250, 500, 1 gram) Syrup (500/5 cc) Supp	15/kg. for hypnosis; 25/kg./day in divided doses for sedation	Rare excitation. May potentiate other CNS depressants; CI in severe liver, kidney, heart disease
Paraldehyde (Paral)	Caps (1 gram) Inj (1 gm/cc)	2–3 cc i.m.; 1 cap. p.o.	Useful in older patients; CI in hepatic and bronchopulmonary disease; inj. must be given deeply, away from nerve trunks
		STIMULANTS	
Amphetamine (Benzedrine)	Tabs (5, 10) SR (15)	5 morning and noon	CI in psychosis & with MAOI; Insomnia, headache, palpitation, tachycardia, tremor, weepiness, anorexia, g.i. disturbances
Dextroamphetamine (Dexedrine)	Tabs (5) SR (5, 10, 15) El (5/5 cc)	2.5 morning and noon	Same. Afternoon dose may be better if smaller than A.M.
Methamphetamine (Desoxyn, Methedrine)	Tabs (2.5, 5) SR (5, 10, 15)	Similar to above	No advantage over dextroamphetamine
Methylphenidate (Ritalin)	Tabs (5, 10, 20) Inj	5–10 morning and noon with meals or 0.5 mg /kg/dose	Rare rash; insomnia, anorexia, weepiness, irritability; use with great caution in conv. disorders and severe agitation
Deanol (Deaner)	Tabs (25, 100)	200–300 in A.M. (initial); 100/day usual main	Headache, const.; muscle tension; pruritus; rash; rare postural hypotension. No anorexia
		ANTIDEPRESSANTS	

MAOI—NOT RECOMMENDED (Isocarboxazid, nialamide, phenelzine, tranylcypromine)

DRUG NAME	AVAILABLE FORMS	DOSAGE	SIDE-EFFECTS AND COMMENTS
Imipramine (Trofrānil)	Tabs (10, 25, 50) Inj	10 3x/day initially	May activate psychosis, prolong A-V conduction time; photosensitization, hypotension, const., dry mouth, blurred vision, drows., insomnia, rash, EPS, rare jaundice
Desipramine (Pertofrane, Norpramin)	Caps (25)	Adults only	Not recommended for children

TABLE 13–5 (*continued*)

DRUG NAME	AVAILABLE FORMS	DOSAGE	SIDE-EFFECTS AND COMMENTS
Amitriptyline	Tabs (10, 25, 50) Inj	10 3x/day	Similar to imipramine
Nortriptyline (Aventyl)	Caps (10, 25) El (10/5 cc)	10–25 1–3x/ day	Similar to imipramine.
Protriptyline (Vivactil)	Tabs (5, 10)	Not established for children	
		ANTIPARKINSON AGENTS	
Diphenhydramine (Benadryl)	(See under minor tranquilizers)		Excellent i.v.: 25–50 mgm.
Biperiden (Akineton)	Tabs (2) Inj	2 1–3x/day; 2 i.m. up to 4 doses; 2–5 i.v. slowly	Useful in treatment of acute or chronic drug-induced EPS
Benztropine (Cogentin)	Tabs (0.5, 2) Inj	1–2 1–2x/day; 1–2 i.v. for acute dystonia	Same as above
Procyclidine (Kemadrin)	Tabs (5)	2.5 2–3x/day	Same as above
Trihexyphenidyl (Artane)	Tabs (2, 5) SR (5) El (2/5 cc)	1 for initial dose, then increase p.r.n.	Same as above
Orphenadrine (Disipal)	Tabs (50)	50 2–3x/day	May produce cholinergic side-effects. Related to diphenhydramine; not sedative

[9] *Abbreviations used:* Tabs = tablets; Caps = capsules; Susp = suspension; El = elixir; Conc = concentrate; Supp = suppository; SR = sustained release form; Inj = injectable form.
CNS = central nervous system; EPS = extrapyramidal syndromes; CI = contraindicated; conv. = convulsive; const. = constipation; drows. = drowsiness; MAOI = monoamine oxidase inhibitor; occ. = occasional; main. = maintenance
NOTE: Numbers indicate milligrams unless specified. (This is not a complete listing of side-effects.)

inner discomfort and resent drug effects. The benzodiazepines may have very different influences: some children become too stimulated and disorganized, others become sedated, and still others act as if they had received amphetamine. She found that while severely disturbed children can often tolerate as much, or more, than disturbed adults, the less disturbed should be tried first on one-half to one-fifth of the adult dose.

Children treated on an out-patient basis should be started on a low dose. The parents may be told to report to the physician by telephone in the first few days so that dosage may be adjusted, unusual side-effects evaluated, and the family supported over the initial "hump" which often entails transient drowsiness or irritability. If such arrangements are not made, many parents will discontinue medication too soon. It must be emphasized here that the initial explanation to the family often does not suffice to deal with this problem.

Choosing a suitable drug may require consideration of the available drug forms (see Table 13–6). Some children will take pills only with

TABLE 13–6

Drug Forms in Approximate Order of Usefulness

| | ORAL FORMS | | | | |
	PALATABLE LIQUID	CONCENTRATE	TABLETS OR CAPSULES ONLY	INJECTION	SUPPOSITORIES
Major Tranquilizers	Chlorpromazine Haloperidol Fluphenazine Trifluproma- zine Prochlorpera- zine Promazine Perphenazine	Thioridazine Trifluoperazine Chlorprothixene Carphenazine	Acetophenazine Thiothixene	Chlorpromazine Trifluoperazine Fluphenazine Triflupromazine Prochlorpera- zine Perphenazine Promazine Chlorpro- thixene [1]	Chlorpromazine Prochlorpera- zine Perphenazine
Minor Tranquilizers	Diphenhy- dramine Meprobamate Hydroxyzine		Chlordiaz- epoxide Diazepam Oxazepam Tybamate	Diphenhy- dramine Diazepam Chlordiazepox- ide	
Sedatives and Hypnotics	Chloral hydrate		Paraldehyde	Paraldehyde	Chloral hydrate
Stimulants	Dextroamphet- amine		Methylpheni- date Amphetamine Methampheta- mine Deanol	Methylpheni- date [2]	
Anti- depressants	Nortriptyline		All except nortriptyline	Imipramine [2] Amitriptyline [2]	
Anti- Parkinson Agents	Trihexyphenidyl Diphenhy- dramine		Benztropine Biperiden Procyclidine Orphenadrine	Diphenhy- dramine Benztropine Biperiden	

[1] Not suggested for parenteral use under age 12.
[2] Not ordinarily useful in this form for retarded children.
NOTE: Concentrates are usually less palatable than syrups, elixirs, or suspensions.

great resistance; liquid forms may be more palatable than crushed tablets, but disguising them may be difficult in occasional cases of marked negativism and suspiciousness. A few children become quite expert at smelling or tasting drugs hidden in food or drink. Spitting up of medication administered by force may also lead to inaccurate dosage.

Many drug concentrates are unpleasant to the taste and are supplied primarily for institutional use. Haloperidol is unique in that its concentrate is odorless, tasteless, and colorless, permitting administration without the patient's knowledge (0.1 mg. per drop).

Some explanation should be given to children who are able to comprehend and whose fantasies may be involved in affecting drug response. This is often neglected because of unwarranted assumptions that retarded children lack an active fantasy life or will be unaffected by previous medical experiences.

The following general guidelines are based both upon the data reviewed in the first section of this chapter and upon personal experience.

Emergency tranquilization or sedation may occasionally be required, and may be accomplished by means of parenteral chlorpromazine, paraldehyde, or other phenothiazines. Caution should be used in observing blood pressure.

Agitated, hyperactive, psychotic children should be tried first on chlorpromazine or thioridazine; if there is no favorable response within a few days after reaching an adult dosage level, chlorprothixene or haloperidol may be used, followed in order of preference by other members of the phenothiazine group. Lack of response to one member of a drug group does *not* mean that there will be similar refractoriness to others. Adequate trial may require surprisingly large doses before declaring the patient unresponsive to a particular medication.

Withdrawn, hypoactive, psychotic patients may be more responsive to trifluoperazine or others of the piperazine subgroup; the evidence is far from conclusive. Drug treatment of these children is often disappointing.

Depressed children or adolescents may be helped by imipramine or amitriptyline; when considerable anxiety is also present, chlorprothixene may be worth a trial since it is said to lack adverse effects in depressed patients which are reported for chlorpromazine in adults.

Hyperactive, impulsive, aggressive, nonpsychotic children are often classified as brain-damaged, although there is little evidence that they form a homogeneous group (Werry, 1968b). They should first receive a trial of dextroamphetamine or methylphenidate, then diphenhydramine, and if these fail, the major tranquilizers. The object is to find a drug which will suppress the undesirable behavior without "snowing" the patient and interfering with learning.

Highly anxious nonpsychotic children may respond to diphenhydramine (except possibly over age twelve) or the minor or major tranquilizers.

Night sedation, if necessary, may be attempted with chloral hydrate, diphenhydramine, or one of the aliphatic phenothiazines such as promazine, in order to avoid use of barbiturates. The latter, especially in some younger children, may have a paradoxical exciting effect.

Tics, particularly if multiple, may be a target symptom which is susceptible to modification by haloperidol. *Enuresis* may respond to imipramine, as well as other nondrug management methods.

Combinations of psychoactive drugs have been used in an attempt to increase desired effects without adverse reactions, but, as has been pointed out in the section on combinations, there is little evidence that this approach is generally successful. There are situations, of course, in which combinations are found helpful by trial and error. Since there is no substitute for individualized adjustment, no purpose would be served here by trying to accomplish the impossible in specifying criteria for use of such combinations.

With the major tranquilizers, extrapyramidal side-effects are usually most distressing to parents, although rarely serious in themselves. These symptoms may be very effectively treated with intravenous diphenhydramine; relief may take only a minute or two and is often quite dramatic. The physician (and parents) must be aware that such reactions may recur hours or days later, even if the offending drug is discontinued. Oral antiparkinson agents (listed in Tables 13–5 and 13–6) may be necessary if the tranquilizer is to be continued, although there seems to be little basis for their routine use from the beginning. Blood and urine studies should be done periodically when children are receiving long-term or high-dosage-level medication. This is largely for parental reassurance and medicolegal protection since the severe reactions may occur with little warning and be best suspected from constitutional signs (sore throat, fever, malaise, excessive fatigue, sudden change in behavior, and so on). The staff and parents must be constantly aware of the tendency of severely disturbed children and the inability of severely retarded children to signal distress in the usual ways.

Parents should also be cautioned about the possible potentiating effects of some psychoactive drugs when combined with certain other agents. Patent medicines, particularly cold remedies, may be dangerous and should not be given without first consulting the physician managing the psychoactive drug therapy. While a complete dossier of possible adverse effects would scare anyone, those which are most likely should be described to the parents so that less anxiety will be aroused if and when they appear.

The problem of what routine to follow in increasing drug dosage is not settled and is usually handled differently in home and residential settings. In the latter, where constant observation is possible, starting with a moderate or high dose may be justifiable. It would seem unwise to do this with out-patients, however. Knowledge of the usual pattern of onset of desired action may guide the physician here. Antidepressants may require many days or even weeks, so that dosage increase should be infrequent. The major tranquilizers, stimulants, and other drugs should demonstrate some effect within a few days, although if the same dose is continued, there may be reduction (or occasionally increase) in side-effects. A few investigators have felt that the stimulants should be used for more than a week before deciding they are not helpful, while others describe an immediate (same-day) response.

Drugs such as thioridazine and fluphenazine are inherently long-acting and do not need to be given more than once a day after the first few days. Most other drugs require several doses each day. With the stimulants, a smaller mid-day or afternoon dose than the morning one may be sufficient. Some drugs (listed in Table 13–5) are provided in sustained-release forms.

So-called "drug holidays" when children are not attending school (weekends or vacations) may be helpful in preventing the development of drug tolerance and in assessing whether certain symptoms will persist in the absence of the medication. However, the author has found that weekends are often unsatisfactory for this purpose since changed environmental factors may obscure pharmacological differences.

Caution must be used in changing a child from one drug to another, particularly when the drugs are members of different groups. With the antidepressants, the "drying-out" period must be about ten to fourteen days. With most of the other drugs a few days will probably suffice without medication.

Kraft (1968) has divided the possible combinations of drug therapy and psychotherapy into three kinds: (1) "directed drug therapy," which refers to making full use of the pharmacological and placebo effects by authoritative prescription and explanation, as well as continuing support, but without counseling; (2) drug therapy primary and counseling secondary; and (3) psychotherapy primary and medication secondary. The setting, previous training of the therapist, demands and pressures from parents or staff, attitudes of superiors, and the nature of symptomatic behavior and family and community ability to tolerate it will all help determine whether or not drugs are used. Some physicians emphasize the magical role often assigned by the child or parents to a drug. Because of this the therapist may avoid medication.

Those with a psychodynamic orientation may shun drugs as interfering with the therapeutic relationship; those with a behaviorist preference may do the same because they feel behavior modification procedures are more effective. Some physicians who are termed (somewhat disparagingly) "organic" may do little else than "directed drug therapy." Strong feelings are often expressed on these issues, as well as on drug preferences. The latter may be based more upon one's early favorable or unfavorable experiences with a drug rather than upon scientific knowledge.

SUMMARY AND CONCLUSIONS

A baseline period of observation and evaluation is always helpful prior to instituting drug therapy. Many children will do just as well with environmental manipulation, family counseling, or individual attention as with drugs. Unless this is kept in mind, parents' frequent concern that medication is used as a "crutch" may be justified.

Considering that chlorpromazine, imipramine, dextroamphetamine, diphenhydramine, chloral hydrate, and paraldehyde have not been clearly surpassed by more recent arrivals, one cannot help concluding that newer drugs are sometimes used primarily because of an exaggerated hope that they may provide "the" answer in a difficult situation.

Children who are unsuccessfully tried on many medications for short periods of time may be unsuitable subjects for drug therapy, may not have had adequate dosage or duration of treatment, or their life circumstances, feelings, or family involvement may have been neglected in the evaluation. Appropriate attention to these factors might increase drug responsiveness or obviate the necessity for medication entirely. The competent physician will do best when he eschews any single treatment modality as a panacea, and when his actions are guided by regard for the individual through establishment of a positive physician-patient relationship. The psychopharmacology of the disturbed behavior of retarded children is no exception to this general rule.

NOTES

1. Preparation of this chapter was supported by the United States Children's Bureau Grant No. 416, Personnel Training Project for Handicapped Children, to St. Christopher's Hospital for Children, Philadelphia, Pa. This chapter is a modification and expansion of the review article: Drug effects on learning in children. *J. Special Education*, 1966, *1*, 17–44. (Permission of publisher granted.)

2. Released in the United States after the writing of this chapter, as Repoise.

REFERENCES

Abbott, P., Blake, A., & Vincze, L. Treatment of mentally retarded with thioridazine. *Dis. Nerv. Sys.*, 1965, *26*, 583–585.

Adamson, W. C., Nellis, B. P. Runge, G., Cleland, C., & Killian, E. Use of tranquilizers for mentally deficient patients. *A. M. A. J. Dis. Child.*, 1958, *96*, 159–164.

Alderton, H. R. Imipramine in childhood nocturnal enuresis: Relationship of time of administration to effect. *Canad. Psychiat. Assoc. J.*, 1967, *12*, 197–203.

Alderton, H. R., & Hoddinott, B. A. Controlled study of the use of thioridazine in the treatment of hyperactive and aggressive children in a children's psychiatric hospital. *Canad. Psychiat. Assoc. J.*, 1964, *9*, 239–247.

Alexandris, A., & Lundell, F. Effect of thioridazine, amphetamine, and placebo on hyperkinetic syndrome and cognitive area in mentally deficient children. *Canad. Med. Assoc. J.*, 1968, *98*, 92–96.

Allen, M., Shannon, G., & Rose, D. Thioridazine hydrochloride in the behavior disturbance of retarded children. *Amer. J. Ment. Defic.*, 1963, *68*, 63–68.

American Medical Association, Council on Drugs. Phenaglycodol, *J.A.M.A.*, 1957, *165*, 157.

————. Evaluation of two tranquilizers: Acetophenazine maleate, carphenazine maleate. *J.A.M.A.*, 1963, *186*, 943–944.

————. Re-evaluation of tranylcypromine sulfate. *J.A.M.A.*, 1964, *189*, 763–764.

————. Evaluation of a new minor tranquilizer: Tybamate (Solacen). *J.A.M.A.*, 1965, *194*, 223.

————. A new minor tranquilizer: Oxazepam (Serax). *J.A.M.A.*, 1966, *195*, 769.

————. Evaluation of a new antipsychotic agent: Haloperidol (Haldol). *J.A.M.A.*, 1968, *205*, 577–578.

Angle, C. R., & McIntyre, M. S. Persistent dystonia in a brain-damaged child after ingestion of phenothiazine. *J. Pediat.*, 1968, *73*, 124–126.

Asatoor, A. M., Levi, A. J., & Milne, D. Tranylcypromine and cheese. *Lancet*, 1963, *2*, 733–734.

Astin, A. W., & Ross, S. Glutamic acid and human intelligence. *Psychol. Bull.*, 1960, *57*, 429–434.

Atkinson, R. M., & Ditman, K. S. Tranylcypromine: A review. *Clin. Pharmacol. Therap.*, 1965, *6*, 631–655.

Babcock, S. D., & Drake, M. E. A study of the behavioral changes of sixty institutionalized female retardates during a three month course of treatment with monosodium glutamate. *Training School Bull.*, 1967, *64*, 49–57.

Badham, J. N., Bardon, L. M., Reeves, P. O., & Young, A. M. A trial of thioridazine in mental deficiency. *Brit. J. Psychiat.*, 1963, *109*, 408–410.

Bair, H. V., & Herold, W. Efficiency of chlorpromazine in hyperactive mentally retarded children. *A. M. A. Arch. Neurol. Psychiat.*, 1955, *74*, 363–364.

Baldwin, R., & Kenny, T. J. Thioridazine in the management of organic behavior disturbances in children. *Curr. Therapeut. Res.*, 1966, *8*, 373–377.

Barancik, M., Brandborg, L. L., & Albion, M. J. Thioridazine-induced cholestasis. *J.A.M.A.*, 1967, *200*, 175–176.

Barker, J. C., Jan, I. A., & Enoch, M. D. A controlled trial of mebanazine ("Actomol") in depression. *Brit. J. Psychiat.*, 1965, *III*, 1095–1100.

Barker, P., & Fraser, I. A. A controlled trial of haloperidol in children. *Brit. J. Psychiat.*, 1968, *114*, 855–857.

Barsa, J. A., & Saunders, J. C. Tybamate, a new tranquilizer. *Amer. J. Psychiat.*, 1963, *120*, 492–493.

Batterman, R. C., & Lower, W. R. Placebo responsiveness—influence of previous therapy. *Curr. Therapeut. Res.*, 1968, *10*, 136–143.

Baumeister, A. A. Problems in comparative studies of mental retardates and normals. *Amer. J. Ment. Defic.*, 1967, *71*, 869–875.

Bazelon, M. Report in *Pediat. News*, 2(7), 5, July, 1968, of paper presented to the 4th Internatl. Scientific Symp. on Mental Retardation, Chicago, Ill.

Beaudry, P., & Gibson, D. Effect of trifluoperazine on the behavior disorders of children with malignant emotional disturbances. *Amer. J. Ment. Defic.*, 1960, *64*, 823–826.

Beecher, H. K. The powerful placebo. *J.A.M.A.*, 1955, *159*, 1602–1606.

————. Increased stress and effectiveness of placebos and "active" drugs. *Science*, 1960, *132*, 91–92.

Bell, A., & Zubek, J. P. Effects of deanol on the intellectual performance of mental defectives. *Canad. J. Psychol.*, 1961, *15*, 172–175.

Benda, C. Promazine in mental deficiency. *Psychiat. Quart.*, 1958, *32*, 449–455.

Bender, L., Cobrinik, L., Faretra, G., & Sankar, D. V. S. The treatment of childhood schizophrenia with LSD and UML. In M. Rinkel (Ed.), *Biological treatment of mental illness*. New York: L. C. Page, 1966, pp. 463–491.

Bender, L., & Cottington, F. The use of amphetamine sulfate (Benzedrine) in child psychiatry. *Amer. J. Psychiat.*, 1942, *99*, 116–121.

Bender, L., & Faretra, G. Organic therapy in pediatric psychiatry. *Dis. Nerv. Sys.*, 1961, *22* (Suppl. 4), 110–111.

Berger, F. M. Classification of psychoactive drugs according to their chemical structures and sites of action. In L. Uhr & J. G. Miller (Eds.), *Drugs and behavior*. New York: John Wiley & Sons, Inc., 1960, pp. 86–105.

Bergin, J. T. F., & Bergin, M. Use of Sparine in low-grade mental defectives. *J. Irish Med. Assoc.*, 1958, *42*, 29 30.

Berman, H. H., Albert-Gasorek, K. E., & Reiss, M. Gonadal immaturity as an etiological factor in some forms of mental deficiency, and its therapy. *Dis. Nerv. Sys.*, 1959, *20* (Suppl. 5), 106–110.

Berry, R., & Turner, P. The pathology of a cross-over trial (Thiazesim—a new antidepressant drug). *Brit. J. Psychiat.*, 1968, *114*, 203–206.

Berthiaume, M., Baser, T., Desrochers, J., Feldman, N., Hamel, O., Hoc, J., & Moamai, N. L'Halopéridol chez les malades mentaux. *L'Union Méd. Canad.*, 1966, *95*, 195–197.

Black, D. B., Kato, J. G., & Walker, G. W. R. A study of improvement in mentally retarded children accruing from Siccacell therapy. *Amer. J. Ment. Defic.*, 1966, *70*, 499–508.

Boatman, M. J., & Berlin, I. N. Some implications of incidental experiences with psychopharmacologic drugs in a children's psychotherapeutic program. *J. Amer. Acad. Child Psychiat.*, 1962, *1*, 431–442.

Bowman, P. W., & Blumberg, E. Ataractic therapy of hyperactive, mentally retarded patients. *J. Maine Med. Assoc.*, 1958, *49*, 272–273.

Bradley, C. The behavior of children receiving Benzedrine. *Amer. J. Psychiatry*, 1937, *94*, 577–585.

————. Benzedrine and Dexedrine in the treatment of children's behavior disorders. *Pediatrics*, 1950, *5*, 24–37.

————. Characteristics and management of children with behavior problems associated with organic brain disease. *Pediat. Clin. N. Amer.*, 1957, *4*, 1049–1060.

Bradley, C., & Bowen, M. School performance of children receiving amphetamine (Benzedrine) sulfate. *Amer. J. Orthopsychiat.*, 1940, *10*, 782–788.

Bradley, C., & Green, E. Psychometric performance of children receiving amphetamine (Benzedrine) sulfate, *Amer. J. Psychiat.*, 1940, *97*, 388–394.

Burk, H. W., & Menolascino, F. J. Haloperidol in emotionally disturbed mentally retarded individuals. *Amer. J. Psychiat.*, 1968, *124*, 1589–1591.

Burks, H. F. Effects of amphetamine therapy on hyperkinetic children. *Arch. Gen. Psychiat.*, 1964, *11*, 604–609.

Carter, C. H. Prochlorperazine in emotionally disturbed, mentally defective children. *South. Med. J.*, 1959, *52*, 174–178.

———. Isocarboxazid in the institutionalized mentally retarded. *Dis. Nerv. Sys.*, 1960, *21*, 568–570.

———. Carphenazine in mental defectives. *Arch. Pediat.*, 1961, *78*, 349–356.

———. Nortriptyline HCl as a tranquilizer for disturbed mentally retarded patients: A controlled study. *Amer. J. Med. Sci.*, 1966, *251*, 465–467.

Cass, L. J., & Frederik, W. S. Review of the techniques which are followed in double-blind clinical investigations. *Curr. Therapeut. Res.*, 1965, *7*, 417–421.

Castner, C. W., & Noble, R. C. Report on a new drug, captodiamine. A preliminary investigation. *Dis. Nerv. Sys.*, 1959, *20*, 594–596.

Chessick, R. D., & McFarland, R. L. Problems in psychopharmacological research. *J.A.M.A.*, 1963, *185*, 237–241.

Chien, C. P., & DiMascio, A. Drug-induced extrapyramidal symptoms and their relations to clinical efficacy. *Amer. J. Psychiat.*, 1967, *123*, 1490–1498.

Clausen, J., Fineman, M., Henry, C. E., & Wohl, N. The effect of Deaner (2-dimethylaminoethanol) on mentally retarded subjects. *Training School Bull.*, 1960, *57*, 3–12.

Cole, J. O. Evaluation of drug treatments in psychiatry. *J. New Drugs*, 1962, *2*, 264–275.

———. Therapeutic efficacy of antidepressant drugs. *J.A.M.A.*, 1964, *190*, 448–455.

Collipp, P. J., Kaplan, S. A., Kogut, M. D., Tasem, W., Plachte, F., Schlamm, V., Boyle, D. C., Ling, S. M., & Koch, R. Mental retardation in congenital hypothyroidism: Improvement with thyroid replacement therapy. *Amer. J. Ment. Defic.*, 1965, *70*, 432–437.

Connell, P. H., Corbett, J. A., Horne, D. J., & Mathews, A. M. Drug treatment of adolescent tiqueurs: A double-blind trial of diazepam and haloperidol. *Brit. J. Psychiat.*, 1967, *113*, 375–381.

Conners, C. K., & Eisenberg, L. The effects of methylphenidate on symptomatology and learning in disturbed children. *Amer. J. Psychiat.*, 1963, *120*, 458–464.

Conners, C. K., Eisenberg, L., & Barcai, A. Effect of dextroamphetamine on children. *Arch. Gen. Psychiat.*, 1967, *17*, 478–485.

Conners, C. K., Eisenberg, L., & Sharpe, L. Effects of methylphenidate (Ritalin) on paired-associate learning and Porteus maze performance in emotionally disturbed children. *J. Consult. Psychol.*, 1964, *28*, 14–22.

Conrad, W. G., & Insel, J. Anticipating the response to amphetamine therapy in the treatment of hyperkinetic children. *Pediatrics*, 1967, *40*, 96–98.

Corless, J. D., & Buchanan, D. S. Phenothiazine intoxication in children. A report of three cases. *J.A.M.A.*, 1965, *194*, 565–567.

Court, J. H., & Cameron, I. A. Psychomotor assessment of the effects of haloperidol. *Percept. Motor Skills*, 1963, *17*, 168–170.

Cowen, M. A., & Martin, W. C. Long-term chlorpromazine retention and its modification by steroids. *Amer. J. Psychiat.*, 1968, *125*, 243–245.

Craft, M. Tranquillizers in mental deficiency: Hydroxyzine. *J. Ment. Sci.*, 1957, *103*, 855–857.

———. Tranquillizers in mental deficiency: Meprobamate. *J. Ment. Defic. Res.*, 1958, *2*, 17.

———. Mental disorder in the defective: A psychiatric survey among in-patients. *Amer. J. Ment. Defic.*, 1959, *63*, 829–834. (a)

———. Mental disorder in the defective: The use of tranquillizers. *Amer. J. Ment. Defic.*, 1959, *64*, 63–71. (b)

Crane, G. E. A review of clinical literature on haloperidol. *Internat. J. Neuropsychiat.*, 1967, *3* (Suppl. 1), 111–127.

———. Tardive dyskinesia in patients with major neuroleptics: A review of the literature. *Amer. J. Psychiat.*, 1968, *124* (Suppl. 8), 40–48.

Creager, R. O., & Van Riper, C. The effect of methylphenidate on the verbal productivity of children with cerebral dysfunction. *J. Speech Hearing Res.*, 1967, *10*, 623–628.

Cutler, M., Little, J. W., & Strauss, A. A. Effect of Benzedrine on mentally deficient children. *Amer. J. Ment. Defic.*, 1940, *45*, 59–65.

Curry, S. H., & Marshall, J. H. L. Report in *Psychiat. News*, 1968, *3*(8), 5.

Cytryn, L., Gilbert, A., & Eisenberg, L. The effectiveness of tranquilizing drugs plus supportive psychotherapy in treating behavior disorders of children: A double-blind study of eighty out-patients. *Amer. J. Orthopsychiat.*, 1960, *30*, 113–128.

Dabbous, I. A., & Bergman, A. B. Neurologic damage associated with phenothiazine. *Amer. J. Dis. Child.*, 1966, *111*, 291–296.

Daneel, A. B. Neulactil (pericyazine) in the behaviour disturbances of institutionalized mental defectives. *South African Med. J.*, 1967, *41*, 995–998.

Darling, H. F. The treatment of ambulatory adolescent schizophrenia with acetophenazine. *Amer. J. Psychiat.*, 1963, *120*, 68–69.

David, L. Push-button brain. *This Week Magazine*, Feb. 13, 1966, pp. 4–5.

Davies, T. S. A monoamine oxidase inhibitor (Niamid) in the treatment of the mentally subnormal. *J. Ment. Sci.*, 1961, *107*, 115–118.

Davis, J. M. Efficacy of tranquilizing and antidepressant drugs. *Arch. Gen. Psychiat.*, 1965, *13*, 552–572.

Davis, K. V., Sprague, R. L., & Werry, J. S. Stereotyped behavior and activity level in severe retardates: The effect of drugs. *Amer. J. Ment. Defic.*, 1969, *73*, 721–727.

Dehnel, L. L., Vestre, N. D., & Schiele, B. C. A controlled comparison of clopenthixol and perphenazine in a chronic schizophrenic population. *Curr. Therapeut. Res.*, 1968, *10*, 169–176.

Dietze, H. J. Dyskinetic syndrome associated with chlorprothixene. *Amer. J. Psychiat.*, 1963, *120*, 503–504.

DiMascio, A., & Barrett, J. Comparative effects of oxazepam in "high" and "low" anxious student volunteers. *Psychosomatics*, 1965, *6*, 298–302.

DiMascio, A., & Klerman, G. L. Experimental human psychopharmacology: The role of non-drug factors. In G. J. Sarwer-Foner (Ed.), *The dynamics of psychiatric drug therapy*. Springfield, Ill.: Charles C Thomas, 1960, pp. 56–92.

Dinello, F. A., & Champelli, J. The use of imipramine in the treatment of enuresis: A review of the literature. *Canad. Psychiat. Assoc. J.*, 1968, *13*, 237–241.

Dinnerstein, A. J., Lowenthal, M., & Blitz, B. The interaction of drugs with placebos in the control of pain and anxiety. *Perspect. Biol. Med.*, 1966, *10*, 103–117.

Dougan, H. T. Hydroxyzine syrup (Atarax) in the management of pediatric behavior problems. *Med. Times*, 1962, *90*, 551–554.

Edwards, G. Comparison of the effect of imipramine and desipramine on some symptoms of depressive illness. *Brit. J. Psychiat.*, 1965, *111*, 889–897.

Effron, A. S., & Freedman, A. M. The treatment of behavior disorders in children with Benadryl. *J. Pediat.*, 1953, *42*, 261–266.

Eisenberg, L. Role of drugs in treating disturbed children. *Children*, 1964, *11*, 167–173.

———. The management of the hyperkinetic child. *Develop. Med. Child Neurol.*, 1966, *8*, 593–598.

Eisenberg, L., Conners, C. K., & Sharpe, L. A controlled study of the differential application of outpatient psychiatric treatment of children. *Japan. J. Child Psychiat.*, 1965, *6*, 125–132.

Eisenberg, L., Gilbert, A., Cytryn, L., & Molling, P. A. The effectiveness of psychotherapy alone and in conjunction with perphenazine or placebo in the treatment of neurotic and hyperkinetic children. *Amer. J. Psychiat.*, 1961, *117*, 1088–1093.

Eisenberg, L., Lachman, R., Molling, P. A., Lockner, A., Mizelle, J. D., & Conners, C. K. A psychopharmacologic experiment in a training school for delinquent boys: Methods, problems, findings. *Amer. J. Orthopsychiat.*, 1963, *33*, 431–447.

Esen, F. M., & Durling, D. Thorazine in the treatment of mentally retarded children. *Arch. Pediat.*, 1956, *73*, 168–173.

———. The treatment of 14 mentally retarded boys with Sparine. *Arch. Pediat.*, 1957, *74*, 471–474.

Eveloff, H. H. Psychopharmacologic agents in child psychiatry. *Arch. Gen. Psychiat.*, 1966, *14*, 472–481.

Faretra, G., & Gozun, C. The use of drug combinations in pediatric psychiatry. *Curr. Therapeut. Res.*, 1964, *6*, 340–343.

Filotto, J., Bordeleau, J. M., & Tetreault, L. Utilisation du thiothixène dans le traitement de la manie: Etude pilote. *Canad. Psychiat. Assoc. J.*, 1968, *13*, 175–179.

Fine, R. H. Clinical experience with trifluoperazine in the severely retarded. *J. Neuropsychiat.*, 1964, *5*, 370–372.

Fischer, E. Reserpine ("Serpasil") in mental deficiency practice. *J. Ment. Sci.*, 1956, *102*, 542–545.

Fish. B. Drug therapy in child psychiatry: Psychological aspects. *Compr. Psychiat.*, 1960, *1*, 55–61. (*a*)

––––––. Drug therapy in child psychiatry: Pharmacological aspects. *Compr. Psychiat.*, 1960, *1*, 212–227. (*b*)

––––––. The influence of maturation and abnormal development on the responses of disturbed children to drugs. In *Third World Congress of Psychiatry: Proceedings*, vol. 2. Montreal: McGill University Press, 1961, pp. 1341–1344.

––––––. Drug use in psychiatric disorders of children. *Amer. J. Psychiat.*, 1968, *124* (Suppl. 8), 31–36.

Fish, B., Shapiro, T., & Campbell, M. Long-term prognosis and the response of schizophrenic children to drug therapy: A controlled study of trifluoperazine. *Amer. J. Psychiat.*, 1966, *123*, 32–39.

Fish, C. H., & Bowling, E. Stuttering—the effect of treatment with d-amphetamine and a tranquilizing agent, trifluoperazine: A preliminary report on an uncontrolled study. *California Med.*, 1965, *103*, 337–339.

Fisher, G. W., Murray, F., Walley, M. R., & Kiloh, L. G. A controlled trial of imipramine in the treatment of nocturnal enuresis in mentally subnormal patients. *Amer. J. Psychiat.*, 1966, *123*, 32–39.

Fisher, S. (Ed.) *Child research in psychopharmacology.* Springfield, Ill.: Charles C Thomas, 1959.

––––––. On the relationship between expectations and drug response. *Clin. Pharmacol. Therapeut.*, 1962, *3*, 125–126.

Freed, H. Current status of the tranquilizers and of child analysis in child psychiatry. *Dis. Nerv. Sys.*, 1961, *22*, 434–437.

––––––. *The chemistry and therapy of behavior disorders in children.* Springfield, Ill.: Charles C Thomas, 1962.

Freed, H., Abrams, J., & Peifer, C. Reading disability: A new therapeutic approach and its implications. *J. Clin. Exper. Psychopathol. & Quart. Rev. Psychiat. Neurol.*, 1959, *20*, 251–259.

Freed, H., & Frignito, N. Tranquilizers in child psychiatry: Current status on drugs, particularly phenothiazines. *Penn. Psychiat. Quart.*, 1961, *1*, 39–48.

Freed, H., & Peifer, C. Treatment of hyperkinetic emotionally disturbed children with prolonged administration of chlorpromazine. *Amer. J. Psychiat.*, 1956, *113*, 22–26. (*a*)

Freed, H., & Peifer, C. Some considerations on the use of chlorpromazine in a child psychiatry clinic. *J. Clin. Exper. Psychopathol. & Quart. Rev. Psychiat. Neur.*, 1956, *17*, 164–169. (*b*)

Freedman, A. M. Drug therapy in behavior disorders. *Pediat. Clin. N. Amer.*, 1958, *5*, 573–584.

Freedman, A. M., Effron, A. S., & Bender, L. Pharmacotherapy in children with psychiatric illness. *J. Nerv. Ment. Dis.*, 1955, *122*, 479–486.

Freedman, A. M., Kremer, M. W., Robertiello, R. C., & Effron, A. S. The treatment of behavior disorders in children with Tolserol. *J. Pediat.*, 1955, *47*, 369–372.

Freeman, H. The therapeutic value of combinations of psychotropic drugs: A review. *Psychopharmacol. Bull.*, 1967, *4* (1), 1–27.

Freeman, R. D. Drug effects on learning in children: A selective review of the past thirty years. *J. Special Education*, 1966, *1*, 17–44.

––––––. The home visit in child psychiatry: It.: usefulness in diagnosis and training. *J. Amer. Acad. Child Psychiat.*, 1967, *6*, 276–294.

Friend, D. G. Antidepressant drug therapy. *Clin. Pharmacol. Therapeut.*, 1965, *6*, 805–814.

Frommer, E. A. Treatment of childhood depression with antidepressant drugs. *Brit. Med. J.*, 1967, *1*, 729–732.

Fuller, J. L. Effects of drugs on psychological development. *Ann. N.Y. Acad. Sci.*, 1962, *96*, 199–204.

Fuller, J. L., Clark, L. D., & Waller, M. B. Effects of chlorpromazine upon psychological development in the puppy. *Psychopharmacologia*, 1960, *1*, 393–407.

Furst, W. Therapeutic re-orientation in some depressive states: Clinical evaluation of a new monoamine-oxidase inhibitor (W–1544–A, phenelzine, Nardil). *Amer. J. Psychiat.*, 1959, *116*, 429–434.

Gadson, E. J. Glutamic acid and mental deficiency. *Amer. J. Ment. Defic.*, 1951, *55*, 521–528.

Galambos, M. Long-term clinical trial with diazepam on adult mentally retarded persons. *Dis. Nerv. Sys.*, 1965, *26*, 305–309.

Gallant, D. M., Bishop, M. P., Timmons, E., & Steele, C. A. Trifluperidol: A butyrophenone derivative. *Amer. J. Psychiat.*, 1963, *120*, 485–487.

Gardner, W. I. Occurrence of severe depressive reactions in the mentally retarded. *Amer. J. Psychiat.*, 1967, *124*, 386–388.

Gardos, G., DiMascio, A., Salzman, C., & Shader, R. I. Differential actions of chlordiazepoxide and oxazepam on hostility. *Arch. Gen. Psychiat.*, 1968, *18*, 757–760.

Garfield, S. L., Helper, M. M., Wilcott, R. C., & Muffly, R. Effects of chlorpromazine on behavior in emotionally disturbed children. *J. Nerv. Ment. Dis.*, 1962, *135*, 147–154.

Gatski, R. L. Chlorpromazine in the treatment of emotionally maladjusted children. *J.A.M.A.*, 1955, *157*, 1298–1300.

Geiger, L. A., & Lesser, L. I. Ocular side effects of chlorpromazine in a child. *J.A.M.A.*, 1967, *202*, 916.

Gelfand, S., Clark, L. D., Herbert, E. W., Gelfand, D. M., & Holmes, E. D. Magnesium pemoline: Stimulant effects on performance of fatigued subjects. *Clin. Pharmacol. Therapeut.*, 1968, *9*, 56–60.

Geller, S. J. Comparison of a tranquilizer and a psychic energizer used in treatment of children with behavioral disorders. *J.A.M.A.*, 1960, *174*, 481–484.

Gerle, B. Observations on use of haloperidol following 3 years' experience. *Act. Psychiat. Scand.*, 1963, *39* (Suppl. 169), 348–350.

Giannini, M. J. Hydroxyzine hydrochloride in treatment of behavioral disturbances in mentally retarded children. *N.Y. State J. Med.*, 1964, *64*, 1721–1723.

Gillie, A. K. The use of Pacatal in low-grade mental defectives. *J. Ment. Sci.*, 1957, *103*, 402–405.

Gilmour, S. J. G. Clinical trial of mebanazine—a new monoamine oxidase inhibitor. *Brit. J. Psychiat.*, 1965, *111*, 899–902.

Gombos, G. M., & Yarden, P. E. Ocular and cutaneous side effects after prolonged chlorpromazine treatment. *Amer. J. Psychiat.*, 1967, *123*, 872–874.

Goodman, L. S., & Gilman, A. *The pharmacological basis of therapeutics* (3rd ed.). New York: The Macmillan Company, 1965.

Grant, Q. Psychopharmacology in childhood emotional and mental disorders. *J. Pediat.*, 1962, *61*, 626–637.

Greiner, A. C., & Berry, K. Skin pigmentation and corneal and lens opacities with prolonged chlorpromazine therapy. *Canad. Med. Assoc. J.*, 1964, *90*, 663–665.

Guey, J., Charles, C., Coquery, C., Roger, J., & Soulayrol, R. Study of psychological effects of ethosuximide (Zarontin) on 25 children suffering from petit mal epilepsy. *Epilepsia*, 1967, *8*, 129–141.

Gupta, J. M., & Lovejoy, F. H., Jr. Acute phenothiazine toxicity in childhood: A five-year survey. *Pediatrics*, 1967, *39*, 771–774.

Guy, W., Gross, M., & Dennis, H. An alternative to the double blind procedure. *Amer. J. Psychiat.*, 1967, *123*, 1505–1512.

Hackett, E., Gold, R. L., & Kline, N. S. A comparison of open-study and double-blind study evaluations of the antidepressant activity of thiothixene ("Navane"). *Psychosomatics*, 1968, *9*, 103–108.

Haefner, D. P., Sacks, J. M., & Mason, A. S. Physicians' attitudes toward chemotherapy as a factor in psychiatric patients' responses to medication. *J. Nerv. Ment. Dis.*, 1960, *131*, 64–69.

Hagberg, B. The chlordiazepoxide HCl (Librium) analogue nitrazepam (Mogadon) in the treatment of epilepsy in children. *Develop. Med. Child Neurol.*, 1968, *10*, 302–308.

Hagopian, V., Stratton, D. B., & Busiek, R. D. Five cases of pigmentary retinopathy associated with thioridazine administration. *Amer. J. Psychiat.*, 1966, *123*, 97–100.

Hanlon, T. E., Michaux, M. H., Ota, K. Y., Shaffer, J. W., & Kurland, A. A. The comparative effectiveness of eight phenothiazines. *Psychopharmacologia*, 1965, *7*, 89–106.

Hare, E. H., & Willcox, D. R. C. Do psychiatric in-patients take their pills? *Brit. J. Psychiat.*, 1967, *113*, 1435–1439.

Harman, C., & Winn, D. Clinical experience with chlorprothixene in disturbed children—a comparative study. *Internat. J. Neuropsychiat.*, 1966, *2*, 72–77.

Hartlage, L. C. Effects of chlorpromazine on learning. *Psychol. Bull.*, 1965, *64*, 235–245.

Heaton-Ward, W. A. Inference and suggestion in a clinical trial (Niamid in mongolism). *J. Ment. Sci.*, 1962, *108*, 865–870.

Heaton-Ward, W. A., & Jancar, J. A. A controlled clinical trial of meprobamate in the management of difficult and destructive female mental defectives. *J. Ment. Sci.*, 1958, *104*, 454–456.

Helper, M. M., Wilcott, R. C., & Garfield, S. L. Effects of chlorpromazine on learning and related processes in emotionally disturbed children. *J. Consult. Psychol.*, 1963, *27*, 1–9.

Heninger, G., DiMascio, A., & Klerman, G. L. Personality factors in variability of response to phenothiazines. *Amer. J. Psychiat.*, 1965, *121*, 1091–1094.

Hesbacher, P. T., Rickels, K., & Weise, C. Target symptoms: A promising improvement criterion in psychiatric drug research. *Arch. Gen. Psychiat.*, 1968, *18*, 595–600.

Himwich, H. E., Costa, E., Rinaldi, F., & Rudy, L. H. Triflupromazine and trifluoperazine in the treatment of disturbed mentally defective patients. *Amer. J. Ment. Defic.*, 1960, *64*, 711–712.

Hoffer, A. Theoretical examination of the double-blind design. *Canad. Med. Assoc. J.*, 1967, *97*, 123–127.

Hollister, L. E. Complications from psychotherapeutic drugs—1964. *Clin. Pharmacol. Therapeut.*, 1964, *5*, 322–333.

———. Antidepressants—a somewhat depressing scene. *Clin. Pharmacol. Therapeut.*, 1965, *6*, 555–559.

Hollister, L. E., & Overall, J. E. Reflections on the specificity of action of antidepressants. *Psychosomatics*, 1965, *6*, 361–365.

Hollister, L. E., Overall, J. E., Bennett, J. L., Kimbell, I., Jr., & Shelton, J. Triperidol in schizophrenia: Further evidence for specific patterns of action of antipsychotic drugs. *J. New Drugs*, 1965, *5*, 34–42.

Horenstein, S. Reserpine and chlorpromazine in hyperactive mental defectives. *Amer. J. Ment. Defic.*, 1957, *61*, 525–529.

Hornsby, L. D., Bishop, M. P., & Gallant, D. M. Suggestibility and placebo response: Further positive findings. *Curr. Therapeut. Res.*, 1967, *9*, 46–47.

Houze, M., Wilson, H. D., & Goodfellow, H. D. L. Treatment of mental deficiency with alpha tocopherol. *Amer. J. Ment. Defic.*, 1964, *69*, 328–329.

Hunt, B. R., Frank, T., & Krush, T. P. Chlorpromazine in the treatment of severe emotional disorders of children. *A. M. A. J. Dis. Child.*, 1956, *91*, 268–277.

Hunt, P. V. A comparison of the effects of oxypertine and trifluoperazine in withdrawn schizophrenics. *Brit. J. Psychiat.*, 1967, *113*, 1419–1424.

Hunter, H., & Stephenson, G. M. Chlorpromazine and trifluoperazine in the treatment of behavioral abnormalities in the severely subnormal child. *Brit. J. Psychiat.*, 1963, *109*, 411–417.

Inouye, E., Kamide, H., Ihda, S., Izawa, S., Takuma, T., Masaki, T., Morishita, H., Eto, M., Umegaki, M., & Kada, M. Effect of bovine brain hydrate on mentally retarded children: A multidisciplinary clinical experiment using co-twin control. *Progr. Brain Res.*, 1966, *21 B*, 1–39.

Ison, M. G. The effect of Thorazine on Wechsler scores. *Amer. J. Ment. Defic.*, 1957, *62*, 543–547.

Jacobs, R. Erfahrungen mit Haloperidol in der pädopsychiatrischen Anstaltspraxis. *Prax. Kinderpsychol. Kinderpsychiat.*, 1966, *15*, 67–70.

Jacobsen, M. The use of rating scales in clinical research. *Brit. J. Psychiat.*, 1965, *111*, 545–546.

Jaquith, W. L., Nail, H. R., Smith, B. S., & Taylor, M. R. Perphenazine therapy among outpatients. *Amer. J. Psychiat.*, 1967, *123*, 1023–1025.

Jensen, O. Haloperidolbehandling af psykotiske andssvage patienter. *Ugesk. Laeger*, 1962, *124*, 1138–1141.

Johnston, A. H., & Martin, C. H. The clinical use of reserpine and chlorpromazine in the care of the mentally deficient. *Amer. J. Ment. Defic.*, 1957, *62*, 292–294.

Jonas, A. D. *Ictal and subictal neurosis: Diagnosis and treatment.* Springfield, Ill.: Charles C Thomas, 1965.

———. The emergence of epileptic equivalents in the era of tranquilizers. *Internat. J. Neuropsychiat.*, 1967, *3*, 40–45.

Jones, D. Psychopharmacological therapy with the mentally retarded. *Ment. Retard. Abstr.*, 1966, *3*(1), 21–27.

Kamm, I. Control of sexual hyperactivity with thioridazine. *American J. Psychiat.*, 1965, *121*, 922–923.

Kamm, I., & Mandel, A. Thioridazine in the treatment of behavior disorders in epileptics. *Dis. Nerv. Sys.*, 1967, *28*, 46–48.

Kanner, L. *A history of the care and study of the mentally retarded.* Springfield, Ill.: Charles C Thomas, 1964.

Katz, B. E. Education of cerebral palsied children—the role of meprobamate: A preliminary evaluation. *J. Pediat.*, 1958, *53*, 467–475.

Kent, L. R. The use of tranquilizers in the treatment of stuttering. *J. Speech Hearing Disorders*, 1963, *28*, 288–294.

Kinross-Wright, J. The current status of phenothiazines. *J.A.M.A.*, 1967, *200*, 461–464.

Kirk, D. L., & Bauer, A. M. Effects of reserpine (Serpasil) on emotionally maladjusted high grade mental retardates. *Amer. J. Ment. Defic.*, 1956, *60*, 779–784.

Kirkham, J. E., Jr., & Kinross-Wright, J. A clinical evaluation of piperacetazine in the treatment of chronic schizophrenia. *Amer. J. Psychiat.*, 1964, *120*, 900–902.

Klein, D. F., & Greenberg, I. M. Behavioral effects of diphenylhydantoin in severe psychiatric disorders. *Amer. J. Psychiat.*, 1967, *124*, 847–849.

Kline, N. S. On the rarity of "irreversible" oral dyskinesias following phenothiazines. *Amer. J. Psychiat.*, 1968, *124* (Suppl. 8), 48–54.

Klingman, W. O. Clinical use of pipradrol. In J. H. Nodine & J. H. Moyer (Eds.), *The first Hahnemann symposium on psychosomatic medicine.* Philadelphia: Lea & Febiger, 1962, pp. 588–594.

Klotz, M. The history and pharmacology of the ataractic drugs. *Dis. Nerv. Sys.*, 1959, *20*, 365–369.

Knobel, M. The environmental "antidrug" effect. *Psychiatry*, 1960, *23*, 403–407.

———. Psychopharmacology for the hyperkinetic child. *Arch. Gen. Psychiat.*, 1962, *6*, 198–202.

Knobel, M., & Lytton, G. J. Diagnosis and treatment of behavior disorders in children. *Dis. Nerv. Sys.*, 1959, *20*, 334–340.

Knobel, M., Wolman, M. B., & Mason, E. Hyperkinesis and organicity in children. *A. M. A. Arch. Gen. Psychiat.*, 1959, *1*, 310–321.

Koch, R., Graliker, B., Bronston, W., & Fishler, K. Mental retardation in early childhood. *Amer. J. Dis. Child.*, 1965, *109*, 243–251.

Kordas, S. K., Kazamias, N. G., Georgas, J. G., & Papadokostakis, J. G. Clopenthixol: A controlled trial in chronic hospitalized schizophrenic patients. *Brit. J. Psychiat.*, 1968, *114*, 833–836.

Kosman, M. E., & Unna, K. R. Effects of chronic administration of the amphetamines and other stimulants on behavior. *Clin. Pharmacol. Therapeut.*, 1968, *9*, 240–254.

Kozinn, P. J., & Wiener, H. Oculogyric crisis after a small dose of perphenazine: Case report of an eight-year-old girl. *J.A.M.A.*, 1960, *174*, 304–305.

Kraft, I. A. The use of psychoactive drugs in the out-patient treatment of psychiatric disorders of childhood. *Amer. J. Psychiat.*, 1968, *124*, 1401–1407.

Kraft, I. A., Ardali, C., Duffy, J., Hart, J., & Pearce, P. R. Use of amitriptyline in childhood behavioral disturbances. *Internat. J. Neuropsychiat.*, 1966, *2*, 611–614.

Kraft, I. A., Marcus, I. M., Wilson, W., Swander, D., Rummage, N., & Schulhofer, E.

Methodological problems in studying the effect of tranquilizers in children with special reference to meprobamate. *South. Med. J.,* 1959, *52,* 179–185.

Krakowski, A. J. The role of the physician in the management of the emotionally disturbed child. Part IV. Management. *Psychosomat.,* 1963, *4,* 270–278.

————. Amitriptyline in treatment of hyperkinetic children: A double-blind study. *Psychosomat.,* 1965, *6,* 355–360.

————. Treatment of psychosomatic gastrointestinal reactions in children. *Dis. Nerv. Sys.,* 1966, *27,* 403–408.

Krupanidhi, I., Gowda, K. A., & Nirmala, N. S. The use of nialamide in mental retardation in childhood. *Ind. J. Pediat.,* 1964, *31,* 351–354.

Kugel, R. B., & Alexander, T. The effect of a central nervous system stimulant (deanol) on behavior. *Pediat.,* 1963, *31,* 651–655.

Kugelmass, I. N. Psychochemotherapy of mental deficiency in children. *Internat. Rec. of Med.,* 1956, *169,* 323–338.

————. Chemical therapy of mentally retarded children. *Internat. Rec. Med.,* 1959, *172,* 119–136.

Kurland, A. A. Placebo effect. In L. Uhr & J. G. Miller (Eds.), *Drugs and behavior.* New York: Wiley, 1960. Pp. 156–165.

Kurland, A. A., Dorf, H. J., Michaux, M. H., & Goldberg, J. B. Cypenamine treatment of mentally retarded children. *Current Therapeutic Research,* 1967, *9,* 293–295.

Kurtis, L. B. Clinical study of the response to nortriptyline on autistic children. *Internat. J. Neuropsychiat.,* 1966, *2,* 298–301.

Laird, D. M., & Hope, J. M. Dartal in treatment of hospitalized schizophrenic patients. *Dis. Nerv. Sys.,* 1959, *20,* 302–307.

Laufer, M. W. Personal communication, February 2, 1968.

Laufer, M. W., & Denhoff, E. Hyperkinetic behavior syndrome in children. *J. Pediat.,* 1957, *50,* 463–474.

Laufer, M. W., Denhoff, E., & Solomons, G. Hyperkinetic impulse disorder in children's behavior problems. *Psychosomat. Med.,* 1957, *19,* 38–49.

LaVeck, G. D., & Buckley, P. The use of psychopharmacologic agents in retarded children with behavior disorders. *J. Chron. Dis.,* 1961, *13,* 174–183.

LaVeck, G. D., de la Cruz, F., & Simundson, E. Fluphenazine in the treatment of mentally retarded children with behavior disorders. *Dis. Nerv. Sys.,* 1960, *21,* 82–85.

Leestma, J. E., & Koenig, K. L. Sudden death and phenothiazines: A current controversy. *Arch. Gen. Psychiat.,* 1968, *18,* 137–148.

Leger, Y. A four-year appraisal of thioridazine. *Amer. J. Psychiat.,* 1966, *123,* 728–732.

Lehman, E., Haber, J., & Lesser, S. R. The use of reserpine in autistic children. *J. Nerv. Ment. Dis.,* 1957, *125,* 351–356.

LeVann, L. J. Thioridazine (Mellaril), a psychosedative virtually free of side-effects. *Alberta Med. Bull.,* 1961, *26,* 141–144.

————. Clinical comparison of haloperidol with chlorpromazine in mentally retarded children and adolescents. Paper presented at the meeting of the New York State Medical Health Officers' Association, Rochester, N. Y., June, 1968. (*a*)

————. Haloperidol in the treatment of behavioral disorders in children and adolescents. Paper presented at the Canadian Psychiatric Association Meeting, Regina, Saskatchewan, June, 1968. (*b*)

————. A new butyrophenone: Trifluperidol. A psychiatric evaluation in a pediatric setting. *Canad. Psychiat. Assoc. J.,* 1968, *13,* 271–273. (*c*)

Levy, J. M., Jones, B. E., & Croley, H. T. Effects of methylphenidate (Ritalin) on drug-induced drowsiness in mentally retarded patients. *Amer. J. Ment. Defic.,* 1957, *62,* 284–287.

Lewis, I. Trial of diazepam in myotonia. *Neurology (Minneapolis),* 1966, *16,* 831–836.

Liberman, R. A criticism of drug therapy in psychiatry. *A. M. A. Arch. Gen. Psychiat.,* 1961, *4,* 131–136.

————. An analysis of the placebo phenomenon. *J. Chron. Dis.,* 1962, *15,* 661–783.

Life Magazine, Sept. 29, 1967.

Lindholm, O. A clinical study of Esucos in a mentally retarded clientele. *Internat. J. Neuropsychiat.,* 1967, *3,* 209–218.

Lipman, R. S., Cole, J. O., Park, L. C., & Rickels, K. Sensitivity of symptom- and nonsymptom-focused criteria of out-patient drug efficacy. *Amer. J. Psychiat.*, 1965, *122*, 24–27.

Litchfield, H. R. Clinical evaluation of meprobamate in disturbed and pre-psychotic children. *Ann. N. Y. Acad. Sci.*, 1957, *67*, 828–831.

———. Clinical pediatric experience with ataractic agent in less severe emotional states. *N. Y. State J. Med.*, 1960, *60*, 518–523.

Livingston, S. Diphenylhydantoin in emotional disorders. *J.A.M.A.*, 1968, *204*, 549.

Logothetis, J. Spontaneous epileptic seizures and electroencephalographic changes in the course of phenothiazine therapy. *Neurology (Minneapolis)*, 1967, *17*, 869–877.

Logue, D. S., & Bessman, S. P. Psychopharmacologic agents. In S. S. Gellis and B. M. Kagan (Eds.), *Current pediatric therapy—3*. Philadelphia: Saunders, pp. 64–72.

Lombard, J. P., Gilbert, J. G., & Donofrio, A. F. The effects of glutamic acid upon the intelligence, social maturity and adjustment of a group of mentally retarded children. *Amer. J. Ment. Defic.*, 1955, *60*, 122–132.

Lourie, R. S. Psychoactive drugs in pediatrics. *Pediatrics*, 1964, *34*, 691–693.

Louttit, R. T. Chemical facilitation of intelligence among the mentally retarded. *Amer. J. Ment. Defic.*, 1965, *69*, 495–501.

Low, N. L., & Myers, G. G. Suvren in brain-injured children. *J. Pediat.*, 1958, *52*, 259–263.

Lucas, A. R. Gilles de la Tourette's disease in children: Treatment with phenothiazine drugs. *Amer. J. Psychiat.*, 1964, *121*, 606–608.

———. Psychopharmacologic treatment. In C. R. Shaw (Ed.), *The Psychiatric disorders of childhood*. New York: Appleton-Century-Crofts, 1966, pp. 387–402.

———. Gilles de la Tourette's disease in children: Treatment with haloperidol. *Amer. J. Psychiat.*, 1967, *124*, 243–245.

Lucas, A. R., Lockett, H. J., & Grimm, F. Amitriptyline in childhood depressions. *Dis. Nerv. Sys.*, 1965, *26*, 105–110.

Lytton, G. J., & Knobel, M. Diagnosis and treatment of behavior disorders in children. *Dis. Nerv. Sys.*, 1958, *20*, 1–7.

MacColl, K. Chlorpromazine hydrochloride (Largactil) in the treatment of the disturbed mental defective. *Amer. J. Ment. Defic.*, 1956, *61*, 378–389.

Maddock, R. K., Jr. Patient cooperation in taking medicines: A study involving isoniazid and aminosalicylic acid. *J.A.M.A.*, 1967, *199*, 169–172.

Madsen, H. Tindal as an aid in the treatment of a psychotic child. Unpublished manuscript, 1965 (available from Schering Laboratories).

Malitz, S. Drug therapy: Antidepressants. In S. Arieti (Ed.), *American handbook of psychiatry*, Vol. 3. New York: Basic Books, 1966, pp. 477–512.

Malitz, S., & Hoch, P. H. Drug therapy: Neuroleptics and tranquilizers. In S. Arieti (Ed.), *American handbook of psychiatry*, Vol. 3. New York: Basic Books, 1966, pp. 458–476.

Mattson, R. H., & Calverley, J. R. Dextroamphetamine sulfate-induced dyskinesias. *J.A.M.A.*, 1968, *204*, 400–402.

McConnell, T. R., Jr., Cromwell, R. L., Bialer, I., & Son, C. D. Studies in activity level: VII. Effects of amphetamine drug administration on the activity level of retarded children. *Amer. J. Ment. Defic.*, 1964, *68*, 647–651.

McCray, W. E., Hawkins, W. A., Kirkpatrick, W. L., & McGovern, W. J. Long term drug treatment of psychiatric out-patients. *Dis. Nerv. Sys.*, 1963, *24*, 167–172.

McDermott, J. F. A specific placebo effect encountered in the use of Dexedrine in a hyperactive child. *Amer. J. Psychiat.*, 1965, *121*, 923–924.

McGaugh, J. L. Reported in *Medical World News*, May 24, 1968.

McKenzie, M. E., & Roswell-Harris, D. A controlled trial of prothipendyl (Tolnate) in mentally subnormal patients. *Brit. J. Psychiat.*, 1966, *112*, 95–100.

McLaughlin, B. E., Duffy, R. E., & Ryan, F. R. Chemotherapy as adjunctive treatment for emotionally disturbed children. *Dis. Nerv. Sys.*, 1962, *23*, 95–98.

McLaughlin, B. E., Duffy, R. E., Ryan, F. R., & Drucker, T. Chemotherapy for emotionally disturbed children: A follow-up report. *Dis. Nerv. Sys.*, 1964, *25*, 735–738.

Mebane, J. C. Use of deanol with disturbed juvenile offenders. *Dis. Nerv. Sys.*, 1960, *21*, 642–643.

Meier, C. W., & Huff, F. W. Altered adult behavior following chronic drug administration during infancy and prepuberty. *J. Compar. Physiol. Psychol.*, 1962, *55*, 469–471.

Mellinger, T. J., Mellinger, E. M., & Smith, W. T. Thioridazine blood levels in patients receiving different oral forms. *Clin. Pharmacol. Therapeut.*, 1965, *6*, 486–491.

Miksztal, M. W. Chlorpromazine (Thorazine) and reserpine in residential treatment of neuropsychiatric disorders in children. *J. Nerv. Ment. Dis.*, 1956, *123*, 477–479.

Millon, R., Delolme, E., Chambon, P., & Billaud, R. Utilisation du nialamide chez les enfants mentalement retardés. *Lyon Méd.*, 1965, *213*, 1621–1625.

Mitchell, A. C., Hargis, C. H., McCarry, F., & Power, C. Effects of prochlorperazine (Compazine) therapy on educability in disturbed mentally retarded adolescents. *Amer. J. Ment. Defic.*, 1959, *64*, 57–62.

Molitch, M., & Sullivan, J. P. The effect of Benzedrine sulfate on children taking the New Stanford Achievement Test. *Amer. J. Orthopsychiat.*, 1937, *7*, 519–522.

Molling, P. A., Lockner, A. W., Sauls, R. J., & Eisenberg, L. Committed delinquent boys. *A. M. A. Arch. Gen. Psychiat.*, 1962, *7*, 70–76.

Morris, J. V., MacGillivray, R. C., & Mathieson, C. M. The results of the experimental administration of amphetamine sulphate in oligophrenia. *J. Ment. Sci.*, 1955, *101*, 131–140.

Moskowitz, H. Benzedrine therapy for the mentally handicapped. *Amer. J. Ment. Defic.*, 1941, *45*, 540–543.

Nash, H. The design and conduct of experiments on the psychological effects of drugs. In L. Uhr & J. G. Miller (Eds.), *Drugs and behavior.* New York: John Wiley & Sons, Inc., 1960, pp. 128–155.

———. The double-blind procedure. *J. Nerv. Ment. Dis.*, 1962, *134*, 34–47.

Newcombe, D. S., Shapiro, S. L., Sheppard, G. L., & Dreifuss, F. E. Treatment of X-linked primary hyperuricemia with allopurinol. *J.A.M.A.*, 1966, *198*, 225–227.

Niswander, G. D., & Karacan, I. Clinical experience with fluphenazine. *Dis. Nerv. Sys.*, 1959, *20*, 403–405.

Oettinger, L. Meratran: Preliminary report on a new drug for the treatment of behavior disorders in children. *Dis. Nerv. Sys.*, 1955, *16*, 299–302.

———. The use of deanol in the treatment of disorders of behavior in children. *J. Pediat.*, 1958, *53*, 671–675.

———. Chlorprothixene in the management of problem children. *Dis. Nerv. Sys.*, 1962, *23*, 568–571.

Oettinger, L., & Simonds, R. Thioridazine in the treatment of behavior disorders in children. Scientific exhibit, American Medical Association Meeting, Denver, Colorado, November 27–30, 1961.

Oltman, J. E., & Friedman, S. Pargyline in the treatment of depressive illnesses. *Amer. J. Psychiatry*, 1963, *120*, 493–494.

Ostow, M. Method and madness: A critique of current methodology in psychiatric drug research. *J. New Drugs*, 1965, *5*, 3–8.

Overall, J. E., Hollister, L. E., & Dalal, S. N. Psychiatric drug research: sample size requirements for one vs. two raters. *Arch. Gen. Psychiat.*, 1967, *16*, 152–161.

Pallister, P. D., & Stevens, R. R. Effects of Serpasil in small dosage on behavior, intelligence and physiology. *Amer. J. Ment. Defic.*, 1957, *62*, 267–274.

Paredes, A., Gogerty, J. H., & West, L. J. Psychopharmacology. In: J. H. Masserman (Ed.), *Current psychiatric therapies*, vol. 1. New York: Grune & Stratton, 1961, pp. 54–85.

Pasamanick, B. Anticonvulsant drug therapy of behavior problem children with abnormal electroencephalograms. *A. M. A. Arch. Neurol. Psychiat.*, 1951, *65*, 752–766.

Pellet, J., Dumas, R., Cotte, M. F., & Beaupère, A. Utilisation du 8089 CB en neuropsychiatrie infantile. *Lyon Méd.*, 1967, *217*, 825–831.

Peppel, H. H., & Joynes, T. Study design for clinical evaluation of phenothiazine derivatives. *Amer. J. Psychiat.*, 1963, *120*, 497–499.

Philips, I. Psychopathology and mental retardation. *Amer. J. Psychiat.*, 1967, *124*, 29–35.

Pilkington, T. L. Prochlorperazine (Stemetil) in mental deficiency. *J. Ment. Sci.*, 1959, *105*, 215–219.

————. Comparative effects of Librium and Taractan on behavior disorders of mentally retarded children. *Dis. Nerv. Sys.*, 1961, *22*, 573–575.

————. A report on "Tofranil" in mental deficiency. *Amer. J. Ment. Defic.*, 1962, *66*, 729–732.

Piuck, C. L. Clinical impressions of hydroxyzine and other tranquilizers in a child guidance clinic. *Dis. Nerv. Sys.*, 1963, *24*, 483–488.

Poussaint, A. F., & Ditman, K. S. A clinical trial of protriptyline in childhood enuresis. *Psychosomatics*, 1965, *6*, 413–416.

Poussaint, A. F., Ditman, K. S., & Greenfield, R. Amitriptyline in childhood enuresis. *Clin. Pharmacol. Therapeut.*, 1966, *7*, 21–25.

Pratt, J. P., Bishop, M. P., & Gallant, D. M. Trifluperidol and haloperidol in the treatment of acute schizophrenia. *Amer. J. Psychiat.*, 1964, *121*, 592–594.

Pregelj, S., & Barkauskas, A. Thioridazine in the treatment of mentally retarded children (A four-year retroactive evaluation). *Canad. Psychiat. Assoc. J.*, 1967, *12*, 213–215.

Price, S. A., & Spencer, D. A. A trial of beclamide (Nydrane) in mentally subnormal patients with disorders of behavior. *J. Ment. Subnormal.*, 1967, *13*, 75–77.

Rajotte, P., Bordeleau, J. M., & Tétreault, L. Étude comparative de la butapérazine et de la prochlorpérázine chez le schizophrène chronique. *Canad. Psychiat. Assoc. J.*, 1965, *10*, 25–34.

Rapoport, J. Childhood behavior and learning problems treated with imipramine. *Internat. J. Neuropsychiat.*, 1965, *1*, 635–642.

Reiss, M., Wakoh, T., Hillman, J. C., Pearse, J. J., Reiss, J. M., & Daley, N. Action of anabolic steroids on the metabolism of mentally retarded boys. *Amer. J. Ment. Defic.*, 1966, *70*, 520–528.

Renard, P., Bicheron, C., & Morin, Y. Quelques résultats de l'utilisation de l'halopéridol dans un institut médico-pédagogique. *Rev. Neuropsychiat. Infant.*, 1965, *13*, 587–597.

Resnick, O. The role of diet in psychopharmacology. *Psychiat. Opin.*, 1965, *Fall*, 14–17.

Rettig, J. H. Chlorpromazine for the control of psychomotor excitement in the mentally deficient: A preliminary study. *J. Nerv. Ment. Dis.*, 1955, *122*, 190–194.

Rickels, K. Psychopharmacologic agents: A clinical psychiatrist's individualistic point of view: Patient and doctor variables. *J. Nerv. Ment. Dis.*, 1963, *136*, 540–549.

Robinson, J. T., Davies, L. S., Kreitman, N., & Knowles, J. B. A doubleblind trial of oxypertine for anxiety neurosis. *Brit. J. Psychiat.*, 1965, *111*, 527–529.

Rosenblum, S. Practices and problems in the use of tranquilizers with exceptional children. In: E. Trapp & P. Himelstein (Eds.), *Readings on the exceptional child*. New York: Appleton-Century-Crofts, 1962, pp. 639–657.

Rosenblum, S., Buoniconto, P., & Graham, B. D. "Compazine" vs. placebo: A controlled study with educable, emotionally disturbed children. *Amer. J. Ment. Defic.*, 1960, *64*, 713–717.

Rosenblum, S., Callahan, R. J., Buoniconto, P., Graham, B. D., & Deatrick, R. W. The effects of tranquilizing medication (reserpine) on behavior and test performance of maladjusted, high-grade retarded children. *Amer. J. Ment. Defic.*, 1958, *62*, 663–671.

Rosenthal, R. Covert communication in the psychological experiment. *Psychol. Bull.*, 1967, *67*, 356–367.

Roswell, H. F. Clinical experience with trifluoperazine in the severely retarded. *J. Neuropsychiat.*, 1964, *5*, 370–372.

Rudy, L. H., Himwich, H. E., & Rinaldi, F. A. A clinical evaluation of psychopharmacological agents in the management of disturbed mentally defective patients. *Amer. J. Ment. Defic.*, 1958, *62*, 855–860.

Salzmann, M. M. A controlled trial with trimipramine, a new anti-depressant drug. *Brit. J. Psychiat.*, 1965, *111*, 1105–1106.

Satanove, A., & McIntosh, J. S. Phototoxic reactions induced by high doses of chlorpromazine and thioridazine. *J.A.M.A.*, 1967, *200*, 209–212.

Schmidt, M., & Daudet, G. Action du Benzpéridol (8089 CB soluté buvable dosé à 0.2 mg/ml) sur les troubles du comportement d'un groupe d'enfants suivis dans un service de débiles profonds. *Ann. Médico-Psychol.*, 1968, *126*, 113–119.

Schulman, J. L., & Clarinda, S. R. The effect of promazine on the activity level of retarded children. *Pediatrics*, 1964, *33*, 271–275.

Segal, L. J., & Tansley, A. E. A clinical trial with hydroxyzine (Atarax) on a group of maladjusted educationally subnormal children. *J. Ment. Sci.*, 1957, *103*, 677–681.

Shaw, C. R., Lockett, H. J., Lucas, A. R., Lamontagne, C. H., & Grimm, F. Tranquilizer drugs in the treatment of emotionally disturbed children in a residential treatment center. *J. Amer. Acad. Child Psychiat.*, 1963, *2*, 725–742.

Shapiro, A. K., & Shapiro, E. Treatment of Gilles de la Tourette's syndrome with haloperidol. *Brit. J. Psychiat.*, 1968, *114*, 345–350.

Sherwin, A. C., Flach, F. F., & Stokes, P. E. Treatment of psychoses in early childhood with triiodothyronine. *Amer. J. Psychiat.*, 1958, *115*, 166–167.

Silberstein, R. M., Cooper, A., Miller, L., & Mandell, W. Avoiding institutionalizing psychotic children. *Internat. J. Neuropsychiat.*, 1965, *1*, 144–148.

Simmons, J. Q., Leiken, S. J., Lovaas, O. I., Schaeffer, B., & Perloff, B. Modification of autistic behavior with LSD-25. *Amer. J. Psychiat.*, 1966, *122*, 1201–1211.

Smith, E. H., & Gonzalez, R. Nortriptyline hydrochloride in the treatment of enuresis in mentally retarded boys. *Amer. J. Ment. Defic.*, 1967, *71*, 825–827.

Soblen, R. A., & Saunders, J. C. Monoamine oxidase inhibitor therapy in adolescent psychiatry. *Dis. Nerv. Sys.*, 1961, *22*, 96–100.

Solomons, G. The hyperactive child. *J. Iowa Med. Soc.*, 1965, *55*, 464–469.

Spencer, S. M. The pill that helps you remember. *Saturday Evening Post*, 1966, *87*, pp. 64–68.

Splitter, S. R. Comprehensive treatment of office patients with the aid of a new psychophysiologic agent, opipramol (Ensidon). *Psychosomatics*, 1963, *4*, 283–289.

Splitter, S. R., & Kaufman, M. A new treatment for underachieving adolescents: Psychotherapy combined with nortriptyline medication. *Psychosomatics*, 1966, *7*, 171–174.

Sprague, R. L., Barnes, K. A., & Werry, J. S. Methylphenidate and thioridazine: Learning activity and behavior in emotionally disturbed boys. Unpublished manuscript.

Sprague, R. L., & Werry, J. S. (Eds.) *Survey of research on psychopharmacology of children.* Champaign, Ill.: Children's Research Center, University of Illinois, 1968 (processed).

Sprague, R. L., Werry, J. S., & Scott, K. C. Effects of dextroamphetamine on activity level and learning in retarded children. Paper presented at the meeting of the Midwestern Psychological Association, Chicago, Ill., May 5, 1967.

Sprogis, G. R., Lezdins, V., White, S. D., Ming, C., Lanning, M., Drake, M. E., & Wyckoff, G. Comparative study on Thorazine and Serpasil in the mental defective. *Amer. J. Ment. Defic.*, 1957, *61*, 737–742.

Sugerman, A. A., & Herrmann, J. Molindone, an indole derivative with antipsychotic activity. *Clin. Pharmacol. Therapeut.*, 1967, *8*, 261–265.

Tarjan, G., Lowery, V. E., & Wright, S. W. Use of chlorpromazine in 278 mentally deficient patients. *A. M. A. J. Dis. Child.*, 1957, *94*, 294–300.

Thal, N. Cumulative index of antidepressant medications. *Dis. Nerv. Sys.*, 1959, *20*, 197–206.

Timberlake, W. H., Belmont, E. H., & Ogonik, J. The effect of reserpine in 200 mentally retarded children. *Amer. J. Ment. Defic.*, 1957, *62*, 61–66.

Turner, W. J. Therapeutic use of diphenylhydantoin in neuroses. *Internat. J. Neuropsychiat.*, 1967, *3*, 94–105.

Ucer, E. Pilot study of Ro 5–4556 in emotionally disturbed retarded children. *Curr. Therapeut. Res.*, 1968, *10*, 187–195.

Uhlenhuth, E. J., Canter, A., Neustadt, J. O., & Payson, H. E. The symptomatic relief of anxiety with meprobamate, phenobarbital and placebo. *Amer. J. Psychiat.*, 1959, *115*, 905–910.

Usdin, E., & Effron, D. H. Psychotropic drugs and related compounds. Washington: Public Health Service (pub. No. 1589), U.S. Dept. of Health, Education, and Welfare, January, 1967 (available through U.S. Government Printing Office).

Vogel, W., Broverman, D. M., Draguns, J. G., & Klaiber, E. L. The role of glutamic acid in cognitive behaviors. *Psychol. Bull.*, 1965, *65*, 367–382.

Waites, L., & Keele, D. K. Fluphenazine in management of disturbed mentally retarded children. *Dis. Nerv. Sys.*, 1963, *24*, 113–114.

Walker, C. F., & Kirkpatrick, B. B. Dilantin treatment for behavior problem children with abnormal electroencephalograms. *Amer. J. Psychiat.*, 1947, *103*, 484–492.

Wapner, I., Thurston, D. L., & Holowach, J. Phenobarbital: Its effect on learning in epileptic children. *J.A.M.A.*, 1962, *182*, 937.

Wartel, R. Intérêt du 8909 R. P. dans une collectivité d'arrierés profonds. *Ann. Médico-Psychol.*, 1966, *2*, 689.

Weir, T. W. H., Kernohan, G. A., & MacKay, D. N. The use of pericyazine and chlorpromazine with disturbed mentally subnormal patients. *Brit. J. Psychiat.*, 1968, *114*, 111–112.

Weiss, B., & Laties, V. G. Enhancement of human performance by caffeine and the amphetamines. *Pharmacol. Rev.*, 1962, *14*, 1–36.

Weiss, G., Werry, J. S., Minde, K., Douglas, V., & Sykes, D. Studies on the hyperactive child. V. The effects of dextroamphetamine and chlorpromazine on behavior and intellectual functioning. *J. Child Psychol. Psychiat.*, (in press).

Werry, J. S. The effects of methylphenidate and phenobarbital on the behavior of hyperactive and aggressive children. Paper presented at the annual meeting of the American Psychiatric Association, Boston, Mass., May 15, 1968. (In press, *Amer. J. Psychiat.*) (*a*)

——. Studies on the hyperactive child. IV. An empirical analysis of the minimal brain dysfunction syndrome. *Arch. Gen. Psychiat.*, 1968, *19*, 9–16. (*b*)

Werry, J. S., & Quay, H. C. Observing the classroom behavior of elementary school children. Paper presented at the annual meeting of the Council for Exceptional Children, April 1968. *Except. Child.*, (in press).

Werry, J. S., & Sprague, R. L. Hyperactivity. In C. G. Costello (Ed.), *Symptoms of psychopathology*. New York: John Wiley & Sons, Inc., in press.

Werry, J. S., Weiss, G., Douglas, V., & Martin, J. Studies on the hyperactive child. III. The effect of chlorpromazine upon behavior and learning ability. *J. Amer. Acad. Child Psychiat.*, 1966, *5*, 292–312.

Williams, E. J. Protriptyline: A double-blind clinical trial. *Med. J. Australia*, 1968, *1*, 537–540.

Wolf, S., Doering, C. R., Clark, M. L., & Hagans, J. A. Chance distribution and the placebo "reactor." *J. Lab. Clin. Med.*, 1957, *49*, 837–841.

Wolf, S., & Pinsky, R. H. Effects of placebo administration and occurrence of toxic reactions. *J.A.M.A.*, 1954, *155*, 339–341.

Wolfson, I. N. Clinical experience with Serpasil and Thorazine in treatment of disturbed behavior of mentally retarded. *Amer. J. Ment. Defic.*, 1957, *62*, 276–283.

Wolpert, A., Hagamen, M. B., & Merlis, S. A pilot study of thiothixene in childhood schizophrenia. *Curr. Therapeut. Res.*, 1966, *8*, 617–620.

Wolpert, A., Sheppard, C., & Merlis, S. An early clinical evaluation of clopenthixol in treatment-resistant female schizophrenic patients. *Amer. J. Psychiat.*, 1967, *124*, 702–705.

Wolpert, A., Sheppard, C., & Merlis, S. Thiothixene, thioridazine, and placebo in male chronic schizophrenic patients. *Clin. Pharmacol. Therapeut.*, 1968, *9*, 456–464.

Wright, W. B. Azacyclonol in mental deficiency practice: A preliminary report. *J. Ment. Sci.*, 1958, *104*, 485.

Yuwiler, A., Greenough, W., & Geller, E. Biochemical and behavioral effects of magnesium pemoline. *Psychopharmacologia*, 1968, *13*, 174–180.

Zigler, E. Familial mental retardation: A continuing dilemma. *Science*, 1967, *155*, 292–298.

Zimmerman, F. T., & Burgemeister, B. B. Action of methyl-phenidylacetate (Ritalin) and reserpine in behavior disorders in children and adults. *Amer. J. Psychiat.*, 1958, *115*, 323–328.

——, & ——. A controlled experiment of glutamic acid therapy. *A. M. A. Arch. Neurol. Psychiat.*, 1959, *81*, 639–648.

Zrull, J. P., Westman, J. C., Arthur, B., & Rice, D. L. A comparison of diazepam, d-amphetamine and placebo in the treatment of the hyperkinetic syndrome in children. *Amer. J. Psychiat.*, 1964, *121*, 388–389.

———, ———, ———, & ———. An evaluation of methodology used in the study of psychoactive drugs for children. *J. Amer. Acad. Child Psychiat.*, 1966, 5, 284–291.

Zubin, J., & Katz, M. M. Psychopharmacology and personality. *Internat. J. Psychiat.*, 1966, *2*, 640–675.

Zukin, P., & Arnold, D. G. Comparative effect of phenaglycodol and meprobamate on anxiety reactions. *J. Nerv. Ment. Dis.*, 1959, *129*, 193–195.

: 14 :

Psychopharmacology as a Treatment Adjunct for the Mentally Retarded: Problems and Issues

Dorothy Colodny and LeRoy F. Kurlander

INTRODUCTION

CONTROVERSY over the effectiveness, wisdom, morality, and meaning of psychotropic drugs in the therapy of the mentally retarded makes it hard to study the subject and to attempt a treatment that at times seems quite useful and safe. But it is possible to lessen the hazards of both the drugs and the atmosphere surrounding them by examining the issues and the anxieties that obscure them. Of course, there are legitimate differences of opinion in this matter, as in all crises in scientific progress. But a remarkable intensity of feeling—fervent support or fanatical opposition—is often evoked by the simple question: Can drugs be of any help to the mentally retarded? This passionate mood suggests that, in addition to the rational arguments on both sides in the dispute, there is another component—an irrational bias—probably out of awareness. A principle on which most modern psychiatrists agree is that the demonstration of irrational attitudes can lessen their destructiveness. In this brief discussion we shall try to describe some of these hidden forces as well as the more conscious intellectual considerations.

Psychotropic drugs were first used as supplements to other types of care of the mentally ill, and much that is said here about problems regarding medication in mental retardation applied first and equally to the chemical treatment of mental illness. But the reports of success in mental illness have not been matched in mental retardation. So far, no specific medication for retardation has been found. Optimistic trials of glutamic acid, deanòl and—most recently—magnesium pemoline have proved disappointing. To be sure, thyroid for cretins and the special diet for phenylketonuria (P.K.U.) are spectacular preventive measures, but these have been in the province of pediatric medicine and have escaped the taint of "psychiatric" drugs.

LIMITATIONS AND EXTENSIONS OF DRUG USAGE

In another chapter of this volume Roger D. Freeman discusses drug therapy in some detail. It is important here to review the fact that while no known drug can "cure mental retardation" now, there are a good many medicines that can significantly improve the life of the mentally retarded patient. Counselors of the families of the retarded know that the initial pain at the news that a child is retarded can be allayed after a time of grieving. Parents can learn to acknowledge a child's present limitations and limited future, and the child himself can often come to terms with it. Harder to live with from day to day is the expression of developmental disorder in behavior, all the way from the syndrome we know as minimal cerebral dysfunction—which we used to call "brain damage"—to gross mental illness. These are the symptoms which may respond well to medication, with a number of positive effects it seems cruel to deny to a child and his family.

The child who is hyperactive and distractible cannot acquire even those academic and social skills for which his capacity is intact. In this group are many of the "pseudoretarded" children whose observable and measured abilities soar when the hyperactivity syndrome is treated. In the genuinely retarded, with a ceiling on academic progress, it still seems well worth seeking partial improvement, which may return an excluded child to school or promote one from the trainable to the educable class, or which may simply make schoolwork easier and pleasanter for pupil and teacher.

Though there may be little gain in academic skills or none at all, a very important benefit may be the change in the child's conduct, relationships, and experience of himself. Various associations of parents have perhaps overemphasized the distinction between mental retardation and mental illness and have overstressed the fact that many of the retarded have sweet, placid natures with good mental health. Many children are more disabled by mental illness, mild or severe, than by the mental retardation itself. Frequently the mental illness is progressive and related to progressive failures in achievement; to the patient's constitutional irritability and his own discomfort with it; and to the family's understandable exhaustion and intolerance of an intolerable child. When he is still quite young, the patient can learn to believe that he is "dumb and bad." Then his mounting anxiety and depression increase his anxiety and disturbed behavior. He develops seriously maladapted psychological defenses, and soon both he and his family will regard him as "dumb and bad and crazy." If at the earliest diagnosis of hyperactivity, irritability, or poor control or abnormal physiological patterning he is given a fair trial of medication for these symptoms, he is freer to develop as a retarded child classified "without mental illness." His self-esteem is protected, and the image he sees reflected in the eyes of his parents will be that of a composed and willing child able to do his own best.

Sometimes, as in P.K.U. and the other more severe retardations, as well as in retardation with uncontrolled epilepsy, the patient's neuropathology itself produces an organic psychosis. The major tranquilizers may offer marked relief of such illness, preventing or shortening hospitalization.

When institutionalization is inevitable, the merciful prescription of adequate drugs may lighten the burdens of a family waiting for a hospital bed or still unready to accept the placement plan. This is clearest when the patient is sleepless or self-destructive, or absorbs the entire time and attention of the mother who has other children as well.

Medications used for these purposes are relatively new. However, as workers correlate symptoms with the most effective drug and dose, some specificity emerges. It is understood that drugs are usually more useful when they are combined with other helpful measures: physical, psychological and social.

ISSUES IN CLINICAL PSYCHOPHARMACOLOGY
FOR CHILDREN

Medical Rationale

The genuinely responsible physician, in general practice, pediatrics, or psychiatry, is in a position to ask, as he would in any other disorder: Is there a drug to alleviate any of the retarded patient's complaints? Is this a suitable patient for such a drug? What is the best drug and how should it be combined with other modes of treatment? In another disorder he could peacefully assess, prescribe, and observe the results. In mental illness and mental retardation he must first search his own soul and then confront his patient, the patient's immediate family, the extended family, the consultant physicians from many specialities, the paramedical aides, school teachers, clergymen, counselors, neighbors, and the general public. He, himself, and each one of those who take an interest in the child, has a background of information, accurate or not; attitudes, rational or not; reservations, realistic or not; and some core of conviction that it is right or is wrong to help a child's or an adult's mind by giving him medicine.

These contenders have all been exposed to discussion of psychotropic drugs in the lay press, and many also have professional knowledge bearing on the issue. Among them are many thoughtful people who are not partisan at all, but consider the merits of the patient's case and favor whatever treatment seems to offer him most help. But there are uncritical advocates of drug therapy of all sorts. They credulously read the miracle cures printed prematurely in new magazines. They are sanguine types who find it hard to concede how partial is our knowledge and control of nature. Sometimes they are seekers for the quick and easy way. They may prefer a hasty prescription to an evaluation of the complex problems of relationship and emotion which surround the failure of a human being to develop like most of his peers. Some of these enthusiasts think that every retarded child should be on drugs.

Objections to Drug Usage

Those opposed to use of any drugs at all have many objections. They start with very valid ones. They emphasize the side effects of medication, realistically citing the danger of the severe reactions. In the doses used outside hospitals these effects are rare. The opponents of medication usually also refer to "clouding of consciousness," "snowing" a child, transforming him into a "zombie." These charges blur the past and the present, the transient and the fixed. Until about thirty years ago, effective tranquillization could be obtained only with sedatives such as barbiturates and bromides, often necessary to control agitation or seizures; but these drugs produced drowsiness and confusion. In contrast, properly adjusted dosage and combinations of modern drugs rarely cloud consciousness, except perhaps briefly while the individual optimum dose is sought. During this time, it seems, a good many articulate critics observe the patient either "glassy-eyed" as they say, or in their other colorful phrase "all hopped up." Another authentic grievance is against the gross misuse of drugs. One must admit frankly that abuses occur in this field as in any other. Outright quacks exist, but they are far less numerous than the zealots who are delighted with some success in treatment prescribing excessively, sometimes carelessly; they are irresponsible and dangerously inexcusable, but probably not malicious or even consciously greedy. They are accused of acting as "fronts" for the commercial schemes of some pharmaceutical houses by publishing speedy, glowing reports of a limited number of cases. Efforts to deny the existence of these lamentable practitioners inflame those who fear them into a blaze of blame, so that they regard all those who use psychotropic drugs as dishonest, subsidized, or stupid.

Such diffuse fears draw some strength from the chemical disasters of recent years. The tragedy of unborn babies deformed by thalidomide, when the public had become so casual about sedatives, was a shock. This drug quoted a frightful price for a night's sleep in the damage done to future generations. It reinforced suspicion in those already suspicious of drug-merchants; it reminded those who doubted their physicians that carelessness is as dangerous as knavery; and it came at a time when it was becoming the style to debunk the medical profession in books and cabarets. Important as this crisis was, it shed little light on the subject to which it is applied here. Reputable physicians are careful to research the known effects of the drugs they use; in the United States thalidomide never was approved. Yet this episode aroused in those susceptible to apprehension, irrational fears beyond those which were appropriate or led to proper action. One cannot completely reassure such questioners that any medication, or for that matter, food and drink—which, to their amazement, also consist of "chemicals"—may not have remote effects we cannot foresee.

During these same years, the grave discouragement of both parents and professionals with their inability to deter or even really understand the young people who have turned to narcotic and psychedelic drugs has inspired distrust for all chemical agents with mental or emotional effects. The distinction is somehow lost between what is an illegal, dangerous substance, of questionable provenance, self-administered in excessive amounts by disturbed youths and a therapeutic medicine, in the legitimate pharmacopeia, prescribed by a licensed physician for a specific purpose after a careful diagnosis.

As we can see, at one end of the scale each of the realistic recommendations or objections can be refuted, to some extent reasonably, so that a reasonable choice remains. Yet, at the other end of the scale, each of these positions can be diffused into an anxious, illogical, arbitrary obstruction.

The same is true of the more theoretical polemic. Since scientific medicine began, therapeutic purists have fought empiricists, quarreling over whether asepsis or aspirin was sufficiently soundly based to be used at all. In the treatment of mental retardation today, purists decline to employ measures insufficiently proven, basic, molecular; or insufficiently demonstrated to their satisfaction by controlled experiment. Opposed to these purists are practical minds who claim that "nothing is lost" by a therapeutic trial. Because of the centuries of despair regarding the retarded, there is still a remnant of irresponsibility toward them—"What have we to lose?" on one side; "Why bother to try at all?" on the other. Underlying the respectable and thoughtful debate is still the influence of individual temperament polarizing the choice. We see the therapeutic nihilist, often academic, perfectionistic, hard to convince except by mathematical proof, cool, seeing values as absolute; and the warmhearted, pragmatic practitioner, less intellectual in disposition, sometimes more intuitive, more willing to be mistaken now and then if he can bring some consolation—even relative —to his patient who is suffering *now*.

Moral Implications

Similar to the foregoing dispute is the battle over the morality of medicating the poorly functioning personality and the limited mind. Without stressing its meaning to theology and our ideas of free will, we observe that most of us seem to lean one way or the other. We may share the conviction that a human being, however frail, must find inner discipline without outside aids; that it is spiritually degrading to "rely on drugs" that are progressively weakening to the human being to use this "crutch"; that artificial intervention impairs the benign forces of nature. Dr. J. B. de C. M. Saunders has referred to tranquilizers as "the painless concentration camp of the mind." However, we may recognize the apparent threat to individual integrity and creativity in the chemical control of mental processes and still be more convinced that, if we have access to means to free the anxious or hyperactive or otherwise incapacitated patient from the misery that preoccupies his mind and body, we may help him to be more moral and constructive in the end.

There is a subtle shift from the moralistic absorption with self-reliance to a very uneasy suggestion that psychotropic drugs are not so much a weakness as a weapon, that these drugs represent less a failure of self-control than an opportunity for unscrupulous men— irresponsible physicians, selfish relatives, lazy attendants—to take advantage of helpless patients. Szasz (1957) has talked about "chemical strait-jackets" and others have referred to "chemical warfare against children," as though the motive to employ drugs is not to reduce suffering but to subdue others' souls and to make less trouble for those who can dispense pills and hold the syringe. True, in under-budgeted, overcrowded hospitals, where mental disorder offers real dangers to staff and to patients, control by drugs has actually replaced control by strait-jacket and isolation rooms. It is a sad fact that this chemical calm may then justify further reduction in budget and staff. One cannot cease to protest against this misinterpretation of the role of medication, even though many of the more indignant objections are genuinely humanitarian pleas for more active, dynamic treatment of the mentally ill and the mentally retarded.

An article by Marmor et al. (1960) shows that very often the fear of control by chemical agents—fluorides, preservatives, tranquilizers and so forth—occurs in an anxious and suspicious personality equally fearful of other external controls—governmental, social, or personal. He may be merely eccentric or else fervidly paranoid about it. This is only one of many correlates, it is true, but we can support the findings of these authors by our own clinical impression that the greatest opposition to medication comes from parents and physicians who are most alarmed by the influence of government or of the school system; by those who find it hard to accept any kind of external aid; by those who, usually after an hour or two, freely inquire whether their child will be poisoned, whether his thoughts will be controlled or his will will be enslaved. Not everyone who objects to drugs is mentally ill or a fanatic, but a mental sufferer, already insecure, can easily regard any drug as an attack on the integrity of his body and mind.

Another issue is the implication of chemical intervention in both mental illness and mental retardation. It is often said that, if one accepts the psychoanalytic or the environmentalist view of mental illness, regarding it as the outcome of early abnormal life experiences, then only a corrective experience of these early events can reverse the process. Some proponents of this view feel strongly that those who prescribe drugs dispute this belief. Similarly, some students of mental retardation who emphasize that it is a "condition" rather than a "disease" resentfully infer that offering medicine implies sickness—possibly "mental sickness" at that. More often, it is understood by workers in both fields that very complex interactions between the physical constitution and the life experience of the mentally ill and the mentally retarded have produced the current pattern of adaption, and that chemical intervention in the present may shift an equilibrium favorably but does not necessarily change one's view of the etiology.

Psychoanalytic Viewpoints

The history of psychiatric thought in this century sheds some light on this interesting inference. Until about twenty-five years ago, the prescription of drugs was the preference of those psychiatrists who opposed the new understanding of psychic and personal phenomena on which modern psychiatry is based. The only drugs available were the sedatives, and they were not very helpful. One attributed to these older psychiatrists then (as we still do to those who depend on drugs exclusively) unwillingness, anxiety, or dislike of coming to grips with the intensity of their patient's feelings or with their own limitations. Quite freely then and with a sense of real progress, many psychiatrists gave up a part of our identity as physicians—the prescribing part—to devote themselves to the therapy of the patient's unhappy inner life. At a time when the multidisciplinary approach in the child-guidance movement was a refreshing inspiration, psychiatrists learned to rely on paramedical personnel who were able to carry out with talent and enthusiasm the therapy of feelings and attitudes. Social workers and psychologists worked well with the medically trained psychiatrists in clinics and private practice but when the new drugs appeared, these specialists without a medical license were not qualified to prescribe and often not eager for others to do so. It was the era of revelation in the purely psychic phenomena, and the discoveries of this era are still priceless. The young psychiatrists of those days invested long years, great zeal, and much money (long before grants were available to them) in special training in psychoanalysis. The psychoanalytic institutes were rigorous in reliance on purely verbal tools, teaching their candidates to regard drugs as they regarded the lobotomies of the forties—as brutal and punitive. These institutes religiously believed that psychoanalytic insights and methods would soon reverse mental illness, would perhaps prevent it entirely, and would maybe even prevent some mental retardation. Real pride in this enlightenment and in the future of psychoanalysis unfortunately became a fixed stake in a single method of treatment. The "Psychoanalytic Movement" did not sound as strange as the "Penicillin Movement" would have sounded. Some psychoanalysts even now cannot give up that old, rather romantic point of view; they speak and write as though they would lose a hard-won position or long-sought identity if they branched out into more varied therapeutics. But, they have been criticized and ridiculed harshly for their unfamiliar style of thought, for their techniques and their reports of striking psychological events in treatment. Hence, it is no wonder that their self-defense has crystallized into rigidity. At present fewer young psychiatrists seek training in formal psychoanalysis, and the psychoanalytic institutes themselves are becoming diversified and discuss new techniques, including drugs, though still in faintly condescending tones. The young psychoanalysts generally assign certain hours of the day to analysis and practice more flexibly the rest of the time.

Unfortunately the residue of our previous orientation remains, if not with the more progressive psychiatrists, at least with those psychoanalysts who still believe they should be concerned only with the "unconscious mind" and with the lay public. Many patients who have been exposed to the popular version of psychiatry seek psychiatric help only after concluding that psychotherapy is all we dispense, just as they think a surgeon spends all of his time in the operating room. What is more, having been "oriented" to the idea of this kind of care, few patients escape an orientation to a value system that, as Hollingshead and Redlich have shown, is partly based on class values. But just as their study in New Haven unearthed the fact that individual deep psychotherapy is most often assigned to the upper social classes and most effective there, the patients have discovered the same truth. They are willing to make the same sacrifices for high-class psychotherapy as they would for orthodontia or a college education to enable their children to have equal opportunities for "the best"—"the best" meaning that psychoanalysis is better than psychotherapy, and psychotherapy is better than medication. Some tendency to establish a corresponding hierarchy among the practitioners of these ranked skills seemed to reach its peak in the early 1950's and is now yielding to a trend toward an academic aristocracy. In this new order, a psychiatrist of any standing may use drugs without risking his prestige.

Whether he chooses to do so is probably related to his personal preference. Until very recently, physicians who chose to specialize in psychiatry were those who were more at ease with speculative pursuits rather than with the active life of the other specialties. But within psychiatry, a further division remains: (1) There are those who are eager to achieve rapid psychological change in their patients and believe that it is their responsibility to do so, that relief of symptoms and betterment of living need not be accompanied by total metamorphosis or total insight, that they should use any means including drugs. (2) There are those who are more comfortable unraveling the minutiae of their patient's feelings and the genesis of those feelings, who— to be truthful—regard the mere relief of symptoms with some disdain. Some psychiatrists are delighted to rejoin the mainstream of medicine now that there are so many relevant discoveries in genetics and developmental neuropsychiatry. Many psychiatrists are eager to give up the old dualism and treat the patient's mind and body together. But it is not so easy to change one's thinking: by making a gigantic effort, many of our colleagues had finally accepted the image of the passive, verbal, and drugless psychiatrist; now they find it a bit difficult to try again for a new image.

Some psychiatrists subscribe to the new treatments against their inclinations. Temperamentally suited to the role of "invisible listener," they may be persuaded to prescribe medication by statistical reports, economic pressure, or the insistence of the patient. Regrettably, these are the members of the profession who report consistent treatment failures in this medium. Then they are quick to proclaim that, since the drugs failed (though they lacked faith all the while), the successes must have been "faith cures" or "placebo effect." The opposition counters that there is another explanation than that of suggestion and bedazzlement: the reluctant prescriber can choose an ineffectual drug, or the wrong one; can admit defeat prematurely; can refrain from trials of alternate drugs; can prescribe in insufficient dosage (especially if he is afraid of drugs); or can fail to convey to the patient or his family the importance of regular and proper administration. The reluctant practitioner can also, like those he impeaches, impart to his listeners his own doubts—"I don't really think it will help, but let's give it a try"—or unspoken signs, which can neutralize chemicals in an amazing way. This practitioner may, as his opponent may, distort the findings by selective inattention or wishfulfilling fantasy.

Thus each side can produce the results it prophesies. This risk, we hasten to add, is no more prevalent in psychiatry than in other fields.

For years, most psychiatrists not working in institutions have been reluctant to treat mental retardation at all. During the flowering of the psychoanalytic movements, mentally retarded patients were not deemed suitable subjects for analysis. It has since been shown that these patients respond well to certain forms of psychotherapy; yet many therapists continue to mistake the "mind" for the "soul," and "verbal agility" for "comprehension." Along with obstetricians, pediatricians, and general practitioners, psychiatrists have felt the impact of the dismay and the demands of the unhappy parents of the retarded as well as the dilemma of their own inability to console or satisfy these parents. Many physicians shun mental retardation if it is chronic and baffling; it is so much easier to dismiss the patient to the educators than to alleviate his condition with medication. This is an incompatible task for psychiatrists overtrained in making verbal contact with patients. For, although the mentally retarded patient is often sensitive and may be very garrulous, he rarely obeys the special rules of our talking game. And before we can help him with drugs, we must complete our confrontation of his retinue; and before we can do that, we must overcome our reluctance to be involved.

Chapter 15 in this volume discusses the medication of the hospitalized mentally retarded patient, a task quite unlike that of treating him in his own home and community. The first goal in the hospital must be safety and the relief of the most severe symptoms. The drugs are more powerful, the dosage is higher, and the side-effects are more common. But medication is easier in one way: once the release forms for treatment are signed by the legal guardians of the patient, the responsibility for treatment is in the hands of the authority administering the release. The physician who prescribes can write explicit orders and can closely oversee the staff who carry them out and can record the response. He, himself, can check his patient at any hour and in many activities. On the whole, in a good institution the success of the medication depends mainly on the quality of the pharmacological action. Side-effects can be discovered in time, and drug changes can be made routinely and objectively.

ATTITUDES OF OTHERS CONCERNED

Outpatient Implications

Drug administration on an outpatient basis by psychiatrists is quite unlike the elaborate diplomacy required in the medication of patients in the usual outpatient pediatric clinic or private practitioner's office. Different specialists approach the matter differently. More mentally retarded patients are under the care of family physicians or pediatricians than of psychiatrists. These physicians have the opportunity, if they are willing, to prevent the secondary mental illness of the retardate which may require psychiatric care. But it is the domain of us psychiatrists to emphasize the need to scrutinize our own motives; this very willingness is a prerequisite to success in any therapy. Whether one is willing, as well as able, to diagnose retardation or cerebral dysfunction is obviously a forerunner to treating it. In addition to the reluctance to make the diagnosis of mental retardation or convey bad news, the temptation to procrastinate in the hope that the child will outgrow his "lag," we are tempted to interpret as volitional or "emotional" a good many genuine disabilities. Our recent style of psychiatric orientation leads to hints that the patient refuses to perform because of faulty attitudes in his parents. Consequently the child may be deprived of understanding and treatment and the parents' feelings may be cruelly, gratuitously hurt. In autism (which we regard as a special form of retardation), the withholding of drugs and of charity by psychiatrists (and others) is particularly likely, and in this peculiar syndrome the parents seem least willing or able to resist. Although we have no statistics to support it, we have the impression that once willing to do so, family physicians prescribe drugs with considerable vigor while pediatricians use the mildest drugs in the lowest dosage. Shortage of time may defeat both groups. To evaluate and adjust the psychotropic drugs in practice takes longer than we expect. We have not even a familiar idiom in which to teach the anxious parent how to dose and what to note, or how to tell us what has happened.

The Family

Once the physician has decided he will use medication, and once he is convinced that he is acting as consciously and conscientiously as

possible, his meeting with the patient or the patient's family needs unusual tolerance and tact. We know of no other medical circumstance in
which families who have been properly referred to reputable professionals (known to have sworn the oath of Hippocrates), ask candid
questions that are so insulting; for example, "Won't it hurt him?" "Won't
he be a dope fiend?" or "Are you using him for a guinea pig?"

The parents of retarded children who seek a psychiatrist's help
have already had an unhappy experience with a physician, whether he
broke the sad truth roughly or gently, or refrained from doing so.
They may have fought both the diagnosis and the physician. By the
time they seek more help, their child has shown his limitations. They
come, if they have had no previous help, in a state of feeling their own
failure; having failed to produce an entirely normal child, they have
again failed in being unable to make him behave or to make him
happy. The counselor knows that, until the family has made some adjustment to the disability, they may resist or misinterpret help of any
kind. This is not a refusal of psychotherapy or speech lessons or
drugs, but a rejection of the diagnosis itself—especially of a distorted
and hopeless view of the diagnosis.

Some professionals feel that the family must verbally accept the diagnosis before they are entitled to help from agencies dedicated to the
handicapped. Another view, more humane, is that a small proof of
progress, no strings attached, may dissolve the anxiety behind the
stubborn rejection of the diagnosis. Medication is one of the simplest
procedures for a family that cannot yet confide in those willing to
help, just because it can be undertaken by the family physician in his
office—quietly, without any pitched battles over terminology. Is that
physician then fostering illusions and reinforcing neurotic denial? One
answers this question in keeping with one's own beliefs. Is the wind to
be tempered to the shorn lamb? Do we believe that our patients can
grow into their burdens slowly? What is the price we exact for help?
Are we free to set such a price on our services?

Sometimes a family is too eager to seek medication, perhaps in
order to pretend that the disorder will be cured by it. They may become pugnacious if medication is denied, or may seek another physician. Ought we to prescribe as a bribe or as a lesson?

Parents are usually allowed and encouraged to ask questions and
these oddly naive inquisitions, sometimes from very sophisticated people, usually prove to be expressions of deeper fears. "Will he still be on
it when he grows up?" may be a screen for "Will he grow up?" "Will it
hurt his mind?" may conceal the dread that his mind is already hurt
beyond repair. Repetitive or persistent concern about one aspect of

the problem (often speech or locomotion) may be an obsessional diversion for much greater uneasiness about the more profound questions of the future: "How helpless will the patient be?" "What is his fate?" "How far can he go?" "Will the drug harm him in any way?"—these questions may reflect a wistful worry, "Have we already harmed him?" Clinical judgment alone determines when it is possible to respond to the hidden questions and when one should answer the questions at the level of the manifest content. The only sure disaster is to be drawn into a wrangle. As in any other obsessional provocation, one must change the subject from the repetitive questions (doubtless already answered repeatedly) and state clearly, firmly, exactly what we know the drug may do for the child and which of his symptoms will probably remain unchanged.

Drug Administration

Parents express their mixed feelings about drugs in many ways: blunt refusal to discuss the subject—"You're the doctor," a shift of responsibility from one to the other parent, turning the issue back to the referring physician who "doesn't believe in drugs," or, saying "you said you would prescribe." These seemingly unreasonable maneuvers may express an intense anxiety lest the medication be begun and fail and worse hopelessness ensue. Sometimes parents feel unable to justify the procedure to other members of the family and one can offer to help them do it. Some parents, having already proved themselves unable to control the child, are certain they cannot make him take his pill and refuse to face further humiliation. Success in treatment also offers a risk. If slight improvement makes a patient manageable but not quite acceptable, does he lose his actual or moral eligibility for an institution? Or, if he improves a great deal, how can his family face without agony the years in which they may have regarded him as incurable and doomed? For each family there are constellations of issues sufficient to explain why a very mundane situation, a very practical choice—pill or no pill—makes them so anxious, so immature, so unreasonable.

Parental behavior takes odd forms. After prolonged discussion of the danger of drugs, they may treat the actual medication very casually. For one thing, psychotropic drugs, especially if prescribed by a psychiatrist, are not regarded in a class with "real" drugs prescribed by "real" physicians. They are given and taken erratically, although if we inquire whether insulin or antibiotics would be given as directed, there is no hesitation at all. Together with contempt for the drug and carelessness in its use there is also an inconsistent overreaction to side effects, whether they are mild or severe. This may be related to the elective nature of the prescription and the fact that parents are allowed the option of medication, although they would not be allowed to participate in another technical decision. If the parent has consented only because he feels trapped or intimidated, he can easily sabotage the project. He can forget, misplace, or misuse the drug; can underdose, overdose, or distort the plan. Deliberately or not, he can falsify his report. The physician then may decide how far to pursue the matter and how to do it, either by patience, for example, sitting out this resistance, or by impatience, such as direct confrontation. Each of the two sometimes works.

Evaluation of Treatment

It is particularly hard to judge the results of chemotherapy in practice, when other concurrent treatments contribute so much to the effects. Parents find this especially hard. When they are in conflict, reports are conflicting, too: "The medicine is doing no good." "Very well, let's stop at once." "Oh, I couldn't let him go back to the way he was." We hear glowing reports of a child who stands before us in as pathetic a state as ever, but a state the parent would rather deny than discuss or finance by offering the child psychotherapy, which they regard as the next step after this failure. For these reasons one must consider the possibility of collateral information from a teacher or a public health nurse.

The patient's siblings may be a source of excellent information and also in need of involvement; even very young ones can sometimes verify a change. "He talks better now," or "He doesn't hit me so much." These siblings have other worries about the family member who needs pills, about his handicap and the likelihood that they or their children will suffer, too. Quite clearly these questions go far beyond the issue of the treatment, but they are basic to the issue of the disorder. But sometimes the extended family may phrase their feelings about mental retardation in terms of any current measures taken. Immature parents may focus their uneasiness about the whole subject on what the grandparents may think about the medicine, projecting their own inner strife. Controlling grandparents may either negate or undermine the physician, or may give him great support.

Attitudes of Psychiatrists and Other Therapists, Teachers, Clergymen, and the Treated Person

Psychiatrists and Other Therapists

Since the retarded patient often has associated physical disabilities, he is under the care of specialists of many kinds. Rarely does the colleague who examines the eyes or feet refrain from comment on the drugs that treat the mind, his remarks reflecting his personal bias and his date of graduation. If antagonistic comments are reported back to the prescriber, it is not easy to avoid a posture of self-defense, which is embarrassing or confusing to the listener, or an apology, which may weaken the patient's trust. Paramedical personnel—counselors, physiotherapists, occupational therapists, therapists of speech and hearing, and so on may feel very strongly one way or the other. They may have referred the patient for treatment in the anticipation of a very different treatment. Nonmedical psychotherapists are challenged by this new development on the edge of their own territory. Sometimes they simply treat the patient within the parameters of their own discipline and discourage any assessment of the value of drugs for him; sometimes they actively oppose medication with all the psychological power they can muster; and sometimes they ask for medication by a physician while they continue to work within their competence. Some very subtle and puzzling undercurrents in both treatments may develop, but with sufficient *good will* all round the patient may still benefit.

Teachers

Teachers of the mentally retarded are in a difficult position. Many have years of experience, have spent hours each day in close contact with their pupils; their stake in a given child may be very great. They may be quite uneasy about drug therapy, especially until the school's health administration or the physicians in the community share information with them, explaining the rationale of chemotherapy in general and giving some specific data regarding each child's treatment. These teachers often express two special fears: That the child will be too "drugged" for classroom learning, or that he will have a "reaction" in the classroom. In addition, a possessive teacher may resent the physician's place in the educational process, may share any of the prejudices described earlier, and usually has free access with these opinions to the parent's ear. Conversely, a teacher may be the first to identify the child's precise disabilities, may urge a parent to seek medical care for the child, and may even advocate medication. Some physicians regard this as intrusion. At worst, this interdisciplinary rivalry may obstruct our treatment. At best, an educator is the physician's strongest ally, a professional trained in estimating a child's ability to obtain and use knowledge of all kinds, a person able to perceive any difference in the child, and to convey both to the physician and to the child himself any positive change. Sometimes these teachers are more willing than the parents of retardates to share with the physician any negative change. The teacher can add an essential dimension to our work, since the mental and emotional conditions necessary for productive learning and socialization are not always quite the same as those for life at home.

The Clergyman

Often the clergyman is included in the care of a retarded person. He may simply perform his duties of ministering to the parents, helping them to accept a dispensation so hard to understand. But currently many clergymen obtain formal training in counseling as well as in theology, and the minister's role and reactions may resemble those of any other nonmedical therapist. His attitudes toward medication reflect his particular philosophical and psychological principles. The range of possibility is extremely wide, and it is well for members of other disciplines to explore the clergyman's actual position before taking one for granted.

Further counsel, supportive of or opposed to treatment, comes from skilled and unskilled friends and neighbors or proselytizing strangers in the supermarket. Evaluation of variables in this work must take them all into account.

The Treated Person

The opinion of the patient himself, whether child or adult, although often the most important, is sometimes the least considered. We progress in our awareness that mental disability is not a total thing; that sensitivity, acuteness, and responsiveness to the thoughts and moods of others may be at a very high level in the presence of a very low measured IQ or very infantile conduct. Young patients; very disabled patients; and old, docile, very resigned patients may not show their awareness, curiosity, or anxiety about the medicine they must take. But if he is encouraged to express his feelings and if he can talk, the patient himself—surprisingly—may be the only one to ask sincerely, "Will it help?"

IMPLICATIONS FOR TREATMENT

It seems as though the sum of all the attitudes already described, the amount of genuine healing intent, compared to neurotic power drives or anxious evasions, can be gauged by the *manner* in which medication is offered to the patient, however young and however retarded. Is the patient's interest enlisted, his responsible cooperation obtained, his dignity protected, in so far as possible? We have long known that psychotherapy is usually unsuccessful unless a patient is more willing than not. One of the obvious advantages of drugs in psychiatry is that the patient need not be so willing, that he can be medicated initially against his will if necessary. Too often, however, the very simplicity of coercion can be a temptation to continue to coerce. Education of the mentally retarded is usually judged by how well it helps each patient to become as self-reliant as possible. One should at least raise the question of the patient's right to be as actively involved in his own medication as in his other therapies. A patient can be medicated forcefully, his pills can be concealed in his food or offered as "candy" or "vitamins." But if he is one of the majority who can understand simple language, he can instead be granted the courtesy of knowing that his doctor and his family are willing to help him and to let him help himself, too. If the patient is forced or tricked, he cannot feel any power over himself at all. He must realize that in some way he is being changed by another's will. It is true that a retarded person's independence must be limited, but we ask if it should be unnecessarily limited. The patient can usually learn that when he takes his medicine willingly and regularly, he may feel better, learn better, please his family more, have better control of himself. He must be shown that the pill cannot do these things for him, but that it will make it much easier for him to do them. If he has stopped trying to learn or behave because he has failed so many times, he may find that one more try, after all those fruitless ones, will now bear fruit. He can take some pride in what he has helped to do for himself. Just as we all sometimes overlook a retarded child's or adult's sorrow over his shortcomings, his shame at failure, his humiliation at his bad conduct, his discouragement at being himself, we may disregard his wish to be better and the joy he feels when he can make some progress. If progress of this kind is impossible, we should try not to raise his hopes.

In sum, the feelings and attitudes and conflicts of all those concerned with the medication of the mentally retarded must be seriously explored before one can tell whether it should be done at all, how it should be done, and whether it can meet with success.

═══════════

REFERENCES

Appleton, W. S., & Chien, C. P. American pharmacology: Second class status? *Brit. J. Psychiat.*, 1967, *113*, 637–641.

Borgatta, E. The new principle of psychotherapy. *J. Clin. Psychol.*, 1959, *15*, 330–334.

Clements, S. D., & Peters, J. E. Minimal brain dysfunction in children. Washington, D.C.: Department of Health, Education, and Welfare, 1966.

Eaton, L., & Menolascino, F. J. Psychotic reactions of childhood: A follow-up study. *Amer. J. Orthopsychiat.*, 1967, *37*, 521–529.

Eisenberg, L. Role of drugs in treating disturbed children. *Children*, 1964, *2*(5), 167–173.

Farber, S. M., & Wilson, R. H. L. (Ed.). *Control of the mind.* New York: McGraw-Hill, 1961.

Fish, B. Drug theory in child psychiatry: Psychological aspects. *Compr. Psychiat.*, 1960, *1*, 212–217.

———. Drug therapy in child psychiatry: Pharmacological aspects. *Compr. Psychiat.*, February, 1960.

———. Drug use in psychiatric disorders of children. *Amer. J. Psychiat.*, 1968, *124*, (8), 31–39.

Freedman, A. M. Drug therapy in behavior disorders. *Pediat. Clin. North America*, 1958, *5*(3), 573–594.

Gross, M. *The doctors: An analysis of the american physician.* New York: Random House, 1966.

Hammond, J. E. Drugs for treatment of children with behavior disorders. *Med. Times*, 1964, *92*, 421–426.

Hellmuth, J. (Ed.). *Learning disorders.* Seattle, Wash.: Hellmuth & Straub, 1966.

Kurlander, L. F., & Colodny, D. Panacea, palliation or poison: The psychodynamics of a controversy. *Amer. J. Psychiat.*, 1965, *121*, 1168–1170.

Leo, J. Psychoanalysis reaches a crossroad. *New York Times,* Sunday, Aug. 4, 1968.

Marmor, J., Bernard, V. W., & Ottenberg, P. The psychodynamics of group opposition to health programs. *Amer. J. Orthopsychiat.*, 1960, *30*(2), 330–345.

Robinson, H., & Robinson, N. M. *The mentally retarded child.* McGraw-Hill, New York, 1965.

Szasz, T. Some observations on the use of tranquilizing drugs. *A.M.A. Arch. Neurol. & Psychiat.*, 1957, *77*, 88–92.

Talalay, P. (Ed.). Drugs in our society. Baltimore, Md.: Johns Hopkins University Press, 1964.

Talland, G., & McGuire, M. T. Tests of learning and memory with remoline. *Psychopharmacol.*, 1967, *10*, 445–451.

Uhr, L., & Miller, J. J. (Eds.). Drugs and behavior. New York: John Wiley & Sons, 1960.

: 15 :

The Use of Psychopharmacological Agents in Residential Facilities for the Retarded

Ronald S. Lipman

INTRODUCTION

SINCE the introduction of chlorpromazine in 1952, there has been a marked increase in the number, variety, and usage of psychotropic drugs for the treatment of mental illness and behavioral and emotional disorders.[1] Although the literature indicates that psychotropic drugs are being employed in institutions for the mentally retarded, it does not reflect either the extent or pattern of drug usage. The purpose of the present study is to illuminate this area by presenting the data of a psychotropic-drug survey. These data, along with the relevant literature, particularly as it pertains to the pharmacotherapy of children, will be considered in an attempt to highlight research methods and directions that might profitably be pursued.

Table 15–1 indicates institutions that were sent psychotropic drug-usage questionnaires and data on returns. As can be seen in this table, 173 institutions were invited to participate in this survey. These institutions, selected from the Directory of Residential Facilities for the Mentally Retarded, included all 142 state and 31 private institutions. Thirteen of these institutions, mainly private, were later deleted from the survey since they were not primarily for the retarded, were not operational, employed the services of noninstitutional physicians, and so forth. A few institutions that completed the survey were also excluded since we were unable to make sense of their returned data. We have currently received 109 usable returns from 100 state (representing 74 per cent of those surveyed) and 9 private institutions (representing approximately 33 per cent of this sample).

TABLE 15–1

Drug Survey Statistics

Total number of questionnaires sent		173
A. Inappropriate institutions	13	
B. Appropriate institutions		160
1. Refusals	27	
2. No response	19	
3. Outstanding	2	
4. Returned (data not usable)	3	
	51	
C. Returned data used in survey		109
1. State institutions	100	
2. Private institutions	9	
Percentage of usable returns in appropriate institutions	68.1%	

PRESENTATION OF SURVEY RESULTS

Before proceeding to substantive findings, I would like to qualify these data. Certain drugs were omitted from the survey: Benadryl, for example, was not included; nor were the butyrophenones and drug combinations such as Triavil or Deprol. Ideally, we should have made a distinction between patients currently on psychotropic drugs and patients who had received psychotropic drugs but were no longer on medication. We thought, however, that even a gross survey that attempted to obtain "ball-park" information on drug usage and dosage and information on duration would be pushing the limits of institutional tolerance.

Against this background the major results of drug usage are presented in Table 15–2. The data in this table are organized by drug class—major tranquilizers, minor tranquilizers, and antidepressants —and within the tranquilizer groups, phenothiazines are distinguished from nonphenothiazines. The two most striking features of these data are (1) the extensive use of psychotropic drugs, 51 per cent, and (2) the fact that two of the sedative-type phenothiazines— thioridazine (Mellaril) and chlorpromazine (Thorazine)—account for roughly 58 per cent of all drug usage.

In Table 15–3 it can be seen that either chlorpromazine (Thora-

TABLE 15–2

Psychotropic Drug Usage

I. Major tranquilizers		(39.19%)
(a) *Phenothiazines*		
Mellaril	15.50	
Thorazine	14.25	
Stelazine	2.62	
Sparine	1.55	
Vesprin	1.38	
Trilafon	1.25	
Miscellaneous	1.53 [1]	
(b) *Nonphenothiazines*		
Miscellaneous	1.11 [2]	
II. Minor tranquilizers		(8.12%)
Valium	2.23	
Librium	2.20	
Miltown	1.62	
Miscellaneous	2.07 [3]	
III. Antidepressants and energizers		(3.80%)
Tofranil	1.16 [4]	
Miscellaneous	2.64	

NOTE: These percentages are based on a total population of 148,371 retardates in 109 institutions. Drugs received by less than 1% of the sample have been grouped under the "Miscellaneous" category.
[1] Compazine, Permitil and Tindal.
[2] Taractan and Reserpine.
[3] Vistaril, Atarax, Serax, Ultran and Phenergan.
[4] Elavil, Aventyl, Norpramin, Ritalin, Dexedrine and Benzedrine.

zine) or thioridazine (Mellaril) is the "drug of choice" in 91 per cent of our institutional sample.

Table 15–4 presents data on chlorpromazine dosage. Typically, chlorpromazine is given in doses of between 75 and 300 milligrams

TABLE 15–3

Chlorpromazine and Thioridazine Usage [1]

	MOST FREQUENT		SECOND MOST FREQUENT	
	N	%	N	%
Chlorpromazine	44	40.37	41	37.61
Thioridazine	55	50.46	32	29.36
	99	90.83	73	66.97

[1] N = 109 institutions.

daily, which would be considered in the low range using adult inpatient schizophrenics as the yardstick, but it can also be seen that some very high dosing is also employed, 2,000 milligrams a day being considered a very high dose for adult psychotics.

T A B L E 15–4

Maximum and Typical Daily Dosage
of Chlorpromazine

Maximum daily dose: (*N* = 103) [1]
    Range   40–3000 mg.
    Median   600 mg.

Typical daily dose: (*N* = 95) [1]
    Range   10–600 mg.

Dose (mg.)	Frequency	Percentage
10 to 50	6	6.32
75 and 100	17	17.89
150	19	20.00
200	16	16.84
225 and 300	24	25.26
400	8	8.42
450 to 600	5	5.27
	95	100.00

[1] Of the 109 participating institutions, 105 (96.33%) reported chlorpromazine usage. However, 10 of the drug-using institutions failed to indicate a typical daily dose and 2 failed to indicate a maximum daily dose.

Table 15–5 presents comparable dosage information for thioridazine. As with chlorpromazine, thioridazine is most frequently given in a daily dosage of between 75 and 300 milligrams, but again maximum dosages well above the manufacturer's recommended dose of 800 milligrams for schizophrenics are being used.

T A B L E 15–5

Maximum and Typical Daily Dosage
of Thioridazine

Maximum daily dose: (*N* = 100) [1]
    Range   25–1800 mg.
    Median   400 mg.

Typical daily dose: (*N* = 91) [1]
    Range   30–400 mg.

Dose (mg.)	Frequency	Percentage
30 and 50	8	8.79
75 and 100	24	26.37
150	19	20.88
200	16	17.58
300	17	18.68
345 and 400	7	7.70
	91	100.00

[1] Of the 109 participating institutions, 103 (94.50%) reported thioridazine usage. However, 12 of the drug-using institutions failed to indicate a typical daily dose and 3 failed to indicate a maximum daily dose.

Table 15–6 shows typical and maximal duration of chlorpromazine and thioridazine administration. The most interesting aspect of these data is the significant proportion of very chronic use. Roughly 25 per cent of patients *typically* receive these drugs for four or more

TABLE 15–6

Typical and Maximal Duration of Drug Administration

	MAXIMUM DURATION		TYPICAL DURATION	
	CHLORPROMAZINE (N = 93) [1]	THIORIDAZINE (N = 89) [1]	CHLORPROMAZINE (N = 78) [1]	THIORIDAZINE (N = 77) [1]
	%	%	%	%
Less than 1 year	19.36	22.47	55.13	54.55
1 to 2 years	13.98	21.35	11.54	14.29
2 to 4 years	20.43	15.73	7.69	6.49
More than 4 years	15.05	7.87	2.56	2.59
Indefinite	31.18	32.58	23.08	22.08
	100.00	100.00	100.00	100.00

[1] Of the 109 participating institutions, use of these drugs was reported as follows: Chlorpromazine: 105 institutions (96.33%)—12 failed to indicate maximum duration and 27 failed to indicate typical duration.

Thioridazine: 103 institutions (94.50%)—14 failed to indicate maximum duration and 26 failed to indicate typical duration.

years. It should be indicated that the use of the term "indefinite" in Table 15–6 is the respondents' and not a term superimposed on the data by the author.

A similar analysis of dosage and information on duration was made for two additional phenothiazines, Stelazine and Sparine, and for the two most frequently used minor tranquilizers, chlordiazepoxide (Librium) and trifluoperazine (Valium). In general, these data fall into the same usage pattern as for chlorpromazine and thioridazine. Again, typical dosage falls within the range employed with other patient populations while maximum dosage rises above usual limits. Duration of usage also reveals a significant proportion of very chronic administration.

Tables 15–7 and 15–8 illustrate, respectively, dosage and duration of usage for the psychic energizer dextroamphetamine, which was employed in 0.80 per cent of the present sample.

This dosage pattern of dextroamphetamine seems quite conservative, since the recommended dose ranges from 0.1 to 0.4 milligrams per pound of body weight a day (Fish, 1967). Again, as with the duration pattern of other drugs, one cannot help but wonder how rational a basis there is for the "indefinite" usage of this drug? Have patients been challenged by drug withdrawal, or have initial orders been "automatically" continued?

TABLE 15–7

Maximum and Typical Daily Dosage
of Dextroamphetamine

Maximum daily dose: $(N=58)$ [1]
Range	5–60 mg.
Median	15 mg.

Typical daily dose: $(N=54)$ [1]
Range	5–25 mg.

Dose (mg.)	Frequency	Percentage
5 and 75	12	22.22
10	19	35.19
15	18	33.33
20 and 25	5	9.26
	54	100.00

[1] Of the 109 participating institutions, 62 (56.88%) reported dextroamphetamine usage. However, 8 of the drug-using institutions failed to indicate a typical daily dose and 4 failed to indicate a maximum daily dose.

Unfortunately, our survey format does not permit an identification of the number of patients receiving a particular drug dosage, nor does it permit us to cross-tabulate dosage by length of administration, age, sex, or reasons for administration. We did, however, relate drug usage to institutional size. At the extremes of resident population, that is, below 500 and more than 3,000, there was some tendency for the larger institution to use drugs more freely and on a more chronic basis. These differences were not very pronounced, and this trend was quite weak over the full range of institutions.

While the *pattern* of drug usage was highly consistent in the sense of chlorpromazine and thioridazine being most frequently used, there

TABLE 15–8

Typical and Maximal Duration of Drug Administration

	DEXTROAMPHETAMINE	
	MAXIMUM DURATION $(N=49)$ [1]	TYPICAL DURATION $(N=42)$ [1]
	%	%
Less than 1 year	42.86	61.91
1 to 2 years	16.33	9.52
2 to 4 years	14.28	7.14
More than 4 years	2.04	2.38
Indefinite	24.49	19.05
	100.00	100.00

[1] Of the 109 participating institutions, 62 (56.88%) reported dextroamphetamine usage. However, 13 of the drug-using institutions failed to indicate a maximum duration and 20 failed to indicate a typical duration.

was considerable variability in the total amount and duration of drug usage from institution to institution. The variability in drug usage is shown in Table 15–9.

This concludes the reporting of survey results. The remainder of this article will focus on implications for research which have developed from this survey, the psychotropic drug literature, and personal communications with administrative and professional staff concerned with the treatment of mentally retarded patients.

TABLE 15–9

Percentage Drug Use by Institutions

PERCENTAGE OF RESIDENTS RECEIVING DRUGS	NUMBER OF INSTITUTIONS (%)	
80 or more	18	(16.5)
60–79	12	(11.0)
40–59	13	(11.9)
20–39	51	(46.8)
19 or less	15	(13.8)
	109	

IMPLICATIONS FOR RESEARCH

Unless the writer's radar equipment has seriously failed, it would seem that, to an overwhelming degree, psychotropic drugs instead of paraldehyde and camisoles are being used for controlling the behavior of the aggressive, assaultive, difficult-to-manage hyperactive patient. Given these survey results, it behooves us to ask: (1) What is the evidence to support the efficacy of chlorpromazine and thioridazine for controlling the difficult-to-manage patient? (2) What do we know of the effect of chronic phenothiazine treatment on the intellectual and physical development of the mentally retarded child? (3) What evidence is there to indicate that sedative phenothiazines should be the drugs of choice for this type of patient?

The large double-blind collaborative studies conducted by the Veterans Administration and the National Institute of Mental Health (Goldberg et al., 1965; Lasky et al., 1962; National Institute of Mental Health, 1964) have, of course, proved the phenothiazines to be of significant value in the treatment of acute schizophrenia. It is not scientifically justifiable, however, to generalize these findings to a different population in whom these drugs are being used for a very different clinical purpose.

When one turns to review articles dealing with the efficacy of different psychotropic drugs for the treatment of both retarded and emotionally disturbed children, it becomes clear that the state of the art leaves much to be desired. Grant (1962) characterized the scientific quality of studies in this field as "parlous," and this theme of research inadequacy is also echoed in the review by Copeland (1965) and the very excellent review by Freeman (1966). The overwhelming majority of drug studies in this area lack adequate controls, appropriate statistical analysis, or both. Nevertheless, most reviewers agree that chlorpromazine and thioridazine are effective in the treatment of the behavior disorders.

In reading the chlorpromazine and thioridazine literature with both retarded and behaviorally disturbed children, the author found approximately three dozen noncontrolled positive reports and fourteen more or less controlled studies—some positive, some negative.

Given these data, it would be possible to prepare a contingency table comparing positive and negative findings versus controlled and noncontrolled studies and reach the conclusion that chlorpromazine and thioridazine were ineffective compounds since positive findings were disproportionately associated with noncontrolled studies. This is essentially what Astin and Ross (1960) did in their review of glutamic acid. I think this is patently unfair, however, since it seems to be part of the sociology of publication that noncontrolled reports see print when they are positive, whereas controlled studies are published regardless of outcome. In essence, this approach to the evaluation of almost any psychotropic drug would yield the same negative conclusion.

In terms of behavior management, controlled studies were more likely to be positive (Adamson et al., 1958; Allen et al., 1963; Horenstein, 1957; Hunt et al., 1956; Hunter & Stephenson, 1963; Shaw et al., 1963; Werry et al., 1966) than negative (Craft, 1957; Garfield, Helper, Wilcott & Muffly, 1962; Lane et al., 1958; Wardell et al., 1958) in outcome. Moreover, results in controlled studies may reflect such factors as small and heterogeneous samples, insensitive assessment instruments, inadequacies of drug dosage and duration, and the application of weak or inappropriate statistical procedures.

When the influence of these phenothiazines on cognitive behavior is examined, results of controlled studies are equally distributed between reliably negative outcomes (Werry et al., 1966; Helper et al., 1963; Moore, 1960)—that is, placebo patients perform reliably better than drug patients—and outcomes in which no significant drug-placebo differences were found (Adamson et al., 1958; Craft, 1957; Ison, 1957).

My synthesis of the literature, in regard to the first question raised is that the sedative phenothiazines are effective in improving the behavior of the "acting-out" child, but—probably—at the price of reduced alertness and cognitive efficiency.

Let us now turn to the second and third questions. Unfortunately, there are no data available on the long-term effects of phenothiazine usage despite the warning issued by Tarjan, et al. (1957): ". . . care should be exercised, not to use chlorpromazine on a prolonged basis in young patients until more is known about the long-range effect of the drug . . ." There are also few controlled drug versus drug trials, with the exception of chlorpromazine-reserpine comparisons, to suggest that the sedating phenothiazines should be the drugs of choice for the aggressive-hyperactive child.

On the basis of the available literature, other potentially promising drug candidates for behavioral control are: (1) The stimulants such as amphetamine and methylphenidate (Ritalin), (2) antihistamines, particularly Benadryl, (3) the newer group of butyrophenones, particularly haloperidol, which has just received Food and Drug Administration approval, (4) chlorprothixene (Taracton), and finally, but perhaps least promising, (5) the more stimulating piperazine phenothiazines such as trifluoperazine (Stelazine).

It is clear that the medical practitioner is faced with a bewildering array of psychotropic drugs and very little in the way of conclusive evidence to guide his choice of treatment.

In considering the relative efficacy of chlorpromazine versus other possible therapeutic agents for the hyperactive-destructive child, Weiss et al. (1969) reached the same opinion as this writer: "The evidence supporting the efficacy of the dextroamphetamine is both historically older and equally, if not more, extensive."

When evidence regarding the influence on cognitive behavior of chlorpromazine versus the amphetamine-like drugs is examined, it seems clear from the excellent studies of Conners (1965; 1966), Conners and Eisenberg (1963), and Conners et al. (1964), Conners et al. (1969) at Johns Hopkins and the well-controlled studies of Weiss et al. (1969), Helper et al. (1963), Garfield et al. (1962), and Moore (1960) that amphetamine tends to enhance learning and performance on many tasks, whereas chlorpromazine tends to interfere with certain types of learning and performance. In a recent review article, Hartlage (1965) summarized the effects of chlorpromazine on learning as follows: "Results of studies involving a number of animals, normal subjects, and psychiatric patients tend to show a linear decline in learning with increased dosage levels."

In evaluating the overall efficacy of psychotropic drugs for the hyperactive child, one should weigh the influence of the drug on educability as well as on behavior.

When one examines progress made in the pharmacotherapy of schizophrenia and depression, it is evident that greater therapeutic advances have been made in these areas. In the treatment of acute schizophrenics, for example, the emphasis has shifted from the more general approach of demonstrating the effectiveness of psychotropic drugs to the more refined question of selecting the right drug for the right patient. In this connection, selecting the "right" phenothiazine as contrasted with the "wrong" phenothiazine results in as great a difference in therapeutic improvement as the therapeutic difference between modal placebo and modal phenothiazine response (Goldberg et al., 1967).

It is my firm conviction that these advances have resulted from the large-sample placebo-controlled, double-blind collaborative study in which the talents of professionals from many disciplines, as well as computer facilities, have been brought to bear on the problem. Such studies are, of course, both time consuming and expensive and have required financial and logistic support from federal agencies.

In commenting on the status of drug research in the area of mental retardation, Copeland (1965) points out that

. . . over 75% of the published research in this area was initially financed by grants-in-aid from the pharmaceutical houses. Consequently, a review of the literature provides a fairly accurate calendar account of the succession of new preparations on the market. . . . It seems safe to say that satisfactory and adequate replication will not occur until financial support is as readily available from other sources as it is from the drug companies.

The conclusion to be drawn from this statement is rather self-evident.

SUMMARY

A survey of psychotropic drug usage in institutions for the mentally retarded revealed a relatively high proportion (51 per cent) of patients receiving drugs and a very consistent pattern of drug usage. The sedative phenothiazines—chlorpromazine and thioridazine—were overwhelmingly the drugs of choice.

The implications of this pattern of drug usage were discussed in terms of the available literature, and directions for future research were suggested.

———

NOTE

1. The author would like to express his appreciation to the many people who found time in their busy schedules to participate in this survey and thereby make this study possible, and particularly to Dr. Max Reiss of Willowbrook State School, N.Y., who originally stimulated his interest in this area. Portions of this chapter were presented at the 91st Annual Meeting of the American Association for Mental Deficiency in Denver, Colo., May 19, 1967. The opinions expressed in this chapter are those of the author and do not necessarily represent any official position of the National Institute of Mental Health.

REFERENCES

Adamson, W. C., Nellis, B. P., Runge, G., Cleland, C., & Killiam, E. Use of tranquilizers for mentally deficient patients. *A.M.A.J. Dis. Child.*, 1958, *96*, 159–164.

Allen, M., Shannon, G., & Rose, D. Thioridazine hydrochloride in the behavior disturbance of retarded children. *Amer. J. Ment. Defic.*, 1963, *68* (1), 63–68.

Astin, A. W., & Ross, S. Glutamic acid and human intelligence. *Psychol. Bull.*, 1960, *37* (3), 429–434.

Conners, C. K. Effects of brief psychotherapy, drugs, and type of disturbance on Holtzman Inkblot scores in children. *Proceedings of 73rd Annual Convention of the American Psychological Association*, 1965, pp. 201–202.

———. The effect of Dexedrine on rapid discrimination and motor control of hyperkinetic children under mild stress. *J. Nerv. Ment. Dis.*, 1966, *142* (5), 429–433.

Conners, C. K., & Eisenberg, L. The effects of methylphenidate on symptomatology and learning in disturbed children. *Amer. J. Psychiat.*, 1963, *120* (5), 458–464.

Conners, C. K., Eisenberg, L., & Barcai, A. The effect of amphetamine on children with learning disabilities and behavior problems in the classroom. *Arch. Gen. Psychiat.*, 1969 (in press).

Conners, C. K., Eisenberg, L., & Sharpe, L. Effects of methylphenidate (Ritalin) on paired-associate learning and Porteus Maze performance in emotionally disturbed children. *J. Consult. Psychol.*, 1964, *28* (1), 14–22.

Copeland, R. A critical review—Psychopharmacological experimentation with the mentally retarded. In James O. Smith & Tom C. Lovitt (Ed.), *Selected papers: Medical aspects of mental retardation and neuromuscular dysfunction*. Lawrence, Kan.: University of Kansas Press, 1965.

Craft, M. Tranquilizers in mental deficiency: Chlorpromazine. *J. Ment. Defic. Res.*, 1957, *1* (2), 91–95.

Fish, B. Drug use in psychiatric disorders of children. Presented at the American Psychiatric Association, Detroit, Mich., May, 1967.

Freeman, R. D. Drug effects on learning in children: A selective review of the past thirty years. *J. Spec. Educ.*, 1966, *1* (1), 17–44.

Garfield, S. L., Helper, M. M., Wilcott, R. C., & Muffly, R. Effects of chlorpromazine on behavior in emotionally disturbed children. *J. Nerv. Ment. Dis.,* 1962, *135* (2), 147–154.

Goldberg, S. C., Klerman, G. L., & Cole, J. O. Changes in schizophrenic psychopathology and ward behavior as a function of phenothiazine treatment. *Brit. J. Psychiat.,* 1965, *111* (471), 120–133.

Goldberg, S. C., Mattsson, N., Cole, J. O., & Klerman, G. L. Prediction of improvement in schizophrenia under four phenothiazines. *Arch. Gen. Psychiat.,* 1967, *16,* 107–117.

Grant, Q. R. Psychopharmacology in childhood emotional and mental disorders. *J. Pediat.,* 1962, *61,* 626–637.

Hartlage, L. C. Effects of chlorpromazine on learning. *Psychol. Bull.,* 1965, *64* (4), 235–245.

Helper, M. M., Wilcott, R. C., & Garfield, S. L. Effects of chlorpromazine on learning and related processes in emotionally disturbed children. *J. Consult. Psychol.,* 1963, *27* (1), 1–9.

Horenstein, S. Reserpine and chlorpromazine in hyperactive mental defectives. *Amer. J. Ment. Defic.,* 1957, *61* (3), 525–529.

Hunt, B. R., Frank, T., & Krush, T. P. Chlorpromazine in the treatment of severe emotional disorders of children. *A.M.A.J. Dis. Child.,* 1956, *91,* 268–277.

Hunter, H., & Stephenson, G. M. Chlorpromazine and trifluoperazine in the treatment of behavioral abnormalities in the severely subnormal child. *Brit. J. Psychiat.,* 1963, *109,* 411–417.

Ison, M. G. The effect of "Thorazine" on Wechsler scores. *Amer. J. Ment. Defic.,* 1957, *62,* 543–547.

Lane, G. G., Huber, W. G., & Smith, F. L. The effect of chlorpromazine on the behavior of disturbed children. *Amer. J. Psychiat.,* 1958, *114,* 937–938.

Lasky, J. J., Klett, C. J., Caffey, E. H., Bennett, J. L., Rosenblum, M. P., & Hollister, L. E. Drug treatment of schizophrenic patients: A comparative evaluation of chlorpromazine, chlorprothixene, fluphenazine, reserpine, thioridazine and triflupromazine. *Dis. Nerv. Sys.,* 1962, *23,* 698–706.

Moore, J. W. The effects of a tranquilizer (Thorazine) on the intelligence and achievement of educable mentally retarded women. *Dissert. Abstr.,* 1960, *20,* 3200.

National Institute of Mental Health, Psychopharmacology Service Center Collaborative Study Group. Phenothiazine treatment in acute schizophrenia, *Arch. Gen. Psychiat.,* 1964, *10,* 246–261.

Shaw, C. R., Lockett, H. J., Lucas, A. R., Lamontagne, M. D., & Grimm, F. Tranquilizer drugs in the treatment of emotionally disturbed children: 1. Inpatients in a residential treatment center. *J. Amer. Acad. Child. Psychiat.,* 1963, *2,* 725–742.

Tarjan, G., Lowery, V. E., & Wright, S. W. Use of chlorpromazine in two hundred seventy-eight mentally deficient patients. *A.M.A. J. Dis. Child.,* 1957, *94,* 294–300.

Wardell, D. W., Rubin, H. K., & Ross, R. T. The use of reserpine and chlorpromazine in disturbed mentally deficient patients. *Amer. J. Ment. Defic.,* 1958, *63* (2), 330–344.

Weiss, G., Werry, J., Minde, K., Douglas, V., & Sykes, D. Studies on the hyperactive child: V. The effects of dextroamphetamine and chlorpromazine on behavior and intellectual functioning. Presented at the International Congress of Child Neurology, Prague, Sept., 1965.

Werry, J. S., Weiss, G., Douglas, V., & Martin, J. Studies of the hyperactive child: III. The effect of chlorpromazine upon behavior and learning ability. *J. Amer. Acad. Child Psychiat.,* 1966, *5,* 292–312.

: 16 :

Methodological Considerations in Evaluating the Intelligence-Enhancing Properties of Drugs

Wolf Wolfensberger and Frank J. Menolascino

HISTORICAL AND THEORETICAL BACKGROUND

MENTAL retardation is widely conceptualized as a disease.[1] For instance, the handbook on mental retardation recently issued by the American Medical Association (1965, pp. 47, 98) refers to retardation as "illness" and "disease." Retardates are frequently labeled as "patients" in the literature, and 39 per cent of American public institutions for the retarded have the term "hospital" in their official name.

Many diseases can be cured, and some diseases considered incurable at one time eventually become curable as new treatments are discovered. It is, therefore, not surprising that many laymen as well as professionals should look forward to the discovery of "cures" of mental retardation. This hope often takes the form of a search for a drug. People who conceptualize mental retardation as a disease usually also conceptualize a potential drug cure to be very similar to, say, the cure of an acute episode of bacterial tonsillitis by means of antibiotics. The person giving the treatment administers the drug to the sick and passive patient, who soon improves and eventually "takes up his bed and walks." As far as mental retardation is concerned, an analogous treatment expectation would be to see an eight-year-old severely retarded nonverbal, nonambulatory child suddenly bursting forth into talking, walking, and doing the things one would expect an average eight-year-old to do. Not only laymen and parents, but even professional workers may, even if only semiconsciously, hold to such a conceptualization of a potential drug cure of mental retardation which Yannet (1957) has labeled the "magic bullet" theory. Evidence that the "magic bullet" analogy is neither farfetched nor specific to retardation is provided by a recent article (Anonymous, 1966), which advocated greater use of rifles and pistols that fire tranquilizing darts.

Without explicitly and consciously articulating the "magic bullet" theory, a researcher may adopt an experimental design that clearly implies it. Thus, a number of glutamic acid studies reviewed by Vogel et al. (1966) had placed retarded subjects on the experimental drug for such short periods (one to two months) that effects upon global intelligence would have had to be very dramatic to reach statistical significance. Burns et al. (1967) conducted a study of the effects of a single dose of magnesium pemoline on learning. The relevant question here is not so much whether drug effects were then actually reported, but why investigators choose to adopt designs that would only assess quick and dramatic, but not gradual and developmentally equally important, effects. Use of adult subjects rather than of children also carries with it the flavor of "magic bullet" expectations. Children generally are believed to be much more plastic than adults, and one can easily conceptualize a significant increase in their developmental rate. In adults, however, a drug effect is difficult to conceptualize except in terms of either performance enhancement or "cure."

The field of mental retardation has witnessed many attempts to improve cognitive functioning by means of drugs, and a number of models of drug action can be discerned. These attempts can be classified as springing from three theoretical models, to be outlined briefly below.

Unblocking model. Within this model, drugs are employed to treat conditions which interfere with the full use or development of intelligence. Examples are the allaying of anxiety by means of tranquilizers; the control of seizures with anticonvulsants; and the diminishing of activity level with motor retardants. Especially in psychiatrically oriented circles, the term "unblocking" may actually be encountered in this connection.

Energizing model. This model implies the use of drugs to stimulate the central nervous system in an effort to improve alertness and performance, thereby hopefully maximizing those intellect-related behaviors that might not even be fully utilized by a well-functioning person. Amphetamines, strychnine, and celastrus paniculata have been used in this fashion (see reviews by Freeman, 1966; and Louttit, 1965).

Direct-action model. Whereas the two models just discussed imply an indirect drug effect, some drugs are employed in the hope that they affect cognitive processes directly. However, within this model, drugs can be perceived as having a number of possible modes of action. Earlier investigators posited a somewhat vaguely conceptualized expansion of consciousness or awareness (for example, Zimmerman et al., 1949), or an equally vaguely defined improvement in higher cognitive processes. A recent and more sophisticated conceptualization envisions improvement in learning and memory processes. Glutamine and glutamic acid (Louttit, 1965; Vogel et al., 1966), vitamins (House, et al., 1964), sicca-cell treatments (Goldstein, 1956), and combination treatments such as Turkel's (1963) "U series" of forty-nine drugs have been used within the framework of the direct-action model.

While none of the pharmacological agents mentioned here has been convincingly demonstrated to improve the intelligence or intellectual development of retardates, some of the so-called replacement therapies that aim at the amelioration of specific metabolic syndromes associated with retardation have been effective. For instance, thyroid preparations have been shown to be effective in selected cases of hypothyroidism, and several other metabolic disorders (for example, phenylketonuria) are treated dietetically and apparently with at least some success (see Kirman, 1965; Waisman and Gerritsen, 1964). However, although many investigators appear to view replacement therapies as essentially constituting "unblocking," agreement as to the most appropriate model or mode of drug action in these therapies appears to be lacking. On one point there has been widespread agreement: the success of replacement therapies appears to be correlated negatively with subjects' age; that is, the older the subject, the less success.

It is crucially important to be aware of certain other conceptualizations and attitudes that can affect designs of drug studies in subtle and detrimental ways. For example, a curious phenomenon can be discerned in the way people may view attempts to improve the intelligence of retarded as against nonretarded individuals. A "pill" to enhance the intelligence of a college student would probably be expected to improve his learning, memory, and general performance. A moderate and gradually accumulating effect would be considered quite desirable and acceptable. However, with a retarded person, a drug may be scorned if it produced anything but a complete and perhaps even rapid "cure"; that is, unless it produced "normality." Similarly, nonpharmacological treatments of mental retardation have often also been interpreted as medical therapy and have been expected to lead to complete cures. Operations to increase the arterial blood flow to the brain (revascularization) and operations designed to prevent the early closure of the cranial sutures in primary microcephaly are typical examples.

Deep-seated unfavorable or conflicting attitudes toward mental retardation may underlie differential expectations regarding the role of drugs in normal persons and retardates. Unconsciously, and often consciously, many people measure the worth of an individual by his intelligence and achievement (see Mead, 1942, pp. 89–90, 107, 109; Stone, 1948), and a "subnormal" person may thus be viewed as also "subhuman" or "nonhuman." Although such attitudes usually remain unverbalized, they are occasionally openly formulated as when retardates are referred to as "monsters," "vegetables," or "vegetative." At any rate, there appear to be individuals who perceive a qualitative difference between normality and subnormality, and who view subnormality as a unitary construct. From such a viewpoint, it makes little difference whether a retardate has an IQ of 20, 40, or 60; he is still not normal. Therefore, a treatment (drug or otherwise) that significantly improves a retardate's intelligence may be dismissed as ineffective because it did not "cure." Examples of this view can be found in the proceedings of the Association for Research in Nervous and Mental Disease (1962, p. 302) and in Birch and Belmont (1961).

Recently, the hope to enhance intelligence chemically has been rekindled by reports that RNA and drugs believed to facilitate the metabolism of RNA in the brain (for example, magnesium pemoline, registered as Cylert by Abbott Laboratories) result in improved retention or perhaps even acquisition of information in animals and human beings. Other potentially intelligence-enhancing or development-enhancing drugs on which there has been widespread recent publicity include 5-hydroxytryptophane. Research on such drugs has now moved from animal to human trials, and both popular press and serious scientists are emitting optimistic forecasts with increasing frequency and publicity. Krech (*Washington Report,* 1968, Volume IV, No. 2) gave such optimistic testimony before a Congressional Committee; Linus Pauling (1968) has recently jolted the field by forecasting an era of "orthomolecular psychiatry" where drugs play a large role in behavior maintenance and enhancement; and Arthur Koestler (author of *Darkness at Noon*) has recently (1967) joined the ranks of prominent writers anticipating a drug-based utopia.

Inevitably, the question of the "cure" of mental retardation by chemical agents has arisen. At this point, it may be timely to recall the past so as not to repeat its errors.

METHODOLOGICAL CONSIDERATIONS

What we would like to attempt in this chapter is to discuss a series of issues that should be considered before embarking upon research designed to assess the ability of drugs to enhance cognitive functioning or development of retarded individuals. Some of these issues are of a theoretical nature and have to do with the role drugs reasonably can be expected to play in the enhancement of intelligence. Other issues are purely methodological, having more obvious implications for the design of relevant experiments than the theoretical issues mentioned.

A basic assumption throughout the remainder of this chapter is that we are discussing studies employing a placebo control group and other features of well-designed drug experiments. While there may be a role for uncontrolled exploratory work, we are committed to the view that the power of the placebo effect has been so convincingly demonstrated (for example, Shapiro, 1960) that no drug should be accepted as possessing development-enhancing properties unless it has undergone the most rigorously controlled tests.

We also wish to emphasize that we are not particularly concerned with those pharmaceutical agents which result in improved performance (for example, central-nervous-system stimulants) or alleviation of secondary conditions (for example, hyperkinesis, seizures, and emotional disturbance) that interfere with intellectual efficiency and development. The focus in this paper is primarily on drugs purported to improve cognitive functioning or development directly. When speaking of drug-effectiveness studies, it is to this type of drug we refer.

General Considerations

The first goal of a study designed to assess a drug's ability to accelerate development should be to explore whether the drug has *any* developmental effect. To demonstrate such an effect is difficult enough without getting involved in tests of sophisticated and advanced hypotheses, or comparisons of several unproved drugs at the same time.

Since attempts to explore the potential effectiveness of drugs are difficult and demanding of time, money, and other resources, experiments should be designed to maximize the ascertainability of a potential effect. Above all, a study should be designed in a way that guarantees a fair test of the drug. Many studies in the past have failed in this regard, and whatever the merit of the drug may have been, such studies were simply irrelevant. The history of the field contains instances in which respected and qualified workers enthusiastically embraced belief in the curative action of a drug that later was generally rejected as ineffective, even though neither the original positive nor later negative studies may have constituted adequate tests of the drug's potential effects. Freeman (1966), in an excellent review of studies of drug effects upon learning in children, has pointed out that after twenty-five years of work with glutamic acid and its derivatives and thirty years of work with amphetamines, we still do not possess adequate empirical evidence regarding the behavioral effects of these drugs. Perhaps the same can be said about the use of thyroid preparations with mongoloids.

Failure to consider certain principles and facts of child development and experimental design account for many erroneous or unpromising research strategies. Much of the remainder of this chapter will concern itself with such considerations.

Fallacy of the "Magic Bullet" Theory

One consideration of crucial importance is that mental retardation is not a disease, and that the "magic bullet" model is not appropriate to the drug treatment of mental retardation. Let us recall the example of the severely retarded eight-year-old boy. Even if it were possible to restore him instantaneously to normal learning capacity, he would, in all likelihood, have to pass through the developmental stages every normal child goes through. Turning, crawling, sitting, standing unsupported, walking, and running would probably have to be developed sequentially. There is even reason to believe that some behavior skills (for example, in the areas of speech, language, and perceptual development) may rarely, if ever, be mastered unless they are acquired during sensitive, or prior to critical, periods of development. Thus, instead of having a "magic bullet" effect, a development-enhancing drug is more likely to work gradually, additively, directionally, and selectively.

Definition of Drug Effect

Once we have emancipated ourselves from the "magic bullet" model, we can address ourselves more productively to the question of when a drug (or any treatment) can be considered to have been effective. As mentioned earlier, one orientation encountered in the field of mental retardation is that, if a treatment does not cure, or at least result in spectacular effects, it is not worth considering. At this point it is important to recall that even very small changes in behavior, or in rate of development, can have major implications to ultimate functioning and to social and management costs. Thus, a real and permanent change in developmental rate equivalent to only seven IQ points will mean a difference of about one year of developmental maturity in adulthood.[2] Being or not being toilet trained can mean a difference of two hours' work a day to a mother, and this, in turn, can mean the difference between the child's remaining in the home or his placement into an institution at great cost to the child, his family, and society. Since relatively small developmental changes even in just one behavior area can have very significant implications for care and management, the effectiveness of a drug should not be assessed by its ability to "cure," but on the basis of its having any effect that would not have been achieved, or not achieved as efficiently, without the drug. Any drug treatment that makes a "just noticeable difference" (Blackman, 1957) in a positive direction should be considered to be effective.

Nature of the Experimental Variable

A common error in the conceptualization of drug effects and, consequently, in the design of relevant experiments is associated with failure to appreciate the nature of intellectual growth. Some traditional theories of child development have held that behavior essentially unfolds automatically, like a predictable sequence of development in an embryo; one only had to sit back and wait for certain behaviors to emerge at specific, almost predetermined, ages, and usually little advantage was seen in developmental exercises, drills, activities, and so forth.

Today a different view prevails. While it is granted that there is a genetic upper limit to development, it is generally believed that a child's current developmental stage is a better predictor of the next milestone to be attained than his chronological age. A child who holds up his head, turns, crawls, stands with support, and walks while being held by one hand is generally ready to learn to walk unsupported, no matter whether he is eight or twenty-eight months old. However, it is also generally believed that a normally endowed child can become retarded if his perceptual, motor, linguistic, and social world is severely restricted. Ordinarily, we would not expect an otherwise normal three-year-old child to walk if he had never been allowed to leave his crib.

Adherence to most contemporary theories and facts of child development would thus lead us to postulate that the effectiveness of a drug in accelerating development cannot be demonstrated, or only very poorly so, unless the child is exposed to an environment and to experiences that are stimulating and appropriate to his developmental level. This means that drug effect must be tested at the interface of readiness and experience. Indeed, the entire concept that the drug is the experimental variable in drug-effect studies should be abandoned. The interaction between drug and experience should be considered to be the crucial experimental variable.[3] An instance where this principle emerged during the dietary treatment of phenylketonuric children was mentioned by Umbarger (1960).

Since any factor which jeopardizes the drug-experience interaction may invalidate a study as a fair test of drug potential, we must clearly identify those factors which can have their locus in the subject, the drug, or the structure that governs the interaction between the medicated subject and the environment. In what follows, each of these potentially limiting factors will be discussed.

Limiting Factors in the Environment

LACK OF APPROPRIATE DEVELOPMENTAL STIMULATION

A common feature of drug studies such as those which involved glutamic acid was the use of perceptually and socially deprived subjects. Thus, residents of institutions appear to have been the main source of subjects to date for many drug-effectiveness studies in mental retardation. Retardates living at home in a stimulating environment and engaged in intensive developmental programs would have constituted a more appropriate subject population.

ENVIRONMENTAL EFFECTS

If institutional or deprived subjects are used, but are placed in stimulating environments for the purpose of a drug study, a special problem must be kept in mind. We must not only expect an ordinary placebo effect in the control group, but a genuine and substantial acceleration of development due to the nonspecific environmental treatment component. Thus, the experimental subjects must not only improve greatly, but must improve significantly more than the control subjects who may improve significantly themselves.

The principle of drug-experience interaction is not restricted to intelligence-enhancing drugs. For instance, there have been attempts to assess the effects of muscle relaxants on ambulatory development of nonambulatory children with cerebral palsy kept under very deprived conditions in an institution. Such designs may have made no provisions for increased stimulation or opportunities, the apparent assumption being that as long as the potential for ambulation was somehow restored, a child *will* learn to walk if he *can* learn to walk.

Limiting Factors in the Subject

HANDICAPS OF SUBJECT

There are certain conditions within a person which can constitute limits to the drug-experience interaction. Emotional disturbance; severe seizures; sensory impairment; and orthopedic, esthetic and health handicaps are of this nature. It therefore follows that an optimal subject group, at least during the early phases of research with a drug, should be free of such limiting conditions.

OPTIMAL FUNCTIONING OF SUBJECT

It is conceivable that some drugs might have an effect only in persons who previously have not functioned near their capacity, while little or no effect might be observed on those persons who are already functioning efficiently. Such a drug effect that can be conceptualized rather readily on the theoretical level is one that would counteract or dissipate neural inhibitory processes. Thus, it is possible that some drugs may be more effective in retardates than in normal persons, and the use of retarded subjects may be a better strategy than the use of normal or even superior subjects such as college students. An analogous phenomenon has been reported by McGough (see Krech, 1968) in mice, where maze-dull strains profited more from metrazol injections than maze-bright ones.

AGE OF SUBJECTS

The subjects' age must be considered to be a limiting factor in drug studies. The rate of mental development is generally accepted to be a positive decelerating function that flattens out in the mid-teens. There is strong reason to believe that most of the growth potential that is not realized during childhood is lost and cannot be recaptured even with intensive stimulation in adulthood. It follows that the younger the child, the more effective a drug-experience interaction should be in promoting development. Conversely, this interaction should decline in effectiveness as the child gets older.

To underscore these points, the negatively decelerating curve in Figure 16–1 illustrates the approximate gain in IQ if one added a constant amount of mental age at different chronological ages to a child of a given base-line IQ. For instance, if we assumed a base-line IQ of 50, adding six months of mental age would raise the IQ to 75 if it were done at the age of two years, while at the age of ten years it would raise the IQ to only 55.

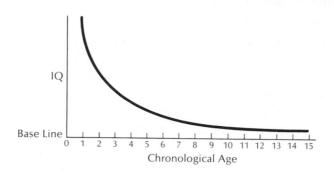

FIGURE 16–1   *Approximate Increase above a Given Base-Line IQ upon Adding a Fixed Amount of Mental Age at Various Chronological Ages*

There is a further implication. A normal rate of mental growth consists of one year's gain in mental age in one chronological year. Even if we could, overnight, restore a retarded child to a normal rate of mental growth, he would still be subaverage at the usual age of maturity. We could expect a negative correlation between his level of adult functioning and the age at which the normal growth rate was instituted. This point is illustrated in Figure 16–1 generally and in Figure 16–2 specifically. For instance, if a ten-year-old child with an IQ of 50 and a mental age of five suddenly attained a normal rate of development, he would gain approximately five years' mental age in the next five years, after which additional growth in mental age could be expected to be small. This means that at the age of fifteen, his mental age would be ten years and his IQ 75. A five-year-old child with an IQ of 50 and a mental age of two years and five months restored to a normal growth rate would gain ten more years by the age of fifteen years and his IQ would then be 83. Complete normality could only be attained if the treatment-induced growth rate during childhood exceeded that of average individuals, or if growth after about the age of fifteen years continued longer in retardates than it does in the general population. While neither alternative is inconceivable, either is un-

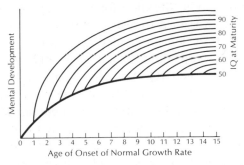

FIGURE 16–2 *Schematic Illustration of Effect of Changing Mental Growth Rate at Various Ages from 50 Per Cent to 100 Per Cent of Normal*

likely. Growth rates above average have been observed in retarded children under intensive treatment, but usually such rates have been sustained for only brief periods. Continued growth in adults has been reported for retardates, but is also expected to some degree in normal persons. Be this as it may, one would think that it would be most satisfying to see a person with a previously markedly subnormal growth rate attain an average rate of growth. On the other hand, expectancy for sustained supranormal growth appears to approach the unreasonable.

The preceding considerations imply that a drug-effectiveness study is more efficient to the degree that it uses younger subjects. If it takes six months to raise the IQ of a five-year-old child by 10 points from 50 to 60, it will take twelve months to raise the IQ of a ten-year-old child by the same amount if we assume equivalent rates of growth. Drug and treatment studies on children of the chronological age of twelve years and over thus are implying expectancy for a dramatic treatment effect. Even in the presence of a strong drug effect, a study of several years' duration would be required to obtain a difference that is significant, keeping in mind that one has to contend with both error of measurement and likely improvement in the control subjects. No matter how well they may have been designed, the many negative drug studies that have used older children can thus be considered to have been inadequate tests of drug effectiveness unless they extended over two to three years.

An insight into the advantages of using younger subjects brings with it a dilemma that is due to limitations in assessment techniques for children of low mental age. Instruments and techniques designed to assess global development are very inadequate for children below a mental age of about two years. Even between the mental ages of two to five years, few global tests are available, and some of these leave much to be desired. The situation for this range of mental age is even more problematic in regard to tests of part or underlying functions of intelligence (attention, learning, memory, and so forth). This means that even with children eight to ten years old, we would have the greatest difficulties if their IQ's were below about 40 to 50. The horns of the dilemma are thus constituted of the need for a group young enough to profit considerably from a drug-experience interaction, and the need for children whose mental age is high enough to permit application of appropriate available assessment techniques. Until more and better techniques applicable to subjects of a lower mental age are developed, we propose that the optimal solution to the dilemma is to use mildly retarded (IQ 50 to 80) children between the ages of five to ten years.

Limiting Factors in the Drug

SIDE-EFFECTS

An agent may have toxic or other undesirable side-effects, or may be difficult to administer. Further, potentially effective drugs may only be effective if they are available to the nervous system during the learning process, in which case drug administration must be planned with drug characteristics in mind. For instance, a potentially effective drug may be rapidly absorbed and metabolized. An experimental design involving drug administration upon rising at six in the morning and upon retiring at nine at night, may not constitute a fair test of that drug because the child may not be exposed to highly stimulating activities until mid-morning, and to none at all at night. One must thus draw a distinction between the administered and the effective dose, and some drugs may have to be administered in timed-release capsules or frequent doses. For this reason, the drug-absorption rates should be carefully considered.

Further, it is important that drugs that have been shown to be active be given in doses high enough to demonstrate their potential effectiveness. Particularly with new drugs, information about desirable and tolerable doses may be scanty, and pilot studies to explore upper dosage tolerance may be indicated.

The need to give drugs in dosages large enough to be effective creates problems in research, since many drugs given in active dosages have side-effects that may reveal the identity of experimental subjects in studies with double-blind or triple-blind controls, thereby destroying the utility of these controls. For this reason, some drug studies employ a uniform dosage for all experimental subjects, hoping that drug effectiveness, if any, will manifest itself sufficiently in at least enough subjects so as to yield a statistically significant group difference. Such a design preserves technical purity but has at least two drawbacks: it may require a large sample before an effect can be accepted as having been adequately demonstrated, and it ignores certain pharmaceutical facts. Thus, the common dosage may be set too low to have a positive and measurable effect on most subjects, or it may be so high as to produce toxic effects that can lead to loss of subjects, or, again, to their identification by the personnel involved. Only a few subjects are likely to receive a dose optimal to them; that is, a dose individualized to their tolerance, sensitivity, metabolic rate, and so forth.

This dilemma was recently highlighted in a review of the literature on the effect of glutamic acid on cognitive behavior. The reviewers (Vogel et al., 1966) concluded that current evidence favors a positive effect. However, rather embarrassingly, the positive evidence came mostly from studies that were either uncontrolled or used individual dosaging techniques that make a double-blind or triple-blind design virtually impossible to maintain. On the other hand, the negative evidence was derived primarily from controlled studies employing uniform dosages. A crucial question thus arises: Are the positive results due to the powerful effects of individualized dosaging, or are they due to a placebo effect resulting from loss of subject identity that might have occurred during dosage determination?

Some researchers have attempted to solve the dilemma by separating the clinical management of the subject from the evaluation of drug effect. However, in the light of past experience, one can raise serious doubts about the adequacy of such a technique in maintaining rigorous blind conditions.

FOUR-STEP INDIVIDUALIZED DOSAGING TECHNIQUE

In the paragraphs that follow, we are outlining a procedure that will permit—with at least some drugs—the use of the individualized dosaging technique, while, at the same time, preserving subject identity and thus safeguarding a double-blind design.

The first step of our proposed method is to select pairs of matched subjects. Secondly, *all* subjects are placed on the drug to be studied so as to determine the optimal individualized dosage for *each* subject. Depending on the nature of the drug, this process may take up to several weeks. All involved personnel should know that all subjects are on the same active drug. However, for the purpose of the experiment, observation, reporting, and rating should concern itself only with toxic or otherwise unpleasant or undesirable effects. Thirdly, all subjects are taken off the drug for a period long enough for drug effects, if any, to dissipate. Again, depending on the drug, this may take a few days or several weeks.

The fourth step is to assign members from each pair of subjects randomly into experimental and control groups. The experimental subjects are placed on their previously determined individualized dosages of the experimental drug and control subjects on an appropriately disguised placebo. Neither the subjects, clinically involved personnel (caretakers, behavior observers and raters, ward physicians, and others) nor the experimenter should know whether a subject is on drug or placebo. The behavior ratings relevant to drug effectiveness can now be instituted as both individualized dosages and high "blind" standards have been achieved.

An additional control may be indicated in the occasional instance where apparently toxic or otherwise alarming effects are manifested in a subject despite individualized dosaging. The code for that subject may be broken with maximal secrecy, and if he is revealed to have been an experimental subject, he should—again secretly—be placed on placebo and should continue to participate in every aspect of the experiment as if he were still an experimental subject. However, both he and his matched control subject, if any, should be eliminated from the analysis of results. If the subject displaying alarming signs turns out to have been in the control group, he should similarly be continued on placebo, and his results and those of his matched experimental partner, if any, should also be sacrificed. The purpose of maintaining the appearance of continued participation of subjects is to minimize the likelihood that personnel associated with the study will draw conclusions as to drug identity or effects which may influence their ability to report behavior objectively.

The four-step procedure just outlined implies an assessment of the criterion measures during or after the fourth phase. Where before-and-after assessment is desired, the base-line measurement might be conducted at the end of phase three. If there exists the possibility that the drug has long-lasting effects, base-line measurement can also be conducted prior to phase two. However, in such cases the design may be less powerful, and the use of a second control group receiving placebos in both phases two and four may well be indicated.

The proposed procedure has limitations and will not be universally applicable. For instance, with some drugs, effectiveness may only be achieved when the agent is administered in dosages at which side effects must be expected. With other drugs, toxicity and side effects may not be a significant problem. In such cases, one technique of dosage determination used in the past has been to adjust dosage until a "clinical effect" was believed to have been achieved. The obvious drawback of such a procedure is that fortuitous improvements, or effects due to other agents and factors, may be ascribed to the drug under investigation and may result in a determination of drug dosage which is actually unrelated to drug action. This technique, of course, is also objectionable because of its lack of "blindness." However, the four-step procedure outlined by us can be adapted to this situation. Instead of assessing toxicity and side effects in phase two, clinical effects can be observed and reported on all subjects until the dosage level appears satisfactory. Again, all subjects are taken off the drug for a period, after which experimental subjects are placed back on the drug and the controls receive a placebo under rigorous blind conditions. Only data collected after this point should be used in the analysis of results.

AN ETHICAL QUESTION CONCERNING ENROLLMENT

A question may be raised in regard to an ethical problem: how can informed consent to participate in a study be obtained if the identity of experimental and control subjects cannot be revealed prior to the experiment? We suggest that all subjects be recruited (1) for the projected duration of the study, (2) on the assumption that they will be on a presumably active drug initially, and (3) on the assumption that they may later continue on the same drug. We believe that this procedure is consistent with the regulations of the Food and Drug Administration, as well as with other guidelines recently proposed (Wolfensberger, 1967). A problem less easily solved is the fact that the proposed procedure is more suitable to "captive populations," such as residents of institutions, than to community retardates who, for reasons discussed later in this chapter, must be considered a more appropriate subject population for drug-effectiveness studies.

There are formidable problems associated with achieving a well-controlled experimental design that uses individual dosaging techniques. However, the importance of such designs was recently underlined in a study by McGough (see Krech, 1968), who found that a drug (metrazol) that appears to facilitate learning in mice can have learning-inhibiting effects when administered in high doses. More importantly, the optimal dosage was found to be higher in dull than in bright strains of mice.

Other Considerations of Experimental Design

It is desirable that a research design be efficient as well as appropriate. First, let us consider that drug-effectiveness studies, by their very nature, must be longitudinal. Experimental and control groups are assessed, a treatment is administered, and then both are reassessed. A statistical design typical for such a study is variously referred to as "repeated measurements of several independent groups" (Edwards, 1950, p. 288 ff.), or a "mixed factorial Type I" design (Lindquist, 1953, p. 267 ff.) In such a design, the crucial statistical test of the drug-experience effect is not of the difference between groups after treatment, but of the statistical interaction between groups and time, that is, the differential rate of change.

Secondly, the efficiency of an experiment is generally related inversely to its duration. Given a potential effect, that design which permits the most rapid demonstration of this effect is, other things being equal, the most efficient one. The adequacy, appropriateness, and efficiency of a drug experiment can be affected by many variables, some of which we shall discuss immediately.

Sample Size

In regard to sample size, we need to recall that the larger the experimental and control groups are, the less of a difference between the means of their criterion scores is usually required for statistical significance. Since we have stipulated a gradually additive drug effect over time, larger groups will usually permit a shorter study. One can estimate the approximate minimal duration of an adequate experiment for various assumed improvement rates if one knows the distribution of the "before" scores. Conversely, if one decides to run a study for a given period, say one year, one can estimate the approximate minimal change needed for statistical significance.

Distribution of the Criterion Scores

In regard to distribution of the criterion scores, we know that the steeper and more narrow the distribution curves are, the less of a change in means is needed to obtain significance, and the less time is needed to demonstrate an existing effect. This principle is illustrated in Figures 16–3 and 16–4. In both figures, the difference between the means (x and y) of the experimental and control groups are identical. However, the distributions in Figure 16–3 have much larger standard deviations and greater overlap than they do in Figure 16–4. Thus, if the differences in means had been due to a drug effect, the difference in Figure 16–3 would have been much less likely to be significant than the difference in Figure 16–4.

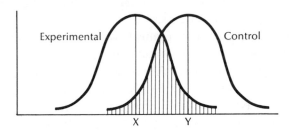

FIGURE 16–3 *Discrimination of Groups with Large Standard Deviations*

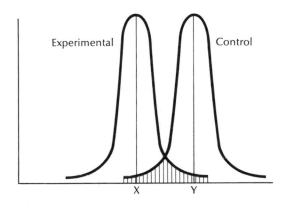

FIGURE 16–4 *Discrimination of Groups with Small Standard Deviations*

Controls

If there is one thing we should have learned from the history of medicine and psychology generally, and the history of the management of the retarded specifically, it would be to insist on the most rigorously controlled studies of a new treatment before it is accepted as effective (see Shapiro, 1960). One may speculate that the common failure to employ controls, or adequate controls, in treatment studies in retardation may, in part, have been due to the investigators' conceptualization of retardation and its treatment. If one views retardation as a static, hitherto "incurable," condition that will only yield to "magic bullet" therapy, then controls may appear to be unnecessary because no improvement would be expected unless the magic bullet had, indeed, been found, in which case the improvement would be expected to be a drastic and self-evident one. For instance, Zimmerman et al. (1949) omitted a placebo control group in their glutamic acid study on the assumption that their retarded subjects were not capable of responding to placebo effects.

The better controlled the control variables are, and the more sources of error variance are eliminated, the more efficient a design becomes. For this reason, matching of subject pairs, though more difficult, appears to be preferable to equation of subject groups. When groups are merely equated (often erroneously referred to as matched), the means of the equated variables are essentially identical, but there may not be a 1:1 correspondence of relevant characteristics between pairs of subjects, and error variance is likely to be higher.

If the design just discussed is employed, care should be taken that the matching does not violate the assumptions that underlie the design. More complex cross-over or Latin Square experiments are frequently employed in drug research, but, requiring double the length of time of the above design, they appear more suitable for drugs where fast and strong rather than slow and cumulative effects are anticipated. Particularly where age and treatment effect are expected to interact, a long-term cross-over experiment has an additional shortcoming: the placebo subjects who cross over into the drug condition will be older than the original drug subjects were when they were first placed on the drug. Thus, the two groups will no longer be comparable in age, and if an age-treatment interaction exists, the group that had been placed on the drug later will show a smaller effect, or none at all.

Diagnostic Homogeneity

The preceding considerations underline the desirability for homogeneity of certain variables. However, some investigators have committed an error in strategy by pursuing homogeneity of variables that should not be homogeneous. For instance, researchers characteristically aspire to set up subject groups with the same clinical diagnoses (for example, mongolism). Thus, in their review of glutamic-acid studies with retardates, Astin and Ross (1962, p. 432) expressed preference for diagnostic (mostly etiologic) homogeneity. Such diagnostic homogeneity is appropriate when there is reason to believe that the drug treatment is of greater benefit in one syndrome than in others. If there is no reason for making such an assumption, diagnostic homogeneity is at best irrelevant and wasteful; at worst it may be destructive to the experiment, for at least two reasons. In some syndromes in which biochemical function is disturbed, the drug may be metabolized in atypical fashion and thus may not act as it ordinarily would. For example, Rogers and Pelton (1957) have raised the question whether certain types of retardates are capable of metabolizing glutamic acid in the usual manner. In other syndromes, the structure of the brain may be characteristically atypical, and those areas in or upon which the drug may ordinarily act may be impaired. In either instance, there is an increased likelihood that a general effect that might have been observed in a diagnostically heterogeneous group may not take place or may not become measurable. Thus, the experiment would not constitute a fair test for the drug and might lead to its premature rejection.

In addition to these more clinical considerations, there is a statistical problem to be considered. Homogeneity of the characteristics of subjects implies a restriction of the range of these characteristics. This restriction, in turn, may prevent the demonstration of existing relationships. Such a situation is illustrated in Figure 16–5, which shows a hypothetical scattergram of the correlation between two variables. The distribution shown in the left half of the figure would result in a high correlation coefficient. However, if only the data in the reduced range of the small box (enlarged in the right half of the figure) had been collected, an almost random scatter of scores and a low correlation would have resulted.

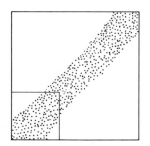 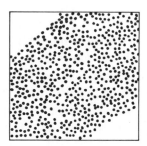

FIGURE 16–5 *The Effect of Constriction of Measurement Range*

Shortcomings of Criterion Measures

A common but questionable feature of drug and other treatment studies has been reliance on assessment of global or very complex behavior. The use of intelligence tests such as the Stanford-Binet, Wechsler and other tests is of this nature. This may have been a poor strategy. Global intelligence reflects years of learning and experience and is modified relatively slowly. Lengthy experiments are likely to be necessary to demonstrate changes adequately. A more promising strategy appears to be the assessment of behavior processes that underlie global intelligence, such as arousal, perception (for example, attention), learning, and retention. For instance, it is conceivable that within a few days or weeks a drug could have measurable effects on vigilance, conditioning speed, or short-term memory, while it might take months and years before such effects are translated into statistically significant improvements on global IQ tests. This point is particularly important if, as suggested by Krech (1968), and as appears reasonable, drugs are more likely to have selective effects on specific conative or cognitive processes.

If underlying processes do not show any change, no change is likely to occur on the global level. On the other hand, once underlying processes have shown improvement, it is timely to design "second generation" experiments that may involve more global measures.

Personnel Variables

One problem in the design of drug and other treatment studies is rarely mentioned. It has to do with the fact that the before-and-after measurements are often made by technicians or other personnel who do not have a high degree of competence with the assessment technique, or who have not developed a consistent assessment style. For instance, a junior psychologist may be hired to give intelligence tests to subjects before and after administration of the treatment. The examiner may only have had experience in testing a small number of individuals with the particular test involved. Thus, he may improve in competence during the "before" assessments, and may obtain systematically higher or lower scores on the "after" assessments on the basis of his increased skills alone. "Improvement" then may be ascribed erroneously to the treatment, and "loss" to detrimental drug effects or to subject characteristics. While such a potential source of error can be handled statistically by having a control group, it is important even then that the order in which experimental and control subjects are tested be random or counterbalanced, so that the examiner's learning process is not confounded with a particular type of treatment or subject. Even if this problem is handled statistically, it is still likely that lack of competence, experience, or consistency in assessment will introduce a variability that detracts from the efficiency of the design. Much better than statistical handling of the problem would be to ascertain that the assessors have reached a high and stable level of performance. This might be accomplished either by using individuals of high skill, or by training less experienced and skillful personnel on a pilot basis to such a (asymptotic) level of performance.

CONCLUSION

In concluding, we would like to return to the distinction made earlier between direct and indirect effects of pharmacological agents. In the light of the foregoing discussion, it is conceivable to us that this distinction may have limited utility. The difference between such potential agents may lie not so much in their effects as in their mode of action—at least as long as children were used as subjects, and as long as they were exposed to intensive environmental enrichment while on the drugs. Also, we emphasize that we have taken no stand in this paper in regard to two issues relevant to drug research in retardation: (1) What is the theoretical likelihood that intelligence in retardates generally can be significantly improved by a pharmacological agent? (2) What emphasis should be given to research of this nature with a global strategy in mental retardation and/or pharmacology? The stand we *have* taken is that, if studies of the intelligence-enhancing effects of pharmacological agents are to be conducted, they should be so designed as to constitute an adequate, fair, and efficient test of such an effect.

SUMMARY

A great deal of effort has been expended in search of pharmacological agents that will improve intelligence or intellectual development of mentally retarded individuals. Regardless of the merit of agents that have been purported to have such an effect, few studies, whether positive or negative in outcome, have constituted an adequate test of drug efficacy. A number of theoretical and methodological issues that underlie adequate design of studies of purportedly development-enhancing drugs were discussed. It was concluded that, if the effect of drugs on cognitive growth of retarded individuals is to be studied, the optimal target group should consist of mildly retarded children with mental ages above two to three years and chronological ages near or below six years who are heterogeneous in regard to etiologic categories, free of secondary handicaps, and exposed to intensive environmental stimulation during the course of the study. It was proposed that the experimental variable in the study of purportedly intelligence-enhancing drugs is not the drug itself, but the interaction between drug and experiential stimulation. These conclusions call for experimental designs substantially different from those typically employed in the past.

_____

NOTES

1. This chapter was written with the support of U.S.P.H.S. Grant No. HD–00370 from the National Institute of Child Health and Human Development, Washington, D.C. It is based on an earlier and briefer article by the same authors (1968) in the *American Journal of Mental Deficiency*, Vol. 73, a journal of the American Association on Mental Deficiency. We gratefully acknowledge permission to reproduce parts of this article here.

2. In discussing intelligence and intelligence tests throughout this paper, we are not proposing to defend the construct of intelligence as an entity, beliefs in constancy of IQs, or discontinuance of mental growth in the mid-teens. Although our language may appear to imply such notions, this is only in an effort to discuss parsimoniously principles and paradigms important to drug effectiveness studies.

3. While true with development-accelerating drugs, this may not apply to other drugs such as tranquilizers where drug effects tend to be inversely related to the intensity of other types of therapeutic programs (Klerman, 1966).

REFERENCES

American Medical Association. *Mental retardation: A handbook for the primary physician.* Chicago, 1965.

Anonymous. *Frontiers Hosp. Psychiat.,* 1966, *3* (23), 3.

Association for Research in Nervous and Mental Disease. *Mental retardation: Proceedings of the association, December 11 and 12, New York, N.Y.* Baltimore: Williams & Wilkins, 1962.

Astin, A. W., & Ross, S. Glutamic acid and human intelligence. *Psychol. Bull.,* 1962, *57,* 429–434.

Birch, H. G., & Belmont, L. The problem of comparing home rearing versus foster-home rearing in defective children. *Pediatrics,* 1961, *28,* 956–961.

Blackman, L. S. Toward the concept of a "just noticeable difference" in IQ remediation. *Amer. J. Ment. Defic.,* 1957, *62,* 322–325.

Burns, J. T., House, R. F., Fensch, F. C. & Miller, J. G. Effects of magnesium pemoline and dextroamphetamine on human learning. *Science,* 1967, *155,* 849–851.

Edwards, A. E. *Experimental design in psychological research.* New York: Rinehart, 1950.

Freeman, R. D. Drug effects on learning in children: A selective review of the past thirty years. *J. Spec. Educ.,* 1966, *1,* 17–44.

Goldstein, H. Sicca-cell therapy in children. *Arch. Pediat.,* 1956, *73,* 234–249.

House, M., Wilson, H. D., & Goodfellow, H. D. L. Treatment of mental deficiency with alpha tocopherol. *Amer. J. Ment. Defic.,* 1964, *69,* 328–329.

Kirman, B. H. Metabolic syndromes. In L. T. Hilliard & B. H. Kirman (Eds.), *Mental deficiency* (2nd ed.). Boston: Little, Brown, 1965, pp. 486–526.

Klerman, G. L. The social milieu and drug response in psychiatric patients. Presented at the annual convention of the American Sociological Society, Miami Beach, Fla., 1966.

Koestler, A. *The ghost in the machine*. New York: Macmillan, 1967.

Krech, D. The chemistry of learning. *Saturday Review*, 1968, January 20, pp. 48–50, 68.

Lindquist, E. F. *Design and analysis of experiments in psychology and education*. Cambridge, Mass.: Riverside Press, 1953.

Louttit, R. T. Chemical facilitation of intelligence among the mentally retarded. *Amer. J. Ment. Defic.*, 1965, *69*, 495–501.

Mead, M. *And keep your powder dry*. New York: Morrow, 1942.

Pauling, L. Orthomolecular psychiatry. *Science*, 1968, *160*, 265–271.

Rogers, L. L., & Pelton, R. B. Effects of glutamine in I.Q. scores of mentally deficient children. *Texas Rep. Biol. Med.*, 1957, *15*, 84–90.

Shapiro, A. K. A contribution to a history of the placebo effect. *Beh. Sci.*, 1960, *5*, 109–135.

Stone, M. M. Parental attitudes to retardation. *Amer. J. Ment. Defic.*, 1948, *53*, 363–372.

Turkel, H. Medical treatment of mongolism. In O. Stur (Ed.), *Proceedings of the Second International Congress on Mental Retardation, August 14–19, 1961*. Basel, Switzerland: S. Karger, 1963, pp. 409–416.

Umbarger, B. Phenylketonuria—treating the disease and feeding the child. *Amer. J. Dis. Child.*, 1960, *100*, 908–913.

Vogel, W., Broverman, D. M., Draguns, J. G., & Klaiber, E. L. The role of glutamic acid in cognitive behaviors. *Psychol. Bull.*, 1966, *65*, 367–382.

Waisman, H. A., & Gerritsen, T. Biochemical and clinical correlations. In H. A. Stevens & R. Heber (Eds.), *Mental retardation: A review of research*. Chicago: University of Chicago Press, 1964, pp. 307–347.

Wolfensberger, W. Ethical issues in research with human subjects. *Science*, 1967, *155*, 47–51.

Wolfensberger, W., & Menolascino, F. Basic considerations in evaluating ability of drugs to stimulate cognitive development in retardates. *Amer. J. Ment. Defic.*, 1968, *73*, 414–423.

Yannet, H. Research in the field of mental retardation. *J. Pediat.*, 1957, *50* (2), 236–239.

Zimmerman, F. T., Burgemeister, B., & Putnam, T. J. The effect of glutamic acid upon the mental and physical growth of mongols. *Amer. J. Psychiat.*, 1949, *105*, 661–668.

[C]

GROUP APPROACHES

: 17 :

Group Therapy Approach to Emotional Conflicts of the Mentally Retarded and Their Parents

Marian H. Mowatt

INTRODUCTION

THE tremendous emotional impact upon parents of the knowledge that their child is defective is widely recognized. In looking forward to the birth of a new baby, the parents' fantasies can be an unverbalized mixture of wishes for the perfect child and hopes that he will enhance the parents, will make up for their deficiencies, and resolve old conflicts. When the wish for a perfect child is thwarted, either suddenly after his birth, or later, as his defectiveness is gradually realized, the disappointment, helplessness, and sense of failure can be overwhelming (Solnit and Stark, 1961). The mother may feel damaged and defective herself, guilty and self-blaming, angry at the loss, humiliated and alone. She may counter her grief and defeat by denial, overdevotion to the child, and an endless search for a "cure." Ross (1964), Mandelbaum and Wheeler (1960), and Cohen (1962) have pointed out the importance of helping such parents work through the load of depression and negative feelings, over and over, through counseling, so as to restore their self-esteem and put their dealings with their handicapped children on a more realistic basis.

SELECTIVE REVIEW OF THE LITERATURE

Most of the counseling reported in the literature takes place with parents in the early years of the child's life, when the diagnosis of retardation, brain damage, or some other defect is made and when plans are worked out for his care. But what becomes of these families after the initial adjustment and planning phase? The majority of retarded children grow up at home, but surprisingly little appears in the literature about the day-to-day, year-in, year-out problems and frustrations of these families as they carry on the unremitting job (usually without help) of bringing up these children. Exceptions are the revealing articles of Holt (1958) and Begab (1966), whose studies of what it means to live with a retarded child may be recommended to all those who see such families only during office hours. Begab emphasizes the difficulties for parents which are caused by the retarded child's low frustration tolerance, his demands for immediate attention, his temper tantrums, and his obliviousness to dangers. His inability to identify with a social group not only makes the child withdraw, but keeps him at home, often unhappy and a burden to his parents. To teach a retarded child takes a good deal of patience, and the parents often are confused as to how much to expect from their retarded child. Neighbors may be aloof, and the unwillingness of sitters to come or of the parents to ask them gives the mother no relaxation or relief.

Holt (1958) listed in detail the restriction in the activities of 201 families of the severely retarded. It proved difficult to take these children on a holiday trip, or even a simple shopping trip. Mothers constantly had to watch or fence in the children. Many were wakeful at night. The mothers were exhausted, burdened with extra expense, neglectful of the other children in the family, and often totally without relaxation. Some of Holt's retarded children made sudden attacks on their siblings, who nevertheless were required to spend a good deal of time helping to care for the retarded one. Many of the neighbors restricted their children from playing with the impaired child, and even the most helpful neighbors offered to "spell" the mother only in caring for the normal, never the retarded child. Many of the parents never went out together, and a good many of the siblings were ashamed and resentful. Most of the families were socially isolated. None of them, Holt concluded, were leading normal social lives in their communities. The despair, misery, and unrelenting need for practical help for these families are graphically conveyed by Holt's dry and objective statistics.

Families, of course, react differently to the presence of a retarded child, as Farber et al. (1960) have pointed out. Many variables influence the family attitudes, among them the sex of the child, the number of siblings in the family, the marital integration of the parents, and their religious ties. A retarded boy, for example, appears to be more difficult than a girl for parents to adjust to. A family that stresses intellectual achievement may be more disappointed than others, and families that are large and happy and have a secure place in the community can absorb the difficulties more easily than most. In fact, the amount of disruption in a family depends not on the degree of the child's retardation, but on the parents' emotional resources, as Fabrega and Haka (1967) have pointed out. They found that emotionally well-balanced parents could adapt to and accept their retarded children more easily than emotionally driven, grieving parents, so preoccupied with the liabilities and stigma surrounding mental retardation that they could not be as responsive to the needs of the child. These authors found that the type or degree of mental retardation and the age of a child were not significantly related to his parents' attitudes. Instead, the mere existence of the handicap, in whatever degree, and its symbolic meaning to the parent may be the crucial factor.

Even less information can be found in the journals about the problems of living with these children after they grow into adolescence and adulthood. Very little help is apparently available for aging and less energetic parents who still must go on providing for the now older retardate at home.

NATURE OF THE GROUPS

This writer had a unique opportunity to study family problems of the kind just described when she led a series of discussion groups for mothers of handicapped older adolescents and young adults at the Cerebral Palsy Center in Seattle, Washington, followed by a similar series for the young people themselves (Mowatt, 1965). The Center is a sheltered workshop for people over the age of eighteen years, where cerebral palsy patients too handicapped to hold regular jobs are accepted. People with other handicaps, such as epilepsy, brain damage, multiple sclerosis, and mental retardation may attend provided no other agency is available to them; some were both physically handicapped and mentally retarded. The enrollees may work five days a week at paid jobs for local industries or attend academic classes; or they may work at speech therapy, physical therapy, or arts and crafts. The mothers' unit, which asked for the discussion groups, helps to provide recreation activities, fund-raising help, publicity, and transportation.

Each group had an average of twelve members and met for an hour every other week over a period of about two months. Attendance was entirely voluntary.

Further observations of retarded children and their parents in psychotherapy, an opportunity to give psychodiagnostic tests to twenty-five mentally retarded young adults for the Washington State Department of Vocational Rehabilitation, and talks with their mothers who brought them to the testing appointments all revealed that the parents' feelings, the children's responses, and the family interactions were surprisingly similar to those in the families of the physically handicapped. In this chapter, clinical impressions of family conflicts will be discussed, with emphasis on the problems of the mentally retarded.

The families studied by this writer may or may not have been more troubled than most. They needed help, but all were taking steps, through various agencies, to find it. In any event, some generalities emerged. Many a mother seemed ambivalent with regard to her child, particularly about his growth toward independence, and tended to be overinvolved, hovering, and protective. In several ways these mothers resembled the 240 mothers studied by Cummings et al. (1966), who found that, when compared with the mothers of ill and neurotic children, the mothers of retardates showed the highest level of preoccupation with the child, as well as of possessiveness and depressive feelings. The mothers of the retarded tended to derive less enjoyment from the child and to feel less competent as mothers. Of the retarded young people seen by this writer, many reacted with passive-aggressive, noncooperative maneuvers and overdependency. Their parents responded resentfully; resentment led to guilt feelings; guilt kept the mothers overinvolved; and thus the vicious cycle kept going, with turmoil and friction constant in many of the homes.

Parent Group Processes

At the first meeting of the mothers' group, many expressed strong feelings of being trapped in a ceaseless care-taking job, with no end to look forward to, as one can with other children who eventually leave the nest. Yet in spite of this strongly voiced discouragement at being perpetually "tied down," few of the mothers had made plans for alternative forms of care for the child, such as plans for either a temporary "breather" or the long-term future. They brought out their worries about what would happen to the child after the parents were gone, and discussed nursing homes, foster homes, and institutions. But mainly the mothers spun fantasies about a wonderful building that would appear some day when money was available, to house their offspring and permit proper care for the child. When the leader suggested that parents' vacations would be a good time for a trial run to prepare the children for eventual change, it turned out that many of the parents had not had a vacation in years. Like the mothers studied by Holt (1958), the mothers in this study found it difficult and embarrassing to take their children on trips and at the same time were afraid these children would feel rejected if left behind. Nursing homes, boarding homes, sitters, and even swapping with each other for short vacations were resisted as unsuitable. It was clear that most of these mothers felt very guilty over their resentment at their unceasing job, and that this guilt made it difficult to "let go" of the child for even a few days. As one mother expressed it: "But you can't resent a helpless child!"

It was hard for the mother to separate from the child, but sacrificing her own freedom only increased her negative feelings toward him, thereby compounding the guilt. If she could permit herself a vacation, as one mother did midway in the series of group meetings, there might be a small break in the cycle. This mother returned, radiant, to the group after her first out-of-town trip in years. The group had helped her to realize that she *could* visit her married daughter in another state, as she had longed to. She was surprised to find that the other members of her family and her retarded son got along very well without her. Possibly helped by his mother's more positive feelings, the son showed progress from an embittered silence on the fringes of his group to active participation.

Without question, some of the mothers were finding rewards as well as annoyance in their overmothering activities. Some drove their moderately retarded children many miles to and from their workshop every day rather than permit them to take busses, a task the children were capable of learning. At the same time, a few mothers refused to drive their adolescents to visit friends on weekends—a potential step toward independence, as well as a potential free period for the mother. Many a mother seemed puzzled as to how to assess just how much her handicapped child could do, but did not set up a series of tasks to find out. One mother assumed that her mildly retarded twenty-year-old son should not go to the city alone on public transportation because he could not obey traffic lights, but she had never gone to a busy corner with him to try to teach him the rules. No doubt, with his normal need for self-preservation, he could have learned as well as any elementary-school child. The amount of protecting apparently had more to do with the mother's anxiety about separating than with the young person's own learning ability.

Although it was rarely stated, fears about sexual encounters no doubt entered into the mother's attitude toward her son's or daughter's traveling alone in the city. The concerns of the mothers' group about sexuality came up in connection with a recent episode: two enrollees had been found embracing on the grounds of the Center. The first reactions were indignation and a call for restrictions to prevent future occurrences of this conduct. It is possible that vague fears and fantasies were present, which linked handicapped and retarded people with other deviants who might be sexually uninhibited, strange, and out of control. Two mothers had refused to let their handicapped daughters accept movie dates, much to the girls' chagrin. Rather than rejoicing in this small social success, the mothers feared that the men would take advantage of the handicapped girls. To teach the girls how to conduct themselves on a date and how to handle possible emergencies was perhaps more threatening to the mothers as a step toward independence than as a sexual hazard. As they discussed the problem further and recalled their own adolescent fun, the mothers began to see their children's sexual impulses in a more positive light, to look at their young people as adults with needs of their own, and to think of ways in which marriage might be possible.

One mother (not in the group) whose retarded daughter had become romantically involved with a fellow worker, withdrew the thirty-year-old daughter from a workshop for retardates when one of the supervisors suggested birth control pills for the young woman. The mother was willing to consider marriage of the two retardates, but the father would not allow them to live at home, and no other living arrangement seemed feasible. Thus the daughter ended up at home, without her job and without her sweetheart, a living reproach to her guilty and confused mother. This problem highlights the parents' need for help with their feelings about their children's (and their own) sexual needs, if they are to be able to give constructive and practical guidance to the handicapped and retarded young people.

The attitude of the public toward handicapped people was another area explored by both groups. Some mothers were uncomfortable in public with their children and wondered whether and how they should tell people that their child was retarded. Some, fearing to expose their children to the curiosity, patronizing attitude, or cruelty of the public, kept the son and daughter close to home. Whether or not the mothers were projecting their own feelings on to others, the result was to cut off another avenue toward growth and independence.

The young people, on the other hand, both physically and mentally handicapped, wanted to go out more and wanted more contacts with normal people. On the whole, their attitude toward the public's reactions was more casual, sometimes even amused.

Perhaps the most significant aspect of the day-to-day transactions to come out in the mothers' discussions was the difficulty in setting reasonable limits on the children. Probably because of their uneasy guilt feelings, many mothers tended to give in when the children became negativistic. In testing retardates, this writer found that they tended to suffer from feelings of helplessness, dependency and devalued self-image. Other investigators have pointed out that such a child, unable to compete successfully, is often frustrated, and may express his rage in tantrums (Begab, 1966). But he is no different from a normal child in wanting to get parents to do what *he* wants. While he may find less varied methods of arousing parental response than a bright child, his ways may be equally effective and more exasperating to boot. In many of the families retardation apparently did not prevent the young people from manipulating their parents unmercifully, since exaggerated helplessness and loud demands always brought swift parental attention.

One mother described her twenty-one-year-old daughter's tears and crankiness if the parents wanted to go out for the evening. To avoid a scene, this mother, who was far from unique, stayed home, suppressing her resentment and, of course, reinforcing the girl's demanding tactics. This set the stage for more testing for limits that were never set. On the one hand, the joyless victory did nothing to build the daughter's self-esteem; on the other hand, the mother, defeated and deprived, could scarcely show positive feelings for the girl. Apparently the mother's guilt over her very natural resentment perpetuated her overinvolvement with the girl. The mother's inability to express her anger freely and to enforce discipline only deprived the child of an opportunity to win approval through more independent and acceptable behavior. As Adams (1967) has pointed out, feeling sorry for a child can interfere with setting sensible controls and thus will prolong infancy. It is realistic to expect children to be angry at restrictions and parents to be angry at "balky" youngsters. But giving in on rules and holding back the expression of parental wrath cuts off the cues by which a child learns what behavior is socially acceptable (Cohen, 1962).

Corroborating this impression, Weiss and Weinstein (1968) in a recent experiment have shown that mentally retarded children living at home tend to ask for what they want and expect to be given in an infantile manner, while institutionalized retardates have made progress in learning to reciprocate, take turns, and share. These experimenters asked the children what they would do and say to get what they wanted in various situations; for example, what they would say and do if another person were looking at a television program they wished him to change to a different channel. Most of the home-raised children felt that simply wanting and asking for the preferred program should oblige the other person to meet their request. More realistically, the institution children were able to use some reciprocity, such as offering to trade, share, and take turns with the other person—tactics virtually unmentioned by the children living at home. The latter had not learned to be aware of other people's needs and wishes—facts of life which are perforce made clear to any child in a boarding school. As the child grows, his mental age slowly increases, so that he can learn to become more sensitive to social situations. Weiss and Weinstein suggest that, because of their need to protect the retarded child, parents do not increase their demands as the child grows, but tend to let him remain at the level of a dependent infant.

In several of the households, disruption seemed to spread among the members. As it became more difficult to leave the child with anyone, the father, alienated by the child's demanding and unattractive behavior and prevented from enjoying recreation with his wife, tended to withdraw from her as well as from his offspring. This deprived the mother of needed support, both for her own needs and for disciplining the child. Several of the mothers expressed a wish for an evening discussion group to include fathers, who were sometimes seen as rejecting the child when they criticized the mothers' overprotection, or when they tried to impose limits. In several cases the needs of fathers and normal siblings had been sacrificed, more than was necessary, to the needs of the defective child as perceived by the mother. It is not surprising that marital conflicts sometimes ensued, or that in Holt's (1958) group the presence of a retarded child was given as the cause for several separations.

This writer saw none of the siblings in her group, but other investigators have pointed out that siblings, too, may need help with their resentful and ashamed feelings about the retarded brother or sister (Begab, 1966; Farber et al., 1960). Discussion groups for siblings would doubtless uncover a good deal of affect in areas such as having to help care for the retarded sibling and interference with dating and bringing friends into the home.

Group Processes in the Young Adult Clients

The discussions with the enrollees usually began with practical problems about the programs at the Center. Many of the young people had speech handicaps. Some communicated only with grunts and through facial expressions. Others, virtually unintelligible to the leader, were listened to attentively by the group and translated by the first member to understand. In spite of speech impediments and the incredibly intense muscular effort of speaking, most of these young people were eager to talk, and often several started to talk at once. A few preferred not to contribute, but listened with obvious interest. Thus neither inability nor unreadiness to talk was a contraindication for group treatment.

The unusual combination of mentally and physically handicapped in the same group led to some advantages. The brighter patients drew out and encouraged the retarded ones, and it was the alert group members, rather than the leader, who most often made suggestions and offered insights to their retarded colleagues. The latter seemed to appreciate this interest and seemed to gain some feeling of worth as they helped the crippled patients, picking things up for them and making room for wheelchairs. The handicapped apparently did not resent these ministrations as they did the patronizing assistance of normal people (one of the targets of group contempt).

After the warm-up on practical matters, the group gradually brought out deeper concerns. They spent a great deal of time ventilating their resentment about the restrictions placed on them by their parents and enthusiastically advocated more freedom for themselves. They blamed their parents for keeping them at home and not allowing them as many privileges as their normal siblings. Various members wanted to ride busses, to take trips with the family, to visit friends, to have dates, or to try living away from home. Only one member reported the opposite situation—a mildly retarded, crippled, and speech-handicapped young woman. Her father had insisted that she learn to cook and keep house and had deliberately sent her on difficult errands and bus trips, to prepare her for eventual life on her own. Now living in her own apartment after both her parents are dead, she expressed real gratitude for what her father had taught her.

The physically handicapped and the retarded alike felt more capable of handling themselves than their parents gave them credit for and, justifiably, considered their mothers overprotective. As one wheel-chair-bound enrollee thoughtfully phrased it, "It's harder for us to get along by ourselves, so we need *more,* not fewer chances to learn than normal people do." The retarded people, who could not have expressed it as well themselves, agreed enthusiastically.

Their own part in the infantilization—the demanding, petulant tactics so irritating to their parents—was not mentioned by the young people. This suggests that joint meetings of children with parents would clarify some of the areas of conflict through direct confrontation.

Sexuality came up early in the young people's discussions, with giggling references to pairs, triangles, and crushes on teachers at the Center. Their interest in each other was obvious; a bit of flirting and hand-holding went on in the group. The remark of one physically handicapped member, "We may be handicapped physically, but we have normal emotions!" could equally well be phrased to apply to the mentally retarded. At the last meeting they brought up their concerns about marriage. Many looked forward to it, but were vague as to how they could handle the role. The young men were particularly concerned about how to assume the usual masculine responsibilities, but few had thought about any practical arrangements that might make marriage possible for them. Again, they tended to blame their parents as the source of their limitations, rather than exploring their own potentialities for changing the situation. The opportunity to discuss seriously matters of sex and marriage was both unusual and appreciated. It helped the members talk more freely and confidently with people of the opposite sex.

Five of the enrollees, who lived in a nursing home, seemed to show a more lively interest in the world outside themselves than most of the other members and were free from the constant focusing on conflicts with parents.

DISCUSSION

The most striking difference between the mothers' group and the patients' group was in the atmosphere. Whereas the young people laughed, kidded each other, and expressed anger easily, the mothers—attractive, intelligent women who had accomplished the difficult task of raising a handicapped child—presented a rather restrained and stoical front. Obviously, no one ever *hopes* to have a defective child. As Olshansky (1962) has emphasized, sorrow can be lifelong in a mother, especially with the retarded child at home as a daily reminder of her disappointment. Most of the mothers in the group had never completed the work of mourning the lost dream of having a normal child. Far from being faced, expressed, and assimilated, the painful feelings had been fought and defended against over the years. Denial of negative feelings and undoing them through overinvolvement with the child had led to inhibition of affect and lack of spontaneity in the mothers. But due credit should go to them. For, in spite of their own paralyzing grief and guilt, these mothers had somehow managed to give their offspring more freedom to express themselves and to enjoy life than they allowed themselves. The young adults, although very unsure in their self-esteem, frequently thwarted by realities, and often misunderstood by others, nevertheless revealed themselves in these brief sessions as less conflict-ridden, inhibited, and unhappy than most of the mothers. Born that way, they had no dream to mourn.

Both the mothers and the young people welcomed the opportunity to listen and to be listened to in an accepting peer group with an accepting leader in a way that had never been available to them before. Mutual support, sharing of feelings, and alternative suggestions by peers seemed to relieve anxiety and guilt and to improve self-respect in both groups. Some of the young adults, at the end of the series, remarked that they had come to know and like each other better through the group. Both series were too short to do more than begin the process of change.

Contrary to earlier opinions that the mentally retarded could not respond to therapy, many recent articles show that group therapy or counseling is appropriate and valuable for both mental retardates and their parents. In reviewing the literature, Sternlicht (1966) finds increasing evidence that parents' groups not only provide support and reassurance, but help the parents to feel more relaxed, more optimistic, and more accepting toward their retarded children. The present need in this field, as Ramsey (1967) points out, is for more controlled studies. We do not know the best way to group parents and to structure psychotherapy or discussion groups. We do not know the necessary qualifications for leaders, nor the occasions when group treatment can be most helpful. We do not know exactly what changes take place as a result of group meetings, nor how lasting the changes may be. Carefully planned studies, with control groups, are necessary to supplement the present rather haphazard but uniformly encouraging reports, if parents' groups in the future are to be maximally useful.

Reports of group treatment for retarded children come mainly from institutions, where children have shown beneficial effects through improved communication and social skills, heightened self-esteem, self-control and responsibility, and relief from anxieties (Sternlicht, 1966). But such therapy is rarely provided for those living at home, no doubt because it is difficult to assemble them in groups. Yet their need may well be greater than for those in institutions, for several reasons. Each is living in isolation from his peers, in a home designed for normal people. Social and recreational groups for him are not readily available. And his caretakers, far from being trained and objective professionals, are emotionally involved, often distressed, and sometimes alienated from spouses and neighbors by the continuous needs of the retarded child. By late adolescence, the retardate no longer has a place in the public school nor in a peer group. If employment is not available, he may be spending most of the day in front of a television set. For him, group discussions could fill vital needs for companionship and communication, for an outlet for expression of feelings, and for developing increased confidence and motivation.

For increasing the value of group treatment for such youths and their parents, some directions can be suggested. Retardates can be confronted with their own passive-aggressive contribution to family conflicts. They can be helped to see themselves not merely as helpless pawns of their parents, but as individuals capable of trying out more mature behavior. The mothers and fathers can not only ventilate their feelings, but can learn to avoid reinforcing the infantile behavior they deplore by ignoring it rather than by reacting to it, and can learn to reinforce every sign of acceptable and responsible behavior through approval and other rewards, much in the manner of the reinforcement techniques used so successfully by institutions in improving behavior. As the child's improvement makes possible more positive feelings toward him on the part of his mother, she will be able to let go more easily of her child and will be able to enforce limits in spite of his noisy objections. Like any child, the retardate will feel more comfortable and will be more likeable when his behavior becomes socially acceptable.

CONCLUSION

In looking toward the future, there is no reason why new techniques developed for other populations could not be used to help relieve the emotional conflicts of the mentally retarded and their families. Family group therapy, now increasingly used for the families of schizophrenic, acting-out, and neurotic children, would in many cases be appropriate. Multiple family treatment, in which several families are seen together, might be even more beneficial in providing support and in relieving feelings of isolation and stigma in retardates and their parents and siblings, all of whom would find peers in such a group. The use of video-tape in a group session, played back to enable members to see and hear themselves in action, serves to intensify the "feedback" from the group and to supplement the therapeutic efforts of the leader and group members.

All of these methods offer promising steps in the direction of helping retarded children and their families to work toward a more rewarding life together.

REFERENCES

Adams, M. E. First aid to parents of retarded children. *Social Casework.* 1967, *48,* 148–153.

Begab, M. The emotional impact of mental retardation. In I. Philips (Ed.), Prevention and treatment of mental retardation. New York: Basic Books, 1966, pp. 71–84.

Cohen, P. The impact of the handicapped child on the family. *Social Casework,* 1962, *43,* 137–142.

Cummings, S. T., Bayley, H. C., & Rie, H. E. The effects of the child's deficiency on the mother: A study of mothers of mentally retarded, chronically ill and neurotic children. *Amer. J. Orthopschiat.,* 1966, *36,* 595–608.

Fabrega, H., Jr., & Haka, K. K. Parents of mentally handicapped children. *Arch. Gen. Psychiat.*, 1967, *16*, 202–209.

Farber, B., Jenne, W. C., & Toigo, R. *Family crisis and the decision to institutionalize the retarded child.* Council for Exceptional Children, *National Education Association,* Res. Monogr. No. 1, 1960.

Holt, K. S. Home care of severely retarded children. *Pediatrics,* 1958, *22*, 746–755.

Mandelbaum, A., & Wheeler, E. M. The meaning of a defective child to parents. *Social Casework,* 1960, *41*, 360–367.

Mowatt, M. Emotional conflicts of handicapped young adults and their mothers. *Cerebral Palsy J.,* 1965, *26* (4), 6–8.

Olshansky, S. Chronic sorrow—a response to having a mentally defective child. *Social Casework,* 1962, *43*, 190–193.

Ramsey, G. Review of group methods with parents of mentally retarded. *Amer. J. Ment. Defic.,* 1967, *71*, 857–863.

Ross, A. O. *The exceptional child in the family.* New York: Grune & Stratton, 1964.

Solnit, A. J., & Stark, M. H. Mourning and the birth of a defective child. *Psychoanalyt. Study Child.,* 1961, *16*, 523–537.

Sternlicht, M. Psychotherapeutic procedures with the retarded. *Internat. Rev. Res. Ment. Retard.,* 1966, *2*, 279–354.

Weiss, D., & Weinstein, E. Interpersonal tactics among the mentally retarded. *Amer. J. Ment. Defic.,* 1968, *72*, 653–661.

: 18 :

Group Approaches to Treating Retarded Adolescents

Stanley E. Slivkin and Norman R. Bernstein

INTRODUCTION

SHORT-TERM group psychotherapy offers many possibilities in dealing with the problems related to the care and emotional growth of mentally retarded adolescents.[1] The authors have been interested in group approaches to setting reasonable goals for assisting the return of retarded adolescents from a state-operated training school to the community. Our experience with adolescent retarded groups suggests that the psychiatrist has a great deal to contribute in the area of understanding the consequences of emotionally disruptive tensions in terms of decreasing social, educational, and work capacity.

In recent years, there has been a gradual buildup of demands for new approaches to the treatment of the mentally retarded. Yet, the construction of large, state-supported training schools has not led to the anticipated benefits. Institutional environments have fostered the development of maladaptive patterns of behavior. Mass-production techniques have led to more efficient institutions, but the institutional setting has destroyed the opportunities for fostering the interpersonal relationships conducive to normal personality development. Institutions for the mentally retarded are *countertherapeutic* and particularly dehumanizing, because their physical organization aims at group control and uniformity. The vulnerable retarded inmate yearns for *personal attention.* The institutions provide a large variety of parent surrogates that range from attendants through teachers to administrators. Unfortunately, the interactions that occur are directed toward more standardized operation of the school rather than toward the development of special relationships with the retardates. Personality development and better adaptive behavior require greater stimulation and interaction with parental surrogates. Understaffed institutions dealing with large numbers of retardates cannot serve adequately *in loco parentis.* Individual psychiatric treatment of the retarded in appreciable numbers hardly seems a practical alternative.

In 1942, Frederick Allen wrote about the therapeutic situation as a prototype of other life experiences. Therapy was seen as an opportunity to experience and gain a sense of ownership of the feelings arising from the reality of living, as well as a sense of responsibility for those feelings. Allen conceived of therapy as the alliance with the child to face the exigencies of the real world. Our efforts have been devoted to an attempt to improve preparation of the retardate for his return to the community by means of group therapy.

The authors feel that the skills and techniques of the psychiatrist have wide applicability with mentally retarded adolescents. Although it required a somewhat longer time to develop a group ego with retarded adolescents than with normal adolescents, group psychotherapy diminished hyperactivity in response to emotional stress, so that group members avoided the rejections that previously had impoverished their personalities. Group methods offer an excellent opportunity to learn about basic ego mechanisms in the retarded, especially in the areas of cognitive functioning and group dynamics. As understanding of dynamic considerations increases, the authors feel that better techniques will be developed for the constructive application of group-therapy methods in dealing with the needs of retarded adolescents.

The group therapist who deals with retarded adolescents must be prepared to respond actively and in an uninhibited manner to the affective needs of the group. At the same time, he must be prepared to encourage verbalization of feelings to diminish acting-out behavior.

Since the retarded adolescent has not developed the ego strength required for postponement of gratification and impulse control, the therapist has to attempt to structure a group situation.

The success of the therapy in the groups of retarded boys and girls we studied was, we are convinced, due to the fact that the techniques we employed were similar to the transactions required for group psychotherapy with schizophrenic patients. These techniques involved activity, reality reinforcing, clear limit-setting, and active teaching. However, the ability of the retarded to relate to one another and to test reality is distinctly different from the responses of psychotic individuals. There was no evidence of thought disorder in the interaction of the retarded adolescents studied, although there was hyperactivity and impulsiveness in the early stages of group therapy.

We have found that physicians and psychiatrists are reluctant to treat retarded adolescents. According to Helen Witmer (1946), with children the therapist can use "his own personality assets for effecting friendly relations in a strictly controlled manner, without false or artificial attitudes, strictly conscious of the possible meaning of the behavior to the child." We think that Witmer's ideas can be applied equally to retarded adolescents.

After thorough consideration of the institutional problems involved, we decided to ascertain the potential for group therapy with retarded adolescents. We were cognizant of the ideas of Gunzburg (1958), who pointed out the defect in the selection process for psychotherapy candidates among the mentally retarded. Gunzburg noted that the patients who are selected for therapy are those who create problems due to their aggression, lack of cooperation, withdrawal, or submissiveness. He also felt that therapy should be available to all who have enough insight to be concerned about their failure to adjust. Yet, he recognized the limitations imposed by the existence of organic factors, sensory defects, and very low intelligence. We would like to enlarge upon Gunzburg's ideas by including all mental retardates who are able to communicate with the therapist either verbally or nonverbally in an affective relationship. We used dynamic psychotherapeutic techniques, which were defined quite clearly by Bibring (1955). He referred to technique in psychotherapy as "any purposive, more or less typified, verbal or nonverbal behavior on the part of the therapist which intends to affect the patient in the direction of the intermediary or final goal of treatment." Bibring's techniques distinguish among suggestion, abreaction, manipulation, and clarification. Interpretation (as described by Bibring), the presentation to the patients of unconscious common denominators of their behavior, were hardly used.

Slavson (1952) has stated that the value of group therapy for retardates is "the discharge of emotions through anger, rage, disgust and quarreling" because their inability to express themselves verbally requires the acting-out of their feelings. Our aim in psychotherapy was to produce the patients' better adjustment within the institution as well as to improve their adaptation to the outside environment of the community at large. An additional goal of ours was to cope with the social and personality defects that render the establishment of meaningful interpersonal relations difficult.

EARLY PHASES OF THERAPY

From the earliest sessions with groups of retarded adolescents, it becomes evident that therapists have to play an active role if they wish to diminish disorderliness in the group-therapy situation. Sternlicht (1964) also has noted the need for an active leader because of the high energy level of the mentally retarded in groups. In our experience, activity of the therapist and structuring of the group as much as possible are the two most important needs to be met for developing the early phase of therapy.

It is most frustrating for the inexperienced therapist when he attempts to conduct group therapy with the retarded for the first time. Innovative and imaginative efforts are required for developing any type of therapeutic alliance. The retarded have such a large backlog of mistrust and hostility due to familial and institutional experiences, that it is difficult for them to accept meaningful group therapy; they have been taught to hide feelings by the staff. For this reason, the retarded find it difficult to express feelings verbally in group therapy instead of through hyperactivity or acting-out behavior in the school and training situations. Because of their impoverished ego structures and the restrictiveness of the school environment, the retardates have left feelings unspoken for too long in favor of self-depreciation, hyperactivity, and acting out. The retardates' behavior, in turn, results in increasing efforts at physical control by the institution, with a further impoverishment of the interpersonal transaction so necessary for personality development. The retardates need to be shown that the group leader wishes to manifest firm, understanding control instead of power to exploit them.

Once therapy has progressed slowly through the period of mistrust and testing of the limits, the group members can accept the fact that the therapist is, indeed, interested in their problems. Thus, a therapeutic relationship can grow. The early phases of therapy are marked by an intense blanket denial of problems, coupled with affective isolation. Projective mechanisms of defense are used continually to avoid involvement with the therapist. However, as the relationship intensifies and the therapist remains nonpunitive, the group members are able to encourage one another to ventilate painful feelings. As Dreikurs and Corsini (1954) have stated so well, "the all in the same boat" feeling is one of the most basic in group psychotherapy.

In the early phases of group therapy with retardates, few probing comments are made. Instead, the therapist focuses on catharsis of feeling and a clarification of the issues. These issues at first involve the conscious conflicts with institutional demands—the reality issues. It is a frightening but novel experience for the adolescent to find that someone will listen to their feelings without reacting in a punitive way. Once they have assured themselves that the therapist will not carry tales out of the group to environmental authority figures, the young patients can commit themselves to a deeper type of therapy.

Common dynamic mechanisms seen in our groups were intense sibling rivalry, pairing, and identification with the therapist in the form of "deputy" therapist within the group. High levels of anxiety led to overt fight or flight behavior patterns in the early phases of therapy. Gradually group members were able to give up some of their more primitive behavior and defenses, while encouraging one another to ventilate painful feelings.

In groups of retarded adolescents, much suspiciousness is leveled at the therapist in terms of questioning his identity and purpose in leading a group. With our groups it was the first time they had been involved in a therapeutic situation with a psychiatrist. Much concern was expressed about the psychiatrist's role as a "shrinker," "nutcracker," or "booby doctor." The initial verbal hyperactivity included many statements to the effect that the group members were "slow, but not crazy." We found it extremely helpful to encourage our adolescents to explore their concern that mental retardation was equated with insanity as viewed by the outside world. Many feelings of shame and self-depreciation were verbalized about their limitations.

Derogation of the therapist is an early defense against the need for significant relationships. Considering that adolescents are prone to challenge the establishment under normal circumstances, the need of the mentally retarded to do so is extreme. The fluidity of the adolescent ego owing to biological and emotional stresses, coupled with the intellectual deficits of the retarded, help to prolong the therapist's effort to develop a therapeutic alliance. Derogation of the therapist serves a very useful purpose in that it helps to unite group members against the feared intrusion of the leader.

The beginning of therapy took on an oral, primitive quality. Group members brought food and candy to the meetings, ate with sound effects, jostled one another, played cards, turned on small transistor radios, and made common cause in uniting to ignore the attempts of the therapist to set limits.

Our girls' group exhibited physical destructiveness and hyperactivity to a greater degree than the boys. In the early phases of therapy they threw chairs about the room, destroyed some games and toys, and slammed the door so hard they almost tore it off its hinges. They appeared to be daring the therapist to stop them. The therapist managed to tolerate this behavior for several sessions, but he had to remove all throwable objects after the first session. The girls were puzzled by the failure of the therapist to reject and punish them beyond locking the door on one occasion to stop the overt running away from the session. They mocked the therapist, decried his physical appearance, and reacted angrily to the presence of a female trainee social worker who was serving as an observer. There were times when the intensity of the acting out visibly upset the three more passive members of the group.

In our experience, the two groups reacted similarly in many ways, but the group of girls overreacted to a male therapist despite the attempts to moderate their anxiety by having a female trainee present. For all the girls their contacts were primarily with females within the institution—teachers, social workers, and attendants. The only adult males they had contact with were physicians in an administrative capacity, or for physical examinations. Their contacts with administrators had been generally either overtly or covertly hostile. They were full of concern about real or imagined threats of punishment from the staff. This was the mood of the underlife of the inmates. It was a new experience for them to be permitted to be active and assertive without being punished in some way. Gradually, over a period of several weeks they gave up their disruptive behavior.

TYPICAL MANEUVERS

Faced with initial rejection of his efforts to develop a relationship, the therapist who works with mentally retarded adolescents must seek ways to establish a therapeutic alliance. Candy and food are a great help with the institutionalized retarded. These youngsters are so impoverished because of familial and institutional rejections that gratifying their orality is a way of establishing an initial relationship. The boys liked candy, and the girls reacted positively to the introduction of coffee and doughnuts. The boys were satisfied with any kind of candy, but the girls requested specific varieties of doughnuts. At times the girls appeared to equate their demand for specific kinds of doughnuts with their fears of rejection by the therapist. When on one occasion the therapist deliberately brought doughnuts other than those requested, the girls rewarded him with an outburst of behavior that was rebellious to the point of demanding punishment. The masochism of the retarded adolescent places them in an extremely vulnerable position at all times (Klein, 1944).

The therapist may also assist the development of a group relationship by actively stimulating discussion about reality issues in the institution or else about current events outside. In the case of the boys, an active discussion of the baseball World Series was encouraged. With the girls it was a discussion about the impending Thanksgiving and Christmas holidays that helped to initiate group formation. In both groups there were active discussions of institutional realities and expressions of anger about the degree of oppression they felt.

As previously reported by the authors (1968), a discouraging aspect of inpatient work with the retarded adolescents was the practical difficulty of communicating with appropriate staff members in the effort to coordinate planning. In several instances the therapist was not told when children were moved to other residence halls or to new job and training situations. As a result, the therapist often had to face unexpected reality issues to work on in the group, as when a boy found out with no preparation that he had been transferred to another dormitory and was upset during the group session.

In the case of the group of girls there was a breakdown in communicating to the therapist that one of the group had become pregnant as a result of an incestuous relationship with her father during her Christmas visit at home. During one of the group sessions the therapist was assailed unexpectedly by three of the girls who first jostled him and then began to punch him as hard as they could. He discovered after terminating the meeting abruptly that one of the three girls was pregnant. This belated information was imparted to him when he asked one of the social workers if there was something unusual going on with these three girls. Armed with this information he was able to stimulate a discussion of feelings in regard to the mistrust of parents, and of fathers in particular. In view of the fact that the therapist was a balding, middle-aged fatherly type [2] it seemed clear that the girls were displacing upon the therapist all their own anger at their respective fathers. Of the three girls who punched the therapist, one was the pregnant member and the other two had histories of sexual molestation by a father or a foster father. During the session that followed the assaultive behavior, the pregnant retardate wept copiously and pleaded with the therapist for forgiveness. She described how her alcoholic father had undressed her and had made love to her while her mother was absent from the home. Mixed with her grief and intense anger was a pathetic need to be loved by her father. She described how wonderful he had been when she was younger, prior to her institutionalization. She spoke with intensity about how her father had been a Salvation Army worker who took her to sing with him on street corners. The idyllic relationship she described obviously was nothing but a fantasy or a screen memory. The other girls in the group agreed with her that something wonderful existed in the relationship between father and daughter, despite the evidence to the contrary. The sustaining hope of a loving relationship with their fathers was a need for all of them.

Another intriguing aspect of this was the mutual facilitation of fantasies within the group. Nothing was done to confront them at any time with reality because of the obvious importance of fantasy in making tolerable their institutional experiences. For therapists dealing with institutionalized retardates it would appear to be important not to disturb an important defense mechanism such as this. In more intricate and subtly changing forms these themes are endemic in normal adolescent fantasy. In time, as more feelings are expressed, the retardates themselves are found to relinquish gradually the fantasies in favor of the interactions with their therapist. However, in the early phases all group members went along with the fantasies of the other members, for this was an important part of their impoverished life.

As an example of this phenomenon, there was the case of one boy who always wore a World War II battle jacket to group meetings. He spoke often and lovingly of a heroic army father who was kept from seeing him by military duties in Vietnam. The group of boys encouraged his embellishments of tales of an ideal relationship with his father who would take him home after the war was ended. The therapist did nothing to indicate that his perusal of the patient's record had revealed that he was illegitimate and that his mother had not visited him for several years. The truth came out during one heated discussion about trust in parents, when he blurted out that he had no father. The group was supportive and he did not wear the battle jacket again after this session. The therapist later learned that the patient had obtained the battle jacket as part of a donation of used and discarded clothing.

Another boy spoke fondly of an idealized mother who loved him very deeply. Later sessions revealed that his father was an alcoholic and that his mother had moved to California many years earlier after a divorce from his father. The retardate had not seen or heard from either parent for many years. The only member of the family who had shown any interest in him was his paternal grandmother who died the week therapy was terminated. There was no opportunity to work out the feelings related to this additional loss in the group, but the therapist did have two tearful individual sessions with this patient about his feelings relative to losing the only two people who cared about him, his grandmother and the therapist.

We cannot overemphasize the importance of not challenging the retardate's fantasies. Our patients' fantasies all involved direct attempts to get the group to support an image of the individual patient as worthwhile. Even after the fantasies had been exploded, the mutual good will enabled group members to accept their actual situations better. An active fantasy life is an important medium for embellishing the very sterile realities, and this, too, has its analogies in normal mental functioning.

LEADERSHIP ROLES

An important facet of group therapy with the retarded adolescents was the use of auxiliary leaders within the group. We quickly became aware that in each group there was one boy or girl to whom the group looked for guidance in determining their behavior pattern. Such an auxiliary leader may encourage either cooperation or acting out. It is crucial for the therapist to enlist the aid of this deputy leader in assisting the formation of a group ego. At the same time, the therapist has to support his deputy in every manner possible because derogation of the leader also includes derogation of the deputy leader. Without the therapist's active encouragement and assistance the impoverished ego of the deputy usually was not able to withstand the verbal assault of his peers.

Among the males the oldest member occupied a special position. One boy, P., was a natural leader because he was the only member of the group who had been deemed well enough to be allowed out of the school twice to enter a job situation. Unfortunately, he had failed both times because not enough time had been taken to work through his anxieties about the expectations of prospective employers and fellow employees. On third attempt, the therapist was not consulted about realistic work plans. Thus, when P. was sent out again without enough preparation, he failed dismally for the third time.

Although P.'s job failure was related to a breakdown of communications between his group therapist and the social service department, he was a great success in the group. His natural leadership qualities were of inestimable assistance in controlling disorderly behavior of the other boys. However, the role as auxiliary leader caused a loud eruption of angry feelings to be directed at P. Several of the boys accused him loudly of being "a bed hopper." He became flustered and angry as various group members revealed episodes of mutual masturbation with P. Usually he had been the aggressive partner, with the others as willing or unwilling participants. The therapist maintained an uncritical, accepting role and this facilitated group catharsis of feelings. Encouraged by the therapist's failure to respond in a rejecting or moralistic manner to their revelations, various group members were able to express their individual needs for closeness and had the confidence to tell how masturbatory play demonstrated their fondness for one another. Owing to the therapist's encouragement of verbalization of feelings and his quiet acceptance of their stories, the group evolved a sexual morality of mutual consent. The anxiety level dropped and open discussions developed, which led to the revelation of feelings of guilt and concern about forcing younger boys into sexual compliance.

The auxiliary leader's importance was demonstrated when the therapist acceded to the insistent request of one of the social workers that he accept an additional group member who was badly in need of group psychotherapy. The group members became angry at the intruder and expressed an unwillingness to share their group experience with him. Open hostility was expressed as the group banded together against the new member, as well as against the therapist. However, after the verbalization of hostile feelings the anger dissipated, and P. terminated everyone's hyperactivity by admitting his fondness for the therapist. Several group members expressed concern about how difficult it must be to be a leader and to try to please everyone. This sentiment appeared more openly and quickly than it would have in a group of adolescents with normal intelligence.

The therapist seized upon the group's open concern about leadership and responsibility to set up a system of rotation of leadership among the group members. The thought that the therapist felt that they might have leadership qualities and that they could behave responsibly came as a total surprise to the group members. Many of the boys expressed feelings of self-depreciation and anxiety about the unexpected role of group leadership. At this point, the strongest boy in the group suddenly challenged the therapist to hand wrestle with him. When the therapist accepted the challenge and won the physical contest, the whole group relaxed as though reassured that the therapist could still control their behavior.

Individual responses to the leadership role were as variable as the individual personalities involved. Several group members identified strongly with the therapist, set limits, accepted challenges from peers, and generally acquitted themselves creditably. They supported each other and mutually reinforced their statement of esteem for the therapist who had surrendered his leadership role to them. Each member was leader for one meeting, and each expressed anxiety about his unaccustomed role.

In connection with the leadership rotation, the boys became more deeply concerned about how they would get along outside the training school if they could leave. There was considerable concern about the possibilities of failure and the consequential need for a return to the protected environment of the school. Several of the boys related incidents in which anger or anxiety have led them into difficulties in either school or training classes. There was general agreement that expression of feelings verbally rather than through acting out would be less likely to create problems if they were able to return to the community.

Attempts to enlist an auxiliary leader in the girls' group were only a partial success. C. was the oldest girl, and all the group members looked up to her. She stepped into the role of auxiliary leader for several weeks as though it was meant for her. However, when the group began the usual game of derogation, she could not maintain herself even with the active support of the therapist. It was interesting to take note of the manner in which she relinquished her leadership role. She came in at one meeting and incorrectly announced to the group that she had heard the therapist say he was giving up the group. This announcement led to extreme hyperactivity and agitation among the girls, lasting for several weeks. C.'s unusual type of resignation gave the therapist a difficult time as it rekindled the basic mistrust the group had for authority figures. Although C. tried to be helpful to the therapist at times, it was impossible to interest her again in the auxiliary role.

SEXUALITY OR SEXUAL ISSUES

One major recurrent theme in our experience with group therapy was the entire area of sexuality. In our boys' group much attention was paid to the subject of "bed hopping." This consisted primarily of two boys indulging in mutual masturbation, but oral and anal intercourse were denied. The boys were very much aware of the "Playboy Girl of the Month"; such material served to stimulate masturbatory fantasies. Certain of the older boys introduced the younger adolescents into the intricacies of masturbatory play. This behavior is quite like that of normal adolescent boys. The boys in the group showed great ability to discuss the oral and anal aspects of sexuality in the "dirty talk" that is typical of normal adolescent boys. The institution, however, regarded all such behavior as deviant and dangerous.

Contrary to the expectation that one has with normal adolescent girls that their approach to sexuality will be displaced and romantic, the retarded adolescent girls showed no hesitation in discussing the oral and anal aspects of sexuality. Whenever they wanted to upset the social work trainee observer, they would sing ribald songs. They also accused her of having sexual designs on the therapist and then would describe the type of sex play indicated. Unfortunately, the therapist was not able to learn the actual sexual practices of the girls' group because of the marked embarrassment of the inexperienced female observer.

All levels of sexuality were seen in the group. There was one seventeen-year-old girl, S., who sucked her thumb passively during most of the early sessions. The group obtained from her the interesting information that her father encouraged her to suck her thumb "to make her feel better," and that he encouraged her to wear infantile, shapeless sack dresses. She described how on a recent visit her father had hugged her, but had quickly let her go. Her feelings were hurt by what she saw as father's rejection, but some group members questioned whether father was not surprised to discover she was no longer a little girl. This same girl responded with normal adolescent enthusiasm when the therapist invited two senior medical students to sit in on a group session to obtain some experience with the therapy of retarded adolescent girls. Shortly after their visit, S. was able to give up thumb sucking as the group teased her about being a baby. Several months after this visit, S. asked the therapist when the young doctors would come back "because they both were so cute." Another interesting experience was the reaction of the girls to the pregnancy of the group member who had had the incestuous relationship with her father over the Christmas holiday. Previously we have described how three of the girls assaulted the therapist to whom they displaced their anger against untrustworthy fathers. Another facet of the same situation was the amount of hostility expressed when the pregnant member of this therapy group recently was transferred to a state hospital to await her confinement. Several members of the group denied any feelings about her departure, but when they were pushed they were able to ventilate markedly hostile feelings. They stated that "she was stupid, deserved what she got," and even expressed the angry hope that the baby would be born either deformed or dead. When the therapist managed to probe further, he discovered that the girls understood that the incestuous relationship probably might lead to a deformed or retarded child under the most favorable of circumstances. Then one of the girls said angrily, "What chance will her baby have anyway with her being retarded herself, so I hope she and the baby both die!" The girls flatly refused to accept the therapist's suggestion that they might like to visit her prior to her confinement.

Blos (1962) has described the idealized and eroticized attachment normal early adolescent girls have toward both men and women. He writes: "The object of the crush is loved passively, with the aim of getting a handout of attention or affection or being overwhelmed by all kinds of eroticized or sexualized approaches . . . the masochistic and passive quality of the crush is an intermediary stage between the phallic position of preadolescence and the progression to femininity." Blos further points out that this quality is typical of the intermediary bisexual stage of early adolescence. The girls in our group were very prone to confuse affection and sexuality. Touching or holding the hand of the therapist or of the female observer stimulated pleasure, blushing, and—on occasion—even obvious embarrassment. During one group session one of the girls printed, "I love you" on a piece of paper, handed it to the therapist, and then fled in panic from the room. On another occasion several girls took dares to kiss the therapist on the cheek, blushed, and then ran from the room.

DISCUSSION

Psychodynamically oriented group psychotherapy has a place in the treatment of retarded adolescents who have the ability to relate to the therapist either verbally or nonverbally. In our experience it is important for the therapist to be active, accepting, and relatively uninhibited in his responses. The therapeutic situation has to be structured as much as possible to diminish acting-out behavior. This is in keeping with the need for an active orientation in dealing with schizophrenics as pointed out by Whitehorn and Betz (1960). As we attempted to formulate our thinking about the therapist's role, we were struck by the fact that with retarded adolescents the therapist plays a role similar to that of the therapist who works with a group of psychotic patients. Despite the obvious differences between the two types of patients, the group management is remarkably similar. In both groups it is important not to challenge fantasies directly, be they neurotic or psychotic in origin. Group process in itself leads to the development of more realistic thinking.

As in every other modality of treatment, the role of the group leader is crucial. We find ourselves in agreement with Orr (1954), who discussed the difference in attitudes that may evolve in therapists. These differences may be both conscious and unconscious, positive and negative. Orr has described the varying differences and attitudes toward transference and countertransference phenomena in terms of identification with patients, hostility toward them, and the special attitudes toward the whole or parts of the patient.

We believe that, in dealing with the retarded, there are conscious and unconscious countertransference problems for psychiatrists. There are glaring errors of teaching about the retarded, such as the allegations that all "mental defectives" are alike and that the organic etiology is central, irreversible, and permanent. This concreteness of attitude works against a dynamic interpretation of the behavior of the mentally retarded. It is not seen then as part of a situation, as a pattern of interpersonal relationships, or as a sociocultural pattern. Perry (1966) has described these conceptual aspects most comprehensively.

There is a general cultural attitude toward mental retardation, which appears to be most especially held by educated people, that the retarded are innately inferior because they have the least amount of educated intelligence. This particular bias seems to be held strongly by psychologists and psychiatrists who feel that, by definition, an interesting and challenging patient is one who has a high intelligence or high intellectual potential. For the psychiatrist, the psychotic child will often present a challenge in spite of the poor prognosis, because the therapist feels that years of work with this type of patient will reveal the most basic mental processes. This is often true and we commend this dedication. However, the mental processes of the retarded also will reveal a great deal to the psychiatrist if he can conquer his negative countertransference attitudes.

Once the therapist begins to work with the retarded he will find that it is quite possible to identify with them and with their plight. He then can begin to see how the institutionalized retarded are victimized by institutional life quite above and beyond their innate deficiencies. Goffman (1961) has described very graphically the development and perpetuation of the institutional personality. This pattern is similar for individuals in total institutions—be they state hospitals, state schools, or prisons. However, the reactions to institutionalization do not deny that the retarded show a variety of special styles of behavior (Shapiro, 1965). The life style of the mentally retarded is related not only to their life experiences but also to their problems in learning (Zigler et al., 1958, 1961, 1962).

Retardates have a great need to learn how to verbalize feelings rather than act them out. They need to be assisted in fostering identifications that are better than their degraded self-image. There is also an aspect in them of innate autism which Webster (1963) described. They tend to give up in learning situations more quickly than other children, as has been discussed by Zigler. Once caught in the vicious cycle of failure and rejection, the retardate has no outlet for inexperienced anguish other than withdrawal or hyperactivity and increased inability to adjust to the demands placed upon him by his environment.

Grunebaum (1962) wrote about groups that "the strategy of group psychotherapy is that the leader does not gratify the infantile needs of the members but rather gives to them increased understanding through clarification and interpretation of their feelings towards each other and towards the leader. This therapeutic aim can only be attempted in a context of a strong alliance between the group and the leader." This general statement is applicable to group psychotherapy with the retarded also, although their reality deprivations and the limitations of their comprehension make it necessary to be somewhat more directive with them. Interactions within the group permit the active exploration of reality issues and neurotic trends including fantasy production, as well as an opportunity to explore the root causes of antisocial behavior in the institutional setting. Our views approximate that of O'Connor and Tizard (1956), who stated that "too often a defective's current manner and behavior is accepted as permanent" and also that "constitutional factors operate but they will not necessarily be the whole determinants of behavior."

The importance of efforts directed at restoring retarded adolescents to community life cannot be overemphasized. Their emotional adjustment comprises a large part of the determinants for a successful life in the community. Dexter (1964) has pointed out important comparison studies on mentally deficient persons matched with controls with reference to age, sex, nationality, background, religion, and father's occupation. The intelligence of the subjects in both groups as determined by IQ test ratings was the only variable that differed. Whereas the IQ of the retardates ranged from 50 to 75, that of the controls ranged from 75 to above. In most respects the differences in economic measurements between subjects and controls were insignificant. In terms of the expected norms of the community—supporting a family; being law-abiding; causing little if any serious trouble for self, family, and community—the subjects generally met the norm of expectation. Dexter (1964) concluded that "it may be that some tests now existing can predict great success in life or in school; what is certain is that failure in life cannot be predicted accurately either on the basis of failure in school or because of low standing in tests which measure ability for school."

We believe that the negative countertransference of the psychiatric community is best handled by contact with these retardates. We have found, along with Philips (1966) and others, that sympathy and interest are quickly aroused, and this leads to concern with the psychodynamics of these children and to active therapy with them. This sympathetic interest reawakens consideration of the mind-body problem and appears to be a most effective way of teaching about the societal aspects of personality functioning through an understanding of the familial and environmental plight of mentally retarded children.

Sarason (1957) has suggested that the therapist of the retarded should be free to make time available for the children, and that the retardates should be allowed to see the therapist whenever they wished. He felt that it should be demonstrated clearly that the therapist does not have a punitive role. While all of these features are ideal, they are not feasible in most schools for the retarded where the psychiatrist functions as a part-time therapist and consultant. We limited our role to being people outside the administrative structure of the institution who made a special alliance with the children and who had a particular attitude toward them and their secret thoughts and hopes. This was especially so in the area of sexual activity and fantasy, in which the institutional staff—despite lectures and conferences about sexuality and children—had a repressive, moralistic, and fearful attitude toward the sex play of the retarded adolescent. The institutional personnel tended to have a fearful attitude toward sexual matters in general, either reacting morally or trying to ignore them when confronted with them. In one session the adolescent girls described an incident in which one of the group was confined to her room for being seen rubbing her genitals. Psychotherapy offers a different attitude, one that helps these adolescents to handle these feelings, an attitude of special acceptance. However, it has to be shown to the groups that this acceptance *is* special, that it cannot be expected from everyone with whom they will be in contact.

Wolberg (1967) states that group therapy gives the patient a chance to see that he is not alone and the opportunity to break down his tendency to assault himself. Group therapy also affords the patient the opportunity to correct his own misconceptions, by listening to others and by studying how others act. Further opportunities are available to patients in groups to modify their own destructive values and deviances by conforming to a group norm. Tension is relieved by openly expressed thoughts, and the individual has a chance to see his own rivalry openly in the group and to gauge his own hostility. Group therapy presents interactions that permit getting from and giving support to others, as well as renewed transactions that help break down social fears and barriers. This in turn permits the development of new interests, friends, and modes of identification. Here, then, is a chance for the retardate to enter into productive social relationships with the group, which acts as a bridge to the world. Wolberg (1967) notes that high intelligence is not positively correlated with good results in therapy, although verbal skill and self-understanding are favorable ingredients. However, he also says that borderline or defective intelligence will make it difficult to use any other technique than that of being supportive. This latter statement is not consonant with our own experience with retarded adolescents. We have found it quite possible to obtain insight and behavioral change with the help of group-ego development.

In view of our own enlightening and informative experiences in dealing with groups of retarded adolescents, we think that for a psychiatrist to be able to function effectively in programs for the mentally retarded, he must have this type of practical experience to draw upon. There is no substitute for practical experience with this group, considering the many misconceptions about mental retardation—both published and unpublished—which prevail. The retarded are as challenging as any other group of adolescents with whom the psychiatrist becomes involved.

Short-term group psychotherapy presents an opportunity for adaptive change in retarded adolescents. This change will be reflected not only in improved relationships within the training situation, but also in terms of a better adjustment when the retarded person returns to community living. Hyperactivity and acting out in response to emotional tensions are major problems for the retarded adolescent because of the resultant concomitant rejection by significant environmental figures, which further impoverishes an already weakened ego structure. This process engenders a vicious circle of tension, acting out, rejection, and increased tension—with self-depreciation of major proportions as the final result.

Our groups of male and female mentally retarded adolescents contrasted sharply with groups of normal adolescents, in which the boys have a greater ability to discuss oral and anal aspects of sexuality and the girls are more mercurial, verbal, and romantic in their speech. With help, the adolescent retarded girls were able to discuss oral and anal aspects of sexuality in the same terms as both normal and retarded boys, despite the rigid institutional morality. However, unable to verbalize freely, the retarded girls frequently confused affection with sexuality in their desperate hunger for affective relationships. It was notable that in cases in which the families were not continuously involved in relationships, there was a tendency to keep the retarded adolescent in a helpless, infantile role. This was demonstrated clearly in the case of a seventeen-year-old girl whose father was happy while she sucked her thumb and dressed in "little girl" clothes. However, when he hugged her recently and found she had matured into a young woman, he felt very threatened. Her simplistic explanation was, "My Daddy loves to baby me," so as to hide her obvious concern about the sexual threat she posed to her father. Yet, this is the same girl who expressed so much interest in the two senior medical students who visited our group.

In this era of enlightened community psychiatry, it will become increasingly important for psychiatrists to be involved in a more significant way in community programs for the retarded which offer outpatient or day-hospital care. Since there are both conscious and unconscious countertransference problems for psychiatrists in dealing with the retarded, there is fundamentally no more constructive way for a psychiatrist to deal with this aspect of successful therapy than to be involved in a training school that reflects the reality situations of the retarded.

The therapist who works with groups of retarded adolescents has to be an active leader while structuring the group situation as much as possible. This is very similar to the role of the therapist who deals with schizophrenic groups, although there is clearly a difference in the way in which the retarded relate and test reality. The use of auxiliary leaders within the group was found to be a generally helpful technique.

Our most striking finding was that the groups of retarded adolescents (male and female), with IQ's running from 45 to 75, could respond to a formal psychotherapeutic approach. This suggests that the skills and techniques of the psychiatrist have wide applicability with the retarded. Group psychotherapy diminishes hyperactivity in response to emotional stress, thus helping the retarded to avoid the rejections that further impoverish their personalities. This approach warrants further application to other groups of retarded individuals by psychiatrists in training schools as well as in community mental health programs.

NOTES

1. The Psychiatric Training Program is supported by the National Institute of Mental Health, Grant 5 TOI MHO5331–15.
2. According to the consensus of his colleagues.

REFERENCES

Allen, F. *Psychotherapy with children.* New York: Norton, 1942.
Bibring, E. Psychoanalysis and the dynamic psychotherapies. *J. Amer. Psychoanaly. Assoc.,* 1955, *2,* 745–769.
Blos, P. *On adolescence.* Glencoe, Ill.: The Free Press, 1962.
Dexter, L. *The tyranny of schooling: An inquiry into the problem of stupidity.* New York: Basic Books, 1964.
Dreikurs, R., & Corsini, R. Twenty years of group psychotherapy. *Amer. J. Psychiat.,* 1954, *110* (8), 567–573.
Goffman, E. *Asylums.* New York: Doubleday, 1961.
Grunebaum, H. Group psychotherapy of fathers. *Brit. J. Med. Psychol.,* 1962, *35,* 147–156.
Gunzburg, H. C. Psychotherapy with the feebleminded. In A. M. Clarke & A. D. Clarke (Eds.), *Mental deficiency: The changing outlook.* Chicago, Ill.: The Free Press, 1958.
Klein, M. The development of conscience in the child. In S. Lorand (Ed.), *Psychoanalysis today.* New York: International Universities Press, 1944.

454   Group Approaches to Treating Retarded Adolescents

O'Connor, N., & Tizard, J. *The social problem of mental deficiency,* London: Pergamon Press, 1956.

Orr, D. W. Transference and countertransference: A historical survey. *J. Amer. Psychoanal. Assoc.,* 1954, *2,* 621–670.

Perry, S. E. Notes for a sociology of mental retardation. In I. Philips (Ed.), *Prevention and treatment of mental retardation.* New York: Basic Books, 1966.

Philips, I. (Ed.), *Prevention and treatment of mental retardation.* New York: Basic Books, 1966.

Sarason, S. *Counseling and psychotherapy with the mentally retarded.* In C. L. Stacey & M. F. DeMartino (Eds.), Chicago, Ill.: Free Press, 1957.

Shapiro, D. *Neurotic styles.* New York: Basic Books, 1965.

Slavson, S. R. *Child psychotherapy.* New York: Columbia University Press, 1952.

Slivkin, S. E., & Bernstein, N. R. Goal-directed group psychotherapy for retarded adolescents. *Amer. J. Psychother.,* 1968, *22,* 35–45.

Sternlicht, M. Establishing an initial relationship in group psychotherapy with delinquent retarded male adolescents. *Amer. J. Ment. Defic.,* 1964, *69,* 39–41.

Webster, T. Problems of emotional development in young retarded children. *Amer. J. Psychiat.,* 1963, *120,* 37–43.

Whitehorn, J. C., & Betz, B. Further studies of the doctor as a variable in the outcome of treatment with schizophrenic patients. *Amer. J. Psychiat.,* 1960, *117,* 215–219.

Witmer, H. *Psychiatric interviews with children,* Cambridge, Mass.: Harvard University Press, 1946.

Wolberg, L. R. *The technique of psychotherapy.* New York: Grune & Stratton, 1967.

Zigler, E. Social deprivation and rigidity in the performance of feebleminded children. *J. Abnormal Soc. Psychol.,* 1961, *62,* 413–421.

———, Hodgen, L., & Stevenson, H. The effect of support and non-support on the performance on normal and feebleminded children. *J. Personal.,* 1958, *26,* 106–122.

———, & Unell, E. Concept switching in normal and feebleminded children as a function of reinforcement. *Amer. J. Ment. Defic.,* 1962, *66,* 651–657.

[D]

FAMILY DIMENSIONS

: 19 :

Counseling Parents of the Retarded:

The Interpretation Interview

Gerald Solomons

INTRODUCTION

MENTAL retardation is not a disease. It is a symptom complex with more than 200 listed causes. Breakthroughs in the field of mental retardation occurred only once the philosophy had emerged that one discipline in and of itself could not accept responsibility for all aspects of this tremendously complex condition. The multidisciplinary team approach then came into being. Initially, the team approach was marred because each discipline focused narrowly on a limited portion of the disabled child's total being (Rembolt, 1961). There was undue emphasis on the handicap rather than on the total child, with a consequent downgrading of the child's self-concept which was quite out of proportion with the way others perceived him. Currently, the sophisticated team evaluates the total child, with disciplines overlapping and giving *opinions* rather than pronouncements. The function of the team moderator is to coordinate all opinions into an understandable report; a report understandable not only to the disciplines that have evaluated the child, but to all disciplines and agencies that will be involved with him in the future.

However, as new terminology, attitudes, and remedial procedures multiplied with the addition of each professional to the team, the multidisciplinary approach has brought about complications. Although team evaluation has added a great deal to the knowledge of the patient's specific problems, it has also complicated both the interpretation of the findings and the communication of these findings to the retardate's parents.

In those cases of mental retardation in which the causes are clearly evident, such as phenylketonuria (P.K.U.) and Downs Syndrome, the task of the interpreter is simplified to a great degree, and the broad statements concerning the condition are accepted by the parents. However, the President's Panel on Mental Retardation (1962) states that, "In 3 out of 4 mentally retarded persons, the causes are not yet clearly known." Therefore, 75 per cent of the time the explanation of their child's problem must be hedged by the parents' confessions of ignorance regarding etiology. If, as is often the case, the physical examination of the patient reveals nothing, the parents of a retarded child begin to find themselves in a nightmarish, will-o'-the-wisp environment in which diagnoses are made, in which programs are authored and futures are planned with no concrete knowledge of what is wrong with the patient other than that he is "slow" or "retarded."

ISSUES IN THE INTERPRETATION INTERVIEW

The fundamental problem of the parents of mentally retarded children is fear that decisions affecting their child's future happiness and livelihood are being made on what appear to be totally inadequate grounds. If the professional can understand this state of affairs, he can empathize better with the parental hostility and denial of retardation which often ensue after the interpretation interview.

It is sad but true that the majority of parents of retarded children do not understand the total problem as it affects their child. The definition of mental retardation or the relationship of the child's intelligence level to the level of intelligence of other children has not been made clear to them. Nor do they know what could have been the possible causes of their child's handicap, or what effect his impaired intellectual level might have on his future educational program. Is it any wonder, then, that the constant rejoinder to the question, "What have you been told?" is, "Nobody told me anything."

The reasons for blame must be distributed equally among the family physician, the school, and the parents themselves.

The Family Physician

The average practicing physician is not happy treating the retardate. He may either resent the amount of time necessary for counseling, be unfamiliar with the role of a team moderator, or have no experience in being on a team. If a physician has either no empathy for or experience with the mentally retarded, his recommendations reflect this. His uncertainty and discomfort are sensed by the parents, who then react with antagonism and denial of the diagnosis.

Because the physician believes that he must have "all the answers" and must do something about the problem "now," he often gives dogmatic advice and opinions that are based on his desire to be rid of the whole problem instead of on his will to initiate a long-term program for the child and his family. In many cases, on the other hand, the physician identifies with the parents and concludes, without justification, that to retain a child in the home will be an intolerable burden for the family. Although identification with the family is important to some extent, the unrealistic attitudes of the physician must not be allowed to influence the therapeutic program. Furthermore, in contrast to his attitude toward the severely retarded, the family physician may tend to overestimate the intelligence of children functioning subnormally (Korsch et al., 1961).

For some unknown reason, the medical practitioner is resistant to educational recommendations, particularly if made by a school psychologist. This may be due to the fact that some psychological tests can suggest evidence of neurological impairment, even when the physical and neurological examinations are negative. The physician then feels that the psychologist is overstepping the bounds of psychology and encroaching on the medical domain. Because of the physician's attitude, the psychologist often becomes defensive. When this happens, communication between the two professionals is carried on by means of lengthy and erudite, but complicated, reports in mutually incomprehensible terminology, with subsequent lowering of the frustration threshold of the communicators, until communication virtually ceases. There is much to be said for both sides. The psychologist should not jump to conclusions without adequate data, and his report to the physician should be couched in plain, straightforward language that explains technical jargon that cannot be omitted. In addition, the psychologist should be extremely hesitant to make grave diagnostic and prognostic announcements to the parents of a mentally retarded child, unless his findings and interpretations are indisputable. The physician, on the other hand, should realize that he can no longer be the sole arbiter of an individual's future, and that he must rely on other disciplines for information he was not trained to collect.

Most often the physician is unaware of the criteria for special educational placement. He should, therefore, be exceedingly cautious in giving advice in this regard. It is very easy for a physician to sabotage a program of special education by simply implying to the parents that nothing wrong can be found with the child and that he obviously is not "stupid." This inadequate advice can start a feud with the relevant school authorities which is never resolved without a great deal of harm to the child. The parents may win a social promotion, but their child may lose his chance to catch up. The physical examination of a child with a learning problem contributes only part of the picture, and the physician should refrain from passing judgment on the impressions of other disciplines, particularly if his experience in those areas is somewhat limited. Many children with average and superior intellectual ability are problems in school and may require placement in special classes because of learning disabilities, emotional problems, or minimal cerebral dysfunction. Negative physical and neurological evaluations do not necessarily rule out the need for a special school program. The physician's resistance to educational recommendations only underscores the social stigma already attached by society to the "slow learner" and the mentally retarded.

Many physicians are aware of their inadequacies in the field of mental retardation and refer their patients appropriately. Others continue to counsel, unaware of the effects their own emotional reaction to the condition may have on the family.

The School

The child functioning in the range of mild mental retardation may never be detected until starting school, sometimes not until the first grade if his poor performance in kindergarten is attributed to "immaturity." It is understandable, therefore, that "mild mental retardation" suddenly diagnosed at the age of six years, can cause more impact and disruption in a family than severe intellectual impairment apparent since infancy. The school authorities are often oblivious to the effects of this element of surprise and unwittingly heighten the parents' reaction by a peremptory handling of the situation.

The child who is having trouble in school is a problem, either by being slow in learning, indulging in disruptive behavior, or both. The school psychologist may have seen the child and, after consultation with the teacher and the school principal, may have recommended a course of action. This is conveyed to the parents in a conference with the school psychologist; often the school principal and the child's teacher also are present. If the diagnosis is mental retardation, the question of placement in a special education program is discussed. Unfortunately, this decision is communicated in different ways according to the attitudes of the school personnel. It can range from a brusque statement on a postcard that the child will be placed in a special-education class as of a particular date (as happened in one of my cases) to a well-conducted case conference with full explanation, understanding, and warmth. In many communities, placement in special education is contingent on the approval of the parents. If this is not given, the child is "socially" promoted and the basic reasons for the recommendation are ignored. The parents feel vindicated, but the youngster gets farther and farther behind in his knowledge, and concomitant anxieties and frustrations tend to lower his already poor academic performance even more.

There is a tendency on the part of some school authorities to imply that the child is being placed in special education because he is causing difficulty in the regular classroom and is disrupting or impairing the work of the class. The implication is that the child has to be removed from the regular classroom because he cannot measure up to the requirements and is impeding the progress of the other pupils and taking too much of the teacher's time. Consequently, he must be demoted into an inferior setting.

Not enough school authorities "sell" special education as a profitable move for the retardate who has difficulty learning in the regular classroom. The regular class teacher is burdened with large classes and a firmly fixed curriculum and has little time to spend on an individual child. The special education teacher, however, has small classes (as delineated by law in most states), has time to spend on each child, and is trained in specific educational methods for children with learning problems. In the special class, the burden of competition is removed, and each child progresses at his own rate, with consequent diminution in anxiety and frustration. If the school authorities were aware of the magic of good public relations, there would be fewer disgruntled parents.

A large number of children are referred to child development clinics, because these facilities will act as referee in a conflict between the school and the parents. That the school is rarely wrong in its recom-

mendations does not mitigate the problem or soothe the parents' ruf-
fled feelings.

Sometimes, in an effort to soften the blow or because the parents
have not listened attentively to the explanation, the placement in a
"trainable" or "educable" class is considered only temporary. The
parents know that "trainable" is a lower class than "educable." Somehow, by implication or desire, they infer that the ultimate goal is
graduation from "trainable" to "educable," and from "educable"—
hopefully—to "normal." Failure to clarify that placement in a special
class is long term and often permanent, produces hostility and recrim-
ination against the child's teacher for not doing her job properly.

In some communities the program of special education is either nonexistent or exceedingly poor. The age span among the children in the
same class may be great and the degree of their retardation variable.
The trainable class, particularly, can produce an adverse reaction in
parents whose child may be merely "trainable" according to intellectual ability, but is considered by them to be superior to the children
presently in the class because of his good socialization experiences
and grooming. The parents may then express the fear that their child
will regress in such an environment. This reaction is reasonable and
should be recognized as such. An alternate educational program, if
available, should be outlined to the parents. Whoever recommends a
program of special education to parents of a retarded child should be
completely knowledgeable of all aspects of that program and should
under no circumstances embellish the facts or portray the future un-
realistically.

The Parents

People are not happy with things and circumstances over which
they have no control and which they do not want, particularly sickness and handicaps. The acute illness is a transient, annoying, uncomfortable episode. The chronic ailment, in contrast, is a lifetime of
frustrations, financial commitments, evaluations, and interviews end-
ing in multifarious advice, some of which is impractical and much of
which is conflicting.

There is an optimum time to discuss a child's deficiencies with his
parents. Unfortunately, this time is difficult to gauge accurately. Parents with a handicapped child go through three emotional stages in
their interaction with the physician (Denhoff and Robinault, 1960):
first, hostility; second, shopping from doctor to doctor; and third, ac-

ceptance. Until this final stage is reached, no therapeutic program is even considered.

The situation of parents who have a retarded child is succinctly outlined by the Group for the Advancement of Psychiatry (1963):

The physician is dealing with parents who have a multifaceted problem: 1. They may not have fully accepted the diagnosis of mental retardation. 2. They have varying degrees of guilt feelings about their possible role in the causation of the child's condition. 3. They resent the fact that this has happened to them and tend to try to find some outside influence on which they can blame the problem. 4. They hope for a magical solution. 5. They have a wish, usually unconscious, to be rid of this burden. 6. They have come seeking advice. Each of these factors deserves separate consideration by the physician who must realize that he himself will have certain reactions to the child's condition and to the parents and their emotional problems.

There are other considerations which affect the parents in their acceptance or denial of their child's problem. As a generalization, the parents of children with familial retardation are more accepting of their child's intellectual impairment. This is engendered by their own inadequate school performance, poor motivation and often antagonistic attitude toward education and the school authorities. At the lowest end of the social scale, maternal rejection, depression and helplessness, inadequate income, crowded home conditions, lack of family ties, absence of stimulating material, and even paucity of conversation further aggravate the total situation. However, in the same social class, these deleterious factors are tempered because the child is allowed to progress at his own speed, meets with less criticism, and—in some instances—learns how to fight for survival.

Middle- and upper-class families place a greater emphasis on intellectual endowment and academic prowess. These parents are more sensitive to social stigma and often exert pressure on their child for unrealistic achievement levels. This is frequently manifested by the purchase of toys, books, and musical instruments or by encouragement of the child to pursue hobbies clearly above his mental age. Although encouragement and support are major necessities for optimum achievement, there is a point of no return when undue pressure produces an additional emotional burden that further impairs the child's performance.

The first duty of the counselor is to listen. Without knowing the concern of the parents he is in no position to advise them. Much of the benefit obtained by a team evaluation must be ascribed to the opportunities the parents have to tell several professionals the things that bother them about their child. When allowed to unburden themselves in this way, the mental catharsis can be extremely beneficial in itself.

It is mandatory to find out why the parents have come for help. Often they do not ask the questions that are particularly bothering them. The physician tacitly assumes that he has answered their questions when he delineates the findings of his evaluation and his recommendations. Nothing could be further from the truth. The problem, as the physician sees it, might be severe brain damage due to anoxia at birth with severe mental retardation, but the parents are there to find out why their child is not talking. They might accept the motor retardation and realize that the child is mentally retarded, but that is not their main concern. Their main concern is that their child is not talking and that, because he is not talking, he cannot make his wants known to them. Therefore, they should be asked specifically, "Why are you here?" or "How can we help you?"

As the parents unfold their story in detail, often for the first time, the physician can gauge their sophistication, their realistic or unrealistic appraisal of their child's handicaps, their hostility to the school or the former physician, their unanimity or conflict in handling the child, and the effect of the child's disability on their marital relationship. The impression obtained will, of course, color the emphasis and interpretation of the findings that must be determined on an individual basis.

Evaluation Parameters

The work-up of the mentally retarded child should be as complete as possible, even if the diagnosis is fairly obvious and there have been many previous examinations by many physicians. The mere fact that a child has been seen by several other physicians is a testament to the parents' dissatisfaction. A thorough evaluation will drive home test by test and point by point the previous findings to skeptical parents and will also rule out the possibility of a previous error in diagnosis. This may end the phase of "shopping around," which is the usual precursor of acceptance of the child's problem. Some may argue that such an elaborate work-up is purely academic and places an unnecessary financial burden on a family that is destined to have heavy, long-term medical expenses. This is not borne out by experience, particularly if the various procedures have been discussed beforehand.

Many parents ask for specific tests, such as an electroencephalogram (EEG), if they have not already been done. Unfortunately, there is the connotation to many that the EEG is somehow therapeutic. The lesson to be learned is that all procedures, including laboratory and X-ray reports, should be reviewed in detail afterwards. There is a paradoxical twist to the concept that laboratory procedures should only be undertaken when they have an almost certain chance of being positive. Parents have a right to be antagonistic if, after an expensive series of laboratory and investigative procedures, the sum total is dismissed with: "our tests showed nothing." When the physical examination likewise shows nothing and then opinions are given on the basis of the completely negative evidence, it is understandable why the experts are mistrusted. The report of the full evaluation, presented with the findings of normality in many areas, can be music to the ears of parents who have wallowed in the dirge of funereal pronouncements. Parental guilt feelings must be assuaged by convincing them that "everything possible has been done," and a detailed report of an extensive work-up is of great therapeutic value. Where possible and practical, any positive X-ray films or abnormal EEG tracing can be shown to the parents to impress on them visually the extent of the involvement of the various organ systems.

THE INTERPRETATION INTERVIEW

When first sitting down to discuss the evaluation, it is helpful to ask the parents not to interrupt until you are completely finished, because many of their questions will probably be answered as you report and frequent interruptions will only complicate and confuse the presentation. Tell them they will be able to ask all the questions they wish to ask at the end.

The findings should be presented in logical sequence as follows:

Review of the Patient's History

It is advisable to reiterate the salient points in the child's history. A large wall chart as depicted in Table 19–1 is of great value in literally pinpointing the pertinent factors in the history and examination if there is any question that the parents have difficulty in understanding. This chart is attached to a bulletin board, and pins with large, red plastic heads are used to delineate those pertinent factors during the recapitulation of the history and the detailing of the examination. At the end of the explanation, the parents can be asked to recount what has been said to them by looking at the chart with its pins.

T A B L E 19-1

Pertinent Factors in the History and Examination of the Mentally Retarded Child

HISTORY

PREGNANCY	DELIVERY	NEWBORN	DEVELOPMENT	ILLNESSES
Normal	Normal	Normal	Normal	Normal
Bleeding	Short	Premature	Delayed	Infections
Toxemia	Long	Breathing Difficulty	Motor	Injuries
Injury	Complicated	Oxygen	Mental	Convulsions
Infection		Convulsions	Speech	
		Congenital abnormality	Hearing	
		Injury		

EXAMINATION

PHYSICAL	NEUROLOGICAL	PSYCHOLOGICAL	SPEECH AND HEARING	LABORATORY
Normal	Normal	Normal	Normal	Urine
Other	Incoordinated	I.Q.	Speech	Blood
	Abnormal	Behavior Problem	Hearing	X-ray
		Perceptual problem		EEG

If no past mismanagement is uncovered on the part of the parents, medical personnel, school authorities, or the various community agencies which have dealt with him, this should be explained thoroughly. The bitter hostility many parents display toward a particular person or group is a common emotional defense reaction and should be negated whenever possible. In some cases the criticism may be, on the face of it, justifiable, but no useful purpose is served by permitting such a belief to be perpetuated. Acceptance of a handicap by parents is all the harder when they know that someone may be to blame for it. Special emphasis, whenever possible, should be placed on the following factors: that heredity plays no part in the child's condition; that mental retardation or a handicap in one or the other side of the family may be pure coincidence; and that bleeding or exposure to rubella during pregnancy is something over which a mother has no control. The accusations, often unspoken, between parents with a retarded child can be a pernicious obstacle not only to acceptance of the child, but to marital harmony. The medical negation of such a possibility might bring the first peace of mind to a troubled parent.

Interpretation of the Findings

The usual procedure is to enumerate the positive items found on examination and to apply them as a basis for the diagnosis. Preferably, a further step should be (to paraphrase the song) to "accentuate the negative." The listing of the negative findings is important and can be a welcome relief from the stress of all those that are positive. It is good practice to start with the physical examination, pointing out the obvious strabismus, peculiar gait or stance, incoordination, hyperactivity, and so forth, but it is also necessary to temper these items with statements such as "His height and weight are average," "His lungs and heart are normal," "There is no evidence of trouble with the thyroid," "He has good muscle strength," "There is nothing we can find wrong with his nervous system, speech, or hearing," or whatever the truth may be.

Visual aids are extremely useful in the presentation of the psychological data. Too often the parents are confused by the term "mildly retarded" when the child is performing in the range of "mild mental retardation." Frequently the school term "trainable" or "educable" is used without the least explanation of what this means or, more important, in what way this does relate to other levels of intelligence, and what percentage of the population has a problem similar to that of the child being discussed. It is a simple matter to use a chart as outlined in Figure 19–1 and to point to the place on the chart with the statement that "Johnny is performing somewhere in here," giving the IQ range and the educational definitions of "trainable" and "educable," emphasizing that the first IQ is purely a base line, and that further testing will be needed periodically to determine its reliability. The term "IQ" has come under a great deal of criticism of late. However,

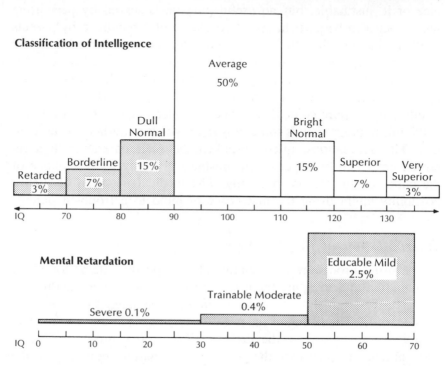

FIGURE 19–1   *Classification of Intelligence*

this is the phrase that parents use most commonly and can be defined as "the level at which a child performs as measured by special psychological tests." It is important to break down the IQ to mental age. During the taking of the history, all parents of retarded children should be asked the question: "At what age level do you think your child is performing?" If the answer is fairly close to that obtained by the psychological examination, this attests to the realistic assessment of their child's capabilities. If the parents' assessment is significantly higher, some denial may be present; if lower, there may be some rejection. All these hints from the parents color and influence the physician's interpretation and presentation of the findings. For example, if a child is chronologically ten years of age and the parents estimate he is functioning at the level of a six-year-old and he is found to have an

IQ of about 65, this is a realistic assessment. It is my impression that these parents are easier to counsel; they accept and follow through on recommendations better, and generally provide a more understanding and supportive environment for the retardate. Those parents whose estimate is markedly higher or lower than that obtained on testing, are harder to counsel, may be antagonistic or hostile to recommendations, and will have difficulty in carrying out a formalized program. Furthermore, their retarded child often has a secondary emotional problem.

Diagnosis

The diagnostic terms used in explaining their child's problem to the parents are extremely important. Unfortunately, these terms are not clearly defined by the various disciplines involved, and classifications of organic and emotional disorders in childhood are controversial and poorly categorized. The generally accepted classification of the American Association on Mental Deficiency (1961) with the main organic term of "encephalopathy" often suggests a progressive neurological disease to many physicians. On the other hand, "chronic brain syndrome" from the *International Classification of Diseases* (1955), used mainly in psychiatric circles, is equally vague and all-inclusive. Similarly, the classification of emotional disorders in children is inadequate and under revision at the time of writing. It is hoped that a new and improved classification will be available in the very near future.

Whenever possible, a diagnosis should be given to the parents. It is amazing how often a specific name for the various signs and symptoms of their child's condition can relieve a great deal of mental anguish on the part of the parents. The lack of a definite diagnosis suggests that the various therapists do not know with what they are dealing and consequently do not know how to treat it. Even when the condition, as is usually the case, has no specific therapy, the parents still feel relieved that at least they do not have to continue to shop around for a diagnosis. Often all they wish is reassurance that "nothing more can be done" than is already being done.

The literature dealing with exceptional children is replete with advice to avoid terms such as "brain damage," "low IQ," "anoxia," and "deficiency," and to substitute more acceptable synonyms such as "cerebral dysfunction," "intellectual level or ability," "lack of oxygen," and "retardation." Strictly speaking, this is academic and with few exceptions, it is unimportant what terms are used providing they

are adequately and concretely explained and—above all—are trans-
parently clear and understandable. Furthermore, the choice of terms
used will vary with the parents' educational level and sophistication.

It is unwise to assume that bright, educated parents have a greater
knowledge of most aspects of mental retardation; they do not. Sometimes they have read so much that they are completely confused.
Their questions may be more sophisticated and their intellectual grasp
of the problem may be more complete, but they still have the same
difficulties in understanding their own emotional involvement and
how it complicates their child's progress.

Parents with limited intelligence should not be burdened with too
much detail. Equivocal findings and interpolations should be avoided.
The chart with pins can be used most effectively in this situation.

Children with subaverage intelligence may have associated neurological impairment. This can range from the severe retardate with severe spastic quadriplegia (cerebral palsy) to the child with mild mental retardation or borderline intelligence with associated minimal
brain damage.

An extremely difficult concept to explain to parents is *minimal
brain damage*. There has been much discussion to abandon this term
and replace it with *minimal cerebral dysfunction* or *minimal brain
dysfunction* as advocated by Clements (1966). It must be remembered, however, that this is a medical diagnosis and is also a symptom
complex with different combinations of varying disabilities such as
coordination, activity, perception, language, and cognition. Educators, on the other hand, are apt to call these symptoms hyperactivity,
learning disability, dyslexia, or the "Strauss Syndrome" (Strauss,
1947).

Irrespective of what it is called, it is extremely difficult to explain
"minimal brain damage" in simple language that can be understood
by the parents of such children. One may start by stating that no evidence of *structural* damage to the brain was found on physical or laboratory examination of the child. Then one should go on to say that
certain facts in the history (incoordination, poor writing, trouble with
geometrical figures, reversals, hyperactivity, short attention span, and
so on) suggest that there is some mild disability, dysfunction, or upset
of the nervous system. This can be likened to a television set whose
picture tube and other tubes are completely intact, but whose picture
is blurred though decipherable because the wire from the antenna on
the roof has not been tightened to the television cabinet. Similarly,
one may liken "minimal brain damage" to a radio that performs fairly
adequately but with a lot of static interference because of a loose

wire. Thus, the patient with minimal cerebral dysfunction has nothing structurally wrong with his brain. His nervous system is "loosely wired," and this may cause him to have difficulty with numbers, poor writing, reversal of figures, and so forth and could account for his hyperactivity and unpredictable behavior. It is very important to emphasize that the patient does not have cerebral palsy, as this conjures up the severely handicapped youngster in braces who commonly appears on the United Cerebral Palsy Association posters and would give a completely wrong interpretation of the problem. It is also wise to stress to the parents at this point that such a child cannot control his behavior, and that he is not to be looked upon as stubborn and recalcitrant, with commensurate punishment. However, the parents should not go to the other extreme and use the diagnosis of minimal cerebral dysfunction as an excuse to abdicate their rights and responsibilities as parents, but should try to maintain consistent discipline in a firm, structured, accepting environment. Describing the problem in such a way, as a definite clinical entity, gives it the status of a disease and therefore makes it acceptable. An understanding of this very often is followed by improvement in parental handling of the child and by relaxation of tensions in the family.

Similarly, explanations of laboratory data should be simple and concrete. It is convenient to describe the EEG as "a tracing of the brain wave" similar to the tracing of the heart on the electrocardiogram. Abnormal foci or patterns can then be called "irregular discharges of bursts of electricity" culminating in seizures or atypical episodes of behavior. Where possible, this should be demonstrated on the tracing or should be drawn.

When a behavior problem proves to be primarily emotional, the explanation should always be preceded by a review of the criteria that have ruled out an organic basis for the condition. Parents may then realize that the physician has given serious consideration to their observation and beliefs before discussing intrafamilial relationships.

Practically every handicapped child has a secondary emotional problem. In the mild retardate this is often due to repeated failure, but may also be due to overprotection, rejection, or pressure from parents or teachers. When present, the behavioral manifestations should be described. It can be pointed out that the child pushed beyond his limitations is apt to be anxious, compulsive, and irritable, and that such manifestations of emotional upset can depress academic performance or even his performance on psychological tests. Explanations should be factual, and jargon should be avoided. Phrases like "Get off his back," and "If you can't praise him, don't knock him," should be used. The child who gives up easily in the face of failure can be called a "born loser." Such phrases are apt to have more impact than esoteric, academic, and professional terms.

Although of no great value from the point of view of treatment, a diagnostic label does contribute markedly to the parents' peace of mind. This applies particularly to the child of school age. Unless the symptoms are severe, the diagnosis of any type of cerebral dysfunction in the first year or two of life may be exceedingly difficult. Practically all impairments, whether purely intellectual or neuromotor, present by delay in development, and only time will clarify the diagnosis. Therefore, general terms such as "delayed motor development," or "psychomotor retardation" should be used, which give the parents the connotation of a specific diagnosis combined with the relative reassurance a label provides.

The patient's history is not always helpful. Even in normal infants complaints of colic, feeding difficulties, irritability, and sleep-reversal patterns are fairly common. Often these symptoms assume only in retrospect the importance of early indications of impaired neurologic function. In these instances one can but record all clinical findings and tentative impressions and follow these by frequent, careful reappraisals.

PROGNOSIS AND TREATMENT GUIDELINES

Once the diagnosis is made, and often before a program of treatment is outlined, the physician is called upon to look into his crystal ball and forecast the future. The objective scientist tends to balk at such a hazardous undertaking; he will sidestep the question and will murmur some such platitude as "time will tell." However, few of us who are treating impaired children can be that blunt or indecisive. Hope is the one commodity that must be dispensed within the bounds of realism, and the amount of hope offered should depend on the age of the child, the extent of the abnormalities, and the outlook of the physician.

It should be realized that instruments used for measuring growth and development, particularly in the intellectual area, are not precise for the child under three years of age, and most psychologists agree that the tests have limited predictive value under the ages of five to six years. The first evaluation done within this age period must be considered a base line for future examinations.

It has also been shown that as the child grows older, the picture of cerebral dysfunction changes to such an extent that an infant diagnosed in the first or second year of life as having cerebral palsy with associated mental retardation may be judged as being within normal limits by the age of three years (Solomons et al., 1963). Consequently, it is wise to be overcautious in the interpretation of psychomotor retardation, particularly in the first year or two of life. The "late bloomer" is a definite entity. Hence, in the absence of definite neurologic impairments, no specific diagnosis should be made. This does not mean that the parents should be reassured that "He'll grow out of it," but rather that they should realize that "He is not performing up to age level at this time," and that there are no apparent pathological reasons for this delay in development. An explanation should be given on the unreliability of testing at such an early age, that many children do catch up, and that a repeat evaluation in six to twelve months would be necessary before a more definitive assessment and prognosis could be given.

In attempting to assess the prognosis, it must always be kept in mind that any child, no matter how much retarded, will improve to some extent with time. The rate of improvement is determined primarily by the degree of retardation, and the prognosis should partially reflect the optimism of the physician. If the retardation is not more than 50 per cent at about one year of age, I tend to leave the parents with a feeling of optimism. When retardation is more pronounced, I find it wiser to be noncommittal. I try to give the impression that the outlook is undecided and that the next evaluation will likely tell us the degree of the retardation we might expect, now that we have a base line for comparison. When the child is severely retarded, performing less than 25 per cent of what is expected at his chronological stage of development, I point out the current developmental age in months. However, even here I mention the unreliability of testing and the possibility of some improvement before the next examination. The physician's degree of optimism should depend to a great extent on the parents' attitude and the home environment. If the parents are sensible, realistic, compatible people with the opportunity and desire to spend considerable time with the child in a warm, accepting home setting, the outlook is good. Rejecting parents with marital and other problems are most unlikely to do a good job even when the handicap is mild. I then tend to paint a blacker picture, in the attempt to motivate the parents to get together to produce the optimum environment for their child.

The attitude of physicians toward institutionalization of the retarded is most peculiar. One study (Olshansky and Sternfeld, 1963) revealed that most pediatricians are not in favor of early institutionalization, and that only a few look upon the decision to institutionalize as belonging to the parents. I personally feel that this decision is purely a family one and never make such a recommendation to parents. In reviewing the management and possible disposition of a patient, institutionalization as an alternative to be considered should be mentioned, but never advocated. On the other hand, once the family decision is made, it should be endorsed by the physician. One way of approaching this exceedingly sensitive aspect of future care is to point out that at the moment this twelve-year-old child is functioning at a specific mental age level, let's say six years; several psychological tests over a period of time have testified to the validity of the test result. It is logical to assume, therefore, that he will function at approximately 50 per cent of his intellectual capacity when he is a young adult (using sixteen years as the cut-off age). It is easy to point out to the parents that if they were no longer around to care for their child, he would require constant supervision because he would be eight years old mentally, and that the only place this could be obtained would be in a residential facility.

In other words, I try to make the parents understand that eventually the child will be institutionalized. The decision as to the best time for that would be entirely up to them, but they should keep in mind the following points:

1. The decision to place the retarded child in an institution should be made not only on the basis of what is best for the handicapped child, but by consideration of all members of the family. The parents must determine what effect keeping this child at home is having on their marriage, their normal children, and the overall family life. Parental guilt feelings should be minimized as much as possible by the physician pointing out that they have done everything possible, but that the circumstances had become such that continued care at home would be detrimental to other members of the family.

2. Sometimes it can be suggested that the child is so severely retarded that he is unaware of who takes care of him; if the care is competent and kindly, this is all that matters. Progressive institutions for the mentally retarded can be described, with emphasis on the fact that children can be sent home for vacations, birthdays, and even weekends. Furthermore, the parents should be advised to visit the prospective institution to see the specific building in which their child will be living. It is important to close this topic by stating that there is no emergency about deciding, and that even if the child were accepted

for admission it would take several months from the time of application. The main theme must be that the decision for institutionalization lies with the parents at whatever time they consider appropriate.

3. By the same token, the decision to have more children rests with the parents, if the handicapping condition of their child has a hereditary basis such as P.K.U. It is the physician's responsibility to explain that an autosomal recessive condition such as P.K.U. carries with it a one-in-four chance that their next child would be similarly affected. He should not sit in judgment or issue edicts concerning future children with complete disregard for the parents' religious and moral beliefs.

Long-term prognostications can be given with some degree of assurance in those children who are in the upper limits of mild mental retardation and the lower limits of the borderline range of intellectual ability. The words of Potter (1964, p. 361) should always be kept in mind:

As a general proposition, mildly retarded children closely resemble rather than differ from "normal" children and significantly differ from, rather than resemble more seriously handicapped and limited mental retardates. Unlike the latter, mildly retarded children seldom have any evidence of retarded development in infancy and the pre-school years; encephalopathy and inborn errors of metabolism are but rarely encountered and all of them are potentially capable of independent living, self-support and socially effective behavior in their adult years. It seems to be the consensus of most sophisticated clinicians that "mild retardation" represents a normal physiological variation in the minus direction on the distribution curve of tested intelligence for any population group. In fact, the only difference between mildly retarded children and children who are not retarded is that the former are, relatively speaking, slow learners in structured educational situations (the classroom) and their capacity for abstract thinking limited.

This happy note can be transmitted to the parents if their child is fortunate enough to function within the range of mild mental retardation and his appearance and temperament are such that he is likely to be accepted by his peers. Many studies point out the fact that the mildly retarded, once the competitive environment of school is over, are likely to be absorbed by the community and are able to function as well as their "normal" neighbors (Kennedy, 1948, 1966; Charles, 1953, 1957; Peterson, 1960).

The team approach to the evaluation of the handicapped child has been stressed repeatedly. Too often the parents are not included as part of the team. At other times they are given too much responsibility. There are some dangers in making parents therapists because, if the treatment fails, they believe it must be the fault of the therapist and thus blame themselves (Freeman, 1967). However, as mentioned previously, without parental help, the outlook for improvement is poor.

Treatment of the retarded, like all treatments, must be understood by parents. This necessitates an explicit, factual explanation that can be simplified by writing out the instructions. Drug therapy, whether for convulsions or hyperactivity, is usually long term with much adjustment of dosage. It is advantageous, therefore, to write down the name of the drug and the strength of each unit dose and have the container labeled accordingly. This prevents panic when medications run out away from home. The need for periodic blood examinations and good oral hygiene when taking certain anticonvulsants should be explained and emphasized. The parents must be made aware that they have the major responsibility in carrying out the program of treatment. Although the family must be given support and direction over the years, the frequency of return appointments should be watched carefully.

SUMMARY

There is the tendency for all problems with mental retardates, however small, to be settled by the physician, and common sense and parental action evaporate as the physician takes over, although the parents themselves should decide the future of their child. Few families start out with the wisdom and fortitude to do this. Only when this ideal state is reached, can the goal of optimal opportunity for optimal potential of the child be attained.

REFERENCES

Charles, D. C. Ability and accomplishment of persons earlier judged mentally deficient. *Genet. Psychol. Monogr.*, 1953, 47, 3–71.
———. Adult adjustment of some deficient American children. *Amer. J. Ment. Defic.*, 1957, 62, 300–304.
Clements, S. Minimal brain dysfunction in children—terminology and identification. NINDB Monograph No. 3. Public Health Service Publication No. 1415, 1966.

Denhoff, E., & Robinault, I. *Cerebral palsy and related disorders.* New York: McGraw-Hill Book Co., 1960.

Freeman, R. D. Controversy over "patterning" as a treatment for brain damage in children. *J.A.M.A.,* 1967, *202,* 83–86.

Group for the Advancement of Psychiatry. *Mental retardation: A family crisis—the therapeutic role of the physician.* Report No. 56. New York, 1963.

Heber, R. A manual on terminology and classification in mental retardation. Amer. Assoc. on Mental Deficiency, 1961, 2nd edition. No. 65, 499–500. *International statistical classification of diseases, injuries, and causes of death,* (7th Ed.), World Health Organization, Geneva, 1955.

Kennedy, R. J. R. *The social adjustment of morons in a Connecticut city.* Hartford, Conn.: Mansfield-Southbury Social Service, 1948.

————. A Connecticut community revisited. A study of the social adjustment of a group of mentally deficient adults in 1948 and 1960. Connecticut State Department of Health, Office of Mental Retardation, Jan., 1966.

Korsch, B., Cobb, J., & Ashe, B. Pediatricians' appraisals of patients' intelligence. *Pediatrics,* 1961, *27,* 990–999.

Olshansky, S., & Sternfield, L. Attitudes of some pediatricians toward the institutionalization of mentally retarded children. In *Institutionalizing mentally retarded children—attitudes of some physicians.* U.S. Department of Health, Education, and Welfare, Children's Bureau, 1963, p. 5.

Peterson, L., & Smith, L. L. The post school adjustment of educable mentally retarded adults. *Except. Child.,* 1960, *26,* 404–408.

Potter, H. W. The needs of mentally retarded children for child psychiatry services. *J. Child Psychiat.,* 1964, *3,* 352–374.

President's Panel on Mental Retardation. *A National plan to combat mental retardation.* U.S. Government Printing Office, Washington, D.C., 1962.

Rembolt, R. R. The "team" in cerebral palsy. Symposium on cerebral palsy. Thirty-seventh Annual Convention, American Speech and Hearing Association, 1961, pp. 49–53.

Solomons, G., Holden, R. H., & Denhoff, E. The changing picture of cerebral dysfunction in early childhood. *J. Pediat.,* 1963, *63,* 113–122.

Strauss, A. A., & Lehtinen, L. *Psychopathology and education of the brain-injured child.* New York: Grune & Stratton, 1947.

: 20 :

A Theoretical Framework for the Management of Parents of the Mentally Retarded

Wolf Wolfensberger and Frank J. Menolascino

Webster's Dictionary defines management as "judicious use of means to accomplish an end." For the purposes of this chapter,[1] we will define a concept of "human management" or "human management services" as "entry of individuals or agencies, acting in societally sanctioned capacities, into the functioning spheres of individuals, families, or larger social systems in order to maintain or change conditions with the intention of benefiting such individuals, their family social systems, or society in general." Thus defined, human management practices would subsume case evaluation, psychotherapy, counseling, guidance, education, supervision, correction, and many other activities. Obviously, psychiatry is a significant human management profession, and according to the above definition, management of the families of the retarded would include many activities that a psychiatrist might perform.

Human management practices in any field or area are determined by the way a problem is perceived, conceptualized, and interpreted. In this chapter, we will briefly review some major conceptualizations of the management of parents of the mentally retarded and then add a new conceptualization to the existing ones. This new conceptualization is a revision of one first presented in an earlier attempt to review and integrate the voluminous literature on the dynamics and management of parents and siblings of the mentally retarded (Wolfensberger, 1967).[2]

A REVIEW OF MANAGEMENT FRAMEWORKS

Early conceptualizations of parental response to a retarded child were heavily influenced by psychoanalytic thought. Major emphasis was placed on the role of guilt, which was seen as a near-universal phenomenon in parents of all types of handicapped children. These parents were commonly viewed as conflicted and almost certain to engage in defense mechanisms such as denial and projection, and it was expected that such defenses would be of neurotic proportions. Virtually everything the parent did was interpreted as constituting "rejection" or "nonacceptance" of the child, and parental behavior that had positive elements was, at worst, labeled as reaction formation or, at best, as ambivalence.

The psychoanalytic interpretation reached its apex with two elaborations. One of these was by Beddie and Osmond (1955) who equated parental response to a retarded child as equivalent to a "child loss" (death of a normal child) resulting in grief that required "grief work" in order to be overcome. Institutionalization was seen as a "death without the proper rites." The other elaboration by Solnit and Stark (1961) coined the term "chronic mourning" for the "object loss" to which the advent of the retarded child was equated. This grief motif became widely accepted (for example, Thurston, 1960; Baum, 1962; Cohen, 1962; Tisza, 1962; Dalton and Epstein, 1963; Roos, 1963; Goodman, 1964; Owens, 1964).

Management derived from psychoanalytic concepts tended to incorporate several elements: (1) The parent was placed into the role of a psychiatric patient, which the parent was expected to accept if he was to be helped. (2) Help consisted primarily of therapeutically oriented individual or group counseling which explored the parent's feelings about his own parents, as well as about the child and his condition and problems. (3) The parent was encouraged to express his deep-seated feelings of responsibility for the child's condition and was provided interpretation, reassurance, and support in an effort to dissipate guilt.

Usually, management did not go much beyond this because, on the one hand, parents were now assumed to be able to make the best adjustment possible under the circumstances and, on the other hand, there prevailed a very pessimistic—almost treatment-nihilistic—view about the retarded child. Thus, there seemed to be little to do in a concrete way except perhaps to recommend institutional placement and to make the necessary arrangements.

More recently, stress has been placed on the realistic demands and burdens that parents of retarded children often bear. Parents were seen as being under a great deal of situational and external stress, and symptoms of such stress were perceived as essentially normal or at least expected under the circumstances.

The neurotic interpretation of parental reactions was specifically attacked and rejected by Olshansky (1962, 1966). He pointed to certain social factors of our culture which induce parents to feel devalued for having a damaged child and to other co-existing factors which inhibit his ability to externalize this sorrow so as to dissipate it. Such a conflict was seen as apt to result in long-term internalization of a depressive mood which Olshansky termed "chronic sorrow"—"an understandable nonneurotic response to a tragic fact" (Olshansky, 1966, p. 21).

The management suggested by Olshansky emphasized ventilation of parental feelings, readiness on the part of the professional to act scapegoat-like as a focus of anger to the parent, and provision of concrete services such as nursery schools, special classes, sheltered workshops, and guidance with practical problems of child rearing.

Farber (1960*a*) advanced a sociological and relatively sophisticated theory of parental response to a retarded child. Briefly, parental conflicts were seen to spring from two types of "crisis" situations: a "tragic crisis" occurs when a parent's expectancies in regard to the family's future are demolished; and a "role organization crisis" occurs when parents are unable to cope with a retarded child over a long period of time. This theory has given rise to a number of studies by Farber, his students, and others, but since the main interest in this work has been theoretical, there has been little elaboration in regard to management implications.

A NEW MANAGEMENT FRAMEWORK

Each of the conceptualizations discussed in the above review has made some contribution toward a better understanding of families of the retarded. However, the approaches have suffered from emphasizing only limited aspects of either the problem or the possible management options. We will attempt here to unify some of the thinking and to propose a framework that may be adequate to handle a wide variety of problems and situations, and that may provide a means for a more judicious selection of management options. Our greatest theoretical debt is probably to the theories of Farber (1960a).

It is proposed that parental management needs arising from the advent or presence of a retarded child tend to have three major sources: *novelty shock,* which results when parental expectancies are suddenly shattered; *value conflicts* due to culturally mediated attitudes toward defect or deviance; *reality stress* resulting from the situational demands of raising or caring for a retarded person. Each of these sources will be discussed in detail below.

Novelty Shock

Novelty shock is a very natural response that occurs when parents learn precipitously that their expectations and perceptions in regard to their child deviate substantially from reality. Novelty shock may occur when a parent of an older child learns relatively suddenly that the child is or may be retarded. However, most commonly, novelty shock occurs upon the birth of an obviously atypical child, such as a child with Down's Syndrome.

Parents usually have great anticipations as to what the prospective baby may be like. Most immediately, there are certain basic normative expectations as to the size and weight and that the baby will have similar racial characteristics as the parents. Aside from these basic normative characteristics, parents—especially if they have not had children before—are apt to idealize the expected baby. As Solnit and Stark (1961) have stated so well, parents often do not merely expect a typical infant but a perfect one.

Aside from expectations as to the qualities of their baby, parents have expectations in regard to the future. In our culture, most parents strongly expect their children to pursue an education, to marry, and to practice an occupation. Some parents not only establish college education funds for children that are not even born yet, but they may even have picked—at least in their fantasies—the college their child is to attend and the occupation he is to assume.

The time of birth itself is, under the best of circumstances, a time of severe physical and emotional stress for both mother and father, accompanied by uncertainty and emotionality. Any additionally stressful events superimposed on such a state of vulnerability and depletion are apt to cause bewilderment, confusion, disorganization, regression to increased dependency upon others, and maybe even temporary psychosis. Obviously, an unexpected and stressful event associated with the occasion itself, such as the birth of a grossly atypical child, is particularly apt to induce such a state, conceptualized here as novelty shock.

Actually, the fact that the child is damaged and likely to be retarded may not be the critical issue. The general disruption of expectancies may be more traumatic than the specific nature of the reality. For illustration's sake, we might say that novelty shock might be equally severe whether the baby is diagnosed as Down's Syndrome, or whether it is 3 feet long, very premature, has purple horns or unexpected racial characteristics, whether it is healthy but dies unexpectedly, or whether the baby turned out to be more than one baby. Often it is not even the unexpected event that induces shock as much as the way the event is interpreted by all involved, including the medical personnel. Imagine an authoritarian medical figure towering over a depleted, lonely, perhaps half-conscious mother, booming dramatically: "Madam, you have just given birth to a mongolian idiot who should be institutionalized immediately!" Incidents of this nature have by no means been rare and are well-documented in the literature (for example, Aldrich, 1947; Holt, 1958; Tizard and Grad, 1961; Zwerling, 1954; Waskowitz, 1959).

The literature also documents that parents can go into novelty shock merely on the basis of the awareness that some terrible event has happened even when they lack all understanding of the terminology that is thrown at them or of the nature or meaning of the event.

McDonald (1962) documented a case where a father walked the streets in confused agitation for two nights and a day after being told that his baby had a cleft palate; he came back asking what a cleft palate was. Kramm (1963) told of a mother who was informed that her child was a mongoloid and who then set out with the help of neighbors and dictionaries to find what a mongoloid was, eventually concluding that it was something kindred to a mongrel dog. Other parents have been known to have been kept from seeing their child or to have been induced into not wanting to see it. One such family finally came in fear and apprehension to see their institutionalized baby which, on the basis of the guidance they had received, they had pictured as an unspeakable monster—and instead found a sweet, beautiful mongoloid baby that they would probably have taken home, loved, and raised if there had been better interpretation earlier.

It is apparent that management for novelty shock must often undo the damage wrought by others who were on the scene earlier. What parents in novelty shock need first and foremost is gentle, undramatic interpretation of the facts, provided in an atmosphere of maximal emotional support. Reading matter and audio-visual devices might be highly useful. Also, interpretation should stress those elements which are realistically positive, such as the positive aspects of likely child development and the availability or expected availability of services and resources. To cope with their grief, parents should be helped to get to know fellow parents who have experienced similar traumas and who have made model adjustments. Where a newborn baby is involved, management should not terminate when the mother leaves the hospital but should continue as needed.

In order to be able to provide facts and information to the parents, it is necessary to assess the condition of the child. However, a comprehensive assessment may be neither possible nor desirable at that time: on the one hand, recognition of certain clinical syndromes permits one to make a number of probability statements about the child; on the other hand, since parental novelty shock occurs almost invariably either at the child's birth or during his first years, one must postpone many judgments until one has had the opportunity to see the child respond to environmental conditions and services.

Thus, it is important to incorporate into the fact-oriented management approach a reasonable balance of caution, uncertainty, and positive elements. Assessment of the child should not attempt to attain a certainty that is not attainable at that time; instead, assessment must be viewed and interpreted as a time-bound process. Such emphasis upon the uncertainty of the future should not be mistaken as merely a device for softening the emotional impact upon the parents; uncertainty is valid even in some very clear-cut and relatively homogeneous syndromes such as Down's and others where occasionally remarkable deviations from typical syndromic expressions may occur.

The benefits of an early, sudden, and somewhat dramatic diagnosis appear to have been greatly exaggerated. Such a "diagnosis-compulsion" on the part of the manager may often be detrimental rather than beneficial (Wolfensberger, 1965a, 1965b).

From the literature, it appears that parents in novelty shock tend to become very inward-directed, usually in a selfish and self-pitying manner. Successful adaptation often requires that the parent broaden his concerns to the spouse and the child. Thus, management that emphasizes future assessment of the child's progress can help the parent to move from a helpless, disordered dependency to a more adaptive concern about maximizing the child's development. One might say that it is better for the parent to move toward a reality stress situation than to remain in novelty shock.

The novelty shock reaction is likely to be well circumscribed and definable, and the management implications tend to be rather clear. However, such reactions—though perhaps memorable because of the extremity of parental response—are relatively rare. In a few instances, an unexpectedly atypical child is born and recognized at birth. In a few other cases, a child is suddenly recognized as significantly atypical sometime after birth. But in the vast majority of cases, recognition comes mercifully slow or some events prior to or associated with pregnancy have sensitized the parent to the possibility that the infant may be atypical.

Reality Stress

Even to rear a child that is gifted, healthy, and beautiful is a tremendously demanding task, and we can see everywhere in the world around us how easy it is for relatively normal adults to fail in the task of rearing children who initially at least were rather typical infants. We therefore should realize that the task of rearing an atypical child is very likely to constitute such a demand that typical parents cannot be expected to manage adequately without being provided with extraordinary resources and services.

It is to be expected that parents of retarded children will increasingly present themselves to human managers such as psychiatrists and to human management agencies such as psychiatric clinics in search of help. While the parents may display signs of stress and occasionally even psychopathology, we must recognize that such symptoms may be no more than normative reactions to situational stress. It is important to realize that crises or conflicts due to excessive reality demands are essentially normal and are only to a limited degree under the control of the parents.

Psychiatric management of families of the retarded has sometimes ignored the realistic burdens associated with rearing an atypical child and instead has tended to be preoccupied with parental psychopathology. Indeed, in the literature one can find endless examples where parents are stereotyped as guilty, rejecting, unaccepting, where they are viewed as "the patient," and where excessive faith is placed on therapeutically oriented counseling rather than on education or provision of concrete relief measures. The physical demands made by a hyperactive child can rarely be handled by counseling alone, and the demands of caring for three children still in diapers are not lightened by probing the mother's anal fixations and deep-seated feelings about feces. If any kind of counseling for such a mother is appropriate, it is of the type that introduces her to operant behavior shaping, but a didactic approach accompanied by home visits would probably be optimal.

All professionals who participate in the management of families of the retarded should be sensitive to the temptation to provide management that might be provided better by others. Instead of maintaining management dominance while doing something that they have been trained to do but that is irrelevant in the specific case, a management professional would do better to act as an effective advocate or aggressive referral and follow-up agent in seeing to it that somebody will provide the management that is appropriate and needed in a given case.

Measures of major and most poignant relevance to the relief of situational burdens are the following: concrete and direct services, such as obtaining acceptance of a child in a day-care or special education program or inclusion of an adult in a vocational training or sheltered-work program; seeing to it that homemaker, visiting nurse, or home economist services are initiated; getting the family enrolled in appropriate clinics and health services; initiating casework to obtain public assistance for which the family may be eligible; exercising advocacy functions to safeguard rights and prevent exploitation, especially of the poor and disadvantaged; providing the family with education in regard to problems of child care, especially feeding, dressing, and toileting the handicapped child; providing the family with equipment (perhaps on a loan basis) that facilitates child care or accelerates child development, for example, walkers, standing tables, toilet chairs, feeding aides; helping find competent baby sitters; assisting in arrangements for residential placement; and so on.

Value Conflicts

Clinicians tend to be more adept at tracing individual psychopathology to pathogenic events and patterns in persons' backgrounds than in dealing with the powerful effects of social and subcultural values and attitudes which are transmitted in relatively "normal" fashion and which may rule a person's behavior.

In our society, there are many perceptions and interpretations of mental retardation that have been transmitted to us from the past. We must recall that, by definition, retardation is a deviancy. In other words, retarded persons are significantly different from others, and in our society the difference is generally negatively valued. Thus, common historical role perceptions of the retardate have included the retardate as a menace, as subhuman (animal-like or even vegetative), as an object of ridicule, and as an object of pity (Wolfensberger, 1969a). Some role perceptions have been more common in some of our subcultures than others. For instance, Catholics appear to be more accepting of retardation than Protestants or Jews, and Hutterites are so accepting that they will not institutionalize any retarded member of their community (Eaton and Weil, 1955; Farber, 1959, 1960b; Kramm, 1963; Stone and Parnicky, 1965; Zuk, 1959; Zuk et al., 1961).

Many well-known books and articles written by parents of retarded children (for example, Abraham, 1958; Buck, 1950; Frank, 1952; Gant, 1957; Junker, 1964; Logan, 1962; Rogers, 1953; Stout, 1959) strongly reflect value conflicts and both adaptive and maladaptive ways of responding. There have been numerous reports of parents who were well equipped with intelligence and resources who found themselves blocked by inner value conflicts from raising or relating to their retarded children; other families have struggled hard against poverty and situational burdens and managed to succeed in raising retarded children to productive citizenship.

It follows from the above that many parents must have conflicts about a retarded child not because the child is an extraordinary burden of care but because they intensely disvalue the meaning (Ryckman and Henderson, 1965) which the child represents. Thus, a value conflict is a very subjective thing but no less real or necessarily less stressful to one family than the burdens of care are to another.

A parental value conflict may result in various degrees of emotional and physical rejection of the retardate. When mild, it may be manifested by ambivalence and overprotection; when severe it is inclined to eventuate in the child being discarded—usually by means of institutionalization—and perhaps even in his existence being completely denied. Unless a parent is exposed to existential management experiences or spontaneously undergoes existential growth experience during the course of his life, the value conflict is likely to last a lifetime.

Appropriate existential management may include psychotherapy, but other measures may be more effective as well as efficient. One of these is counseling that is not oriented toward psychodynamics and unresolved childhood fixations but toward the meaning of life and its ultimate values. Various schools of existential thought specialize in this type of counseling, for example, the school of logotherapy.

Another and very underutilized measure is religious counseling. Much, of course, depends on the selection of an appropriate pastoral or religious counselor, but most religions permit multiple positive interpretations of a retarded child (for example, Eaton and Weil, 1955; Hoffman, 1965; Zuk, 1959). Some persons, though actively involved in a religion or church, are not aware of these interpretations. However, a person is likely to accept them when exposed to them in the proper context because these interpretations, although perhaps inconsistent with other values he may hold, are consistent with the large and deeply meaningful values and beliefs that are mediated by his religion.

The rationale for a third measure of assisting parents of retarded children was apparently first fully elaborated by Weingold and Hormuth (1953). They pointed out that since value conflicts are mediated by a process of socialization involving various groupings of society, a very promising management should be group-derived resocialization. While group techniques had been used earlier, Weingold and Hormuth were the first to present a truly systematic rationale for the use of group counseling with parents experiencing conflicts in attitudes.

If this rationale is valid—and it has much face validity—congregational support should be one of the most powerful management options because it can combine group-mediated resocialization with adaptive religious interpretation. Congregational support implies that a parish, church, or church group show its acceptance —or continued acceptance—of a family with a retarded child in a

TABLE 20-1

A Theoretical Framework for the Management of Parents of the Retarded

	SOURCES OF PARENTAL MANAGEMENT NEEDS		
	NOVELTY SHOCK	VALUE CONFLICT	REALITY STRESS
Normative initial parental responses	Confusion Disorganization Helplessness Dependency Anguish Anger	Profound existential pain and insult to ego Ambivalence about acceptance of facts	Stress symptoms Deterioration of health Family tension
Management needs	Immediate supportive counseling to realign expectancies Medical-diagnostic interpretations that are realistic yet focus on positive developmental expectancies Preparation of parents for planning and utilization of services Provision of societal and peer support, as by referral to parent groups	Existential type of therapy or counseling (for example, pastoral counseling) Resocialization, as with group counseling, congregational support Finding a niche for the child in the parental value system Exposure of parents to models of positive conflict resolution, as in the parent movement	Correct assessment of reality-based family needs Knowledge of and rapid provision of concrete services that relieve situational demands
Adaptive parental adjustments	Acceptance of reality factors Seeking or acceptance of guidance Realignment of expectations and plans	Resolution of existential parental quandary Value change Investment of value in the child Empathy for the child	Search for resources Utilization of resources Participation in the creation of needed resources and services Placement of child outside the home where appropriate
Maladaptive parental adjustments	Rejection of child Inappropriate discarding of child Precipitous institutionalization Denial of reality Surrender to irrational guilt Conflicted management of child Withdrawal Irrational affixing of blame	Rejection of child Inappropriate institutionalization Denial of child or his condition Severe and continued ambivalence Shopping for invalid diagnoses and cures Reaction formation Conflicted management of child Sense of unfulfillment Chronic sorrow Prolonged emotional disorder	Rejection of child Premature separation from child Unnecessary institutionalization Family dissolution Passive surrender to situational demands

number of ways, both large and small. This would include friendly and frequent socialization with the family, offers of baby-sitting and other assistance, active expression of interest by the pastor, and so on. A major manifestation of congregational support would be the operation of Sunday School classes or day-care services for retarded children, with active voluntary participation on the part of church members.

There are, of course, other alternatives. The important thing for the manager is to understand the principles and processes involved in a value conflict and then to invoke management alternatives flexibly, creatively, and in ways which take account of local and specific circumstances.

In Table 20–1, we have summarized the theoretical framework in regard to the sources of management needs. Some normative behaviors of parents in novelty shock, in value conflict, or under reality stresses are listed; some major management measures for each of the three sources of management needs are given; and positive and negative parental adjustments are indicated. We will now proceed to present a management strategy that is based on this management framework, and that provides practical guidance in individual cases.

PROGRAMMING THE MANAGEMENT PROCESS

We propose that family managers explore a general strategy of management which appears to have high parsimony and to be consistent with decision theory by exploring and meeting family-management needs in a rank order of immediacy of the problems, by minimizing superfluous or irrelevant assessments, and by investing management options selectively so as to maximize the probability of their effectiveness. This strategy involves three stages, which will be discussed below and which are summarized in Fig. 20–1.

Stage 1

Immediately upon referral, the manager should ascertain whether the parents appear to be experiencing novelty shock. If so, emotional support as well as information, education, facts, and reading matter should be provided, and the child's condition should be interpreted in a way that places a realistic emphasis on positive developmental expectations and resources likely to be available in the future. Also,

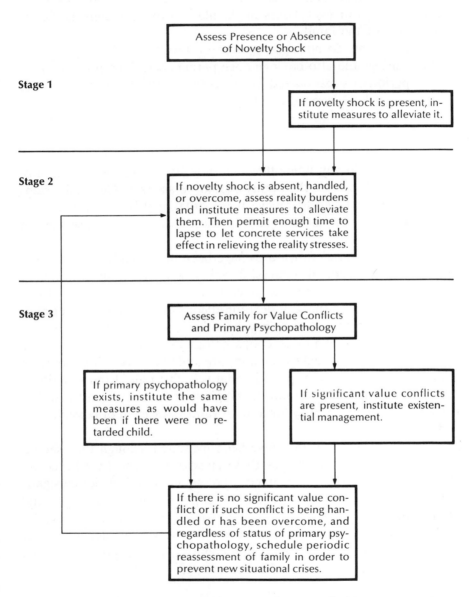

Stage 1

Assess Presence or Absence of Novelty Shock

If novelty shock is present, institute measures to alleviate it.

Stage 2

If novelty shock is absent, handled, or overcome, assess reality burdens and institute measures to alleviate them. Then permit enough time to lapse to let concrete services take effect in relieving the reality stresses.

Stage 3

Assess Family for Value Conflicts and Primary Psychopathology

If primary psychopathology exists, institute the same measures as would have been if there were no retarded child.

If significant value conflicts are present, institute existential management.

If there is no significant value conflict or if such conflict is being handled or has been overcome, and regardless of status of primary psychopathology, schedule periodic reassessment of family in order to prevent new situational crises.

FIGURE 20–1   *A Suggested Approach to Family Management*

joining of the parent movement should be encouraged, and the necessary names, addresses, phone numbers, brochures, and so on should be provided. Such help should be delivered as speedily as possible; a matter of days or even hours might make a difference in the future life course of the family.

If the parents do not appear to be in novelty shock, stage 2 is invoked; this should also be done once parents pass from novelty shock into a period of stress caused by awareness of the realistic burdens of caring for a handicapped child.

Stage 2

For parents in any state other than novelty shock, the realistic situational demands upon the family should be assessed. Generally, steps should then be taken to relieve these situational burdens. This may imply a number of measures such as those discussed in the section on reality stress.

Until concrete relief measures have been instituted in order to alleviate the immediacy of a stressful reality, it is ordinarily senseless to be concerned with problems of real or suspected psychopathology. Here, it is useful to think in decision-theory terms: alleviation of reality demands might alleviate psychopathology, no matter whence its source, but alleviation of psychopathology might be either impossible or of little benefit if reality demands are still excessive. Thus, concrete and direct measures that provide relatively fast relief from situational stresses not only may accomplish the greatest benefits at least cost, but also may open up the way for a more valid assessment of possible psychopathology.

Once concrete measures have been instituted, enough time should be permitted to lapse so that those stresses that can be relieved by these measures may have a chance to dissipate or at least lessen significantly. During this time, it can be expected that those signs and symptoms of family stress that can reasonably be assumed to have resulted from the situational demands will dissipate enough to permit the assessment of more deep-seated conflicts. At this point, it is time to move to the third stage of management.

Stage 3

Once it is reasonably certain that the parents are no longer in novelty shock and that the family has found some relief from the burdens of a demanding reality, the time is optimal to assess the following:

"primary psychopathology," that is, problems of personal adjustment which may be aggravated by the presence of a retarded family member but which basically have their origin elsewhere; and personal and social values and attitudes relative to retardation which interfere with adaptive behavior.

Primary psychopathology can be managed much as it would be if the retarded family member were not retarded. Value conflicts would be managed as indicated in the earlier section on value conflicts.

General Remarks about the Management Cycle

No matter what problems existed, what management was conducted, or what results were obtained, families should be scheduled for periodic reassessments. Novelty shock due to retardation is almost always a nonrecurring event of short duration. Value crises tend to be long-term, but once resolved they are not likely to again become a major source of conflict. However, reality demands are likely to move from cycle to cycle and from crisis to crisis as the retarded child and his family pass through various developmental life stages. Thus, reassessment should be oriented primarily toward situational stresses. Reassessment may take place at regular intervals or during those developmental phases most likely to be fraught with stress. At any rate, we predict that management of families will increasingly be perceived, not as a one-shot effort, but as a life-long process. We will probably see the development of services and service delivery systems more appropriate to such a conceptualization than exist at present (Dybwad, 1969; Nirje, 1969; Wolfensberger, 1969b).

One often hears the cliché that assessment should be a continuing process. From the above, it is obvious that assessment of family functioning is an integral part of the management cycle. One can thus question the meaningfulness of the present custom of conducting the most comprehensive assessment prior to the provision of significant amounts of services. The argument is often advanced that it takes a thorough assessment in order to determine the need for any type of service. We believe this view to be erroneous. Many families are under such obvious environmental stress that needed relief measures can be identified by any intelligent citizen who has a general familiarity with available resources. Perhaps the initial evaluation should be more modest in extent, attempting mostly to ascertain existence of novelty shock, the extent to which the child's condition warrants concern about the future, and the needs for immediate, stress-relieving services. More extensive or at least additive assessments can then be conducted later after concrete services have been initiated, after the crisis atmosphere has dissipated, and after the parents have become more oriented toward problem-solving by means of service utilization.

Most important, the predictive function of assessment probably should be greatly de-emphasized. Instead, assessment of the child should be used more to help select the optimal developmental services and to measure the apparent response to such services. Such a reconceptualization would not only be more practical but would also help in shifting parental concern away from an unpredictable and often distorted view of the future, which is likely to create a feeling of impotence and hopelessness, and toward the generation, obtaining, and utilization of services which have immediate relevance. By intimately tying a theory of parental stress dynamics to a strategy of assessment and management, we feel that we can more confidently answer the old question: Assessment for what?

During any stage of the management cycle, great care should be exercised in the use of referrals to other agencies. Often, such referrals constitute unconscious defensive maneuvers on the part of a human manager or an entire agency and may start a family on the run-about circuit. If referrals appear to be indicated, they should be accompanied by aggressive follow-through on the part of the referring manager or agency until it is ascertained that appropriate services are being provided from another source, or until a conscious and deliberate decision has been reached to terminate or suspend management. Too often, management is not terminated by a conscious decision but is permitted to "fizzle out" and casually drop out of awareness. [3]

CONCLUSION

The provision of services to the families of the retarded can be justified by pointing to three potential beneficiaries of such services. First, there is the retarded person himself, whose life course can be profoundly affected by the services he receives. Often, the only way to help him and to insure that services rendered to him are not wasted is by working with and through the family. Second, services may provide significant or even crucial assistance to members of the family so that they (singly or as a unit) can function in a relatively normal or at least adequate fashion. Third, society itself benefits by preventing individual and family disorganization or the need for even more costly services later.

In this chapter we have presented a broad concept of management, a highly selective literature review, and a theory proposing that management needs of families of the retarded are found in three major phenomena: novelty shock, value conflicts, and reality stresses. We have then proposed a practical management strategy which encompasses a cycle of assessments, decisions, and service provisions.

N O T E S

1. The writing of this chapter was supported by United States Public Health Service Grant No. HD 00370 from the National Institute of Child Health and Human Development, and by Project No. 405 of the United States Children's Bureau, Department of Health, Education, and Welfare.
2. A collection of edited and interpreted key readings in the field (Wolfensberger and Kurtz, 1969) is intended to serve, together with the 1967 review, as a supradisciplinary text on management of families of the retarded.
3. For discussion of some questionable assumptions and practices involving the assessment and referral of families of the retarded, the reader may wish to refer to Wolfensberger (1965*a*, 1965*b*).

R E F E R E N C E S

Abraham, W. *Barbara: A prologue.* New York: Rinehart & Company, Inc., 1958.

Aldrich, C. A. Preventive medicine and mongolism. *Amer. J. Ment. Defic.*, 1947, *52*, 127–129.

Baum, M. H. Some dynamic factors affecting family adjustment to the handicapped child. *Except. Child.*, 1962, *28*, 387–392.

Beddie, A., & Osmond, H. Mothers, mongols and mores. *Canad. Med. Assoc. J.*, 1955, *73*, 167–170.

Buck, P. *The child who never grew.* New York: John Day, 1950.

Cohen, P. C. The impact of the handicapped child on the family. *Soc. Casework*, 1962, *43*, 137–142.

Dalton, J., & Epstein, H. Counseling parents of mildly retarded children. *Soc. Casework*, 1963, *44*, 523–530.

Dybwad, G. Action implications, U. S. A. today. In: R. Kugel & W. Wolfensberger (Eds.), *Changing patterns in residential services for the mentally retarded.* Washington: President's Committee on Mental Retardation, 1969, pp. 383–428.

Eaton, J. W., & Weil, R. J. *Culture and mental disorders: a comparative study of the Hutterites and other populations.* Glencoe, Ill.: Free Press, 1955.

Farber, B. Effects of a severely mentally retarded child on family integration. *Monogr. Soc. Res. Child Develop.*, 1959, *24*(2).

Farber, B. Perceptions of crisis and related variables and the impact of a retarded child on the mother. *J. Health Human Behav.*, 1960, *1*, 108–118. (*a*)

Farber, B. Family organization in crisis: Maintenance of integration in families with a severely mentally retarded child. *Monogr. Soc. Res. Child Develop.*, 1960, *25*(1). (*b*)

Frank, J. P. *My son's story.* New York: Alfred A. Knopf, Inc., 1952.

Gant, S. *One of those: The progress of a mongoloid child.* New York: Pageant, 1957.

Goodman, L. Continuing treatment of parents with congenitally defective infants. *Soc. Work*, 1964, *9*(1), 92–97.

Hoffman, J. L. Mental retardation, religious values, and psychiatric universals. *Amer. J. Psychiat.*, 1965, *121*, 885–889.

Holt, K. S. Home care of severely retarded children. *Pediatrics*, 1958, *22*, 744–755.

Junker, K. S. *The child in the glass ball*. New York: Abingdon Press, 1964.

Kramm, E. R. Families of mongoloid children. Washington: U. S. Government Printing Office, 1963.

Logan, H. My child is mentally retarded. *Nurs. Outlook*, 1962, *10*, 445–448.

McDonald, E. T. *Understand those feelings*. Pittsburgh: Stanwix House, 1962.

Nirje, B. The normalization principle and its human management implications. In: R. Kugel & W. Wolfensberger (Eds.), *Changing patterns in residential services for the mentally retarded*. Washington: President's Committee on Mental Retardation, 1969, pp. 179–195.

Olshansky, S. Chronic sorrow: A response to having a mentally defective child. *Soc. Casework*, 1962, *43*, 190–193.

Olshansky, S. Parent responses to a mentally defective child. *Ment. Retard.*, 1966, *4*(4), 21–23.

Owens, C. Parents' reactions to defective babies. *Amer. J. Nursing*, 1964, *64*(11), 83–86.

Rogers, D. E. *Angel unaware*. Westwood, N. J.: Fleming H. Revell, 1953.

Roos, P. Psychological counseling with parents of retarded children. *Ment. Retard.*, 1963, *1*, 345–350.

Ryckman, D. B., & Henderson, R. A. The meaning of a retarded child for his parents: A focus for counselors. *Ment. Retard.*, 1965, *3*(4), 4–7.

Solnit, A. J., & Stark, M. H. Mourning and the birth of a defective child. *Psychoanal. Stud. Child*, 1961, *16*, 523–537.

Stone, N. D., & Parnicky, J. J. Factors associated with parental decisions to institutionalize mongoloid children. *Training School Bull.*, 1965, *61*, 163–172.

Stout, L. *I reclaimed my child*. Philadelphia, Pa.: Chilton, 1959.

Thurston, J. R. Counseling the parents of the severely handicapped. *Except. Child.*, 1960, *26*, 351–354.

Tisza, V. B. Management of the parents of the chronically ill child. *Amer. J. Orthopsychiat.*, 1962, *32*, 53–59.

Tizard, J., & Grad, J. C. *The mentally handicapped and their families: A social survey*. London: Oxford University Press, 1961.

Waskowitz, C. H. The parents of retarded children speak for themselves. *J. Pediat.*, 1959, *54*, 319–329.

Weingold, J. T., & Hormuth, R. P. Group guidance of parents of mentally retarded children. *J. Clin. Psychol.*, 1953, *9*, 118–124.

Wolfensberger, W. Embarrassments in the diagnostic process. *Ment. Retard.*, 1965, *3* (3), 29–31. (*a*)

———. Diagnosis diagnosed. *J. Ment. Subnormal.*, 1965, *11*, 62–70. (*b*)

———. Counseling the parents of the retarded. In: A. A. Baumeister (Ed.), *Mental retardation: appraisal, education, and rehabilitation*. Chicago, Ill.: Aldine Press, 1967, pp. 329–400.

———. The origin and nature of our institutional models. In: R. Kugel and W. Wolfensberger (Eds.), *Changing patterns in residential services for the mentally retarded*. Washington: President's Committee on Mental Retardation, 1969, pp. 59–171. (*a*)

———. A new approach to decision-making in human management services. In: R. Kugel and W. Wolfensberger (Eds.), *Changing patterns in residential services for the mentally retarded*. Washington: President's Committee on Mental Retardation, 1969, pp. 367–381. (*b*)

Wolfensberger, W., & Kurtz, R. A. (Eds.), *Management of the families of the mentally retarded: A book of readings*. Chicago: Follett, 1969.

Zuk, G. H. The religious factor and the role of guilt in parental acceptance of the retarded child. *Amer. J. Ment. Defic.*, 1959, *64*, 139–147.

Zuk, G. H., Miller, R. L., Bartram, J. B., & Kling, F. Maternal acceptance of retarded children: A questionnaire study of attitudes and religious background. *Child Develop.*, 1961, *32*, 525–540.

Zwerling, I. Initial counseling of parents with mentally retarded children. *J. Pediat.*, 1954, *44*, 469–479.

: 21 :

A Shift of Emphasis for Psychiatric Social Work in Mental Retardation

Marjorie C. Mackinnon and Barbara S. Frederick

INTRODUCTION

AS more psychiatric hospitals and clinics now include services to the mentally retarded and their families, it becomes imperative for social workers to identify the characteristic differences that may exist between parents of emotionally disturbed children and parents of mentally retarded children. In the light of these probable differences, there is a need to re-examine and modify social-work skills in order to more effectively provide services for the latter group of parents. There have been serious repercussions when many of the skills, knowledge, and techniques proven appropriate for work with the families of the emotionally disturbed have been presumed applicable to families of the mentally retarded.

With the recent increase in concern for the problem of mental retardation and the concomitant refinement of skills, there has been a lag in conceptualizing such specific skills into communicable terms. The preponderance of literature on mental retardation relates to the retardate and the family in terms of range of incidence, causative factors, social, cultural, and economic aspects. However, there seems to be a dearth of material focusing on the qualification of the helping professions for providing effective services for this unique population. Therefore, this will be our primary concern: to describe the distinguishing characteristics of families of the mentally retarded, and then to discuss the demand for the professional person to shift his emphasis from other aspects of mental health in ways that will be adaptive and appropriate for families of the mentally retarded. In large measure this will represent a distillation of repeated comments from the parents themselves derived from their experiences with a range of medical and para-medical persons in their quest for meaningful help.

DEVELOPMENTAL OVERVIEW

Until recently the primary source of help for families with retarded children has had to come, not from professionally trained persons who are knowledgeable in human behavior and family dynamics, but instead from the parents of the retarded themselves. Mental retardation was one of the few significant social problem areas in which there were no institutionalized supports in the form of community resources and few professional experts who understood and dealt with their problems. There was no visible effort to educate a misinformed and often rejecting public. It must remain a tribute to these parents and an indictment of neglect of the helping professions that the initial thrust for concern for the mentally retarded generated from these parent groups, the origins of which now exist as the National Association for Retarded Children (N.A.R.C.). From these vocal parent groups have come pertinent suggestions to professionals on how best to utilize their skills and knowledge. They stressed the importance of their need, as parents, to be viewed within the context of their own individual problem framework and not as an extension of another clinically identified group, namely, parents of emotionally disturbed children. Although similarities between these two groups certainly do exist, their particular characteristics must be differentiated.

Emotional Disturbance versus Mental Retardation

One basic assumption in the diagnosis of an emotionally disturbed child is that this child, identified as the "patient," was born without physical or emotional problems and in the course of living within this family system has become emotionally ill. An inescapable difference is immediately apparent in the birth of a mentally retarded child, regardless of when in this development this congenital difference becomes evident, namely, that this problem was introduced *into* the family system rather than resulting *from* the system itself.

Although it is elementary to explore the parent-child, parent-parent, and intra-familial relationships to understand causative factors and to assess strengths and probable sources of infection in the treatment process for emotionally disturbed children, this approach, in this form, is not qualitatively applicable to families of mentally retarded children. The initial focus with parents of a retarded child should shift from one of causation (environmental) to an assessment of the accommodation efforts this family system has made and is making in coping with an introduced stress. This basic difference precludes such premature and unwarranted procedures as viewing the parents of a mentally retarded child as requiring therapeutic programming in response to their request for a limited and realistic service.

It has been our repeated observation at Kennedy Child Study Center and U.C.L.A. Neuropsychiatric Institute that parents have deeply resented, in prior clinical encounters, having their request for information or service shunted into a treatment situation for them. Social workers in psychiatric settings are sensitized to requests from parents of emotionally disturbed children often masking the "real message" which is frequently one of help for themselves. Conversely, parents of mentally retarded children who have experienced having their request for a limited service deflected into premature or intrusive therapy have been universally resentful of this practice. They have been most vocal in their resistance to an intrusion into their feelings and defenses, with the common assumption of guilt, rejection, or hostility. This distinction does not suggest, however, that some parents of mentally retarded children could not benefit from and may, in fact, be asking for therapeutic services for themselves. Such services, of course, should be offered.

We do suggest that the responsibility for distinguishing a request for therapy from a request for information falls upon the diagnostic skill of the professional person. An emotionally disturbed child cannot be treated in a vacuum without the involvement and participation of his parents in order to effect some changes within his environment to enhance his growth. This is a consequence of the emotionally disturbed child emanating from a family system. However, the coping devices of parents with a mentally retarded child may be capable of making a maximum accommodation, and thus they require only factual information for guidance at various life stages. In most instances they can best utilize a partnership with a professional team for on-going intermittent contacts as different life stages of their child present new problems, needs, or resources. As the life-task of the child changes, from preschool to school, or from school to work, the parents often require the knowledge and support of the professional team in order to accomplish a smoother transition from one stage to another.

The Initial Task of the Social Worker

Perhaps the initial task of the social worker who contemplates entering the field of mental retardation should be to examine his own feelings about this commitment and his reaction to mental retardation. Professionals often have deep-rooted attitudes toward defects and intellectual handicaps; these are obliquely transmitted to parents in the form of overobjectivity to maintain distance from the problem or an excessive empathy that belies a personal disdain.

One outstanding characteristic of parents of the mentally retarded is an acute sensitivity to the reactions their child arouses in professional persons as well as others. Often their ears and hearts have been assaulted by professionals using words such as "guilt," "rejection," and "hostility" which, they say, usually betray the attitudes of the therapist rather than accurately reflect parental feelings. It has been our impression that parents of a retarded child describe a deep sense of responsibility, which is not a euphemism for guilt, but rather encompasses the total concept of the child's prolonged and often chronic dependency. Parents report their deep resentment when a professional person makes an interpretation of guilt, and this suggests to them that the professional person has made some kind of judgment regarding their contribution to the existence of the problem. It may be professionally seductive to attempt to work with these feelings, but the temptation is fraught with dangers.

The social worker who is new to this particular problem area will be confronted with his own feelings in working with an irreversible diagnosis, a chronic sorrow that pervades parents as they attempt to cope with an unending dependency. This field requires infinite patience on the part of the social worker to hear and to rehear a chronology of probable causes, probable solutions, and a reporting of a child's newest accomplishment that is often a thinly disguised plea for a more promising prognosis. The social worker needs to be patient with infinitesimal gains over the years and then help to communicate this need for patience to the parents. Unless the professional person achieves a measure of personal comfort in working with an irreversible defect, content with small gains over an extended period of time, he can be most effective by *not* working in the field of mental retardation.

Parents of the retarded have most often experienced nonhelpful to profoundly negative encounters with prior professional persons and agencies, so that it is important that social workers acknowledge these reality-based complaints without becoming defensive. Often there exists an "esprit de corps" among professionals that denies the probability of nonhelpful colleagues. The complaints of parents of emotionally disturbed children might realistically suggest to the therapist that this could represent neurotic resistance, denial, projection, and may raise the question of treatability. Here again, there exists the need to shift the emphasis from one group to another and to be aware that, as a group, parents of the retarded have experienced both isolation and rejection. If they are angry and guarded initially, this could hardly be neurotic. Parents repeatedly report experiences of having their problem met with a stampeding for placement, or have heard professional jargon that mystified rather than clarified. The comment "I know how you feel" suggests to them that they are, in fact, isolated and not understood. It is safer to assume, at least initially, that the negative encounters they report are realistic and unfortunate, and that a certain defensiveness may exist until they are assured of acceptance. This is a time when the parents are taking measure of the social worker as a potentially helpful or nonhelpful person, and they may be unduly guarded and defensive in the early stages of a diagnosis. This period may be exaggerated or extended if their child is more seriously or conspicuously handicapped.

Social workers are aware of a continuing need to avoid stereotyping in their work with parents of the emotionally disturbed. We frequently find that clinical terms, such as "overprotective mothers" and "passive fathers," gradually become judgmental in their connotations. The injunction to resist stereotyping is crucial in work with parents of the retarded. There is a popular label of "shopper" used with these parents, as if this were an indictment of untreatability. Shopping may well represent a healthy pursuit for help with a mystifying problem. It can be a reality-based response to negative experiences with professionals who may have held out vague but unrealistic hope, *or* who may have responded with indirectness that disguises the many unknown dimensions of retardation, *or* who may have been insensitive to the disproportionate length of time parents need to really *hear* verdicts.

It is typical for parents to require an inordinate amount of time to incorporate the impact of the diagnosis and to work toward some measure of "acceptance." Many of the special skills of the professional person will be called upon at the time the diagnosis is related to the parents, and the degree of skill and sensitivity can contribute to a reduction in "shopping." For instance, during the diagnostic phase, we have found it essential to include *both* parents as historians and to

assess these architects of the family as well as the siblings. Historically, the focus has been primarily on the mother, but the exclusion of
the father can do violence to the design of a therapeutic partnership
intended to exist over an extended period of time. Diagnostic findings
are seldom revelations to parents, but rather dreaded suspicions that
are validated. Most sensitive parents have been increasingly aware
that "something was wrong" and that the pediatrician's reassurances
that "he will outgrow it" have corroded over a period of time.

Parents need to clearly understand the terminology and the implications of medical terms and what medical science can and *cannot*
do. They need to know what to expect in both short- and long-range
terms, what caused the condition if this is known, such as Rubella
syndrome, and whether it is safe to have more children. Routinely
parents require another appointment soon after the diagnosis to rehear the findings, as well as to raise questions that occurred when the
initial impact subsided.

Thus the same behavior, that of "shopping," will have distinctly
different diagnostic meanings for these two parent groups, suggestive
of a healthy concern in parents of the mentally retarded and suggestive of questionable treatability in parents of emotionally disturbed
children.

THE DIAGNOSTIC PERIOD

During the diagnostic period, a time when history-taking is a routine
procedure, emphasis must shift again to a more detailed investigation
regarding the pregnancy, delivery, and the developmental landmarks.
Generally, parents of the retarded have experienced this process often,
and the professional person should be aware that parents are keenly
attuned to guilt-provoking questions of attitudes. A skilled and sensitive social worker can elicit the affectual climate and the strengths
and weaknesses of the coping mechanisms of the family, including the
responses of the siblings. This period affords an opportunity to assess
the role the retarded child plays within the family, from one of omnipotent to one of scapegoat. When possible it is important to learn
about the existence of an extended family, particularly grandparents,
who may be resources or deterrents both for the child and the parents.

Often during these initial contacts with the parents there will be an
indication of how well the marital relationship has sustained the impact of a retarded child. That is, it can be learned whether the parents

are able to provide support for one another or whether the birth of this child has proved a greater stress than the marriage can tolerate. Within different cultural groups the impact of a retarded child assumes greater proportions, the sex and sibling order are significant considerations, and the maternal and paternal expectations of a child and their differing disappointment may be apparent. It will be most important to identify where a particular family falls on the social, economic, and cultural scale, as these factors play a significant part in the family's capacity to accommodate a retarded child, as well as being an indication of their reference group as predictably supportive or excluding. For instance, a well-educated upper-middle-class family can accept an emotionally disturbed child with less stress than they can a mentally retarded child, with differential support from their reference group. In the upper-middle-class family, with its inherent emphasis on intellectual achievement and material success, the limited child is a more conspicuous deviation, and the impact of his problem may represent a more severe detriment to family functioning. In a lower-middle-class family there may be more acceptance of a limited work-training program with less difficulty adjusting to more practical aspects in an educational program. But lower-middle-class families have understanding of causation and a decreased ability to work within the long-range framework of clinical goals. Cultural and religious factors will enter into parental attitudes toward defects, particularly in reference to causation and superstitions. An assessment of these factors will be important ingredients in establishing an effective program for both the parents and the child.

FAMILY THERAPY

To achieve an effective diagnostic and treatment program, two techniques which prove useful in work with parents of an emotionally disturbed child are most adaptable, with certain modifications, for families with a retarded child. First, the diagnostic family interview, including the siblings, provides an opportunity to view the interaction of the family with and around the retarded member to discern attitudes, responses, and alliances. Siblings often provide an accurate barometer of the family cohesiveness in coping with a deviant family member, the potential sources of strength as well as their ability to illuminate potential weaknesses.

Second, family therapy, which may or may not include siblings, is readily adaptable for families with a retarded child. This not only emphasizes the importance of each member in problem-solving, but it can operate to document and validate each person's contribution in positive directions, away from causation and toward resolutions. Family therapy may afford permission to express many of the negative feelings that are so often aroused in the presence of slow yielding dependency, disproportionate demands and attention, as well as expense. Family therapy can reduce the guilt that siblings experience when they feel angered or embarrassed by a retarded brother or sister and thus help parents accept such feelings in their normal children.

When family therapy is instituted, should this be indicated and acceptable to the particular family, it becomes increasingly evident that the participation of the father is essential. While he plays a significant role in the treatment process with emotionally disturbed children, his presence and involvement as an active team member for a retarded child must be considered crucial. The shift of emphasis to underscore the importance of the father's contribution is based upon the long-range partnership concept for a mentally retarded child.

In many instances the father proves to be the primary source of nurturing and acceptance for the child and his active participation provides a viable support for the mother. In situations where the father may be aloof or excessive in his expectations for the child, then family therapy provides the mother with immeasurable relief as the child's limitations are clarified for the father and she is removed from the position of primary responsibility. As a continuing participant, the father is included in discussions about recommendations for medical or corrective therapies that may represent an on-going expense, and his responses are valued in the formulation of a treatment program. Again, this relieves the mother of becoming the messenger of factual information and medical proposals concerning their child and spares her the conflictual role of notifying the father of ensuing expenses.

As the therapeutic partnership evolves, the parents of a retarded child find reassurance as they anticipate the problems that arise during the various life stages of beginning school, adolescence, sexual maturation, preparation for work roles, social adjustments, and recreational resources. While chronic dependency does, in fact, exist, it can be molified in many instances with the provision of appropriate training programs directed toward increased autonomy. It is, therefore, incumbent upon the professional person to become knowledgeable about existing community resources for the wide range of treatment and training demands the child will present at various life stages in order that he might achieve his maximum potential. With recent Presidential interest in the field of mental retardation, vast funds have been made available for the development and expansion of services, so that many creative and specific resources are coming into existence each year. The professional person must be constantly alert to these new or expanded programs.

THE DILEMMA OF
INSTITUTIONAL PLACEMENT

In the past, the rush for institutional placement often represented an injury rather than a service to parents. Now, in the light of expanding resources for the mentally retarded, it can represent a serious disservice. Even in situations where the initial appraisal suggests that placement will be an ultimate resolution, the recommendation for a placement, except under medical or emotional urgency, is one that should be approached with extreme caution. Parents are usually aware of swings in professional attitudes, from an historic one of placement to the current one of acknowledging the accruing benefits to a child remaining in his home as long as possible. As the partnership between the parents and the professional team evolves, the subject of placement, when indicated, can be discussed in a more benign atmosphere, frequently introduced by the parents themselves. The consideration of placement generates understandably from parental concern to provide protection for their child beyond their own lifetime.

Professionals, however, should be alert to the implications the subject of placement may have to and from parents. Frequently, the subject is introduced by parents as a consequence of realistic desperation. When the care and supervision of a retarded child results in physical and emotional exhaustion, it poses a genuine threat to the timbre of the marriage itself. The lack of day-care facilities for the mentally retarded imposes a constant task of vigilance on the mother that threatens to bankrupt her energies. Family therapy can operate as an equalizer for delegating supervision and responsibility in order to relieve the mother; in this regard the extended family members may make a significant contribution. Placement will be a less guilt-provoking consideration when its primary goal is for the child's immediate and ultimate benefit rather than for the understandable relief of the family. Premature or unwarranted recommendations for placement fail to take into account the contribution the retarded child makes *to* the family, its values and sense of appreciation.

CONCLUSION

The social worker who has achieved the level of maturity and understanding that is required for working in the field of mental retardation will find there are abundant rewards, a richer philosophy, and a deeper appreciation for fundamental values to be gleaned from an association with these parents and their children.

━━━━━━

REFERENCES

Ackerman, N. W., The psychodynamics of family life. New York: Basic Books, 1960.

Adamson, W. C. Ohrenstein, D. F., Lake, D., & Hersh, A. The separation used to help parents promote growth in their retarded child. Soc. Work, 1964, 9, 60–67.

Appell, M. J. Changes in attitudes of parents of retarded children effected through group counseling. Amer. J. Ment. Defic., 1964, 68, 807–815.

Baker, E. M. Diagnostic and treatment services for the mentally retarded child. J. Child Welfare League Amer., 1960, 8, 369–373.

Beck, H. Casework with parents of mentally retarded children. Amer. J. Orthopsychiat., 1962, 32, 870–877.

Begab, M. J. The mentally retarded child: A guide to service of social agencies. Washington, D.C.: U.S. Government Printing Office, 1963.

Caldwell, B. Factors associated with parental reaction to a clinic for retarded children. Amer. J. Ment. Defic., 1961, 65, 590–594.

Cohen, P. C. The impact of the handicapped child on the family. Soc. Casework, 1962, 43, 137–142.

Dalton, J. Counseling parents of mildly retarded children. Soc. Casework, 1963, 44, 523–530.

Hersh, A. Casework with parents of retarded children. Soc. Casework, 1961, 6, 61–66.

Katz, A. Parents of the handicapped. Oxford, England: Blackwell Scientific Publications, 1961.

Kelman, H. R. Social work and mental retardation: Challenge or failure? Soc. Work, 1958, 3, 37–42.

McDonald, E. T. Understanding those feelings. Pittsburgh: Stanwix House, 1962.

Michaels, J., & Schucman, H. Observations on the psychodynamics of parents of retarded children. Amer. J. Ment. Defic., 1962, 66, 568–573.

Murray, M. A. Needs of parents of mentally retarded children. Amer. J. Ment. Defic., 1959, 63, 1078–1088.

Olshansky, S. Chronic sorrow: A response to having a mentally defective child. Soc. Casework, 1962, 43, 190–193.

Parsons, T. The social system. New York: Free Press, 1961.

Patterson, L. Some pointers for professionals. Children, 1956, 3, 13–17.

Rothstein, J. H. (Ed.). Mental retardation-readings and resources. New York: Rinehart & Winston, 1961.

Schild, S. Counseling with parents of retarded children living at home. Soc. Work, 1964, 45, 93–98.

Slaughter, S. S. The mentally retarded child and his parents. New York: Harper, 1963.

Thurston, J. R. Counseling the parents of the severely handicapped. *Except. Child.*, 1960, *26*, 351–354.

Waskowitz, C. H. The parents of the retarded speak for themselves. *J. Pediat.*, 1959, *54*, 319–329.

Wolfensberger, W. (Ed.). Counseling parents of the retarded. In A. A. Baumeister, (Ed.), *Mental retardation*. Chicago; Aldine Press, 1967, pp. 329–401.

Zwerling, I. Initial counseling of parents with mentally retarded children. *J. Pediat.*, 1954, *44*, 469–479.

PART THREE

Challenges to the
Psychiatrist in Current
Service Systems

[A]

CHALLENGES IN COMMUNITY SERVICES

: 22 :

Community Psychiatry and Mental Retardation

Evis Coda

IN the current psychiatric emphasis on community approaches to mentally handicapped individuals, there has been a slowly increasing interest in mental retardation. It is the purpose of this paper to describe the problems and issues in establishing a multidisciplinary community clinic for the retarded. It is hoped that sharing our experiences and results will act as a stimulus to other colleagues in this dynamic area of community endeavor.

GENERAL CONSIDERATIONS

In October of 1963, the 88th Congress enacted Public Law 88-164, a bill entitled, "The Mental Retardation Facilities and Community Mental Health Centers Construction Act." The broad plan implied that many more of the mentally retarded and mentally ill can be successfully treated in their own communities. Its major programs were comprehensive enough to consider a broad range of services to meet the needs of all age groups. Continuity of care, coordination and integration of existing services, and rapid availability of services were also considered to be major focal points of this bill.

In brief, this particular bill spurred the provision of comprehensive community care for the mentally retarded. The program elements were based on the assumption that most mentally retarded individuals can be successfully treated and cared for in their own communities, and this was considered as desirable by and for the individual and his family.

An opportunity to accomplish much for the retarded was ushered in by this history-making bill. However, there were associated problems: How do you start such services? Will they be effective in providing meaningful alternatives to the current scene? How do you include the need for professional training, and research dimensions? Essentially, these and similar questions demanded the thinking through of short-, intermediate-, and long-range goals.

The short-range goals encompass those services that have the highest priority need, while being consistent with future plans. These short-range goals include planning challenges such as the following: identifying available services; providing missing elements of services —integration of services; and coordination of existing programs (via mergers or affiliations). Concurrently, there must be a system of priorities for these services (for example, preschool programs, those patients who are currently receiving partial or no services, and so on). The short-range goals are usually projected over a two year period. They are intimately associated with intermediate goals, which basically consist of setting up three- to five-year priorities and the further development and extension of the short-term goals. At this stage, the introduction of training programs, evaluation of cost for service benefits, current diagnostic methods, and treatment procedures are also of major importance.

Long-range goals are directly concerned with preventative aspects and the provision of a full spectrum of services for retarded persons within the community where they live. These particular goals demand the continuous evaluation of available services to spur innovation toward new program needs and to modify current programs, emphasizing both their effectiveness and efficiency.

We shall now share our own experiences and results in attempting to implement this national legislative mandate to provide services for our mentally retarded fellow citizens.

EVOLUTION OF A COMMUNITY PROGRAM
FOR THE RETARDED

Multidisciplinary programs for the mentally retarded are of recent vintage. Their inception on a national scale, dates back to the early 1950's. Since that time a variety of models of service have been proposed (Pearson, 1965). However, each such program has tended to be specific to its own unique social-political-geographical needs or methods within the geographical-demographic setting of a large metropolitan area.

The Kennedy Child Study Center has been involved in active programming for mentally retarded children and their families for the past eight years. Psychiatric treatment is considered an essential and integral part of the total service program. The Center serves emotionally disturbed, mentally retarded, and neurologically handicapped children from infancy through age seventeen who reside in the greater Los Angeles area. The total program includes a child guidance service, mental retardation diagnostic and counseling services, cerebral palsy and developmental defects clinic, speech and hearing service, and an observational-therapeutic nursery program for multiply handicapped infants and prekindergarten children. An added feature is a clinic school and day-care program which includes a special class for children with minimal cerebral dysfunction and severe learning disabilities. The total professional staff consists of twenty-six full time and nine part-time members. In addition six full-time aides are assigned to the school and day-care program. The disciplines represented include pediatrics, psychiatry, psychology, social work, education, speech pathology and audiology, and occupational, physical, and recreational therapies. Volunteer staff physicians from the nearby St. John's Hospital in the specialities of pediatrics, neurology, opthalmology, otolaryngology, and orthopedics assist the medical staff in the diagnostic evaluation and counseling service. In addition to direct patient services, the Center provides community education and consultation, training, and study programs.

Historically, one of the first services of the Center was that of the Mental Retardation Team, providing active consultation to the Pediatric Outpatient Department of St. John's Hospital. This service was modeled after a similar one which the author helped establish in 1954 for the Pediatric Outpatient Service at Charity Hospital, Louisiana State University. The initial team at the Kennedy Child Study Center consisted of a psychiatrist, psychologist, and social worker offering diagnostic evaluation and planning consultation for emotionally disturbed and mentally retarded children.

In attempting to establish the major focus of our activities, we have formulated guidelines that had meaning to us in relation to the following: the overall research potential available at the Center, in terms of personnel, skills, special interests, and experience; the community needs, including the types of problems presented at the Center, and the available resources; the task assigned to the Center when it was established, which consisted primarily of direct patient service for training and study projects which were to evolve out of the program.

One of the initial steps was to attempt to meet the community needs, as reflected in the community request for service. As previously noted, since we were situated near a general hospital that wanted rapid diagnostic-counseling services in contrast to long waiting lists, we tended to focus on rapid implementation of the report received from the pediatric clinic of the general hospital. During a series of preliminary conferences, we focused on the most perplexing types of cases, for which consultation was sought, and reviewed methods and techniques for rapid intervention.

The next step was to focus on another major community service request: the local school system. A sampling of the initial cases referred from the school revealed a similarity of complaints: the hyperactive child who literally overwhelms the teacher and is disruptive in the classroom; the withdrawn, noncommunicative child; and acting-out behavior (fire-setters) and "typical" neurotic cases. The number of cases referred prompted us to set aside a block of time to focus only on school referrals.

Our referral sample then evolved from the community at large. Essentially, any parent with any problem which was significantly interfering or interrupting the family-school adjustment potentials was included. Also included in this heterogeneous group was the family that was "shopping" for their diagnostic studies or treatment and also children who presented multiproblems in regard to manifestations of their disorders.

The above-noted set of initial experiences of our clinic clarified the major feature goals of our role in the community. (Essentially we decided to focus on the very young as to chronological age, stressing crisis intervention as to rapidity of services, parental counseling, and continuing the attempt to unify our services to both the parents and the community in regard to initiating the "life plan," as described by Murray. For example, it became clear that our diagnostic and therapeutic role in the community would have to be that of a catalyst for those with disturbed behavior, the young mentally retarded child [especially the moderate, and severely retarded], and the multiply handicapped). Diagnostic services, interpretation of such findings to the parents, parental counseling and specific therapeutic prescriptions as to indicated services became the essential ingredients of this unified approach.

INTERMEDIATE PLANS AND
THEIR IMPLEMENTATION

It soon became apparent that there were a number of cases whose problems were such that services beyond that of diagnostic screening and family counseling would be needed. Requests for psychiatric out-patient treatment for mentally retarded children were repeatedly requested of our Center. Prior to establishing this service, a study of other psychotherapy programs for the mentally retarded (including a review of the literature) was accomplished. These studies and reports quite uniformly suggested that psychotherapy with the retarded can be successful, and the reported treatment results generally pointed toward positive changes in personality characteristics and improvements in behavior. A wide variety of treatment modes and orientations have been utilized, ranging from an occasional report of long-term intensive analytical therapy to a more common brief supportive therapy on an individual group basis. Diagnostic categories included any or all of the major and minor psychiatric disturbances, ranging from psychotic reactions to the relative benign adjustments of childhood: some gave results as beneficial and encouraging, others contradictory and inconclusive. Clear-cut criteria for selection of cases or effectiveness of method of treatment were not apparent.

Despite active involvement of our clinic in the above-noted goals and methods, it soon became apparent that a far more active focus on treatment and other techniques of management were needed. For example, a special psychiatric out-patient treatment program was needed for some of the children referred from the pediatric clinic who appeared in need of services beyond diagnostic consultation. This appeared consistent with staff resources, community need, and assigned tasks. The most frequent cases referred were those in which the retardate had an associated minimal cerebral dysfunction of the impulsive-hyperactive type, resulting in a degree of disturbance and disruption within the classroom or on the playground sufficient to result in either limitation of his day at school or, in some cases, complete exclusion from special classes. Other common complaints included severe disruption of the home situation so that placement was requested, disturbance in the neighborhood, including destruction, sexual activity, stealing and continual wandering off.

Individual psychotherapy was scheduled on a once-a-week basis and later scheduled every two to four weeks. The therapeutic approach varied, depending on the ability of child and parent to involve themselves in a meaningful relationship to begin to examine behavior and attitudes and to attempt to modify maladaptive patterns. In this respect, the child and family did not differ markedly from those seen at the child-guidance treatment program for the nonretardate. Psychopharmacological agents were commonly used as adjuncts to therapy, particularly in the persistent, impulsive, hyperactive child.

Currently, less severe emotional problems are seen routinely through the regular guidance program, with increasing utilization of activity group therapy. The majority of children referred and seen are males, ages eight through eleven, within the upper end of the moderate-to-borderline range of intellectual capacity. Those children with anxiety, shyness, constriction of personality, and acknowledged low self-esteem, as reflected in such spontaneous comments as "I'm in a reject class," "Other kids call me a retardo," or "Who would marry me?" are the ones who seem to benefit the most from activity-discussion group therapy.

As an increasing number of requests for similar services have been received from school personnel, private physicians, and parents through our routine admission and intake service, a comparable program was set up for this group the following year. As staff experience and interest increased, other treatment modalities were introduced, so that at present group and family therapy is utilized in addition to individual methods. Our methods have evolved over the last seven years to include the following direct services to patients and their families.

Parent Orientation-Consultation Service

Orientation services, single sessions for six to eight parents, were scheduled as soon as practical after the initial request for service to acquaint parents with the scope of center activities, treatment philosophy and goals, types of problems studied, duration, and costs of service, etc.

Consultation services, single individual services were given immediately following the orientation. Discussion of specific problems, help sought, appropriateness of referral, preliminary background information, decision made to continue at center or seek appropriate referral elsewhere.

Intake Interviews

These consisted of one to three interviews in which parents were seen individually or conjointly. Further exploration was made of problems and background information—family, social, and school history. Information from outside sources was obtained and reviewed (reports from family physicians, school, previous studies).

Diagnostic Studies

These studies consisted of two or three individual or conjoint interviews of the following: parents, assessment of family; patients (children), two or more individual interviews depending on the nature and complexity of problem; and medical. The medical interviews included: (1) pediatric studies—complete diagnostic history and physical examination, initiation of further diagnostic studies, laboratory x-ray, electroencephalogram, etc., interpretation of treatment program, medication, and recommendations; (2) medical consultations—usually single consultation visits, particularly indicated on medical studies of the multiply handicapped child, including neurology, opthalmology, otolargnygology, and orthopedics; (3) psychiatric studies —one or two examinations including psychiatric history, mental status examination, diagnostic formulation, and recommendations; and (4) paramedical diagnostic studies. The paramedical studies consisted of the following: (a) psychological evaluation (one to three individual interviews-psychometric testing, projective testing, formulations and recommendations); (b) educational evaluation (one-to-one individual interviews or assessments); (c) speech and hearing evaluations (individual interviews with special examination such as audiometry); (d) occupational therapy evaluation (individual interview assessments of areas such as motor skills or impairments and sensorimotor perceptual impairment); (e) physical therapy evaluation (individual interviews, assessment of physical motor handicaps, and recommendations for treatment); and (f) public health nurse evaluation (via home visits).

Following completion of the diagnostic studies, the parents are scheduled for an interpretive process as needed, but the public health nurse acts as a liaison person between the parents and the respective staff members who have examined the child—particularly when parents are unduly anxious, or hesitant to ask questions raised during earlier history taking sessions with the caseworker. It is not unusual for a parent to become anxious to the degree of blocking during these sessions (for example, "After I heard that my child was retarded, I heard nothing the doctor said") and yet not appear so externally. As a consequence many vital questions may go otherwise unasked and unanswered.

Interpretive and Reinterpretive Interviews

A reinterpretive interview at approximately two- to four-week intervals is scheduled with the social worker and parents to review findings and to minimize any inaccuracies and distortions that may have occurred. The social worker, having been present at the initial interpretive interview, is in an excellent position to evaluate these misconceptions and to help in correcting them at this point.

Follow-Up Visits

These visits are necessary for single individual medical and paramedical treatment and to periodically assess treatment-management progress, so as to establish a more definitive prognosis. Schedule at three- to twelve-month intervals as indicated.

Treatment Services

1. Medical: pediatric (single visits at periodic intervals for children receiving medication for metabolic, epilepsy, or similar disorders).
2. Psychiatric and paramedical (individual or group psychotherapy interviews).
   a. Psychological (individual or group psychological counseling and therapy sessions)
   b. Social work (individual or group casework therapy)
   c. Education (individual or group educational therapy)
   d. Speech and hearing (individual or group speech or hearing therapy)
   e. Occupational therapy (individual or group occupational therapy)
   f. Physical therapy (individual physical therapy sessions and programs)
   g. Public health nursing
3. Parents: treatment intervention encompasses individual casework inter-

views with social worker, group therapy by a social worker or psychologist; family therapy by a psychiatrist, or a combination of these disciplines as in conjoint therapy.

RECENT MODIFICATIONS TO MEET
SPECIAL SERVICE NEEDS

Despite the rather extensive program ingredients outlined above, and substantial staff increases, it has become necessary to periodically introduce new service focuses and ingredients. In order to minimize the waiting list for service it was necessary to introduce a system of priorities and modification for treatment approaches. One such priority and modification of service is noted in the following section, entitled Crisis Assistance. Further special subgroups of patients presented such unique therapeutical challenges that new programs had to be created to meet special needs. An example of such groups were the problems presented by the multiply handicapped young retardate and the psychotic retardate. Our recently initiated programs for both of these groups is also described below.

Crisis Assistance

The more severely acting out and disturbed patients, particularly those on a partial or full school exclusion basis are now seen almost immediately in a program aimed at crisis prevention or crisis intervention. Immediate consultation and professional help may determine the difference between psychological health and disintegration of individual and family. For children this is particularly true since the child's own resources are so limited and often a delay in a child's life might be irremediable.

The proposed crisis intervention program offers opportunity for innovative, creative professional action. The clinical team (for example, psychiatrist, psychologist, and social worker) can move into a crisis situation in many ways. Crisis cases may be identified either by a staff member receiving an intake call, by "drop-in" visits of parents who find themselves searching for some professional help, or by school and other local authorities who are seeking specific help for a child. These cases will be scheduled for immediate interview and consultation. Generally, a crisis situation is defined as an occasion when a child is potentially dangerous to himself or others, that is, a situation when family resources are unable to cope with the problem or exclusion from school. The intake interview may indicate the need for immediate action, and treatment can begin immediately. Depending upon the presenting problem, the program may be modified for brief services. These brief services may mean a limited number of visits or a variation in scheduling as needed, such as scheduling one visit monthly, then every six weeks, then every two months.

The crisis team may modify approaches by seeing parents and child simultaneously in the same room in the presence of the psychiatrist and social worker. Built-in consultation programs may be offered by inviting school personnel, law-enforcement authorities, and other significant persons in the environment who have professional interest in the child to participate in diagnostic and treatment processes. In this way the community forces may be mobilized and coordinated to assist the child.

This particular service is especially helpful to those families who find it difficult to relate to a professional setting but who may be reached and assisted if the program for the child can be symptom oriented initially. Thus, regularly scheduled interviews for medication for the hyperactive child, the availability of the professional staff to confer with the school when the need arises, and the availability of some professional person by telephone are important components of this program. The crisis intervention program not only assists in ameliorating the immediate problems of the child, but also assists the parent by providing support and practical aid. It follows that any child seen in one service may be recommended for any of the other services.

A pilot project initiated by the Center focused on an attempt to develop rapid-service approaches to crisis population groups. Brief half-hour consultations were offered at intervals no more frequent than once a month and at least once in eight weeks. The two groups considered to be able to make the most opportune use of these services were the hyperactive children threatened with exclusion or already excluded from school and the smaller group of children with psychosomatic complaints, such as enuresis and soiling, which local casework agencies were reluctant to treat without ongoing medical consultation. It was felt that both groups could be offered medication under the supervision of the child psychiatrist, and that the team of psychiatrist and social worker could also offer directive counseling to parents and a play-activity-therapy experience of brief psychotherapy to the child, depending on his age and needs. As a part of the pilot project, it was decided to offer such services to twenty-five families, scheduling half-hour appointments on a clinic schedule every other Thursday from 9:00 to 10:30 A.M. The psychiatrist's office and adjacent playroom were the facility for the clinic. Of the first twenty-five families referred by the diagnostic teams of the Center, ten referrals were judged inappropriate for the clinic program. These cases were referred back to the teams for further disposition. Of the remaining fifteen, five were referred on to community agencies or counseling within the Center once medication had been prescribed and controlled. Of the remaining ten, sixty-two clinic appointments were made.

In the half-hour consultations, the team of psychiatrist and social worker did not confine themselves to traditional roles regarding treatment of child and parents. Several modalities were used after the psychiatrist's initial diagnostic impression was made. At times the whole family would be seen conjointly or the social worker would engage in an activity or game with the child while the psychiatrist interpreted the child's behavior patterns in vivo to the parents. After the initiation of medication, the parents reported their observations to the social worker, who noted this information in the clinic chart and brought it directly to the psychiatrist's attention. The social worker also used schools as a source of observation of changes in the child's behavior.

Our experiences can be reviewed as follows: (1) *Appropriateness of referral:* As with any new service there was initial difficulty in educating the Center staff as to those children who would benefit from the clinic program. (2) *The defined half-hour period:* Both team members felt some difficulty in altering interview techniques so that they stayed within the model of brief services. (3) *Effectiveness:* While a full research investigation would be needed to measure effectiveness, ten families were sustained with sixty-two hours of service for periods of four to eight months during crisis periods, suggesting an economy of service time and an appropriate supportive approach to the crises of school exclusion and psychosomatic hyperactive syndromes.

In summary, a brief, supportive approach, again utilizing medication as an adjunct, together with environmental manipulation, assistance from school, and other community resources, such as parks, recreations, and volunteer groups, has produced a surprisingly high percentage of success in achieving limited goals. We noted that 85 per cent of the children were reinstated and able to be maintained in school following the reasonably brief period of treatment time. In reviewing this group it is our impression that the rapid intervention, offering supportive and back-up services to school and family, has helped to restore equilibrium and security to the situation.

The Multiply Handicapped Young Retardate

Ironically, in this day of specialization for disorders—diseases and handicaps—often the young child is referred who has a multiplicity of handicaps and literally belongs to no "specialist." We felt that a new program was necessary in order to assure both the availability and continuity of services that such children need. Too often these children have been managed in a symptom-to-symptom fashion, without much concern for their overall (global) needs. The following program was initiated to avoid this pitfall.

The general purpose of our program for these particular multihandicapped young children was to promote the development of each child toward the realization of his own potential in all areas. Specifically, he is helped to improve gross and fine motor skills, to establish needed neuromuscular patterns, to experience creative and imaginative play activities, to be stimulated in both receptive and expressive language, to learn to initiate independent activities, to cooperate in interpersonal activities with peers or adults, and to gain in emotional control. Both regular developmental group staff members and other Center personnel are alert to the opportunity for observation in this setting for the purpose of ongoing diagnosis.

Many of the children who have become involved in this program have mental retardation as the problem of greatest degree in the initial total-weighted multiple diagnosis. All types of cerebral palsied children have participated. Chronic brain syndrome is to be found in many of these children, with attendant problems of hyperactivity, short attention span, and perceptual motor deficits. Language problems vary from unclear speech to total lack of language. Psychiatric disorders range from general immature behavior, to separation anxiety, to autism. However, the philosophical orientation held is that these are first and foremost children who are just beginning to learn about the world and the people in it.

Five main factors must be considered in the group care of these youngsters: the physical setting, the program plans, the therapist-child relationship, the peer group, and the personality of the individual child. The Kennedy Child Study Center nursery room is a large, well-ventilated room with windows along one entire side. A sliding door provides easy access to a fence enclosed play yard with both grass and asphalt areas. Tables, chairs, toilet facilities and counter with sink are all built at the proper height. A large one-way mirror in one wall permits observation by several individuals at once. Play materials and equipment are carefully chosen to meet the special needs of these children.

The program was designed to provide for meeting the goals discussed above. The occupational therapist is concerned with the development of motor skills and self-care activities. She looks for the ways in which the child uses (or fails to use) his hands. Perhaps one hand is preferred or is kept tightly fisted, or perhaps the child over-reaches or cannot grasp or release in a normal manner. Other children simply may not evince any interest in the objects provided. Another child becomes fascinated with colored shapes of circles, squares, and triangles. However, instead of placing these on the flannel board, he finds a small space in the outside fence through which he pokes these objects. The interest is there but it is inappropriately directed. Considerable flexibility is permitted in the activities which the children are allowed to choose or in the selections made by staff members. Simple step-by-step directions are provided with limited goals that permit successful accomplishments. Puzzles of varying degrees of difficulty are provided. A board offers opportunity for free drawing or copying of graphic forms. The child may display an interest in the tricycle, the horse, or the merry-go-round. Rather than lifting him in place, he is helped to feel the desired movements which will achieve his goal. Physical therapist and occupational therapist closely interrelate their efforts in such behavior as this.

This physical therapist utilizes the Rood Method of Sensory Stimulation, which focuses on neuromuscular organization at the reflex level. Thus, the voluntary cooperation requested is minimal, an important factor with the mentally impaired. Coordinated efforts of the physical therapist and speech clinician make progress possible at an accelerated rate. By stimulation of lips, tongue, and other oral mechanisms, the patient gains better control to be used in direct speech training. With one speechless patient, the physical therapist first brushed and iced the tongue. Then she placed a small amount of honey in various locations within the mouth, and the patient had to move his tongue in different directions to obtain it. In this manner, tongue control rapidly improved and the speech clinician's efforts became more successful.

The speech therapist is concerned with providing the proper environment for language growth. She uses materials and other children to assist in stimulating and motivating each child who is in need of speech help. In this situational speech therapy, the goals of physical therapy, and occupational therapy can be incorporated in the speech work. Young children enjoy words and actions that go together. Ball-throwing, marching, and follow the leader all provide large muscle motor activity and also help the child learn to follow simple oral directions and use beginning language. Musical games and rhythms provide experience in listening and making appropriate responses to sounds, as well as developing coordination and awareness of body image. Self-care activities are ideal for building associations between words and objects of practical value to the child. The attitudes of the other children and adults permit practice of the newly acquired verbal skills in an accepting climate.

Educators who are experienced with mentally retarded or slowly developing children recognize that such preschool programs provide an opportunity for the most efficacious academic placement, which will serve to reduce the frustrations and possible emotional scarring of the child. Principles of learning are related to the developmental stages of the particular child. As the child is maturationally ready, those conditions which help in the acquisition of skills conducive to learning are introduced. Each therapist employs the motivating techniques of encouragement or discouragement, of supporting desired values by their behavior, and of accepting the child as he is so that he gains self-assurance and a willingness to try.

The children in the group must be viewed both in terms of their chronological and their mental age. Parallel play may be appropriate, for example, in some of our children, even though chronologically we might expect more social interaction. This also involves the personality factor of the child and the distinct possibility of less than normal opportunity for personal interaction. The life experience the child has had and his own unique personality characteristics as these have been revealed in the diagnostic study largely determine the goals to be set for him in the developmental group.

The mother's group provides an opportunity for interchange of ideas, concerns, and hopes with others sharing a similar problem, specific information to be gained, feedback relative to their own child, and observation of the child. The psychologist who conducts this group attempts to create an atmosphere that encourages free discussion. Certain topics (most frequently toilet-regulation techniques) are presented in an instructional manner. It is also possible to present information concerning the handicaps existing with these children in a general way if the parent is not yet fully ready to cope with the acceptance of the problem on a more personal basis. From the beginning, the mothers are prepared for the eventual "graduation" of their child into the most appropriate available program. In this regard, therapies, schools, and other possibilities are discussed.

The mother's group provides support for individual members who suffer anxieties or depression, whether the reaction is to the initial shock of the discovery of mental retardation or to the recognition of the extent of the problems that they face. Great is the need to reveal to others who really can share their feelings the cruel words of professionals, the blunders by well-intentioned friends and relatives, the doubts, the guilt, the feeling of helplessness and loneliness. Often the mothers have extended their relationships to visits at one another's homes or to social activities which include the husbands. One mother indicated recently that she still meets with mothers from a group that formerly met at the Center nearly two years ago. Fathers occasionally attend the regular group meetings or are active in the once a month night meeting of the parent's group.

From time to time the professionals who work directly with the children will meet with the mothers to report on progress and to answer questions. Each different professional, adding varied points of view which supplement or complement one another, provides greater evidence of the child's abilities or deficits. More formal conferences which include both parents are arranged during the year and at the end of the program for their child. This latter serves as an exit interview to evaluate what the Center has done as well as to assist the parents in the transition to the next phase of care for the child.

One of the most effective techniques with many of the mothers has been the use of the observation room with its one-way mirror. In this manner, they can observe their own child in interaction with other children and adults in a different physical setting. This is done only when a staff member is present and usually with the whole group of mothers. The staff member must be aware of the dynamics in the case and sensitive to the impact on the mother. One mother whose boy was severely handicapped both physically and mentally had built strong defenses to make her adjustment to her son. When she saw him in comparison to other children she was nearly overwhelmed. Another mother claimed that her little girl "could not tolerate being separated" from her mother and was "not sociable at all." When observing through the mirror, she saw her daughter happily engaged in play with another child and with the toys, obviously getting along with no difficulty. This was the opening needed to help her look at her own role in the problem.

In order to deal in greater depth with individual problems, a psychiatric social worker may see a mother alone in addition to the group meeting. The personnel working with the children and those working with the mothers hold weekly conferences to discuss the program. Each child and his mother are discussed, and this information can then be used in subsequent activities in the groups. Administrative details can be considered, such as timing of parent conferences and planning for the future.

In summary, a special developmental program was designed to help children under four years of age who exhibit one or several mental or physical handicaps. Diagnostic procedures rely on multiple-discipline impressions, with varying degrees of weight given to elements within the total composite diagnosis. A group experience provides for serial diagnosis and integration of therapeutic approaches. A concomitant mother's group provides information, support, ongoing feedback, and observations of the child. An exit interview serves to help in the graduation of the child to the next phase of his life and provides significant evidence of the effectiveness of this developmental program.

Programs for the Psychotic Retarded

The psychotic retarded child, with associated schizophrenic reaction or autistic traits, presents a major challenge. The length of psychotherapeutic intervention, the observed level of functioning in the retarded range, and the associated need for ongoing educational programming makes these children problematical as a treatment challenge to a Center such as our own. Following initial evaluation, a therapeutic intervention focuses on individual psychotherapy, family psychotherapy, and frequent utilization of psychotropic medications for the child. It is our policy to include these children in the regular therapeutic educational programs with nonschizophrenic children. It is our impression that placing these schizophrenic children in separate groups severely limits their opportunity for meaningful contacts with peers. Indeed, it has been our experience that such programs tend to provide opportunity for negative reinforcement of the schizophrenic symptomatology. However, when schizophrenic children are placed in a class of retardates that includes a number of reaching-out, friendly children, the socialization process is significantly enhanced. Also, such an educational setting allows placing these children in ongoing educational pursuits, regardless of the stage of remissions as to their clinical symptomatology. Our experiences have been most positive, and we feel that there has not been ample stress placed on the socialization qualities of pure interacting for schizophrenic children.

Utilizing the above-noted therapeutic-management approach, we have been able to successfully provide ongoing services for retarded children who have associate psychotic reactions. Such children are commonly referred from a psychiatric clinic to a mental retardation clinic in the dispute as to who should and "can provide effective services for the child and his family." Our approach avoids this common "musical chairs" approach to troubled children and their parents.

Children's Day-Care Center

It was found that another imminent need was a day-care program for children whose emotional problems preclude their participating in the regular school-social life of their peers. Children who have been in psychiatric hospitals frequently encounter too many problems when they return to home and family life; these may be alleviated by an environment geared to their special needs, a kind of half-way house. Active children, who, because they are withdrawn, antisocial, hyperactive, and overly aggressive, are unable to tolerate the normal school routine. These children are excluded from school on indefinite "medical exclusions." Other children with school phobias and related problems are also at times unable to mobilize themselves for attendance at school. The day-care program established at our Center provides for all such children a therapeutic setting wherein close accepting personal relationships with adults is provided in an educational atmosphere which paces its learning activities to the child's needs.

Under the immediate supervision of a staff psychiatrist, an individually tailored ongoing therapeutic program is arranged for each child. With the consultation of the staff psychologist, developmental goals can be determined for each child in social, emotional, intellectual, and physical adjustment. Thus, a highly individualized program can be developed for each child. Since the child lives in a context bombarded by many social and environmental factors, close liaison with home and family is maintained by the social workers. In addition, programs of parent cooperations are developed which are concomitant with and complement the program designed for the child. These include casework, parent discussion groups, counseling, parent participation, and observation when indicated. Thus, by integrating the activities of the child, his parents, his home, and the day-care center, the child's adjustment potential is maximized. The program is flexible enough to permit the child to grow in self-confidence and self-esteem. Staff members plan and coordinate the daily activities presented by the clinic team. These include individual and group therapies, recreational and occupational therapy, and other specialized therapies as needed. Although academic goals are secondary, the existence of the present Kennedy Center School provides an opportunity for regular classroom instruction as well as for special tutoring. Field trips, hobbies, music therapy, dance therapy, club and social activities are provided and encouraged. Post-school or late-afternoon activities are structured so as to permit other children to come into the program for special activities, such as scouting, group therapies, and scheduled recreational activities.

SPECIFIC TAILORING OF SERVICES

In a recent paper, Wolfensberger (1965) underscored a recurrent problem of clinics for the mentally retarded: excessive diagnosis when minimal activity is requested or needed. We have attempted to avoid such unnecessary diagnostic-therapeutic ventures by specifically tailoring our service to each request for help. One method that has been successfully utilized will be described.

It was recognized that many families applying to the Kennedy Child Center may be helped significantly by providing an immediate and limited type of service. One such situation is that in which a specific school problem exists. We initiated a service which was designed to offer rapid educational and intellectual evaluation to assist the parents and the school in pursuing the best available plan to insure academic adjustment and satisfaction.

This service was intended for the child who appeared to be academically misplaced. Briefly, the criteria considered in selecting a case for rapid screening included the following: (1) children whose difficulties appeared due to possible intellectual inability, especially children for whom intellectual testing was difficult to obtain through the school (for example, parochial school system); (2) younger children—those in third grade or below, including those children already placed in a special training situation (unless such a placement is being questioned as inappropriate), those families in which there is a likelihood of a strong need for ongoing counseling, and those children who appear in need of more formal medical workup (for example, those who have physical complaints, unusual auditory or motor symptomatology, or significant emotional problems).

We attempt to complete this service within two weeks, from initial intake to parent-school conferences on the findings and then treatment implications. The educational and psychological evaluations are accomplished in one- or two-hour visits. An informal staff conference then reviews outside reports and current findings, followed immediately by interpretative conference with both parents. Sending of re-

ports and a telephone call follow-up in two weeks complete this particular special service. Cases are returned to the full multi-
disciplinary-team waiting list if further study is indicated at the time
of follow-up.

It is our impression that much more specific tailoring of services
will be necessary if we are to meet the varied developmental needs of
mentally retarded children and their families.

SUMMARY

This chapter has reviewed two of the trends that have been developed
recently: it discusses a multipurpose child psychiatry out-patient
clinic, the Kennedy Child Study Center, which actively programs
treatment needs for the mentally retarded child (rather than giving the
usual limited diagnostic overview that mentally retarded children received in the past from child psychiatry facilities); it reaffirms the
child-guidance model approach to the mentally retarded child but embraces and helps to establish many of the needed services in the community in a most positive way.

This chapter has also reviewed the wide number of treatment-inter-
vention modalities that are available, including some of the variations
needed for psychotherapy of the mentally retarded. These must take
into account nonverbal dimensions, possible need for psychoactive
drugs, life-planning concepts, and developmental considerations as to
when psychiatric intervention will be necessary and how to do it, and
so on. Some of the realistic dimensions in the treatment of the mentally retarded have been underscored. In the personal encounters with
such patients one is brought face-to-face with personal identity problems, the child's exquisite awareness of how he is viewed by other
members in society (including his peer group), and the problems commonly encountered in working with some parents of mentally retarded
children.

The rather unique program of the Kennedy Child Study Center
stresses community aspects wherein psychiatric services are only a
part of an ongoing out-patient spectrum of services that works closely
with special educational approaches, multigroup-therapy approaches,
and a flexible team approach to the diagnosis, treatment intervention,
and treatment follow-up aspects of this community approach.

Psychiatric out-patient services for the mentally retarded children
have much to offer and receive from both child-guidance clinics and

mental retardation diagnostic and counseling clinics. A considerable number, if not a majority, of child guidance clinics tend to exclude mentally retarded children on the basis that the intellectual limitation precludes successful utilization of psychotherapy. This has not been our experience. We have found that including retardates has added considerably to our differential diagnostic skills. It has also been a challenge to the further development of our therapeutic skills, as well as a more full creative use of the therapist's personality and emotional capacity in direct dealings with children. In our mental retardation diagnostic and counseling service, the inclusion of an ongoing psychiatric program has significantly lowered the incidence of repeated costly diagnostic studies for children who have already been adequately studied but whose parents and themselves are urgently in need of psychotherapeutic help. Such ongoing programs have also substantially added to the prognostic and realistic counseling skills of our staff.

Perhaps more importantly the inclusion of community-wide psychiatric treatment programs for mentally retarded children in child-guidance clinics and mental retardation centers is to be recommended on the basis of its being a useful, much requested, program.

REFERENCES

Pearson, P. H., & Menesee, A. R. Medical and social management of the mentally retarded. U.S. Department of Health, Education, and Welfare, Public Health Service, Divisions of Chronic Diseases, Mental Retardation Branch. From *G. P.,* 1965, *31.*

Wolfensberger, W. Diagnosis diagnosed. *J. Ment. Subnormal.,* 1965, *11,* 62–70.

[B]

CHALLENGES IN
RESIDENTIAL SERVICES

: 23 :

The Psychiatric Consultant in a Residential
Facility for the Mentally Retarded

Edward T. Beitenman

INTRODUCTION

THE need for more extensive psychiatric services in institutions for the mentally retarded is being increasingly recognized and recommended (President's Committee on Mental Retardation, 1968). The general aims and principles required for such services have been established in theory but only to a small degree in practice. Potter (1964, p. 371) accurately summarized the current status of psychiatric involvement in this type of treatment setting: "The groundwork has been laid and now the need is for more application of these principles based upon actual experience in a school for the mentally retarded." The wide gap between these principles and their application is shown by the current paucity of literature on this particular problem.

This chapter will review the writer's five-years' experience as a consultant to a residential facility for the retarded.[1] It will outline the common problems and challenges, both clinically and administratively, which were experienced while providing mental health consultation to such a facility.

ESTABLISHMENT OF A MODEL
OF PSYCHIATRIC SERVICE

Caplan (1964) has written about the needs for preparatory work in order to build appropriate and effective relationships between the consultant, the consultees, and institutional administrative structures. The initiation of the author's consultantship to this particular residential setting for the retarded was facilitated by the fact that the superintendent had not only requested such services but was also able to clearly pinpoint some of the problem areas in which he felt a psychiatric consultant might be helpful. Two of the superintendent's major concerns were: the fact that his facility was receiving, with increasing frequency, young children and adolescents who were admitted solely on the basis of their reported inability to adapt to available community facilities for the retarded; and the changing nature of the family's relationships to the institution.

As to institutional administrative structure, the superintendent felt that the consultant would be most effective in working with the four treatment teams in the institution. Although the team approach for this particular institution has been delineated elsewhere (Pedrini et al., 1967), a brief overview of their structure and function will be described. The treatment team consists of a physician, psychologist, social worker, teacher, recreational therapist, vocational supervisor, nurse, and child-care workers. The team is responsible for the administration of a designated geographical area in which the patients are grouped on the basis of sex, age, and function. Although psychiatric consultation was available previously, this was limited to behavioral emergencies, and the consultant remained outside of the ongoing functions of the treatment teams. The psychiatrist's role had been limited primarily to diagnosis with resultant treatment prescriptions, often with no control or follow-up on his recommendations. The author felt that a continuation of this "inherited" role for psychiatric services would become an endless foray into the area of symptom control and would preclude effective communication with the professional staff.

Accordingly, the author decided to utilize a case-seminar type of consultation, with the goal of improving communication among the staff as well as initiating general management and attitudinal changes. The initial clinical cases, which were chosen by the staff, represented major behavioral problems about which there was a paucity of clinical and personal historical information. It rapidly became evident that it was necessary to develop better methods of obtaining clinical-historical information. More importantly, the team's concept of the psychiatrist's role—that he was to provide direct service with little expectation of change on their part—also had to be modified if effective consultation was to be provided. When the psychiatrist refuses to accept this rather traditional role, then the treatment team begins to reevaluate his role and function and the door is also open for a mutual reassessment of the function and role of each team member. A decade ago, the professional resistance would have been too great to suggest or initiate such reevaluation. However, with the recent increasing reemphasis on education and habilitation of the mentally retarded patient, along with the introduction of new people from professions which are becoming increasingly interested in mental retardation, certain roles are becoming obsolete and others are changing, all with great anxiety to the individuals involved. Moreover, it has been pointed out (Caplan, 1964) that there is a crucial need for the consultant to become acquainted with the organizational structure early in his contact with any institution.

In residential facilities for the retarded, one notes that below the top administration there is a hierarchy of roles based on tradition (as opposed to function) which have to be understood and then clarified. It will now be indicated how some of these critical initial administrative problems in delineating team members' roles (and hence a clearer role for the psychiatric consultant) were clarified.

The Child-Care Workers

These people have been the lowest paid, the lowest in terms of status, and the least listened to, but paradoxically they are in a position to maintain the most personal daily contact with the patient in the least structured setting. Their active involvement in a case seminar is a "must," although it is not an easy task to assure their presence in some. Often case seminar meetings must be transacted on the ward to allow the child-care workers an opportunity to participate. Not only are they the primary sources of information regarding developmental and behavioral aspects of the patient as he functions in daily living skills, but without their cooperation, the implementation of any therapy program is impossible. The importance placed on their attendance at case seminar meetings, as well as their contributions, serves to enhance the child-care worker's self-image, and often they are able to move into a very active position on the team. For example, the author has noted that given such a climate, several child-care workers at this residential facility have become interested and involved in setting up programs of remotivation, behavioral shaping, and instigating physical changes on their wards (for example, decorations, curtains, painting, and many other types of "spruce-up" operations).

As a group, they have been low in the hierarchy traditionally but probably the most important functionally. They are at the "front lines" for both behavioral observation and initiating meaningful interventive treatment approaches. It was necessary to focus attention strongly on the elimination of those aspects of the child-care worker's job duties which traditionally have proven to be major obstacles to utilizing the fullest potential of these personnel. This necessitated administrative changes and expectations as to their previous janitorial duties on the wards. It was decided to reduce the focus on their traditional custodian role and to place major emphasis on their teaching role with the patients. Lastly, there was a clear understanding that their reflections and suggestions for patient management would be both welcomed and listened to attentively.

The Nurse

Traditionally the nurse has been an important person on the team, but functionally the medical role is too constricted and outmoded to allow for full utilization of her professional and personal attributes. Leaders in the field of nursing and mental retardation have recently recognized this problem and suggested remedies (Wright and Menolascino, 1966). This enlightened view strongly suggests that the nurse must function as the chief child caretaker, which consists of providing more for the emotional rather than the medical needs of the mentally retarded patient. Introduction to behavioral-shaping paradigms, alternate use of the nurse as treater or teacher, and coordinator of psycho-social-developmental approaches to helping handicapped patients are prime examples of the new approach. Group-therapy approaches to sex education and personal grooming are also within the realm of the nurse's emerging new role in mental retardation. The psychiatric consultant can capitalize on the nurse's professional training and experiences to establish other specific child-care guidelines for and with her. The nurse can then initiate a supervisory program for aides and attendants aimed at establishing and maintaining meaningful child-care programs which meet the patient's needs and involve the ward personnel to their greatest capacities. These new roles allow the nurse to establish greater and more beneficial channels of communication with both the patients and the professional staff.

The Educational Therapist

As more information about each patient becomes available, a specific assessment of the child's developmental-adaptive status can be obtained, with a resulting individual educational placement. Teachers have tended to identify with their counterparts in public schools, and often only through discussion in the case seminars have they been able to point out or see the need for both separation and continuity within the child's educational experience. Closer planning as to teacher changes (vacations, placement, and so on) and a focus on education as a vehicle for initiating and reinforcing socially acceptable skills and feelings are underscored. The continuity of the teacher is often a major asset, and the teacher's role as a personality model for identification and sublimation is brought into sharp perspective.

For the severely retarded, especially those with associated handicaps (for example, blindness) that tend to elicit autistic postures toward the outside world, the therapeutic-preventative role of preschool programs is stressed. Specific discussions of such teaching challenges allow the educational therapist to extend her sights beyond the usual educational focus on the trainable group of children and into an area of educational therapy that has been woefully neglected, although it represents a literal gold mind 'for treatment intervention.

The Physician

The physician's role is also undergoing a major shift. Psychopharmacological agents are increasingly stressed within the context of the total management approach to the emotionally disturbed mental retardate. The physician plays an important role in the education of the other team members as to the effects and limitations of the various psychoactive drugs. However, a natural widening of the physician's diagnostic horizons to include etiologic, descriptive, and developmental assessments of the adaptive capacities of each patient is a necessity in the evolution of his new role on the treatment team. At times individual preceptorship has been utilized in clinical areas, such as interviewing techniques and issues and goals of supportive psychotherapy for the retarded, and in helping the physician enhance his overall effectiveness on the clinical team.

As with the nurse, the changing role of the physician in mental retardation is expanding far beyond the traditional obsession with diagnosis. For example, attention to the dynamic interplay between the host of factors that eventuate in the "failure-to-thrive" child alerts the physician to the ongoing need such children have for a positive interaction with the outside world. Focus on such issues allows the physician not only to more fully appreciate the role of other team members, but also to systematically reassess the intrinsic-extrinsic complexity of factors that mediate human behavior.

The Psychologist

The psychologist has usually been quite conversant with both historic and current perspectives in the field of mental retardation and has been encouraged as a resource person whose skills and educational background extend far beyond his frequent title of "psychometrician." Psychologists have been actively supported in their efforts to provide continuity and follow-up on specific staff recommendations. Similarly, they have received active guidance in experimental approaches to group psychotherapy, individual psychotherapy, behavioral shaping, and ward-management techniques which were quite innovative.

Of all the team members, the psychologist was most suitably prepared for research approaches to personal-behavioral and family dimensions of mental retardation. His research approach to current treatment-management techniques has been most helpful both to himself (rekindling his interest in areas of especial expertise) and to the staff since it demands a serious review of the efficaciousness of current programs.

The Social Worker

The social worker usually has the first contact with the family and can be utilized to obtain the necessary social history data via a guided developmental-historical method. The social worker also becomes the main figure in maintaining and fostering close family-child communication. Social workers have been encouraged to establish ongoing relationships with the families, placing greater emphasis on recognizing and preventing family distancing devices from the child, optimal timing of a child's vacation schedule, and energetic exploration and activation of placement opportunities. Prevention is stressed in setting up more time for family counseling, especially at times of crisis, such as admission, transitory family-patient interactional problems, and community placement. Social workers are aided in enlarging their professional role horizons to encompass new directions (for example, group care and other therapeutic living arrangements). This necessitates that they leave the cherished one-to-one counseling role and embark on other tasks, such as implementation of a kibbutzim environment of child-care services within the structure of "cottages" that encompass fifty to sixty patients. Attention to programmatic aspects of the life space, grouping by functional levels and personality variables, and group cohesiveness have aided in initiating such a program.

Vocational Rehabilitation

A continual dialogue has been initiated with the vocational rehabilitation staff members. Much consideration is given to the frequently noted apparent conflict between the goals of the patient's current vocational placement in the institutional work force and possible ongoing rehabilitation plans. This demands a closer appreciation of each patient's specific interests and capabilities. The patient's work assignments are reviewed within the context of providing opportunities for self-achievement which would enhance the patient's self-image as well as raise his self-confidence—regardless of whether or not the patient could be autonomously employed in the future. The initiation of direct payment for daily vocational services rendered by the patient has been a major step in achieving this goal.

The meaning and importance of work to the patient's psychic life is stressed. Too often the severely retarded have been viewed as not being suitable for vocational rehabilitation. Discussion of work-activity programs and the need for a closed-end sheltered workshop have resulted in the initiation of work experience for many patients who would otherwise have been left to their self-stimulatory devices and a life of emptiness.

Generic Services

The services of the chaplain, dentist, physical therapist, and speech therapist can add meaningful dimensions to the armamentarium of needed services. However, they are often divorced from day-to-day contacts as well as from direct communications with the other team members. The major goals of staff development in this area have been to stimulate further knowledge and interest concerning the generic services so that the various members of the team can collectively assess and then individually determine the proper timing for the utilization of these particular services in a manner which will enhance the specific planning and individual goals for each patient.

Coordination of Team Members' Roles

As programs for each patient have become more individualized, with new services added and old services expanded, the problem of coordination has become more complex. The understanding and acceptance of the priorities of a treatment program by all team members is the first essential step that must be taken, without which the healthy competitiveness between various disciplines in relation to individual patients may turn into a negative downgrading of all disciplines. Yet there are still certain predictable trouble-prone areas which may well be anticipated when several services are involved in a treatment plan. The presence of such problems is usually confirmed when the consultant receives consistent reports of behavior which are each different and dependent upon who prepares reports. When there is a breakdown in the treatment plan, the most frequent candidates for the scapegoat role are the child-care workers and the social worker. This dynamic interplay is not too unlike that noted in the noninstitutionalized child, as both the child-care worker and the social worker are the most involved in the substitutive or actual parent role.

With the younger child, the teacher and child-care worker often need help in working with each other to determine mutually convenient school hours and to maintain feedback regarding troublesome behavior; it should be realized that the child-care worker can be quite supportive if she is kept informed of the patient's school level and progress. When such collaboration does not occur, the typical school-parent conflict arises with all its well-known ramifications.

In the older patient, the social worker and the vocational rehabilitation counselor may reach an impasse over the timing as well as the choice of placement for the patient, or the social worker may easily end up assuming the blame and responsibility for the lack of appropriate community facilities for the patient.

As our experience increased, it became obvious from a logical standpoint that the overall coordinator selected for each child should be a person not directly identified with any of the four above-named disciplines [teacher, social worker, child-care worker (nurse), and vocational rehabilitation counselor], but rather a physician or psychologist who was not directly involved in the everyday care but still had frequent formal contacts with all of the disciplines involved.

Another major coordinating need is for one person to be assigned the responsibility for integrating the treatment services in each case. Without this, efforts at implementing services are usually doomed to failure, and the major emphasis in the treatment program will depend upon which discipline has the most dominant and aggressive personality.

CONSULTATIVE METHODS

It was recognized early that it is doubtful whether a psychiatric consultant in this particular type of residential setting will ever enjoy the luxury of an exhaustive developmental study. As a result it became necessary to devise certain shortcuts and rather fixed points of reference in collecting such data. Case presentations were used to focus on the pertinent material needed to understand an individual resident and also to demonstrate the necessity of knowledge concerning his previous life experiences and his overall pattern of development. A sequential interview based on the philosophy that developmental outcome is a result of the interaction between the child's constitutional endowment and his caretaking environment was illustrated by tape-recorded interviews with mothers of the children being discussed at the case-centered seminars. This "new-wine-in-old-bottles" approach to the reassessment of the personal historical data and demonstrations on how to obtain it were aimed at both service needs (since the interviews were slanted toward discovering possible areas of treatment intervention) and the previously noted aim of helping the staff to develop their professional capacities on many levels.

The response to this consultative approach was quite dramatic, decreasing the initial negative staff attitudes, enlisting the staff interest in possible new avenues of treatment, and providing an interprofessional forum for the mutual rethinking of the multiple facets and challenges of symptomatic behavior. The most objectively demonstrable change was noted in a more positive attitude toward the patient's family, not only in formulating meaningful treatment considerations and goals, but also in recognizing the importance of the staff's every contact with the patient's family as an opportunity to enhance the overall continuity of communication between patient, family, and staff.

These considerations were pertinent not only for the recently admitted patients, but also for those who had prolonged behavioral problems or whose families had found it most difficult to accept and participate in the ongoing institutional programs for their children. The application of these principles and methods via their translation into actual clinical practice is illustrated in the following case histories.

CASE HISTORIES

The Cultural-Familial Resident

This was a fourteen-year-old, mildly retarded boy who was born of a common-law marriage. His delayed developmental milestones became more obvious as he entered school, where he was noted to have increasing behavioral difficulties; later there occurred a series of minor altercations with the police, culminating in a car theft which necessitated his being removed from the community. His parents had tended to blame the school for his poor performance and maladjustment; his institutionalization was very much against their wishes as they tended to feel that they were being persecuted: "The law is against us." "He is a good boy if other folks will just leave him alone." His adjustment to the home was characterized by frequent temper outbursts when demands were placed upon him. He manifested continual sullenness and failure to involve himself in any of the institution's programs, except to demand that his parents be allowed to visit him weekly. The basic concern was on what methods the staff might utilize to motivate him toward a more active and positive role in his ongoing training program at this residential facility.

In the case seminar, it became apparent that once the boy had been institutionalized, the staff had minimized the ongoing importance of the family's angry attitude toward the institution and the effect of this attitude upon his ongoing adjustment. Collectively, the members of the team provided information from letters, telephone calls, and visits which all had the common theme that the institution was responsible for his placement, with the family not only disclaiming any responsibility but continuing to convey the message, "You can come home whenever they allow you. . . ." Individually, it would have been extremely difficult for any staff member to be aware of the total clinical picture and associated treatment challenges. However, with clarification and direction, they were able to augment some imaginative intervention techniques which would involve many of them individually, as well as collectively. Specifically, in a planned conference with both the parents and the boy, the parents were told that they could take their son home if they desired. The family responded by listing a number of factors which they would have to consider, became quite uncomfortable, and announced that they would telephone the boy their decision. However, when it was insisted that the boy be told of their decision by them and in the presence of the staff, the mother asked the boy to leave the room; she then stated that she couldn't tell him that she didn't want him home because, "He will be mad at me." When the boy was told of the family's decision by the mother, he predictively responded in an angry outburst directed toward the family. In the follow-up plan, the family's visits were restricted with a member of the team present at all times, and the boy's other contacts with the family, such as letters and telephone calls, were controlled. The staff was instructed to meet his angry outbursts with the disclaimer that they were only there to help him and were not holding him against his family's wishes.

The cultural-familial group is almost ten times greater than the combined number of all other cases of retardation, and yet 90 per cent of this group is not institutionalized. Many of the institutionalized children are there for their protection from severe emotional and material deprivation. Unfortunately, these children are usually the last to be identified as mentally retarded and may have spent the formative years of personality development in deprived settings. Not only have they been identified with dyssocial and antisocial pathological living situations, but their personality, attitudes, defenses, and patterns are usually well entrenched by the time of admission. Thus the institutionalized cultural-familial patient probably represents a specific subgroup of community problems within the general classification of cultural-familial retardation. (Benda et al., 1963)

Problems of adjustment to an institution routinely require an assessment of the family's attitudes as they affect the behavior of the child. Even though the institutionalized child is frequently the source of unacknowledged family frictions, as in the above case, these families paradoxically function in a cohesive manner to project hostility on authority figures or representatives thereof, such as the institution. It has been noted that these families are characterized by an inability to look at themselves and an ability to blame others, usually the institution. The child is never allowed to separate from the family, and various atypical methods of intrafamily communication are maintained which keeps these children from investing little in their placement setting except anger.

The Child From The Closely Knit Family

The patient was a ten-year-old boy diagnosed as moderate mentally retarded due to a birth injury. He was the youngest of eight children from a closely knit family of middle-class socioeconomic status. Shortly after admission to this facility, the child refused to eat, became withdrawn, and continued to lose weight to a degree where medically there was concern for his survival. The parents had not visited since the time of admission as they had been advised not to visit until he was adjusted to the institution, which had been the routine practice. In the case seminar the team recognized the need for extensive contact between the family and their boy, including ongoing counseling around the family's own grief. The primary focus of the family counseling was on a gradual separation and realization that a boy such as this does not have the capacity to handle or understand in totality the crisis of separation.

Children from closely knit families represent a different therapeutic challenge and are in sharp contrast to the first case history. They are usually admitted to the institution in late childhood, generally after prolonged and empathic attempts on the part of their parents to help them function effectively within their primary home settings. Often this particular type of family response is of such a marked degree that the total family pattern of functioning is organized around the care of this particular child. The personal and clinical history in such instances contain specific patterns of behavior as well as family responses that provide the alert staff with guidelines for reducing the child's anxiety to a totally different situation, while simultaneously programming a series of gradual, separating experiences. Such cases also serve as an excellent entrée into a review of the admission procedures of this institution.

Psychotic Behavioral Disturbances:

The patient was a nineteen-year-old farm boy who had been admitted to the institution at age seven years because of frequent temper tantrums, noisy screeching, carrying a large screwdriver at all times, and cruelty to animals. At age three, he was considered somewhat precocious by his parents, but was noted to display periodic elective mutism, and a hearing loss was suspected. Shortly thereafter he became mute and there was regression in his intellectual and motor achievements. At the time of admission he was felt to be "different" and "slow" and quite unable to function in the available special education pursuits. The team was concerned about his withdrawal as well as his bizarre behavior, reporting that he watched linoleum tile patterns quite carefully, turning to the right on every twenty-second tile interval. On examination, he grimaced frequently, bizarre hand movements were evident, and he mumbled incoherently to himself. The diagnosis was mental retardation secondary to a major psychiatric disorder (for example, childhood psychosis) (Menolascino, 1966). A treatment plan was devised to include not only the use of psychotropic drugs, but also the need to provide a milieu which focused on closer interpersonal contacts and activities in relationship to this patient.

Despite the available diagnostic techniques, it is not unusual for this type of patient to be institutionalized at a home for the retarded on an expedient basis. The spectrum of treatment modalities that are available for such a patient and their relative value in view of the chronicity of his illness not only allow for the formulation of both general and specific therapeutic guidelines, but also tend to quickly remove the psychiatric consultant from the pedestal of omnipotence.

Idiopathic Retardation:

This is the case of a seven-and-a-half-year-old, moderately-retarded boy admitted two years previously because of marked hyperactivity who was now displaying passive and indifferent attitudes toward involvement in the school program. A review of his past personal history revealed that he was a member of an aggressive and intelligent family, with both parents being college graduates. Pregnancy, birth, and early developmental milestones were described as normal until age nine months. At that time he was placed in a body cast for eleven months as part of the treatment for a hip dislocation. At age three, he was felt to be different, difficult to understand, and overactive.

At the request of the staff, a detailed tape-recorded developmental history was obtained from the mother of this boy. It revealed marked multiple deprivations during the crucial time of his physical immobilization secondary to the hip problem and for some time thereafter. During this time he had been isolated from the rest of the family (on medical advice), and this had been compounded by marital difficulties and the death of several close relatives.

The treatment program originated by the staff underscored the residuals of the multiple emotional deprivations and possible provisions for fulfilling his needs with regard to a school program and close interpersonal contact which focused on identification with maternal figures. Counseling interviews with the parents (which were tape-recorded for further discussion at team conference) began to help him to recognize and work out some of their guilt as well as lessen the competitiveness and distance between the staff and the parents.

Discussion of such cases showed the need for understanding and modifying the passivity of similar children. All too frequently this passivity needlessly progresses into the apathy of the young adult retardate. These cases bring into focus the relatively new dimension of emotional-maternal deprivation as a cause of mental retardation, and thus serve as an excellent instructional model for abnormal child development. Similarly, an alternative in diagnostic-therapeutic intervention is presented—a descriptive view stressing both an operational and descriptive orientation toward such patients. This is in contrast to the traditional "organic" orientation that tends to unduly stress possible etiologic dimensions which conjure up visions of dire prognoses and leave precious little room for positive professional attitudes toward treatment interventions.

CONCLUSIONS

Residential facilities for the retarded are undergoing rapid change. The increasing establishment of community mental retardation facilities has resulted in a very selective type of mental retardee who will enter a residential setting, and the criteria for admission is usually an inability to adjust to a local facility for the mentally retarded. Accordingly, most of the institutionalized children have emotional and behavioral problems associated with their retardation. As a result these residential facilities not only have had to develop new or different programs, but also have had to face the challenge of understanding the child's inner needs to help him benefit from their programs. Such institutions are very much in need of psychiatric consultation.

General principles of mental health consultation, which outline the need for laying the groundwork for consultation and the necessity of knowing the institution and listing the various types of consultation needed, are a helpful sendoff to the psychiatrist. However, if he has had little experience with a residential facility for the retarded, the psychiatrist will find a bewildering array of professional people (many of whom have functional roles that are quite different from the psychiatrist's expectations of same), and he will be given a place in the power structure that is of greater or lesser importance than might be expected.

Members of the treatment team tend to be threatened by the introduction of a consultant psychiatrist, and initially they collectively attempt to place him in a position where he can expect little change in team members' roles. If the psychiatrist resists the maintenance of the team's homeostasis and demands a different role of and from his services, then the opportunity opens up for a reassessment of all treatment team members' roles. Despite the initial resistances, this is not a very difficult task to implement since most residential facilities for the retarded are currently in major crises concerning their future roles and change is more easily implemented during such circumstances.

Case seminars prove to be an effective method for both introducing psychiatric services to the treatment team staff and helping the staff utilize this new service more effectively for both individuals and groups of patients. The seminars have the added benefit of being a learning experience not only for the staff, but also for the psychiatrist! Attendance, however, is a problem in an understaffed institution, but this can be partially solved by holding meetings on the ward. Surprisingly some of the more important team members often have only a minimal amount of information concerning the patient. A thorough discussion of a case in which an adequate developmental history has been obtained and to which individuals can contribute from their ongoing experiences with the family or child has many rewards. Very few of our cases are still diagnosed as "idiopathic mental retardation." Not only is such a consultative technique of value in ascertaining more specific etiologies, but with a better knowledge of the family, the staff's attitude tends to become more positive and less competitive.

The case presentations were selected from a variety presenting psychiatric problems discussed in case seminars. This particular grouping of cases offered a vehicle for discussing family and personality dynamics in the retarded, as well as initiating communication and attitudinal changes in the treatment team. This was possible because, as noted in the case histories described herein, the team was able to feel the satisfaction of having modified undesirable behavior through the use of both newly acquired information and changes within themselves.

NOTE

1. Glenwood State Hospital-School for the Retarded, Glenwood, Iowa. It has a general census of 1,125 residents.

REFERENCES

Benda, C. F., Squire, N. D., Ogonik, J., & Wise, R. Personality factors in mild mental retardation. Part I. Family background and socio-cultural patterns. *Amer. J. Ment. Defic.*, 1963, *68*, 28–40.

Caplan, G. *Principles of preventive psychiatry.* New York: Basic Books, 1964, pp. 232–265.

Pedrini, D. T., Krusen, M., & Lavis, L. Habilitation at a state school for the retarded. *Psychiat. Quart. Suppl.*, 1967, *40*, 37–44.

Potter, H. The needs of mentally retarded children for child psychiatry services. *J. Amer. Acad. Child Psychiat.*, 1964, *3*, 352–374.

President's Committee on Mental Retardation, Second Report. *The edge of change.* Washington, D.C.: U.S. Government Printing Office, 1968.

Rogawski, A. Teaching consultation techniques in a community agency. In: M. Solomon (Ed.), *The psychiatric consultation.* New York: Grune & Stratton, 1968, pp. 65–85.

Wright, M., & Menolascino, F. J. Nurturant nursing of mentally retarded ruminators. *Amer. J. Ment. Defic.*, 1966, *71*, 451–459.

: 24 :

Empty Revolution beyond the Mental

Burton Blatt

OUR so-called "revolution" now being waged on behalf of the mentally retarded is an empty revolution, as were those of its progenitors.[1] It is an inert revolution, a formless revolution, an irrational revolution, and—that which is least justifiable and most irrational—it is a hoax. The fire of its purpose is in its oratory, not its action. This oratorical crusade, this still-mutiny will—if we permit it—cause a reformation to sameness. If we permit it, the revolution will entrench what is; we will have revolted to what we were and are, rather than to what we should become. We will have won the battle for the mentally retarded, but the spoils of our victory will be ashes. For ashes are what we fought for, nothing more, and these we had from the beginning, nothing else.

Our no-change revolution in mental retardation is a random revolution, a random journey where the magnitude and direction of each step of any progress are determined by chance. And, contrary to other forces for change, its leaders are the caretakers of the oppressed, not those who are themselves oppressed; some have conviction for their cause, some are without conviction. I wish I could speak differently today. I wish I could say that "our time has come." I wish I could advise those who have waited so long for so little that now that great progress has been achieved on behalf of the mentally ill, those who have fought that valiant struggle will devote their talents, energies, and resources to the least of the least, the mentally retarded. I want to believe that, in our day, things will be different for the mentally retarded, but my disillusion is deep. The evidence supporting it is like an ideational anchor holding fast in the mire of our history. And, although that history has taught us to crawl when we were not permitted to walk, to be grateful for small gains as we experienced chaos around us, it has also demonstrated the futility of compromise that is resignation, of modesty that is cowardice, of change that is deception, and of responsibility that is irresponsibility. As the world is changing, as the lot of mankind becomes less arduous in our civilization, the condition of the mentally retarded remains what it was in our fathers' time, which is what it was in their fathers' time. And as each seeks to establish his innocence for this condition, each knows the degree of his responsibility—one, because he did little when he should have done a great deal, and another because he did too much of what should not have been attempted.

In other forums and formats, innumerable confrontations, I have presented evidence for everything said here. However, the evidence hasn't been very helpful. That is, it hasn't done very much good. I was troubled about this until I realized that it isn't evidence that you need because you know—almost as well as I do—that I speak the truth. The evidence is all about us. However, for those who really don't know, who need evidence, review the public record. Review and compare the annual budgets for state mental hospitals and state schools for the retarded. Review and compare our community programs for the mentally ill and the mentally retarded. Review and compare the empty beds in our mental hospitals and the human warehouses in our schools for the retarded. Survey the indifference of our medical schools, schools of social work and nursing, and their learned societies toward the mentally retarded, and form comparisons with their involvements with the mentally ill. No new evidence will be presented here. It is fruitless and I see no need for it. The need for such data is long passed. My mission here is to ask you who represent "mental health"—ask you, not tell you, because you are in control—to welcome us as full and equal partners for human welfare or give us our freedom to defend and prosecute for our defenseless and persecuted brothers as you are so successfully defending others in as great need, but fortunately, receiving more of their due.

Our two fields—mental health and mental retardation—have always had a dichotomy of nomenclature as well as objectives, services, and share of the public treasure. The classic differentiation between mental illness and mental retardation is found in the meanings of our traditional terms "dementia" and "amentia," one signifying a loss of mentality and the other that mentality was never present. Beyond that relatively simple discrimination, however, are all the implications and inferences that give true understanding of these terms. Mental illness is a sickness where there is hope and possible cure and is the concern of the physician and the therapist. Mental retardation is a condition which is traditionally without hope, without cure, with little more than the drudgery of day-to-day habit training and the ameliorative effects of prosthesis. It is not an accident that with rendering of the term "mental illness," the corollary "mental health" is either echoed or assumed. It is not an act of forgetfulness or impreciseness that we have no such corollary for "mental retardation." We have no associations for mental adequacy. The chronicity of our charge defeats any optimistic objectives we have for it and almost guarantees the total disinterest of those trained to heal. Consequently, in the light of logic, it is not surprising that organized medicine, social work, nursing, and even government have not shown the same interest and concern for the mentally retarded as they have shown for the mentally ill. Nor, can I say to you that mental retardation is, to a large degree, preventable or, to an undetermined degree, curable. I believe that we are now finding ways of preventing mental retardation and we will find procedures to cure this affliction. However, I would have to reach far beyond the evidence currently available to make such guarantees to you. Neither will I claim any special significance for my personal belief that what was just said concerning the possibilities for prevention and cure for mental retardation can be said—with equal justification—for the mentally ill. That is, my evaluation of the available research and my personal experiences lead me to conclude that mental retardation is no less amenable to prevention and cure than is mental illness. However, the ethos of mental health is one of faithfulness and optimism.

In many ways, our cause has been served by its affiliation, largely unwanted on both sides, with the field of mental health. The term "mental" denotes to the world that the deficiency is in the mind, not the soul or the spirit. Whatever communality we share protects us somewhat from the banalities and stupidities of those who would have us correlate retardation with evil or with the vengeance of Jehovah. Further, it is probable that the "mental" preceding retardation and our company with the field of mental health have helped us to recruit mental health workers, some of whom may not have viewed their affiliations with us as last resorts or testimony to their own failures and incompetencies for employment in their "true" field. But, "beyond the mental" our jointure has been fruitless and, consequently, the revolution in mental retardation has been empty.

For too many decades we have received a disproportionately insufficient share of the mental health treasure. Further, the allocation for mental retardation is made less useful by the encumbrances and "strings" that always appear to accompany it, "strings" that may be appropriate for the alleviation of mental illness but, insofar as mental retardation is concerned, are untenable. We are told, on the one hand, that administrators of public institutions for the mentally retarded must be physicians, at least, and, in the best of all possible worlds, psychiatrists. On the other hand, the medical profession—collectively and in innumerable individual demonstrations—makes it abundantly clear that no self-respecting physician should ever accept a position in a state school for the mentally retarded. The results of this ludicrous contrivance are predictable. We do have administrative shortages in our schools for the mentally retarded; we do have too many foreign physicians, medical failures, and others who are ill themselves mixed in a profoundly complicated juxtaposition with a minority of the most ennobling and dedicated humanists who are consciously sacrificing wealth and prestige to serve this cause for reasons I cannot fully comprehend but for which I am thankful. Add two questions to this problem and then ponder the difficulties created for us, albeit unwittingly, by the field of mental health: In that utopia of all worlds, are physicians most qualified to administer residential facilities for the mentally retarded? In that utopia of all worlds, what is the relative importance of medicine as contrasted with other professions in caring for and treating the mentally retarded?

I don't claim definitive answers to the above questions, although obviously I have my own biased notions concerning what those answers would be if a book of all truth and wisdom were available to us. I do claim that a terrible injustice is being perpetrated in the name of comprehensive mental-health—mental-retardation planning. In other years there were other names proffered in the guise of progress and unity, probably well intentioned, but leading inevitably to dereliction in our responsibilities to the mentally retarded. Nor, as I envision the future from the clouded jaundice of today, will things be different in our children's time. The shibboleths may change, the irrationalizations may be modified or redefined, but if we continue our current course the plight of the mentally retarded will remain invarient from now until then, however long from this time that "then" will be.

Human beings may invent and define words such as "mental retardation" and "progress," but the subtlety and meaning of these words usually escape our full comprehension. These incredibly complex and superior minds that shape language ironically are not equal to utilizing this unique human product in the intended way. We have created a language but are trapped by our own brilliant invention.

There are two human struggles which together parallel the history of efforts to include the mentally retarded within the family of mankind and to give him all the benefits of such inclusion. The disaffection that organized medicine, psychology, social work, and even nursing demonstrate toward the geriatric patient is virtually isomorphic with their interest in the mentally retarded person and for substantially similar reasons. Secondly, the alienation that is felt by people such as myself, as one apart from the mental health movement, and what is hoped will be done about it are strikingly similar to the alienation that the Negro is said to feel and what he hopes will be done about it.

We are asking you to cease thinking of our cause, or any human concern, as a hopeless one that is doomed to failure before it has had a chance to be. We are asking you to integrate us, to make us truly a part of you and you truly a part of us, or to set us free, to separate your mission from ours. We are not certain how well we can exist apart from you; we do know that our situation is now intolerable and will not change as long as our concerns are secondary ones and as long as we are ministered to with the left hand, if at all. As I have stated at the beginning, I will not catalogue for you the almost inexhaustible and unremitting lists of grievances that can be documented concerning the unavailable, inappropriate, abusive, scandalous treatment a family of a mentally retarded child may expect when they place their child in a state residential facility. Nor will I present the abundant documentation clarifying for all but those who do not wish to see that there are no alternatives for the mentally retarded other than institutionalization or, if the child is both lucky and capable, public school special classes. For those who are not eligible for the public schools or who are no longer children, the alternatives to institutionalization are few indeed—if they exist at all in most communities; also, because of the unavailability of community programs and the subsequently large waiting lists for residential placement, institutionalization is often not available as a choice.

In recent years, those of you who call yourselves "mental health workers" have appeared to be seeking a rapprochement with the field of mental retardation. Yet, so it seems to me, and I have participated in attempts toward reconciliation, you have been rebuffed and hurt by the unwillingness of those in the field of mental retardation to trust you or welcome your support as other than a mixed blessing. It is true! We have been distrustful, possibly with good reason. As with Negro-White relationships, for untold years you have denigrated our purpose and have caused the term "mental deficiency" and all of its successors to become pejorative terms. Now, for your own purposes—be they guilt, rescue fantasy, the lure of federal gold, or genuine humanitarian concern and realization of a horrible neglect— you come to save us, bringing your science and your prestige and your power, yet knowing so pitifully little of either whom you will help now or the condition that gave rise to his problems. Those of us who have struggled alone have learned that our ignorance is great concerning the nature and conditions of mental retardation. Those of you who have not given thought to this problem, *because* you have not given thought to this problem, know far less yet behave with a certainty that derives from callowness, naiveté, and a raw opportunism that the superficial and unsophisticated are addicted to. If your true purpose is to join with us in the common struggle for the mentally ill and the mentally retarded, then you must come to be taught as well as to teach, you must come to serve as well as to be served, and you must be humble in a confrontation with uncertainty and complexity. Unfortunately, you must expect abuse from those of your colleagues who have been defamed and those parents whose problems have been ignored. For there is a suspicion among many professionals and parents concerned with the mentally retarded that will not easily permit such offers of friendship and coalescence of values that may come from workers in mental health. If your motives are genuine, you will not permit our rejection to discourage you. You will understand this and allow for it. You will understand that we do not want to be apart from the field of mental health. In fact, we realize that progress for the mentally retarded will never be truly achieved until we have achieved progress for all of the afflicted and burdened and those whom society now derogates.

If it is the true desire of the field of mental health to join as one with the field of mental retardation, mental health—being the more favored and more advanced—will have to treat sympathetically a condition they are at least partially responsible for. For want of a name, as no name for this now exists, I call this condition "oligophrenic racism." By "oligophrenic racism," I mean the attitude expressed by many in my field that the mental health profession should set us free to struggle for ourselves, to find our own way and not be shackled by the restraints that you have placed upon us and the roadblocks you have constructed between our current condition and our envisioned destiny. However, if your purpose is genuine, if you can withstand some initial frigidity and caution in response to your warmth and good will, you will find that we truly want to join you and, in fact, we need you as you need us. On the other hand, if the field of mental health does not view the field of mental retardation as part of a common endeavor, then you *must* permit us to disassociate ourselves from you and join forces with other groups or "go it alone" as we have in the past, but now without the weight of your resistance diluting our efforts and progress.

It has been said that artists distort reality to present reality. Possibly, that which has been presented and certainly that which will be presented are distortions. Nevertheless, they are real. It is real to phantasize a state institution for the mentally retarded as Milton phantasized Pandemonium. It is real to view that necropolis, Pandemonium, as part of the context of a state institution. It may not be accurate to utilize such analogies, but it presents one side of reality that accuracy is unable to present. One does not describe Pandemonium but reacts to it as I have in this presentation. My purpose is plain: to grate on your conscience, to make you aware, to gain your support in a reformation that will return the mentally retarded from the brutality of institutional back wards to the realm of human awareness, compassion, and interrelatedness.

In Pandemonium, there are many aliases:
solitary confinement is therapeutic isolation
restraint is protection
punishment is negative feedback
and indifference to all of these is thoughtfulness.
In Pandemonium, a girl has seven healthy teeth removed to prevent
her from eating the threads of the day room rug.
In Pandemonium, the physically handicapped become more disabled as
          each
   day passes each identical day and as each old contracture is the
   cause of new contractures and as both old and new are the effects
   of indifference and ineptitude.
In Pandemonium, we appropriate such progressive terms as

                                             "comprehensive"
                                             "community"
                                             "regional"
                                             "prevention"
but nothing changes or we wouldn't be in Pandemonium.

In Pandemonium, there is little drug addiction but there is pervasive,
more destructive, environmental addiction with its accompanying with-
        drawal
syndrome and sickness.
In Pandemonium, the cry of the anguished is, "I am here!"
    children are locked and forgotten in solitary confinement cells
    for such things as breaking a window or speaking disrespectfully
    to an attendant.
In Pandemonium, the tunnel is endless, the darkness unendurable
                                the light extinguished.
    Weakness is strength and strength is weakness.
    Power is causing nothing to change.
    Trivial questions are answered erroneously while meaningful ones
    are never asked.
In Pandemonium, Utopia is anywhere else.
In Pandemonium, humanists dislike people.
    both labor and management are represented by one collective
                                negotiator, the devil.
    we find new ways to express horror and debasement.
In Pandemonium, to embrace life is to kiss death.
        the humanists are inhuman
        the theists are atheists
        the lovers are haters.
                    You die before you live; the end
precedes a beginning.
    In Pandemonium, labeling someone or something makes it fact.
    In Pandemonium, the luxury of life is death—
                            you are in the eye
                                of the eye
                        of that mischief, Hell.

Pandemonium is the sophist's paradise.
    disguising inertia as reasonableness.
    demonstrating the tautology of the
            "evil of massive institutions"
    and the non sequitor in
            "excellent large institutions."
Pandemonium is entranced with medical curiosities rather than concerned
with human necessities—a phantasmagoria which is real.
Pandemonium proves the gnostics' thesis that man is wicked and the
                    world is an evil place.
Pandemonians hope for their nightmares to end while knowing their terror
                            is permanent
    waiting for the floods to subside while expecting the deluge.
Pandemonians respect an equality that understands no difference between
                        "he" and "it"

having learned that the next hour will be a greater
                              catastrophe
    than the last.
Pandemonians who are deaf never speak, who are palsied never walk, who
are retarded never think and in Pandemonium,
                              the blind have no eyes and the lame no feet.
Pandemonians know that life is war.
Good works are inherited from evil doings in Pandemonium
                              people are strangers. We are trapped
because the priest *does* practice what he preaches.
The internal vacuum and the external wasteland are the empty looms—
and hollow threads—weaving the fabric—Pandemonium.
When one chooses to die, it is his method to confirm death rather than
                              to reject life in Pandemonium.
    There is no need to talk through one's problem as there is no shade
of difference, just an omnipotent
            MAN
who proclaims what IS in Pandemonium.
    Artists distort reality to present reality; distortion is the reality
                              in Pandemonium.
    Naiveté and innocence cannot survive.
    Subterfuge is the shortest distance between two conspirators in Pande-
        monium.
    One man lives in the future, another in the past,
while no one has either in Pandemonium.
    Nothing ever changes, yet there is an illusion of change, for things
    do not change differently, now from the way they have not changed
    before.
There are many liberals but few equalitarians in Pandemonium.
No one is dehumanized because he is a
            man
but many are dehumanized because they are residents in Pandemonium.
Sick people live in a healthy culture and healthy people live in a sick
culture; the mix is Pandemonium.
                          Today is Doomsday in Pandemonium.
    The concept of Pandemonium is in knowing right and doing wrong
                              thinking well, and behaving poorly,
believing that nothing can be done so nothing need be attempted
                          the system is wrong while we are right.
    The concept of Pandemonium is in treating other humans as if they
                                              weren't
                          then treating ourselves as if we
                                              were.
    The concept of Pandemonium is to promote the administrator's pseudo-
    giftedness while he promotes the patients' pseudo-custodialness,

not believing in the fulfillment of every human being,
denying the poet an opportunity to arrange for a better life.
The concept of Pandemonium relates more to *ahumantia* than to *amentia*,
presenting a public image that disguises closed systems
as open systems.
The concept of Pandemonium unfolds the animal ethos leading the human
spirit.
The concept of Pandemonium is to build
ideational and physical tunnels
to deny man the sensation of natural light and experience,
learning geography while neglecting etiology.
The concept of Pandemonium relies on the truth of its deceit
the courage of its cowardice
and the love of hate.
The concept of Pandemonium is for the state to give the patient
everything
but he gets
nothing.
Pandemoniacs destroy relationships
respecting chaos.
Pandemoniacs build evil
exuding unforgiveness
inducing pain
revolting against competence.
causing mental retardation.
What will the reformation of Pandemonium bring? We will agree that mere
intention is meaningless; mere speech is noise; behavior is character.
And, we will question not only truth but value!
In our affair with humanity, we have learned that
loves penetrates hate
the heart moves mountains while the mind moves only the heart
and the soul is man's ultimate triumph.
The saga of humanity has its glory in the human value
The glory of humanity is its saga of humanhood
In the cause for humanity, we must agree that
all men are human beings
all human beings are valuable
and all the rest is commentary.

―――――

NOTE

1. The author is grateful to Commissioner Milton Greenblatt and other colleagues of the Massachusetts Department of Mental Health, whose support and encouragement caused me to hope that there is hope. At times they have agreed and at other times they have disagreed with my assessment of the nature of things, with my pessimism, or with my optimism. Regardless of how often or how well our views were as one, I was given every opportunity to express my position and advocate its acceptance. This chapter was written during leave of absence from Boston University while I served as Director of the Division of Mental Retardation, Massachusetts Department of Mental Health. It is being published simultaneously in the author's new book, *Exodus from pandemonium: a reformation of residential treatment for the mentally retarded*. Special Child Publications, Seattle, Washington.

: 25 :

Roadblocks to Renewal of Residential Care

Gunnar Dybwad

INTRODUCTION

PRESIDENT Kennedy's message of October 1961 brought to the nation a strong reminder that services to the mentally retarded citizens have been grossly neglected.[1] Since that time, considerable sums of money have been spent on research and training, particularly on planning and constructing large new centers for research and training, and the availability of adequate and appropriate services in communities throughout the country has increased at a slow pace.

As far as state institutions for the mentally retarded were concerned, the 1962 Report of the President's Panel on Mental Retardation (President's Panel, 1962a) described the general level of care provided by them as low. The recent report of the President's Committee on Mental Retardation, "MR67," issued five years later, used much harsher words, saying many of these institutions are "plainly a disgrace to the nation and to the state that operates them."

The facts are plainly established. A continuous series of exposés in state after state and the subsequent investigations clearly indicate that we are not dealing with occasional unfortunate incidents, such as the unrelated actions of single employees, but rather with inevitable consequences of weaknesses inherent in the system. Cruel and unusual punishment, inadequate medical attention, inadequate staffing practices, interference with basic civil rights, exploitation through forced labor, working hours far beyond anything tolerated in the open community, on the one hand, idleness and total absence of activity, on the other, punishment (such as prolonged isolation) rather than treatment for those severely disturbed—all of these occurrences can be documented again and again even in large and well-to-do states which otherwise pride themselves on enlightened health and welfare services.

Yet this, of course, does not tell the whole story. Particularly in recent years outstanding progress has been made throughout the country. Indeed, traveling with a skilled cameraman, one could put together a composite motion picture of, if not an ideal, at least an excellent system of residential care for the retarded. The problem lies in the unevenness of the situation. Examples may be found in one state of excellent community services and yet the most backward residential care, or vice versa; often these are paradoxical variations from state to state and, indeed, within the same state.

Significantly, the amount of overall state expenditures alone is not a helpful index. Of the two largest states, California, according to the latest published federal statistics (National Clearinghouse for Mental Health, 1967), spent $11.41 per diem on its institutions for the retarded but provided only 71.1 beds per 100,000 population, while New York spent only $6.94 per diem yet provided more than twice as many beds—150.2 per 100,000 population. While the lowest-ranking state spent only $2.30 per diem, the highest-ranking state (excluding Alaska because of its special problems) spent $12.18 per diem, or more than five times as much. Yet within this highest-paying state there were very distinct qualitative differences between institutions. As a matter of fact, throughout the country one can find instances of rather satisfactory care given to the less severely retarded, while in the same institution the more profoundly physically and mentally handicapped are grossly neglected and living under intolerable conditions. It is also fair to say that in some states conditions are worsening due largely to overcrowding and the increasing problem of obtaining adequate personnel at the salaries offered.

What are the reasons for this continued deplorable state of affairs in the year 1968, five years after President Kennedy tried to mobilize the nation's conscience on behalf of the mentally retarded? Why is it that methods which have been proved highly successful decades ago in one state are still being ignored in neighboring states? What is the explanation for the fact that New York State already in the early 1930's built modern attractive small cottages in its institutions for delinquent youth, yet in its institutions for the mentally retarded even thirty years later, in the 1960's, continued to use archaic, inadequate, mass-housing designs? How is it possible that year after year, in spite of exposés, publicity, and anguished outcries of concern from professional workers and relatives, conditions continue to exist in our state institutions which would result in criminal prosecution if condoned in a privately owned facility?

Why does this nation, which will unhesitatingly go all out with men, materials, and funds to rescue a little girl fallen into a well and breathlessly await word of her safe return, turn away in disgust or, even worse, diffidence when it reads in the country's largest magazine a documentary article on the purgatory conditions in our state institutions for the mentally retarded?

What *are* the roadblocks in the long-sought renewal of enlightened residential care for the mentally retarded? This chapter will systematically review what are considered to be the major components of these roadblocks.

THE ROADBLOCKS

A Major Roadblock: The Medical Model

There is clear evidence that roadblocks can be found in the way in which the various professions have functioned in the field of residential care, in administrative and legal considerations, and in the basic attitudes toward the mentally retarded existing within the professional community and the public at large.

The majority of institutions serving the mentally retarded in the United States have been fashioned on the medical model, administered and staffed like the traditional hospital for the mentally ill (Wolfensberger, 1969). Both the American Medical Association and the American Psychiatric Association have expressed themselves strongly to the effect that institutions serving the mentally retarded should be directed by physicians and, insofar as the latter association is concerned, specifically by psychiatrists. Very considerable lobbying activity has been carried on in support of these claims.

There is no doubt that with very few exceptions all institutions for the mentally retarded have a large number of residents who have a primary need for acute or chronic nursing care under immediate medical direction. However, it is equally true that for a very large number of residents presently admitted to our institutions the primary need is not for care given by physicians and nurses; rather the primary need is in the broad realm of education, from early-childhood development to schooling, training in activities of daily living, as well as social and work training. As Smith (1968) has pointed out in another context: "The medical language of illness and health, disease and cure, has to be stretched beyond comfortable limits to accommodate these objectives." The focus on pathology which is part of the traditional medical diagnostic approach has resulted in inadequate attention to the educational programming in the institutions (Richardson, 1965).

From the foregoing it might be assumed that at least the medical programs in the institutions are of adequate quality. Unfortunately in many institutions this is not the case, and the record will show that while the professional medical organizations have been vociferous in their demands for control of the institutions, they have shown far less concern for the actual standards of medical attention and nursing services. For instance, even a cursory study of numerous state institutions under medical direction reveals procedures in the use of drugs, in the performance of medical examinations, in the dispensing of medications, and in medical record-keeping (charting) which grossly violate accepted hospital standards. Although there are still numerous states which maintain that the primary physicians in the institutions for the mentally retarded should be psychiatrists, and that the superintendent must have that specialty, in many of these institutions it is hard to discern much that would constitute psychiatric treatment as taught in medical schools or practiced in psychiatric clinics.

A realistic general index of the activities of the medical profession, including the field of psychiatry, is to be found in the articles published in the professional journals and in the papers submitted to large scientific meetings: The number of papers written by psychiatrists over the past ten years on aspects of psychiatric treatment in institutions for the mentally retarded is indeed minimal.

Another indicator of the nature of the major concerns of psychiatry is the testimony given annually at Congressional hearings by outstanding, recognized leaders of the profession on past progress and future planning. Over the past years here, too, discussions of psychiatric procedures in the field of mental retardation have been conspicuous by their absence.

Roadblocks to Institutional Management

If one turns from the specific field of psychiatric intervention to the broader field of institutional management, the picture is similarly disheartening. In the majority of the institutions under psychiatric direction, the lack of application of the principles of dynamic psychiatry in the administrative organization, in interstaff relationships, in the day-to-day care of the residents, and in the relationships with the families is astounding. The management of disciplinary measures and the use of restraint and isolation over prolonged periods, with adults and children alike, are particularly to be noted in this context.

Yet there is, of course, an important, albeit largely unfilled, place for psychiatry in institutions for the mentally retarded: first, in the specific therapeutic intervention with those residents who give evidence of distinct emotional disturbance and, indeed, psychosis; and, second, in promoting a climate of mental hygiene throughout the institution, thereby preventing a considerable amount of disturbed behavior which results from institutional pressures, tension, and neglect. Training schools for juvenile delinquents have demonstrated for many decades the great contribution psychiatry can make in this way, without becoming burdened by the minutiae of the administrative process which is so typical in the institutions for the mentally retarded.

When in 1959 Denmark modernized its system of care for the mentally retarded, a major objective was to achieve a balanced interdisciplinary approach to the problem. Therefore, the traditional position of the medical superintendent was replaced by a directorate of four, namely, the medical director, the director of education, the director of social service, and the administrative manager. From the point of view of effective administration, this innovation constituted a calculated risk, but the experience of the past nine years has shown that the main objective, that of a balanced participation by the various professions,[2] is increasingly being achieved.

It is not here suggested that a similar move should be undertaken in the United States, but somehow we must remove the roadblocks by which the medical model has impeded the contribution of education, psychology, social work, and other nonmedical professions toward meeting the needs of the residents in mental retardation institutions.

Traditionally, under the medical model, psychology has accepted a rather limited role in these institutions, namely, that of testing. In recent years, however, psychologists have made significant contributions in two important areas: psychotherapy (particularly group psychotherapy) and, increasingly, behavior-shaping and operant conditioning. Especially through the latter procedures, psychology has initiated and opened up promising approaches toward lessened dependence of even the profoundly retarded. Yet in many institutions for the retarded the effectiveness of these programs is impeded by the fact that the psychologist can only function through and with the sanction of the superimposed medical structure.

The situation is more complicated in the field of education, which has largely been limited in many institutions to the classroom teaching of children considered by the administration as eligible for schooling. Yet obviously the most significant and vital area for education in the institutions is the day-to-day learning in the elementary tasks of living, which must take place not in the formal atmosphere of the schoolroom but on the wards or in the cottages, in short, in the living units of the residents. Unfortunately, with few exceptions, educators have tied themselves to the classroom routines and have left this significant area of training for the basic life skills to others. The challenge remains, and the question is whether the educational profession will move forward to meet this responsibility outside the classroom.

Anyone acquainted with prevailing practices in institutions for dependent and neglected children in this country is shocked when confronted with the vastly inferior conditions in institutions for the mentally retarded. This is only one of the areas where social work could make a distinct contribution to institutional management. Yet the national professional organization in social work has for years turned a deaf ear when it was urged that it recognize and meet the profession's responsibilities in the area of mental retardation.[3] Introduction of long-established and proven methods of child care into the institutions for the retarded remains an urgent necessity.

Professional Attitudes

The emphasis of the foregoing discussion has been on the professions as such, rather than on the failure of specific members of the profession working in the institutions. The reason for this lies in the fact that the most formidable roadblock toward renewal of residential care for the mentally retarded is tied to the prevailing attitudes toward the mentally retarded which unhappily are as representative of the professional community as they are of the public at large.

Anyone who works in the broad field of human disability is aware of how seriously prejudice interferes in the life adjustment of the affected individuals. Deviance in general is associated by the public with social conduct, yet in our culture social deviance is frequently far more tolerantly accepted than the grosser types of physical deviance, such as the person with severe spasticity. But the most severe consequences are attached to deviance in the realm of intellectual performance, particularly if it is severe enough to require institutionalization.

Much as the past objections on the part of physicians to the use of Negro blood in blood banks was predicated on cultural beliefs taking precedence over scientific evidence, so today certain "medical" decisions in the field of mental retardation, such as the insistence on immediate and permanent separation from the mother of any child born with mongolism, are a clear reflection of social prejudice rather than of the current state of knowledge (Dybwad, 1964; Pearson, 1965).

Similar extreme rejection of the severely retarded individuals can be encountered on the part of educators, psychologists, sociologists, clergymen, and, of course, quite large segments of the public. The extent to which public and professional opinion merge in this area was most recently documented in two parallel articles in *The Atlantic Monthly,* which in essence held that children afflicted with mongolism and other severely retarded individuals were, in effect, nonpersons or subhuman creatures, who should be disposed of by euthanasia or in any case left to die. Nor can the *Atlantic* article be considered an isolated and extremist view. The terms "subhuman," "human vegetables," and "animal level of functioning" can still today be found in printed utterances by physicians and others (*Frontiers of Hospital Psychiatry,* 1968), are frequently encountered in face-to-face discussions, and are clearly reflected in practices found in numerous state institutions for the mentally retarded.

Recently the head of the State Mental Retardation Service of Denmark commented that conditions he encountered on certain wards in a California state institution for the mentally retarded would not be tolerated in his country in the care of cattle. The significant point about his comment is not the severity of criticism by a foreign visitor, but rather that this very same observation has been made for many years by American observers. Indeed identical conditions could be found in the midwest or in the larger sophisticated states of the eastern seaboard.

Two years ago David J. Vail, one of our country's best-known state psychiatric administrators, published a book entitled *Dehumanization and the Institutional Career* (Vail, 1967). It provided a detailed documentation of the many ways in which institutions serving the mentally ill or mentally retarded go about stripping away from the residents their human dignity, identity, motivations, privacy, and basic human rights. Dr. Vail's book underlines cogently that where these conditions exist we are dealing not so much with the incompetence of a superintendent or the malfeasance and misfeasance of employees, but with the viciousness of a system ordained and maintained by official sanction and predicated on the belief that the residents are inferior creatures, devoid of sensitivity, to whom the usual norms of human interaction do not apply. There can be no question but that this type of system produces a setting that can provoke in employees an indifference toward human suffering and a tolerance of cruelty.

As pointed out earlier, there are distinct variations among and within the institutions, and while the process of dehumanization can be observed in many, by no means does it apply to all. But in practically all institutions one can find a process which George Sharman (1966) of Australia has called "dehabilitation." Since the mentally retarded person is presumed a priori to be incapable of acquiring certain skills and knowledge, he is not given the opportunity to learn, and things he could learn are done for him. Jack Tizard's Brooklands film (1960) well documented this at the old Fountain Hospital in London.

Actually the process of dehabilitation is reinforced by a characteristic of the medical model which encourages in the "patient" a dependency (Richardson, 1965) and surrounds him with a highly protective, activity-stifling environment that avoids the "risk" situations that form an important part of the human learning process.

Administrative Roadblocks

In the long-standing dispute about the size of institutions for the mentally retarded, those who are opposed to the large institutions have often pointed to its rigid impersonal administrative structure. Certainly such rigidity is particularly in evidence when we are dealing with the hierarchical system so inherent in the medical model. One way of characterizing the resulting problem is to say that the typical institution for the mentally retarded is administration-oriented rather than client- or resident-oriented. The weight of the decision-making in the administration building, the unusual power of the superintendent (in some states strong enough to successfully contain any meaningful program direction from central state government), the social and professional distance between the concentration of professional staff in the administration building (the "brain trust"), and the low-status, low-salaried personnel in direct contact with the residents have long been recognized as militating against the kind of dynamic, flexible, multifaceted approach which can focus on and respond to the varied needs of the residents in a large institution (Dybwad, 1964*b*).

There is another aspect to the inappropriateness of the medical model as applied to the institution for the mentally retarded: In the general hospital, the care of the patient is predicated on a continuous close interplay between the nursing staff and the physicians, with the supplementary services of various types of hospital aides rigidly circumscribed. But when one views this system as applied to the institution for the retarded, one finds a director of nursing with a very small staff of graduate nurses and a very large low level staff of attendants, aides or so-called "psychiatric technicians" on whom falls the main weight of the care program; the physician is more concerned with general administrative routine than with the specific needs of the individual residents.

This rigid hierarchical pattern, in many instances circumscribed by civil service classifications which were largely written in the image of the state hospital for the mentally ill, is in many states being further solidified through the introduction of employee unions, which have naturally tended to take as a base the status quo and thus tend to reaffirm an existing inappropriate division of responsibility and labor.

Almost without exception, visitors to the Scandinavian institutions for the mentally retarded are impressed by the large number of young staff members who work directly with the residents and for whom this work is a career opportunity (beginning in Denmark with a three-year, fully paid, full-time theoretical and practical training course). In our country we cannot hope to attract young workers unless we not only remove the barriers set by low salaries, but also effect substantial changes in the rigidity of the hierarchical system, thus setting the stage for a different, more dynamic and satisfying functioning of the basic "front-line" staff aides. Much effort has been spent in the United States on developing new and vital staff training materials, and those produced by the Southern Regional Education Board are particularly outstanding (Bensberg, 1964, 1965; Bensberg and Barnett, 1966). But their effectiveness is impeded as long as the general climate in the institution remains stifling to individual initiative and as long as the old-line supervisory nursing staff carries on defensively, on guard against encroachment of the status quo.

One of the most insidious roadblocks to the introduction of a more effective and dynamic program in our institutions is a distortion of the concept of efficiency, namely, efficiency oriented to ease of administration rather than to meeting the human needs of the individual residents (Dybwad, 1969). Thus we have tile on the wall because it is efficient to maintain and large central dining rooms where residents are fed efficiently rather than eating leisurely meals in small groups in their own living quarters. There are efficient assembly-line procedures for bathing, dressing, and clothes' storage, and even for using the toilet. Indeed, in one of our country's newest institutions for the mentally retarded, the toilet facilities have been placed right in the middle of a hexagonal type of "cottage" structure; thus maximum efficiency and accessibility have been achieved by placing the toilet in the center of the child's universe. This type of efficiency in building layout can reach a point where it reduces to a minimum the traffic as well as the child!

Clearly, efficiency of any operation, whether in business and industry or health and welfare, must be oriented to the basic purpose of the operation, and ease of maintenance and administration is certainly not the basic purpose of institutions serving the mentally retarded.

Legal Roadblocks

A major problem in effecting a renewal of residential care rests in the traditional perceptions of the legal status of the mentally retarded. Albert Deutsch (1949) has pointed out to what extent institutionalization of the mentally retarded constituted banishment, a police measure in the interest of public safety. Again, there are wide variations within the United States in the extent to which this historical pattern is reflected in the institutional practices of today. In some cases this refers merely to such matters as extent of mail censorship, restriction of visiting privileges, and so on, while in others it refers in far more serious fashion to denial of rights and to modes of disciplinary punishment which would not be tolerated in the prisons of the same state.

The recent Supreme Court decision (1967) regarding the adverse effect of informal juvenile court procedures and dispositions on the constitutional rights of juvenile offenders foreshadows all too clearly a similar judicial move on behalf of the constitutional rights of the mentally retarded residents of state institutions. While the 1961 and 1963 Hearings of the United States Senate Subcommittee on Constitutional Rights were primarily concerned with the rights of the mentally ill, some of the testimony had direct bearing on the need to safeguard the constitutional rights of the institutionalized mentally retarded.[4]

Architectural-Programmatic Roadblocks

Throughout the world in recent years there has been an effort to re-move architectural barriers impeding the physically handicapped. A similar campaign has recently been launched to remove the architectural barriers which have effectively impeded modern institutional programming (Dybwad, 1967; Architectural Institute, 1968).

More than twenty-five years ago the Connecticut State Institution at Southbury successfully demonstrated the feasibility of an informal type of building plan with small housing units for a relatively large institution serving all types of mental retardation. Almost ten years ago Arkansas, in its first state institution for the mentally retarded, advanced the Southbury model in line with more current architectural design and construction methods. Yet in a neighboring state just a few months ago the state mental health department was prevented only by a veto from the governor from constructing a $17 million single-building monstrosity with dormitories of seventy beds—a building that would have been thirty years out of date on its opening day. Similar horrors are now under construction or on the drawing boards in other states. Obviously the architectural design reflects the two factors which have been highlighted earlier in this paper: on the one hand, the medical model which insists on looking upon all institutional residents as patients, regardless of their actual condition; and, on the other hand, the view of the mentally retarded as a subhuman species for whom commonly accepted standards of comfort, decency, and aesthetics need not be observed.

An additional architectural barrier toward construction that would be both functionally satisfactory and economically sound is created by unreasonable and inappropriate standards set forth by the federal government, by that most powerful semiofficial body, the Board of Fire Underwriters, and by a multitude of rigidly interpreted state regulations, which in turn relate to pressures brought by industrial groups and by building trades' unions. As a result, construction expenses are vastly increased by inappropriate inflexible specifications, elaborate and expensive safety measures, and service facilities which are insisted upon for buildings that house residents who do not require them. Concomitantly, efforts to create attractive, practicable, and comfortable surroundings are defeated. The cost to the nation of all this is staggering, especially when compared to the sums available for such services as day care, and the resulting architecture defeats its own purpose.

IMPLEMENTATION OF THE
FOREGOING GUIDELINES

How can these roadblocks to the renewal of residential care for the mentally retarded be altered or removed, given some of the major care problems that must be managed? This question, usually followed by a direct reference to the "most difficult" residential clients—the severely and profoundly retarded—has often been stated directly or indirectly in the discussions of some of the roadblocks previously reviewed. Accordingly, we will specifically focus on how these roadblocks can be altered so as to implement an excellent program-services approach for the most challenging of our mentally retarded clients who have been institutionalized: the severely and profoundly retarded adults in the "back wards."

The following guidelines are predicated on the conviction that of the present profoundly and severely retarded adult population in current residential facilities, all but a very small minority, with proper staff resources and an improved environment, can be trained to dress themselves, feed themselves, and to engage in simple activities of daily living. Furthermore, a considerable portion of these groups, once they have mastered these basic life skills, can be trained to perform simple work routines, and some will eventually be able to "graduate" into a full-fledged production, sheltered workshop on the residential grounds.

An exception would be those so acutely disturbed as to qualify for admission to a hospital for the mentally ill. If it is decided that these individuals should nonetheless remain at an institution, then obviously they need to be housed and cared for in a facility under immediate psychiatric supervision and designed differently from that which will be proposed here for the rest of the residential facility population. It should be noted, however, that experience elsewhere has shown that once an institutional environment has been improved and the number of persons housed together in a unit has been sharply decreased, behavioral disturbances decrease both in number and degree.

In terms of physical handicaps, only those people would need to be eliminated from the projected new programs and buildings who require acute nursing care. The new design should accommodate persons requiring wheelchairs, crutches, and so on, as long as they can participate in the main activities of the daily program to an adequate degree.

The reference to the residents' capacity for productivity should not be misconstrued to imply that work output per se is the essential program objective. Rather, what is implied here is an insight we have gained, alas, far too late, that the lack of opportunity for productivity (for example, the enforced idleness so typical of the wards for the severely and profoundly retarded throughout the United States) has been a main factor in the process of deterioration. In this, as in so many other aspects, there are distinct parallels between the care of the mentally retarded and the care of the aged in nursing homes. Thus opportunities for productivity are, of course, only one aspect of the programming here envisioned, and they must be supplemented by organized recreation, opportunities for leisure-time activity (or inactivity) of the patient's own choice, and so on.

Past policy in the design of facilities for the mentally retarded prescribed that smaller housing units, and within those units smaller groupings in day rooms and sleeping facilities, be provided for the less severely retarded. Conversely, larger housing units and larger groupings within those units both for daytime activities and sleeping facilities were prescribed for the more severely retarded. Experiments and demonstration projects, both in this country and abroad (particularly in the Scandinavian countries), backed up by research findings, provide compelling evidence for a complete reversal of this policy regarding the severely and profoundly retarded. The evidence is very clear that the large groupings of the severely and profoundly retarded during daytime and at night, resulting in a depersonalized mass regime, have been a primary factor in the steady deterioration of these individuals. This is clearly evident in most residential facilities for the severely and profoundly retarded, the conscientious efforts of the staff to the contrary notwithstanding.

Thus the most basic requirement in the design of facilities replacing such buildings is small housing units. This does not merely mean small dormitories, small dining rooms, small living rooms, and so on. Rather the term "unit" is meant to imply an integral spatial arrangement whereby the main activities of daily living (excluding occupational activity and certain types of recreational activity, in other words, eating, sleeping, toileting, bathing, and normal leisure-time activities) are carried on in a space limited to a small group of people under guidance of staff personnel who are specifically assigned to them. How small a group? Recent suggestions have varied from six to ten. An increase in the size of such a group will result, with the severely and profoundly retarded, in a lessening of the effectiveness of the daily program, which is predicated on close contact with the unit staff who will then be able to carry through training activities to meet the needs of each individual resident.

The concept of "unit" does not necessarily imply a separate building. Where problems such as nighttime staffing require it, the challenge of architectural design is to find ways in which several such units can be combined under one roof without disturbing the program integrity of the individual units, but allowing for basic construction economies in terms of heating, installation of various facilities, and delivery of food, certain central administrative services, such as an office for a group supervisor in charge of several units, space for supporting services, and so on. The crucial point is that each unit be independent of the others, have separate entrances, separate outdoor space, and so on.

Merely to exemplify what is possible here, one can refer to an arrangement whereby one serving kitchen with serving counters on either side (which can be closed at the end of the meal) can accommodate the dining facilities of two separate units. Or a row of separate rooms for sanitary facilities (toilets, washrooms, and showers) could be arranged either back-to-back or with doors which open alternately into the one or the other of two units, thus combining economy of installation with complete separation of the two groups of residents involved. Preference should be given to small houses accommodating just one unit; however, two totally separate units might be constructed back-to-back, side by side, or at an angle, using one foundation, one roof, and one main connection to heat, water, cables, conduits, and so on.

It would seem indicative at this point to emphasize that separation of groups does not mean segregation. During occupational periods, recreational periods, and at least for the more advanced (that is, better-adjusted) residents, interaction between the members of various groups is entirely appropriate and indeed desirable. As a matter of fact, this style of building design even permits a much greater proximity between units for men and for women than has been envisioned in the past, and this, again, would be considered a desirable situation. Furthermore, separation of these units as far as the daily living of the residents is concerned does not preclude intercommunication between the buildings by way of doors which could be left open at night to permit supervision of more than one unit by one staff member.

The establishment of smaller units permits distinct variation not only in activity but also in assignment of staff. With the least-adapted group, immediate full-time supervision during the night may be required at least during the initial stages of the use of such new facilities, whereas units housing residents with a higher level of adaptation should require far less intensive and immediate supervision during nighttime. Obviously lessened supervision must be initiated on a gradual scale as the results of the new program become evident.

The second cardinal principle for the design of these new facilities should be the greatest possible adaptability of space for varied usage. In many ways, the traditional design of institutional space is very wasteful. Large dormitory spaces used only at nighttime and large dining spaces utilized only three times a day for short periods constitute very uneconomical usage. The new design pattern should create adequate space for dining, which at the same time could be used for varied daytime and evening activities appropriate for this type of room and furnishing; hence the need for limited access to the serving kitchen by means of a door and a serving window that can be completely closed off after meal time (and which permits serving meals both "cafeteria style" and "family style"). Also needed is care in selecting small dining tables (preferably seating four only) which can be used for a multiplicity of sedentary activities and yet, by choice of the proper material, can be easily kept clean to meet proper sanitation requirements.

Similarly, bedrooms (accommodating not more than four residents, but preferably only two or one) should be designed to provide for additional furnishings, such as tables, chairs, and shelves so as to create a highly personalized living space, which is perhaps the most crucial requirement in our new design requirements. The extent to which such individualization can be put into effect, that is to say, the extent to which such furnishings actually will be installed, is of course a question of training and development and can be varied from unit to unit. The main point is that the architect needs to envision from the very beginning this type of eventual usage of the space, that he clearly sees that the task is to build a bed-sitting room—not just a new type of dormitory arrangement.

Another basic principle in the design of these facilities is the need to provide a stimulating environment and a space that is meaningful in terms of human functioning and experience, space that aids rather than hinders a crucial point of the programming: the teaching of techniques and activities for daily living.

During a recent staff discussion at a residential facility, which referred to the high incidence of glass breakage as possible contraindication to a less restrictive building design, an aide pointed out that one of the windows that had never been broken in a building for young active boys was one of the few that permitted residents a pleasant and unobstructed view. Dutch architects, in particular, have been most concerned about creating an immediate surrounding for cottages serving severely and profoundly handicapped individuals, which provides an attractive and stimulating view. In the United States this matter is all too often overlooked.

A sense of individuality of oneself as a person, as well as a sense of meaningfully belonging to a group (such as a group of four in a bedroom) and of having meaningful belongings (within one's capacity to perceive), are of crucial significance for the human being. Danish architects, therefore, emphasize that beds should be placed along a wall so that that particular space gives the resident a feeling of identity. They provide on the wall above the bed a simple bulletin board or a strip of soft wood or similar surface which offers a space for some personal photographs or other things of meaning to that particular resident. A simple night table next to the bed and some simple adjacent on wall shelving have been found in other countries to be entirely compatible with the presence of severely and profoundly retarded individuals in such rooms.

The so-called "sanitary installation" of the typical American institution lives up to its name: It is almost the hallmark of a planned program of depersonalization, a place where human dignity as well as conventional behavior is squelched rather than fostered, and a place which, all too often, is the center of disciplinary problems. Regrettably, it is still necessary in this country to emphasize that failure to provide toilet stalls can no longer be justified. If the staff so insists, one might leave off at first the doors to the toilet stalls in the units serving the least-adapted residents, thus providing easier supervision of the toilet training. However, once intensive training has brought the positive results we have reason to expect, on the basis of recent demonstration programs, the doors could then easily be attached to the side partitions which should, in any case, be installed from the very beginning.

While a bathtub should be provided in each unit, the preferred method of bathing should be by shower, which not only provides a better means of teaching the resident proper methods of cleanliness, but also eliminates a lot of time-consuming and back-breaking cleaning of bathtubs by the staff. Details of proper shower construction that can also be utilized by people with a wide range of physical handicaps are now easily available and should be carefully considered.

It is desirable to avoid the construction of the typical "all-purpose" sanitary facilities with toilets, bathtubs, showers, and individual hand-basins all in one room. Again, for the units serving the least-adapted residents such a design may be considered essential by the staff in the beginning, but provision should be made by the architect for an eventual subdivision of this large space through walls and connecting doors. For severely and profoundly handicapped residents, it is important to have toilet facilities not too distant from daily activities; therefore, depending on the layout of the building and the location of the exit leading to the outdoor space, a toilet may have to be located near that exit.

Reference was made earlier to the need of providing a stimulating environment. There is also need to avoid negative overstimulation; in the traditional institution this would refer typically to acoustical overstimulation, in other words, an unduly high noise level. Therefore, it is strongly recommended that throughout all the units care should be taken to select building materials with good acoustical properties. In particular, it is most desirable that in at least one or two of the units, carpeting be provided on a test basis in the day rooms, bedrooms, and hallways. Carpeting once was considered a sure sign of luxury, but now modern manufacturing techniques have produced carpeting which not only is extremely economical in use but also reduces cleaning time and is impervious to damage from spilled food, urine, and so on.

It would be most worthwhile for many states, with view to future building practices in institutions, to have some of the units equipped with acoustical ceilings and no carpeting and some with both carpeting and acoustical ceilings. This would allow the collation of specific data on the effectiveness of the various methods in terms of noise control and the general effect on the resident.

As far as wall coverings are concerned, tile should be avoided except in those areas where they are standard in normal family homes: bathrooms, kitchens, and so on. If possible, a variety of wall coverings is preferable. Beside standard plaster walls, brick walls have added greatly to the warmth of the institutions for the mentally retarded in the Nordic countries (and in some cases in the United States), as has the use of wood and vinyl wall covering, which is available in excellent quality and very attractive colors. Care in construction design (for example, covering the vinyl edges by molding on the sides and by an inset base on the floor) can greatly reduce damage through wear and tear or intentional destruction by residents.

In Danish institutions one frequently observes in bedrooms a fairly heavy multiple railing along the wall below and above the height of the bed. This protects the wall, provides an added attractiveness to the bed space, but is also utilized for hanging night tables. This latter arrangement has two advantages: since the night table thereby does not need to have legs, cleaning is facilitated, and since the night table can easily be taken off or put on the wall railing, it can be eliminated in rooms where residents are not yet ready to properly utilize such equipment.

Window safety has been a major concern in past institutional construction and has resulted in extraordinarily high expenditures. Window safety is a poor excuse for the lack of active programs; moreover, there is strong evidence that where active programming for the residents is combined with quality of design (with the advantages of small grouping and a high degree of individualization, including a sense of belonging and a chance of having personal belongings near him), a resident is less likely to show destructive behavior. Window safety could again be differentiated among the various units.

A question that will need further exploration pertains to the extent to which a small service unit such as projected here needs to include offices and consultation rooms. Obviously, a staff room is indispensable, but with the contemplated small number of residents per unit, records and office supplies will require a minimum of space. It would be desirable, however, to equip the staff room with comfortable attractive furniture so that its primary function could be to serve as a place where a staff member can relax with a cup of coffee or talk quietly with a staff consultant or visitor. Small but attractively furnished staff lounges are an important feature of Scandinavian institutions for the retarded and contribute to the lack of staff strain and tension one notices there.

Arrangements for a dispensary room and for interviewing space for psychologists, social workers, and so on, would depend on the architectural design pattern in combining several of the small units into one building or a complex of buildings. In the latter case one might either construct a separate service building with an office for the supervisor of this group of buildings, interview rooms, rooms for special therapy or instruction, and a small dispensary, or one could add a separate wing to one of the small unit buildings. It would be very important to prepare quantitative and qualitative analyses of the types of ambulatory medical treatment now provided in a given residential building to determine how much of it really needs to be provided within the residential unit itself and what types of ambulatory treatment rooms would be needed.

Inevitably, the question is raised whether single- or multiple-storied buildings should be planned. On the whole, for this type of resident, the single-story building will provide for easier management, unless the advantageous use of available terrain allows for second-story immediate access to the outdoors from the rear of the building. If multiple-story design is deemed necessary (for whatever reason), then only those residents should be placed on the second floor who have the capacity to move about freely. It would also be desirable to have separate entrances to the first and second floors. Dumbwaiters will be needed for the transportation of food and supplies, but the use of an elevator would produce many administrative and program problems, aside from the very high cost of installation and maintenance which is a poor use of building funds (an exception, of course, would be a multistory facility in a densely settled urban area).

It should be emphasized again that the general design on which these guidelines are predicated would provide certain occupational and recreational spaces outside of the buildings which house the residential units. There has been too often a tendency to eliminate having severely and profoundly retarded residents move over longer distances. Progressive thinking rejects this practice (whether based on "protection" of the resident or "efficiency" of staffing) and sees many advantages in an arrangement which makes it necessary for residents to leave their buildings and move, without immediate shelter, to other buildings. Obviously, these occupational and recreational spaces could be used by both men and women, thereby promoting a desirable social interaction which has distinct advantages. Therefore, there is no need in the small living units to have large spaces for special events, such as parties. Where necessary, this can be arranged for in the recreational space, but in general the artificial and all-too-often "stale" parties and entertainments can be replaced by the more intimate, informal, and stimulating day-to-day living in the smaller units.

It hardly needs to be emphasized that successful use of such a new type of facility will only be accomplished if it is put into use gradually, thus permitting the staff and the residents alike to adjust themselves, unit by unit, to the new set of circumstances. Equally obvious should be that once a new building pattern has been selected, an intensive training program needs to be instituted to prepare the residents for the higher demands which the environment of the new units will put before them. This would require some radical changes in the present arrangements and routines in the usual residential facilities for the severe and profoundly retarded, including changes in the present staffing patterns.

In general, when there is discussion of the need to develop new programs for the retarded, reference is made to financing. In this chapter, however, lack of funds has not been singled out as a major roadblock to the renewal of residential care. The existence all over the country of recently constructed institutions, costing hundreds of millions of dollars yet actually decades out of date, testifies to the fact that the availability of money does not necessarily contribute to the advancement of residential care.

CONCLUSION

In 1960 a conference of sociologists, discussing directions of future sociological research in mental retardation, concluded (Farber 1960):

A contention which needs to be tested is that the prevailing practice in most institutions is less related to the scientific body of medical or psychiatric knowledge than it is related to the mass cultural attitudes which are reflected in traditional institutional regimes which have become an accepted stereotype.

Today, this research need is as unfilled as it was then. Moreover, the same would have to be said with regard to existing educational, psychological, and sociological knowledge. The lack of large-scale research findings related to all these factors and specific enough to aid in program development supports the status quo and holds back effective reform measures.

It is safe to predict that the statements put forth in this presentation will be hotly disputed; yet the factual record stands, and the witnesses are ready to testify. It may also be argued that the judgments made here about the problems created by the traditional medical model are too excessive; however, they have been made repeatedly and even more pointedly from within the psychiatric leadership as far as institutions for the mentally ill are concerned.

It will be suggested that it is not helpful to single out misdeeds of individuals; yet what has been pointed out here is the failure of a system and the system's deleterious effects on its agents. The question will be asked, "Why has not equal space been given to the many positive developments in institutions throughout the nation?" But these positive developments have been amply publicized to little avail. More importantly, it is of little use to the parent in a western state, who finds his institutionalized child covered with sores and signs of physical mishandling, that in Connecticut an enlightened administration has greatly advanced the quality of residential care.

One further point needs to be highlighted. Paradoxical as it may appear at first, a definite roadblock to the renewal of residential care is the inadequacy both quantitatively and qualitatively of nonresidential community services. On the one hand, this causes unnecessary, inappropriate institutionalization, and, on the other hand, it prevents the release from the institution of those persons for whom continued residence there is no longer indicated.

The very objective of this presentation has been to explore what keeps us from applying nationwide the advances which have been successfully tested in progressive states. Thus what needs to be done is to attack the system as a whole, and the system is invariably tied to and supported (actively or by acquiescence) by organizations. It is organized medicine that is forcing the medical model on the institutions for the mentally retarded; it is organized psychiatry that carries on the power play for control but fails to insist on programming consonant with its own philosophy and professional tenets. It is organized education that has turned its back on the broad educational responsibility outside the classroom. It is organized social work that has shrugged off its responsibility toward the mentally retarded. Governmental departments and legislative groups are subject to "political realities," but professional associations can apply their wisdom and knowledge in independence and security. It is to them that we must address ourselves.

What has happened to the action groups in this field? The National Association for Retarded Children, in the past the strongest force for change, has sadly failed to live up to its own challenge and has equivocated rather than confronted this nation with the problems of residential care in the kind of straightforward language recently used by the President's Committee on Mental Retardation (1969).

The American Association on Mental Deficiency seems to have decided to approach the problem through the development of standards and the initiation of a process of accreditation, but it has failed to take the essential first step of clearly spelling out the basic faults inherent in the present system. A process of accreditation, introduced prematurely at this stage, can only result in an essential reinforcement of the medical model and other objectionable features of the system.

At the first meeting of his Panel on Mental Retardation, President Kennedy turned to the chairman and said, "Mr. Mayo, what can we learn from other countries that would help us in our work?" This stimulated the panel to send several missions to other countries known for their progressive programs. And when the panel met again with the President at the time the report was submitted, one of his first questions to the chairman was, "Mr. Mayo, what *have* you learned from the visits to other countries?" There was indeed a great deal that had been learned and set forth, particularly in the published mission reports on the Netherlands, Sweden, and Denmark (President's Panel on Mental Retardation, 1962*b*, 1962*c*); yet relatively little use has been made of this foreign documentation. Indeed more recently a distinct chauvinism has been voiced, a kind of "anti-Scandinavian backlash," to the effect that "We can't be as bad as all that." Unfortunately, the facts cannot be waived aside by misplaced patriotic feelings. We *are* as bad as all that, and to the memory of John F. Kennedy and the campaign which he so forcefully initiated we owe determined action in tackling the roadblocks keeping us from a renewal of residential care which will do honor to this nation.

NOTES

1. Portions of this material were presented at the Fourth International Scientific Symposium on Mental Retardation, sponsored by The Joseph P. Kennedy, Jr., Foundation at Chicago, Ill., April 29, 1968. Also portions of this material were adapted from a position paper on residential programmatic-architectural needs for the mentally retarded, prepared by the author at the request of the Walter E. Fernald State School, Waverly, Mass.

2. It was possible, within the realities of developments in Denmark, to have the director of education also responsible for the closely related psychological concerns.

3. It has been reported that a major position statement of mental retardation by the National Association of Social Workers is at last to be published.

4. Of major significance in this context are the Conclusions of the Symposium on Legislative Aspects of Mental Retardation held in Stockholm, June, 1967, by the International League of Societies for the Mentally Handicapped (Sterner, 1967).

REFERENCES

Architectural Institute, Denver, Colo. *Architectural contributions to effective programming for the mentally retarded.* Conference Report. New York: National Association for Retarded Children, 1968.

Bard, B. The right to die—a father speaks. *Atlantic Monthly,* April, 1968.

Bensberg, G. (Ed.). *Recreation for the mentally retarded. A handbook for word personnel.* Atlanta, Ga.: Southern Regional Education Board, 1964.

———. (Ed.), *Teaching the mentally retarded. A handbook for ward personnel.* Atlanta, Ga.: Southern Regional Education Board, 1965.

Bensberg, G., & Barnett, C. *Attendant training in southern residential facilities for the mentally retarded.* Atlanta, Ga.: Southern Regional Education Board, 1966.

Conditioning the retarded may be inhumane procedure. *Front. Hosp. Psychiat.,* January, 1968, *5,* 5.

Deutsch, A. *The mentally ill in america. A history of their care and treatment from colonial time.* New York: Columbia University Press, 1949.

Dybwad, G. Medical needs of the displaced retarded child. 43rd Ross Conference on Pediatric Research, 1962. In: *Challenges in mental retardation.* New York: Columbia University Press, 1964. (*a*)

————. New horizons in residential care of the mentally retarded. 1959 Annual Convention of the National Association of Retarded Children. In: *Challenges in mental retardation.* New York: Columbia University Press, 1964. (*b*)

————. Changing patterns of residential care for the mentally retarded. A challenge to architecture. In: *Proceedings of first congress of the international association for the scientific study of mental deficiency.* Montpellier, France: 1967.

————. Action implications, U.S.A. today. In: R. B. Kugel, and W. Wolfensberger (Eds.). *Changing patterns in residential services for the mentally retarded.* Washington, D.C.: President's Committee on Mental Retardation, 1969, pp. 383–428.

Farber, B. (Ed.). *Directions of future sociological research in mental retardation.* New York: National Association for Retarded Children, 1960.

Fletcher, J. The right to die—A theologian comments. *Atlantic Monthly,* April, 1968.

Mentally handicapped children growing up. The Brooklands experiment. (16mm MP) London: The National Society for Mentally Handicapped Children, 1960.

National Clearinghouse for Mental Health. Provisional patient movement and administrative data—public institutions for the mentally retarded. *Ment. Health Stat.,* January, 1967, Ser. MHB–I–II.

Pearson, P. The forgotten patient: medical management of the multiple handicapped retarded. *Public Health Reps.,* October, 1965, *80,* 10.

The President's Committee on Mental Retardation. *Changing patterns in residential services for the mentally retarded.* Washington, D.C.: author, 1969.

President's Panel on Mental Retardation. *A proposed program for national action to combat mental retardation.* Washington, D.C.: Superintendent of Documents, 1962. (*a*)

President's Panel on Mental Retardation. *Report of the mission to the Netherlands.* Washington, D.C.: U.S. Public Health Service, 1962. (*b*)

President's Panel on Mental Retardation. *Report of the mission to Denmark and Sweden.* Washington, D.C.: U.S. Public Health Service, 1962. (*c*)

Richardson, S. The handicapped child: social obstacles to growing up. *The social and emotional needs of the handicapped child.* Proceedings of an Institute held at Boston University, September 10, 1965. Waltham, Mass.: Florence Heller Research Center, Brandeis University, 1965.

Sharman, G. Do we "de-habilitate" the retarded? *Proc. 5th Ann. Interstate Conf. Ment. Defic.,* Melbourne, Australia, Australian Group for the Scientific Study of Mental Deficiency: 1966.

Smith, B. The revolution in mental health care—a "bold new approach?" *Transaction,* April, 1968, *5,* 5.

Sterner, R. (Ed.). *Legislative aspects of mental retardation. Conclusions Stockholm symposium 1967.* Brussels: International League of Societies for the Mentally Handicapped (12, rue Forestiere), 1967.

Vail, D. J. *Dehumanization and the institutional career,* Springfield, Ill.: Charles C Thomas, 1966.

Wolfensberger, W. The origin and nature of our institutional models. In: R. B. Kugel and W. Wolfensberger, (Eds.). *Changing patterns in residential services for the mentally retarded.* Washington, D.C.: The President's Committee on Mental Retardation, 1969, pp. 59–171.

Human Values as Guides to the Administration of Residential Facilities for the Mentally Retarded

Howard W. Potter

EACH of the preceding two chapters (Chapter 24 by Burton Blatt and Chapter 25 by Gunnar Dybwad) deplores the kinds of lives the mentally retarded live in too many residential centers or institutions. Each finds that in many institutional communities the patient-care staff and even those in posts of responsibility share in common an unhappy sense of defeatism about the mentally retarded.

Both Blatt and Dybwad seem to have a deep-seated conviction that the image of the residential center would be a happier one if physicians, and especially psychiatrists, would renounce their administrative roles in these centers and, like the Arabs, "fold their tents and silently steal away." But according to a recent directory of the American Association on Mental Deficiency (A.A.M.D.), only 19 of 135 institutions for the mentally retarded are administered by psychiatrists. It was not the author's impression that Blatt and Dybwad were writing about only 14 per cent of our residential centers for the retarded. Everyone, including Blatt and Dybwad, knows that ineffective and unimaginative administration of our institutions for the retarded is not a matter of what kind of professional stripes the administrator wears! Nor does the professional allegiance of an administrator guarantee constructive leadership.

Everyone professing an interest in the mentally retarded should read the annals of the A.A.M.D. from the time of its inception in 1876. They would learn that our institutions of the nineteenth century, administered by physicians with a neuropsychiatric orientation, were hives of patient activity, with vigorously pursued programs of training and education. These programs, in turn, had been conceived, formulated, and promoted by Edouard Séguin, a neuropsychiatrist and pupil of Pinel, the Parisian psychiatrist. I wonder how many of the members of the A.A.M.D. have read Séguin's monograph, "The Moral Treatment, Hygiene and Education of Idiots and Other Backward Children," published in 1848?

In that work, Dr. Séguin, who, I repeat, was a psychiatrist, said that education and training of the retarded "consists in the adaptation of the principles of physiology through physiological means and instruments, to the development of the dynamic, perceptive, reflective and spontaneous functions of youth." It is upon Séguin's *principles,* extended and elaborated by educationalists Froebel and Pestalozzi, that most of our present methods as well as those employed by our nineteenth-century neuropsychiatrist administrators *were and are based.* Most of our so-called new and exciting programs of training and education of today are neither new nor novel and were carried out in nineteenth-century institutions with their neuropsychiatric administrators with greater skill and sophistication than exist in most centers today.

Perhaps there are some who do not know that the A.A.M.D. was founded (1876) by seven physicians, each with a neuropsychiatric orientation, and each an administrator of a residential center for the retarded. These founders declared there was a need for an association "to promote the care, training and education of idiots and other backward persons." These founders and most who followed after them appear to have regarded the training and education of the mentally retarded as a primary aim and responsibility.

Contrary to the assertorial position of Blatt and Dybwad that psychiatrists make poor administrators for our mental retardation residential centers, the author ventures a likewise unsupported conviction that our institutions of today might have been better mental retardation communities had more of the psychiatrists of modern times, with their sensitivity to human needs, dedicated themselves to a career in mental retardation. The modern psychiatrist, by virtue of his intensive training in adaptational dynamics and his intimate knowledge of the impacts of constitution and ecology on emotional, intellectual and social development, is admirably well prepared to come to grips with the assessment and treatment of the personality problems and learning impairments of mental retardates.

Beginning in the second and third decades of this century, there has been an ever-growing critical shortage of services for the mentally retarded and their families at both the institutional and community levels. During the first four decades of the twentieth century the mentally retarded were viewed as a genetic menace and a political and social threat to the American way of life. The retarded were regarded as socially irretrievable because a grandfather had bitten the family tree and poisoned it or because some kind of "brain fever" had left its victims with an irreparable "hole in the head." It was believed that the retardation itself carried with it a high probability of social irresponsibility, popularly peddled as "the menace of the feebleminded."

With this as the popular image of the mentally retarded, a great hue and cry went forth which bade "welfare ladies" and "overseers of the poor" to "beat the bushes" in order to identify the retarded and commit them, one and all, to institutions. No one who has not lived through those days (as has this author) can appreciate the nationwide dedication to this policy of identification and institutionalization. It was a patriotic duty! Was not the preservation of American democracy worth this effort? This is not an exaggeration!

Many a retardate was committed to an institution with the conviction that he or she should remain there for the rest of his or her natural life. It was fiscal policy that those committed should earn their board and lodging by "the sweat of their brow." They did so in those years, *and they do today* in some places! Those whose mental and physical infirmities made them unemployable in the institutional community lived out their lives in a bed or wheelchair or on a dayroom bench. They did so in those days, and they do, in some places, today!

Unfortunately, this unhappy and uninspiring image of the mentally retarded persists in too many places today. It is why psychiatrists, pediatricians, psychologists, social workers, and educators have avoided and still avoid mental retardation as a professional career. We are indeed confronted with a herculean job of education about the mentally retarded for all of those professional groups before we can acquire their sorely needed services!

At the risk of being dubbed a reactionary, this author is not convinced and does not believe it is in the best interest of the retarded and their families that most of our established institutions should be abandoned. A new institution, even of optimum size, is no guarantee of optimal services and sophisticated administration. An intimate professional association of nearly fifty years with the retarded and institutions for the retarded has convinced this author that most of our established institutions are here to stay, and that what is wrong with them can be righted provided that those persons holding posts of responsibility and leadership in the administrative hierarchy have the perspicacity to know what is wrong, the courage to admit it to the public as well as to themselves, the wisdom to know what to do about it, and the determination and finesse to get it done. Once a few basic guidelines are rigorously adopted, the *effective* administrator, whatever his professional stripes might be, will find ways and means to implement them. Administration too often loses sight of the needs of those whom it harbors, and focuses its efforts on erecting a hierarchal structure built on maintaining the lowest possible operational costs, "law and order," and avoidance of negative or sensational publicity.

Speaking more specifically about administrators of our institutions or residential centers for the mentally retarded, administration must proceed from a few, basic, self-evident orientations, as follows: (1) Institutions are authorized, planned, erected, equipped and operated to meet the needs of the retarded populations within their respective spheres of influence. Institutions are not, and never were, setup primarily to provide employment and comfortable living for administrators or any other category of institutional personnel. (2) Clinical experience, dating as far back as the dawn of the nineteenth century, has unequivocally defined the needs of the mentally retarded and (at least in general terms and sometimes in a more specific sense) how these needs are to be met.

Some of the more important needs of the mentally retarded should be obvious to any professional who has spent three to five years working with the retarded in a residential facility. The author takes a dim view of the practice, which has become increasingly prevalent, of appointing institutional administrators whose professional involvement with institutionalized retardates has been minimal. A major challenge of any institutional setup is how to carry out its functions without losing sight of the individual patient. Much of the repetitious, narcissistic behavior of the more seriously retarded patients is not in itself an inevitable phenomenon of severe retardation but is undoubtedly a reflection of the failure of institutions to provide suitable activities programs and appropriate housing for these patients. It would seem that this class of patients too often is abandoned as being altogether hopeless and beyond response to efforts to raise their respective levels of physiological functioning and social adaptation.

Among the less seriously retarded patients, the "problem behaviors" of some arise out of the threat of losing their personal identity. Although these are difficulties inherent in "mass care," a perceptive administrator, with inspirational leadership of an alert staff who have a keen appreciation of the human needs of those under their immediate care, has almost unlimited opportunities to materially offset the disadvantages of group living. Any residential center in which the educational, social, and emotional needs of its retarded population are inadequately met will create much in the way of frustration, unhappiness, and anxiety.

Mental retardates of all levels of intellectual subnormality, like all other persons, are human, too. All persons need a sense of security; security as it relates to the family and/or the social group, security as it relates to personal achievement and self-realization, and security as it relates to a person's inner drives and "built-in" controls.

Security needs are fostered by the following: warmth, protection and stimulation of good mothering or other "care" persons; appropriate attention to dependency needs, yet avoiding perpetuation of dependency; warmth, acceptance, and recognition; constructive and meaningful identifications; promotion of welfare emotions—happiness, contentment, consideration, sympathy and love of others; control and guidance; appropriate opportunities for new experience, achievement, and self-realization; stimulating constructive motivation by providing healthy incentives. .

In the writer's opinion, most institutions succeed in promoting the best interests of those retardates within their respective spheres of influence if their administrators, whatever their "professional stripes," have the conviction that the overall functional level of any retardate, no matter how incapacitated he may seem, is susceptible to betterment. The aims and goals of betterment may be stated quite simply: self-help and self-care as the first goal for the helpless and the profoundly and seriously retarded; limited self-direction and "usefulness" within the framework of dependent living for the moderately retarded; self-direction, a belief in oneself, and the "know-how" of gainful employment involved in independent living for the mildly retarded.

The administrator should bear in mind that in principle the admission of any retardate to his institution signalizes a breakdown, failure, or inability to provide for his needs at the family or community level. In most instances, those retardates admitted to residential centers (and other retardates, too) have been subject to personal traumatization such as the following: denial of affection, acceptance, relatedness, belongingness, dependency, recognition, and so on; restriction, rigidity, overprotection; emphasis on personal limitations; frustrations of needs for individuality, achievement, and self-realization; threats to self-esteem; intensification of feelings of guilt, ideas of unworthiness, and fear of failure.

Planning for the care or rehabilitation of any mental retardate without a sophisticated dynamic appraisal of personality structure and function is both capricious and naive. A diagnostic study which fails to illuminate the needs of a mentally retarded child and which fails to highlight those guidelines essential to promoting the best interests of him and his family is an empty gesture. It wastes the time and skills of professional personnel, imposes undue stress upon the child, and is disappointing and irksome to the parents or referring agencies. In too many institutions, the case record comprises an actuarial like case history, a static summary of a physical examination, an IQ report, and a diagnostic classification of more value to some bureaucratic statistician than to the institution's administrator and his staff.

The goal of a comprehensive diagnostic evaluation is to understand the retardate as a human being, to illuminate his ways and means of getting along or failing to get along in the world, and to learn in what ways to help him.

A comprehensive diagnostic evaluation should provide the following: (1) a pool of information about what the child does or does not do, his physical status, his living routines, his relationships and attitudes toward others, his physical, emotional, educational, and social needs, how well or how inadequately these needs are met, his values and identifications, his reactions and levels of intellectual functioning, and his assets as well as his liabilities; (2) a pool of information about where, how, and with whom the child is living, some reasonable sophistication about the impact of life experiences on the physical and mental health of the child, and an evaluation of the child's impact on those with whom he is living.

The institutional community, when suitably constructed, operated, and supervised, can do much for those retardates whose behavioral problems and needs for training and control are beyond the family's capacity to provide, or where family attitudes and intolerances cannot be modified to work toward the best interests of the retardate. In many instances, especially among the mildly retarded, family life is so disorganized and home conditions so substandard that these and other related factors are inimical to the child's best interests and the institutional community can be a constructive force in the child's development.

For retarded children from disorganized homes and blighted communities, institutional life provides the following securities: an ordered way of living; a bed to sleep in; three square meals a day; a school and teacher prepared to make allowance for individual limitations and to stimulate learning; plenty of space for supervised and spontaneous play; a planned recreational and social integration program; social contacts with peer group; medical and health services as needed; responsible personnel to look after them; a kind of overall experience and training that frequently pays off in a much better adjusted and happier retarded boy or girl.

Starting with the level at which one finds a child upon admission to an institution, care should be oriented to the measures needed in the individual case for treatment and development. Treatment should be focused on employing the following: corrective or ameliorative medical, surgical, or psychiatric modalities; psychodynamically oriented case management; and structured systems of training and education. The overall developmental aim should be directed at promoting or strengthening self-assurance and self respect, self-control and tolerance of frustration, social integration, a personal involvement with reality, and the best possible level of performance. The child should be helped to achieve some adequate level of a sense of security; he should be encouraged to acquire such knowledge and skills that will be of use to him and those social qualities essential to interpersonal transactions, self-help, self-care, usefulness, or gainful employment in the community at large.

Not many administrators and other persons involved in services for the retarded are aware of Itard's program for Victor (1800), which embodied the following principles and objectives:

To endear him to social life by making it more congenial than the one he had recently been leading

To awaken his nervous sensibility by the most energetic stimulants and at other times by quickening the affections of the soul

To extend the sphere of his ideas by creating new wants and multiplying his associations with surrounding beings

To lead him to the use of speech by determining the exercise of imitation, under the spur of necessity

To exercise, during a certain time, the simple operations of his mind upon his physical wants, and therefrom derive the application of the same to objects of instruction

In too many institutional communities the hierarchy of benevolent authoritarianism, with its established procedures, rules, regulations, and restrictions, inevitably depresses the retardate's self-respect and sense of being an individual, depreciates his self-confidence, intensifies his feelings of inadequacy, fosters and encourages dependence, and impoverishes affect and emotion.

Residential centers for the mentally retarded *can* and *must* make the best possible contribution to the growth, development, and adaptive capacities of those who require the services that a well-ordered institution should provide. Every institution should have an established overall policy concerning all phases of institutional life based on meeting *four basic psychological needs* of the retardate as a person. These needs are essentially ego-oriented and may be set forth as follows:

1. The need "to be," with the aim to protect, respect, and promote the sense or awareness of being a personal entity.
   a. Comfortable living and sleeping quarters, attractive furnishings and surroundings, lockers for individual use, cubicle wards or four or six bedded rooms, appropriate attention to health, freedom from pain or discomfort, nourishing food well-prepared and attractively served.
   b. Attitudes and behaviors of patient care rehabilitation personnel signifying recognition of the retardate as an individual.
   c. Protection, guidance, supervision, control, and discipline as needed from patient care and rehabilitation personnel.
2. The need "to belong."
   a. Acceptance, consideration, recognition by patient care and rehabilitation personnel.
   b. Promoting constructive identifications with parent surrogate figures among patient care and rehabilitation personnel. The ideal surrogate is one with a "soft heart" and a "hard head."
3. The need "to get."
   a. Promoting a sense of achievement and self-fulfillment through education, social integration, training and recreation within current scope of capacities.
   b. Urge movement from passive receptivity to initiative. Though obedience is an adaptive trait for some retardates, it must be balanced by stimulating his curiosity and helping him to reach out for new opportunities.
4. The need "to create."
   a. Encouragement in self-expression through various modalities with an eye to special interests or tastes.
   b. Incorporation or encouragement of welfare conditions—happiness, sympathy, consideration of others.
   c. Inculcation of desirable aims, goals, and ideals through use of appropriate incentives (often praise or appreciation).

Health, shelter, food, and clothing are as basic to the mentally retarded as they are for other persons. Health, not only in sense, but health as it is translated into comfort and freedom from distress is that which is important to the individual. To be freed from the discomfort of an ingrown toenail, or to be fitted with and wear corrective lenses, hearing aids, dental prostheses, and so on, is, from the retardate's point of view, more important than a series of immunization "shots."

A nutritious, well-balanced diet, with the proper number of calories and an optimum ration of vitamins, is the goal of scientific dietetics. But that which is important from the retardate's point of view as a person is how well his meals are prepared and how attractively they are served. To eat messy-looking unsavory stews day after day, served in aluminum dishes in a huge, plain, undecorated congregate dining hall, seating twelve to twenty persons at a table, amid a near-intolerable decibel level from the clatter of dishes, the scraping of chairs on a terazzo floor, and the shouted orders of attendants is not the way administrators and staff usually dine. Is it really "good enough" for the retarded? Oddly enough, in most institutions, no help or instruction in "table manners" is offered.

Most of us like some choice as to our clothing—its style, color, material, fit, and so on. The visitor to most institutions is usually unhappily impressed by the "dowdy" look of the patients, for example, clothing that is colorless. One female retardate the author has known often appears in a "wrap-around" skirt (many sizes too large around the waist) that falls to the ankles; it is to be noted that she invariably apologizes for her appearance! Another male patient refuses to wear underpants because the waistband is so oversized that they slip down to his knees and hobble him as he goes about his work *for the institution* as a mechanics helper. What has been said about clothing applies equally well to footwear. Observe, if you will, any group of patients —particularly adults—how they limp and waddle as they move about the grounds. These are indications, in most instances, of ill-fitting shoes or uncared-for feet!

Again, so many institutional setups, judged by their interior architecture and built-in facilities, seem to have been planned to rob their patients of self-respect and a sense of individuality and to impress the average retardate with an unhappy self-image. It is indeed amazing how the need for privacy has been so successfully thwarted! If retardates have any considerable psychopathological urges for exhibitionism, many institutional lavatories and shower rooms reinforce these urges. It is amazing, too, how little opportunity there is in many institutions for their retarded populations to have a place to keep their personalized possessions and treasures. How pathetic it is to see patient after patient carrying a paper bag or a shoebox with him wherever he goes, storing it under his bed at night if permitted! Administrators should not tolerate those antiquated space arrangements in long-established buildings that are inimical to the best interests of the retardates who live therein. It is indeed rare that the interior of any well-constructed building cannot be modified and renovated.

SUMMARY

Day by day and year by year we have become more and more sophisticated as to how the administration in residential centers for the mentally retarded and how the manipulation of the residential environment should be geared to meeting basic needs of mentally retarded persons. Health services, shelter, food, and clothing must be provided in accordance with personal needs rather than based on an inhuman per-diem allowance predetermined by some "armchair expert" in the state budget director's office. More specifically, at the institutional level, administration should emphasize that acceptance, recognition, understanding, and warmth are the basic exchange media in interpersonal relationships with the retarded as well as with all people. Administration should recognize and be guided by those well-established needs of the retarded.

Whether or not our "all-purpose" institutions can encompass these larger and more sophisticated responsibilities is open to question and needs serious reconsideration. In the past twenty-five years, there has been a corresponding sharp increase in the demand for admission of seriously and profoundly handicapped retardates. Can the same professional and patient-care institutional personnel meet the needs of severely physically and mentally disabled children and in like manner rise to the challenges posed by emotionally and socially maladapted children who have only a minimum of cognitive impairment? The time is upon us when our administrators can no longer refrain from taking a new look at the institutional community from the vantage point that the retarded, too, are human! This should give impetus to the application of psychodynamics in the management, care, treatment, education, and rehabilitation of all mentally retarded persons, adults as well as children.

[C]

CHALLENGES IN THE
LEGAL SPHERE

: 27 :

Law and the Mentally Retarded

Richard C. Allen

INTRODUCTION

THE Task Force on Law of the President's Panel on Mental Retardation, appointed by President Kennedy in 1961 to prepare a "National Plan to Combat Mental Retardation," began its report with a quotation from an English law book of the early eighteenth century:

> [I]t is most certain that our Law hath a very great and tender consideration for Persons naturally Disabled . . . The Law protects their Persons, preserves their rights and Estates, Excuseth their Laches, and assists them in their Pleadings . . . They are under the Special Aid and Protection of his Equity, who is no less than Keeper of the King's conscience . . .[1]

And on the façade of that magnificent marble edifice which houses the Supreme Court of the United States is a hallowed phrase, which is the keystone of American jurisprudence: "Equal Justice under Law." But for the mentally retarded, these words, on parchment and stone, and spanning three centuries of the most creative epoch of the common law, have brought neither equality before the law nor protection of basic rights.[2]

A century or less ago, when most people, even many in the learned professions, looked upon the retarded as hopelessly incapable, often dangerous, almost subhuman creatures, they were not often thought of as having legally enforceable rights. Indeed, when the term "rights" was used in relation to the mentally retarded, the reference was usually to the prerogative accorded to relatives and creditors to obtain appointment of a guardian or conservator to prevent waste or destruction of any property that might come into the possession of the retardate; or perhaps was to the "right" of society to protect itself against the retardate's derelictions and unwanted offspring by confining and sterilizing him, generally on no more proof than the fact of his intellectual impairment. Today we know that the mentally retarded are far from "hopeless," need be neither dangerous nor promiscuous, can be good citizens and even good parents, and that in most cases they can be trained to become self-sustaining contributors to society rather than burdens upon it.

The author had the great pleasure and privilege of presenting a paper at the Fourth International Congress of the International League of Societies for the Mentally Handicapped, held in Jerusalem in October, 1968. The theme of that meeting, "From Charity to Rights," charts the course which, in the author's opinion, must be taken if the mentally retarded—the inherently unequal—are to enjoy the elemental right of all citizens to equal justice. Improvement of laws and administrative regulations is an important segment of that journey, but far from all of it. Research conducted over the last half-dozen years by the Institute of Law, Psychiatry, and Criminology of The George Washington University has provided ample proof of the aphorism of Spinoza, that "He who tries to fix and determine everything by law will inflame rather than correct the vices of the world." [3] Among the shoals along the way are our prejudices and traditional ways of dealing with the retarded; there is as well the Scilla of "administrative convenience" and the Charybdis of chronic inadequacies in the investment of human and physical resources. And just beneath the surface, and therefore the more hazardous, lie the barriers to effective communication about mental retardation and its associated legal problems.

THE SEMANTICS OF MENTAL RETARDATION

In commenting upon the myriad of terms infesting statutes dealing with guardianship and incompetency, the author observed (Allen et al., 1968*b*):

The cliche, "It's all a question of semantics," is a facile and inaccurate—albeit a convenient—explanation for the vagaries of human interaction. Yet, one is tempted to apply it to the problems and confusions that abound in the area of determinations of civil incompetency. By sheer weight of numbers, the terms which must be contended with pose a formidable communications barrier.

When one adds to the picture the other aspects of legal regulation and the bewildering array of technical, institutional, and colloquial terms which have been applied to the retarded (most of which seem somehow to have found their way into law), both numbers and confusion are compounded.

Most of the communication problems in the world of the mentally retarded and the law are problems of innocence. They are engendered by the ambiguity of words and their reification, by the difficulties of traversing disciplinary and jurisdictional lines,[4] and by the inevitable limitations of both scientific and legal knowledge. But sometimes words are artfully chosen to cloak or distort meaning, as where "occupational therapy" becomes an euphemism for menial housekeeping tasks performed for the benefit of the institution, or "seclusion" for punitive jailing. Again, in one state, the statutes require appointment of an attorney to represent one against whom a commitment is sought, if requested by the alleged retardate, his parent, or guardian. Any such request, however, is met with the response: "But this is a *medical* hearing, and all we are concerned with is the child's *welfare*." The request is usually withdrawn.

The origins of many of the terms in use will, perhaps, never be known with certainty,[5] but not all of them are obscure or ambiguous. The name of one residential care institution still in operation in this country could not more clearly reveal the attitudes of the legislators who established it: "Institution for Defective Females of Childbearing Age."

In 1963, the California State Legislature created a Study Commission on Mental Retardation to conduct research and make recommendations on planning and implementation of appropriate state and local policies and services, including revisions in state law. As its initial task, the Commission compiled and published a compendium of state statutes affecting the retarded, taken from nineteen state codes (including such diverse codifications as Unemployment Insurance and Fish and Game Laws) and covering some twenty-three major topics.

In many respects, the California mental health statutes are better drafted (and contain fewer epithetical anachronisms) than those of many other states. To illustrate, however, the plethora of terms under which legal protections, restrictions, regulations, and services are provided (or withheld) in every state, a "head count" was made. The California laws contain more than fifty different terms apparently intended to include or exclude mentally retarded persons, application of which may control the rendition of a protective service, provide a basis for institutionalization, or determine the existence of jural and civil rights (to make a contract, vote, drive a car, marry, have custody of children, and so on). Some recall older medical nosologies ("idiot," "imbecile"); some have no discernible meaning ("entirely without understanding," "deranged"); and some are inappropriate to the subject matter of the statute (for example, use of the term "incompetent" to describe one found eligible for institutional care); but most are merely ambiguous, leaving it quite uncertain whom the legislature intended to denominate ("mentally irresponsible person," "unsound mind").

Among the findings made by the Institute of Law, Psychiatry, and Criminology in a recent study of state statutes and regulations affecting the retarded and their families (Newman, 1967) are the following:

1. There is no agreement upon a basic generic term descriptive of the class of persons for whom institutionalization, guardianship or other protective service may be appropriate. A number of primary terms are used, which are either undefined in the statute or are defined through use of secondary terms of equally uncertain meaning.
2. In many state institutionalization laws it is quite unclear whether a distinction is made between the mentally retarded and the mentally ill.[6]
3. In 25 states "inability to manage oneself or one's affairs" is the critical determination in an institutionalization proceeding, although such lack of capacity is clearly relevant to a proceeding to determine civil competency and the need for a guardian, and is not apposite to a determination of the need for institutionalization. And the test is the same for children as for adults, although "inability to manage oneself or one's affairs" would be as characteristic of the normal as of the retarded child of tender years.
4. Other definitional criteria, such as "need for care, supervision, con-

trol or guidance," which exist in over half the states, and variously stated social, vocational and educational handicaps (inability to learn, adapt, earn, adjust, support, compete, etc.) also applicable in more than half, are not adequate to distinguish between retarded persons in need of institutionalization and those for whom alternatives to residential care are more appropriate.

5. Statutes and administrative rules regulating marriage and driver's licensure, voting, occupational employment, and the validity of wills, contracts and conveyances, employ equally ambiguous terminology; and often use of identical terms in each of several areas of jural activity results in a presumption of incompetency for *all* purposes when one is found to be in need of a *particular* protective service.

6. Similarly, agency and institutionally applied terms result in unwarranted limitations, as with the child denominated "trainable" who is thereby denied exposure to "educational" programs from which he might well benefit.

Before leaving the subject of semantics, mention should be made of the ubiquitous IQ score as a method of institutional legal, social, and educational classification. Whatever differences of opinion may exist among educators, psychologists, physicians, welfare workers, and institutional superintendents with respect to mental retardation, on two points, at least, there seems to be unanimity: first, that an IQ score standing alone says very little and should never be the sole basis for making critical decisions about a person; and second, that because of the imprecision of definitions and ambiguity of terminology, IQ scores are the only practicable common language. Unfortunately, legal status is too often determined on the basis of a single IQ scoring, despite the reservations expressed by all who participate in the classification process.

INSTITUTIONALIZATION

Institutionalization of Children under Six

First admissions to residential care institutions for the mentally retarded are predominately children. Therefore, as a part of our study of the mentally retarded and the law, the Institute of Law, Psychiatry, and Criminology interviewed obstetricians, pediatricians, psychiatrists, and institutional superintendents in seven states to determine their attitudes concerning institutionalization of young children. Comparing the results with those of earlier studies, we concluded that there is a growing trend favoring home care of very young children whenever possible. However, many, including most of the obstetricians interviewed (who have perhaps least contact with retarded children, but whose opinion may weigh most heavily with parents at that traumatic time of first discovery of an apparent impairment), still urge institutionalization of retarded children under six, even in the face of parental objection (especially in the case of the mongoloid child, whom they view with despairing negativism). In fact, a majority of obstetricians said they would recommend institutionalization of *all* infants recognized as retarded where there are other children in the home. Only 17 per cent of the pediatricians and psychiatrists and none of the institutional physicians would agree.

Our laws seem to operate on the premise that institutionalization is for the benefit of the child; indeed many urge that institutionalization on parental application should be made as easy as possible. Yet, it would seem that a great many children are institutionalized less for their own benefit than for the comfort of others. Because it is believed that the retarded—and retarded children as well—do indeed have "rights," the author would be inclined to differ with the Task Force on Law of the President's Panel on Mental Retardation and require judicial approval in any case in which institutionalization is based not on the needs of the child but on the needs of others, in order that appropriate resolution may be made of the perhaps conflicting interests of the child and his family, and that use of alternatives to residential care may be explored.

Institutionalization Procedures

Where judicial procedures are required for admission to a residential care institution, our researches disclosed that in most courts a petition for commitment is invariably approved. Rarely does a court inquire into the possibility of utilizing community resources instead of institutionalization. Indeed, rarely is the judge even aware of them.

In only one of the jurisdictions in which empirical research was undertaken did the proceedings appear to be an inquiry into the merits of the case. In one of the two courts observed, three of forty petitions were disapproved; and in the second (which required testing of the alleged retardate by its own clinicians), ten of forty-one petitions were disapproved. Of the cases dismissed, four of the children were found not sufficiently retarded to require institutionalization, and nine were found not mentally retarded (one, for example, was found intellectually normal, but deaf).

Our studies disclosed hundreds of "displaced persons"—retarded children and adults in mental hospitals and children with a primary diagnosis of mental illness in schools for the retarded. Admission of the retarded to state mental hospitals is sometimes the result of ignorance or mistaken diagnosis, but more often it is knowingly permitted because of the crowded conditions of state training schools. Some training schools blame the courts for improperly committing mentally ill children to their facilities, but others admit accepting mentally ill children because the state hospital has no facilities for children and they "have no place else to go." Both groups of children suffer as the result of their "displacement."

It has been long known that institutionalization and legal incompetency are quite different, though related, concepts. Thus, a determination that a mentally retarded person is in need of institutional care should not automatically deprive him of his civil rights. Yet in two of the states in which we conducted studies, although the law expressly declares that institutional commitment does not of itself constitute a finding of legal incompetency, other statutes and hospital regulations prohibit *all* residents of institutions for the retarded from holding a driver's license, making a will, marrying, executing a contract (even one involving a small purchase or a magazine subscription), and from having any right of management of property (Allen et al., 1968*b*).

Legal Status and "Treatment" in the Residential Care Institution

In every state there is a need for many more community facilities to serve as alternatives to residential care: day-care centers, sheltered workshops, recreational programs, family casework, job placement, private boarding facilities, developmental centers, and the like. In addition, residential care institutions suffer from severe shortages of funds and trained personnel. At one institution, for example, with a patient population of over 3,500, only four patients have been placed in day work in the community; and at another, with a high proportion of educable patients, there is no educational program at all. In several states little or nothing has been done to develop vocational training, and work assignments are based more on institutional needs than on habilitation of the patients.

The opening sentence in the recently published compendium of policy statements on residential care approved by the Board of Directors of the National Association for Retarded Children (N.A.R.C.) is this indictment of state residential institutions for the retarded (National Association for Retarded Children, 1968): "The failure to eliminate dehumanization in state institutions throughout the United States is testimony that the work of the National Association for Retarded Children is far from finished."

The Task Force on Law of the President's Panel on Mental Retardation urged that ". . . every means should be sought to minimize the need for physical restraint and to scrutinize its use." Most institutions, we found, employ "seclusion" and other restraints as means of protecting patients or controlling their behavior, and in most institutions they are applied humanely and in the interest of the patient. In some, however, discretion to employ them is given to untrained ward attendants, and that discretion is often exercised less for the patient's well-being than for the comfort of the staff. In one institution, seclusion was regularly applied for much longer periods than permitted by hospital regulations and under conditions which would not be permitted in the most repressive penal institution. In another, ward attendants had obtained prescriptions for tranquilizing drugs at one time or another for many of the patients in their wards. Once obtained, these prescriptions are refilled and administered by attendants with no medical control whatever.

Subtler, but perhaps of even more insidious effect, are the intrusions into a patient's dignity as a human being that occur not through malice but for "administrative convenience." The N.A.R.C. policy statement notes (National Association for Retarded Children, 1968):

Lack of privacy, lack of personal possessions, lack of involvement in decisions affecting oneself, lack of praise for a job well done, lack of feeling that someone cares, lack of being recognized as an individual with ability and potential for growth, enforced and unnecessary regimentation, being ignored, living in crowded unattractive wards—these are but a few of the many kinds of conditions which can and do exist in residential facilities and which contribute greatly to dehumanization.

Nor are the effects of such dehumanizing treatment of relevance only with respect to the "educables" and "trainables." Our field investigators observed wards for the profoundly retarded containing "crib cases": children whom the attendants explained to them "don't walk much." The field researchers, unsophisticated in institutional methods, noted also in their reports that in many instances there was nothing to walk *to*—no toys, no playroom, nothing to entice a child from the world of his crib. In one instance, a "nonambulatory" child was taken from such a ward and given special care in a program conducted by a child psychologist and supported by a small grant from the National

Institutes of Mental Health. With weeks of effort and skilled attention, the child did learn to walk. Then, when the grant ran out she had to be returned to the ward, where she is now living—as a "crib case."

Laboring under severe shortages of money and trained personnel, institutional officials express uncertainty as to the objectives their institutions can or should try to meet. Should emphasis be placed upon teaching the educable retardate? Inculcating personal and work skills among the trainables? Providing short-term care during family emergencies or vacation periods for retardates who live at home? Providing custodial care for the severely and profoundly retarded? Offering day-care, vocational placement, and other services? Each of the foregoing? Many institutional personnel expressed to us the view that the residential care facility had become a "dumping ground," enjoined vaguely to accomplish all of these ends, but with insufficient resources to do a good job at any of them. And many expressed doubt that a large, multipurpose residential facility is the appropriate vehicle to accomplish them in any case.

Some of the institutions visited in our study retest all inmates periodically (periodicity ranges from one to five years, with two institutions, in different states, testing at varying intervals based upon age and IQ level); others retest only when change of status is under consideration (for example, placement in a new program, reported evidence of marked progress or deterioration, and so on). In some institutions what testing is done fails to meet even minimal standards of adequacy: in one such institution, the position of psychologist is unfilled and has been for some time, and no testing is being done; in another, the psychologist-resident ratio is so out of proportion that initial testing cannot be carried out for all incoming residents; and in a third, some residents (presumably being prepared for community placement) had not been tested in thirty years!

Periodic staff review of the status of all residents (and, in at least some cases, periodic psychological retesting as well) would seem essential to insure appropriate treatment and release to the community as soon as institutional care is no longer required. Equally important is that staff decision-making be subject to review by some disinterested outside authority. The Task Force on Law of the President's Panel on Mental Retardation recommended a system of guardianship for institutionalized retardates and, in addition, judicial review of the need for continued institutionalization when a resident reaches the age of twenty-one and every two years thereafter. A majority of the judges and half of the institutional administrators whom we interviewed opposed such judicial review (generally on the grounds that it is unnecessary and would be unduly burdensome and expensive). Yet many institutions do not now provide comprehensive staff review on a resident's attaining the age of maturity or periodically thereafter, and for the most part there is no review of institutional decision-making by external authorities (only a small minority of retardates, whether in or out of institutions, have guardians).

The new (1965) New Jersey law, which has been called a "bill of rights" for retardates, requires examination of all institutional residents prior to their reaching the age of twenty-one. If it is determined that a resident will need continued protection and supervision, his parents are notified and asked whether they plan to have a guardian appointed. If a guardian is not appointed at the instance of the resident's parents, the law requires the state to perform "such services for the mentally deficient adult as he may require, and which otherwise would be rendered by a guardian of his person." At the time the Institute was conducting the study, the law was too new for thorough evaluation, but it seems clearly to be a step in the right direction.

Our empirical data indicate that once a retardate enters a public institution, his "status" so far as the institution is concerned is that of "resident," and it makes little or no difference whether he is a minor or adult, or whether he entered voluntarily or was committed. Differences in the treatment of residents with respect to their exercise of jural "rights" (property management, marriage, making purchases, communicating with persons outside the institution, and so on) are based upon institutional judgments about their capacity and on staff practices in a particular ward or cottage, rather than upon the requirements of "law," about which institutional personnel are, for the most part, either uninformed or misinformed (Allen et al., 1968b).

The chief sources of funds of institutionalized retardates are monthly benefit payments (Social Security, Veterans Administration, and so on), small sums provided by parents, earnings for work done in the institution or in the community while living at the institution, and occasionally fairly substantial sums coming to the retardate by inheritance or otherwise. The latter generally leads to a proceeding to appoint a guardian, but the other types of income are routinely received, held, and managed by the institution (with or without statutory authority); indeed, benefit payments are often made directly to the superintendent as "substitute payee." All institutions co-mingle such trust funds, and all apply such funds, at least in part, toward meeting the expenses of the retardate's care. Most allow the retardate to retain some portion of his money for his own use, but there is wide variation in the practices of the institutions we visited. The amounts assessed for cost of care ranged from a token $1 per month to "actual cost," which in one institution was as high as $215 per month.

State statutes are vague, but in most jurisdictions the parents of minor residents are first looked to for payment of the cost of their care (although formal collection procedures are rarely invoked). Perhaps here is an area for "bold new approaches." Why, for example, should not the state training school be considered in the same light as the public elementary school: an economic burden to be shared by all of the citizens of the community in the interest of all, rather than one to be borne only by those with children in need of such care and training? Indeed, why not provide a system of governmental payments *to* parents of retarded children capable of living at home, to enable them to provide the special care and training which might otherwise be available only through placement in a residential care facility?

It is generally agreed that the proportionately small number of residents now returned to the community by residential care institutions could be increased greatly if institutional and community resources were improved. There is some basis for optimism in a slight upward trend in such community placements and in a decreasing rate of return of those conditionally released in recent years. The primacy which should be accorded to habilitation of the resident in every institution is illustrated by the view expressed by a staff member in one institution when interviewed by our staff investigators:

> We aren't too concerned when one of our people on conditional release has to come back. We look on every day outside the institution as a step forward. If somebody has to come back for more training, that's all right. We'll try again and again until he can make it on his own.

Involuntary Sterilization: Is It Legally Defensible?

Today twenty-six of our states have eugenic sterilization laws, twenty-three of which are compulsory. The number of reported sterilizations per year has decreased steadily, from over 1,600 some twenty-five years ago to less than 500 today, a decrease in large part due to the widespread rejection of the view that mental illness and mental retardation are hereditary.

Our empirical studies have shown, however, that the problems associated with eugenic sterilization are not confined to states with compulsory laws. In states with a "voluntary" statute, "consent" is often more theoretical than real. For example, it may be made a condition of discharge from an institution that the patient "consent" to sterilization. And in one state our field investigators observed a "voluntary" sterilization proceeding for a six-year-old boy.

We found further that sterilization operations are conducted outside the institutions in states without sterilization laws. In one state, an institution official told our interviewers that he had performed fifty to sixty such sterilizations during the last two years. If true, his activities alone would give the state a sterilization rate higher than the reported rates of twenty states that have sterilization laws! Another institution physican in the same state told our field investigators: "I, on occasion, have let my knife 'slip' in surgery and cut the tubes, but with most nurses present, I would not do it, as they have large mouths" (Ferster, 1966).

The Task Force on Law and the several state Mental Retardation Planning Committees have equivocated on the matter of involuntary sterilization. The Institute has been unable to find persuasive scientific proof either of the inheritability of the defects for which sterilization is now being imposed, or of the fact that a child—even if of normal intelligence—will be seriously handicapped by the fact of being reared by a retarded parent. With the increasing availability of improved supervision and protective services, and of birth control devices far less drastic and irrevocable than surgical procedures, it is the author's view that there is no sound basis for sanctioning the continuance of involuntary sterilization—under whatever euphemism it may be applied.

The Problem of the Retarded Delinquent

Placement of the delinquent who is retarded is a problem in each of the states we studied. The following summary of a case followed by our field investigators illustrates the plight of the child no one seems to want:

One day in late fall, the police of a large city found a child sleeping on a park bench. He replied to their questions incoherently and they brought him before the juvenile judge that same day. It was learned that he was fifteen years old and had run away from home, and had done so many times before, and that a year earlier he had been before the court on a delinquency charge and had been diagnosed as moderately retarded. At that time a recommendation had been made for foster home placement because of the inadequacy of his home environment . . . but there are no foster homes for retarded teen-aged "delinquents," so he was returned to his home.

The boy was sent to a juvenile detention center to await the court's decision, and while there was retested. The Center's report to the court stated that his IQ was "estimated at 45 as he is below the (WISC) scale." It also stated that he had a speech impediment, "no conception of personal hygiene," and presented marked behavior problems. He was kept at the detention center pending a new hearing.

At the second hearing a month later, the judge announced that he was going to place the child in a residential care institution for the retarded. But in that state commitment by the juvenile court requires consent of the training school (and the judge had been unable to obtain such consent in a dozen similar cases since his appointment a year and a half before). The institution to which the boy was sent confirmed the fact of his retardation, but averred that "no vacancy is contemplated . . . now or at any time in the near future," and recommended placement "elsewhere." A second institution was tried—also unsuccessfully, although the judge found its officials "much more sympathetic."

The boy was released by the court, and two weeks later was picked up by police wandering aimlessly in a bus station. When brought back to juvenile court it was found that he had been missing from home for ten days. Fearing for the boy's safety, the judge hit upon the idea of instituting a commitment proceeding in the probate court, since the statutes are silent as to whether or not approval of the institution is required in such cases. Finally, nearly two years after the first referral to the juvenile court, the boy was admitted under "protest" by a state training school.

The point of the story is not exploitation of a legal "loophole" to gain admission for a child to an institution for the retarded, nor is it to question the wisdom of a law which restricts judicial commitment by requiring institutional approval; rather, it is our failure to create appropriate facilities to meet the needs of the retarded child with associated problems of behavior. In two of the states in which we conducted research, we found significant numbers of retarded children in juvenile correctional facilities, for the most part lacking in resources to meet the special needs of their mentally retarded residents. And in two others, we found new intensive care facilities, offering at last some hope of reaching the institutional outcast—the retarded "delinquent."

GUARDIANSHIP AND PROTECTIVE SERVICES

Guardianship and civil incompetency—including determinations of capacity to contract or convey, to execute a will, to sue or be sued, to drive a car, to marry or have a marriage annulled, to have custody of children, to manage social security or Veterans Administration benefits, to vote, and so on—are the subject of a book recently published by this author and colleagues, which contains a chapter with detailed recommendations for improvement in our present laws (Allen et al., 1968b); therefore these subjects will not be considered in depth here.

Some of the shortcomings of typical state statutes and proceedings are the following: (1) Again the terminology is imprecise, and, as has been pointed out earlier, because of inappropriate use of terms (for example, "incompetent" for one found in need of institutional care), a determination in one area may create the status of general "incompetency." (2) Guardianship proceedings are cumbersome and expensive. (3) Both the terminology employed and the procedures required create unnecessary stigma for the retarded person in need of help and unnecessary pain for parents seeking to insure that he will get it. (4) Institutionalization often creates at least a *de facto* if not a *de jure* incompetency. (5) Most courts do not have facilities for clinical evaluation, nor do they have sufficient staff to oversee the discharge of fiduciary responsibility by guardians or institutional personnel. (6) Often the alleged incompetent is not really represented by counsel, even when the procedure requires appointment of an attorney *ad litem,* and the determination is frequently made *ex parte*. (7) There is great uncertainty as to when a guardian of the person should be appointed and what his duties should be. (8) There is no established procedure for review of the competency of an institutionalized person upon his reaching his majority. (9) Guardians of the person are rarely appointed for those in residential care institutions. (10) Guardianship is an "all or nothing" situation, although in many cases partial or limited guardianship is all that is required. (11) Few states have established a system under which a state agency can assume some or all of the functions of a guardian when there is no one else who can fill this role. (12) In part because of lack of community resources and in part because of misconstructions of existing law and regulations, in some states it is necessary to go through a commitment proceeding to receive needed protective services.

Our field investigators interviewed the parents of more than fifty retarded children and adults in half a dozen states to determine what, if any, planning had been done for the future of the retardate. The interviewees were selected at random, but many of the names came from lists supplied by the National Association for Retarded Children. Hence, as a group they were not representative of all parents of retarded children but rather of those parents concerned enough about the welfare of their own and other retarded children to have become involved in N.A.R.C. activities. Most were middle-class families (with a fair sprinkling of professional persons); half of their retarded children were classified as "educable," and all but thirteen lived at home. Most of them had done, they said, "some thinking" about preparing for their child's future.

We were surprised by what we found. None of the adult retardates had either a guardian of the person or estate, although two had substitute payees for social security benefit purposes. Few of the parents of minor children had made thoughtful plans for the future of their children, and most were ignorant about such important facets of planning as testamentary guardianship, the status of their children on reaching the age of twenty-one, and what can be accomplished through an *inter vivos* trust. Much of their planning was inappropriate (wills out of date or invalid, trust arrangements inadequate), and in several cases children had been in effect disinherited on the erroneous assumption that any estate given to the child would be taken to reimburse the state for the cost of its care.

But fault does not lie exclusively or even primarily with the parents. The inadequacy of community facilities and services, the largely unrelieved financial burden of providing for a retarded child, the fact that hospitalization and health insurance coverage may not include the retarded child, the paucity of comprehensive evaluation and counseling services, the ignorance of most lawyers, physicians, and other family advisors about the problems involved in planning for the retarded, and the stigma and expense of guardianship—all seem to surround the parents with an impenetrable curtain of confusion and frustration, defeating every effort to plan effectively.

In several states there are imaginative new legal approaches: *New Jersey* now requires that all retardates receiving services from the state be examined at age twenty-one; parents or next of kin are encouraged to obtain a private guardian if the retardate needs such help, but if they wish it, the Division of Mental Retardation will perform the functions of a guardian of the person. *Louisiana* has a simple, inexpensive procedure whereby the parent's guardianship (tutorship) of a child may be continued past the child's reaching the age of majority if he is mentally retarded. In *Connecticut* new duties have been reposed in the Office of Mental Retardation, located within the Department of Health, whose records of children in need of services are now fully computerized. *Minnesota* has had for a number of years a system of state guardianship (but cf. Levy, 1965). And *California,* with its emphasis on community-based services, created in 1965 a number of regional diagnostic, counseling, and service centers. In 1968, guardianship services were added to the package, under legislation, similar to the earlier "personal surrogate" bill which failed of passage. Although rarely used, *Washington*'s Co-Custody and Parental Successor laws are worthy of study. And major innovative efforts are under way in *New York, Ohio,* and other states.

The major concern of parents—Will there be someone to "look out for" their retarded child when they are gone?—may be to a great extent relieved if voluntary "retardate trust" plans (now in existence in Maryland, Massachusetts, and Michigan) prove successful. These plans provide limited estate management, but appropriately emphasize personal contact and protection.

Again, passing a law or adopting a "plan" alone will not solve the problem. There must also be: education about the laws and regulations which affect the retarded and their families—for parents, for institutional personnel, for community workers, and for lawyers as well; sufficient funding to provide the differential services needed, preferably within the retardate's own community; and understanding and effective workers to administer the program.

In an earlier paper (Allen, 1968a), the author noted that "protective services" fail to protect:

1. when legal proceedings become routinized and *pro forma,* and decision-makers lose sight of both the nature of the services available and the needs of the people to be served;
2. when there is a lack of adequate staff and physical facilities;
3. when important decision-makers are ignorant of them or their appropriate use;
4. when they impose coercive sanctions unnecessarily, or for longer periods than necessary; or when more appropriate noncoercive measures are available;
5. when the legal provisions under which they may be rendered are phrased in terms, which, because of their ambiguity or inappropriateness, make it difficult to identify the categories of persons eligible to receive them;
6. when custodial care, because of ignorance, or because of its ease of application, becomes the treatment of choice over other protective

services more appropriate to the needs of the retardate (in all too many of the jurisdictions we studied, institutionalization has become the "poor man's guardianship");

7. when they are rendered by a multiplicity of agencies with ambiguously defined, and often overlapping, jurisdiction; and, perhaps most important,

8. when they do not respect the dignity and worth of the individual.

THE RETARDED OFFENDER

Although there is a paucity of factual information about mental retardation and crime, there has been no shortage of opinions about it through the years. About a half-century ago, it was pretty widely believed that every intellectually impaired person was a likely delinquent, and that most criminal offenders were such because of impaired intellect. The polemicists have now come full circle, and it is today just as stoutly maintained by some members of the scientific, legal, and correctional communities that mental retardation bears no causal relationship to crime.[7] Indeed this view is so strongly held in some quarters that when staff members of our Institute have discussed the preliminary findings of our researches, the most strenuous objection has been voiced by persons ordinarily in the vanguard of liberal reform. As the author once noted (Allen, 1966):

. . . in our zeal to dispel the chimeras and rubrics that have existed so long, we may have fallen into another kind of error. There seems to be developing a sort of reaction formation in which it has become fashionable to deny that gross intellectual deficit plays any significant role in producing criminal behavior.

In 1963 a questionnaire survey was made of all correctional institutions in the country, with the exception of jails and workhouses where misdemeanants and minor offenders are confined. Responses were received from over 80 per cent of the institutions contacted, housing some 200,000 offenders, of which number the reporting institutions have IQ records on about half. The following were among the findings made based on analysis of these records (Brown and Courtless, 1967):

1. About 9.5% of prison inmates can be classified as mentally retarded, using IQ 70 as the cut-off point (it is estimated that about 3% of the general population is mentally retarded).

2. Although more than 70% of the reporting Institutions routinely test the intelligence of inmates on admission, a number of different tests are used, and testing procedures vary widely; and several reporting institutions make no effort to test the intelligence of their inmates.
3. Nearly 1500 (1.6%) of the inmates had reported IQ scores below 55, ranging down to a low of 17.
4. There is a general lack of mental health manpower resources within the institutions and consequently virtually no special programs for retarded inmates; 160 institutions with nearly 150,000 inmates, are served by 14 full-time psychiatrists and 82 full time psychologists; and more than half of the institutions reporting offer no program of any kind for their retarded inmates—not even a single special education class.

In the criminal-law–correctional phase of the Institute's study of the mentally retarded and the law, six adult correctional institutions in six different states, each of which had reported housing inmates with IQ's below 70, were selected, taking into account the character of the institution, the availability of records, and geographic location. To each of the institutions was sent a field worker, who compiled from prison records a list of all inmates identified by the institutions as retarded, selected a random sample from this list for retesting, and determined the type and manner of institutional testing and the nature of any educational or other rehabilitative programs provided by the institution for its allegedly retardate population. He also collected detailed sociopsychological, socioeconomic, and criminological data on each of the inmates in the sample.

The sample was then retested by a second member of the team, a clinical psychologist, using the Wechsler Adult Intelligence Scale, Draw-a-Person, and Thematic Apperception tests. The third member of the team, a lawyer, then analyzed the legal data for each case in the sample, including examinations of trial transcripts, and interviews with judges, prosecutors and defense counsel, probation officers, and police personnel involved in each case. In this later facet of the study, we sought answers to such questions as the following: At what point, if at all, was an attorney appointed to represent the accused? Was a confession or other statement to the police offered in evidence, and was objection taken to it? Was the issue of competency to stand trial raised? Was there a referral for an examination or observation? Was the defense of lack of criminal responsibility "insanity" asserted? Was there a presentence investigation? What were the dispositional alternatives available to the court? The primary focus of inquiry was to determine at what point, if at all, significant decision-makers became aware of the fact of the defendant's mental retardation; and, if it was not discovered in the course of the criminal trial, why this was so; and if it was discovered, what effect, if any, it had.

Correctional institutions use a number of different tests of intelligence; some are given to large groups of inmates as part of the admissions procedure, sometimes using other inmates to administer and score them. Surprisingly, despite this fact, we found institutional testing to be a fairly reliable indicator of mental retardation. The mean IQ of the sample of fifty-one inmates whom we retested was 66.0, compared with a mean IQ on institutional testing of 62.4. Further, we found 74 per cent of the sample to fall within the retarded range, with an additional 8.7 per cent testing in the borderline range (IQ between 70 and 74). Of course, disparities were also discovered. In one state the "Otis Quick Scoring Test" is used. On that test the mean IQ of the supposedly retarded inmates was 61.8; our retesting of a sample of that group showed a mean IQ of 77.8, with only one inmate in the sample scoring below IQ 70.

Projecting the percentage of retarded inmates identified by the institutions responding to our initial survey to the total prison population, there are in American prisons today nearly 20,000 adult offenders who are substantially intellectually impaired, some 3,300 of whom are classifiable as moderately to profoundly retarded. But the problems which these offenders present transcend their numbers, and they are rejected at every point where help might be given: by those concerned with treatment for the mentally retarded because they are "criminal" and by corrections because to meet their special needs would exhaust the limited resources of most penal institutions.

The Task Force on Law of the President's Panel on Mental Retardation declared, as though it were axiomatic, that "There is no reason to believe that the small percentage of the mentally retarded who ran afoul of the criminal law are prone to commit crimes of violence." Our findings suggest that this rubric—so long accepted in refutation of the once widely held view that all retardates are potential killers—could bear reexamination.

United States Bureau of Prisons statistics indicate that a little over one-fourth of all inmates of adult penal institutions were sent there for having committed assaultive crimes against other people (as opposed to property and other types of offenses), and that about 5 per cent were convicted of some degree of criminal homicide. The largest single offense category is burglary—breaking and entering, which includes 30 per cent of all inmates.

Of the inmates reported by the institutions responding to the

Brown-Courtless Questionnaire as having IQ's less than 70, a sample of 1,000 was selected with measured IQ's below 55. The proportion of this group who had been committed on conviction of burglary—breaking and entering corresponded closely to the figure cited by the Bureau of Prisons for the total prison population (28 per cent). However, among this grossly retarded group, 57 per cent had been convicted of crimes against the person, and the percentage convicted of homicide was three times as high as that of the total prison population (15.4 per cent). And among the fifty prisoners in the six states selected for further empirical research, 72 per cent of the sample selected for retesting who were found to be retarded had been incarcerated for crimes against the person and 36 per cent for some degree of homicide. Indeed, the most frequent crime committed by inmates identified on retesting as retarded was first-degree murder, which accounted for nearly 21 per cent of the total.

Perhaps our sample of half a hundred inmates is too small for this apparent predominance of violent crimes to have much significance. Perhaps also the proportion of retarded prisoners who have committed such crimes is inflated by the fact that the retardate is more easily apprehended, more prone to confess, more likely to be convicted, and will probably be incarcerated longer than the nonretarded offender. Also, one might assume that some of the retardates who commit non-assaultive crimes are diverted from the criminal trial process and committed to institutions for the mentally retarded (although we found no evidence that this occurs in any of the courts and other agencies in which our researches were conducted). And finally, it may be more accurate to state that both mental retardation and crime are largely products of certain socioeconomic and cultural factors (President's Committee, 1968), than to postulate a causal relationship between the two. But however the results of our inquiries may be qualified in light of these factors, one fact rather clearly emerges—that the special problem of the mentally retarded offender warrants much greater attention than it has ever been given in the past.

There are several points in the criminal trial process at which the defendant's retardation might be expected to be revealed: in determining his competency to stand trial; in considering the admissibility of his confession; in resolving the issue of his criminal responsibility (insanity); or in the course of a referral for mental examination. In fact, however, it is not discovered, or if it is, it plays no significant part in the outcome of the case. An important facet of the problem, of course, is that none of these legal procedures operates automatically; rather, the issue must be affirmatively raised. And the system works in such a way as virtually to insure that the issue will *not* be raised.[8] Another is the lack of opportunity presented by the typical criminal trial for discovery of gross impairment. Most of the prisoners in our sample were poor, most Negro, and most had appointed counsel who spent little time with them. The trial was often little more than a formality; more than 95 per cent of the defendants either confessed or pled guilty, and the entire proceedings—from arrest to incarceration in prison—were often completed in a matter of weeks.

Finally, the following excerpts from our interview data suggest still another dimension of the problem:

From a prosecuting attorney, discussing a subject retested at IQ 57:

. . . we all thought he was dumb, but he was a mean ————, and we all were a little afraid of him.

From a public defender, several of whose clients were identified as retarded in prison:

. . . I don't recall that any of my clients were retarded.

From a judge, said of a retarded defendant convicted of first degree murder:

. . . He did appear somewhat slow, but most of these migrant farm workers are retarded to a certain extent anyway.

And from a psychiatrist, asked to render a report in the only case in our sample in which the accused pled "insanity":

. . . In my opinion he could be certified as a mental defective and committed to an appropriate institution. However, in my opinion he is sane and responsible in law for his actions both at the time of the alleged crime and since.

Several years ago the author suggested experimental establishment of an exceptional offenders court, which suggestion was seconded by Brown and Courtless in their report to the President's Crime Commission (Allen, 1966):

The laws of most states have established special procedures outside the normal processes of the criminal law for defined categories of offenders: juveniles, youthful offenders, sex offenders and defective delinquents, for example. Perhaps the closest conceptual model to the exceptional offenders court, among extant judicial institutions, is the juvenile court, with which there are at least two points of similarity: first, both are concerned with persons who are inadequately equipped to meet certain responsibilities of adulthood—in the case of the juvenile, because of his tender years, and in the case of the mentally retarded, because of his intellectual deficit; and second, like the juvenile court, the exceptional offenders court would have as a primary objective the welfare of retarded persons coming under its wardship, rather than imposing punishment for criminal offenses.

Two determinations would be required for such a court to assume jurisdiction, and in each the due process requirements of notice, confrontation, representation, a fair hearing with full right of appeal, and so on, should be observed: first as to the existence of gross intellectual deficit (under a flexible definition, not bound to arbitrary IQ levels, for example, "substantially impaired in his intellectual capacity to cope with the demands and responsibilities of normal adult life, or to conform his behavior to the requirements of law"); and second as to commission of an act, which if committed by a person of normal intelligence would constitute a felony or serious misdemeanor (Allen, 1966):

The court should have broad supervisory powers over all persons properly coming under its jurisdiction, including authority to commit exceptional offenders to appropriate specialized institutions for indeterminate periods. Institutionalization should, however, be based upon a finding of dangerousness to self or others, and such orders should be subject to periodic review. Where the offender is capable of living in society under supervision, probation should be available, making full use of group therapy, special education, and other techniques.

The court should also have authority to confer powers of guardianship (of the person, of the estate, or both) on the probation officer, where the exercise of such powers is deemed necessary or desirable. Where a guardian had previously been appointed for the exceptional offender by another court, the exceptional offenders court should have authority to intervene in such proceedings, either to make the appointed guardian subject to its supervision, or to terminate the prior order of guardianship.

Following the analogy to juvenile court proceedings, it would perhaps be desirable to confer jurisdiction upon the court in cases of dependency and neglect as well—thus making it a court for exceptional adults rather than an exceptional offenders court. Indeed, such a court could be given exclusive authority over the institutionalization and guardianship of the mentally retarded.

The concept of an exceptional offenders court embraces more than merely adding one more court to the judicial system (indeed it need not require even that; such a court might well be a division of an already existing juvenile or family court). It would not, of itself, supply the differential resources necessary for an effective treatment program, but it would be a start; and a step toward implementation of the recommendation of the President's Commission on Law Enforcement and Administration of Justice (the "Crime Commission") for "early identification and diversion to other community resources of those offenders in need of treatment, for whom full criminal disposition does not appear required" (Brown and Courtless, 1967).

Only a small minority of the mentally retarded get into trouble with the law, but for those who do, the criminal trial process is not equipped to identify them and the correctional system cannot provide rehabilitative care appropriate to their special needs. Our researches have shown that such offenders commit a preponderance of assaultive crimes and have a much poorer record of recidivism than intellectually normal offenders (Allen, 1966):

Historically, society has pursued three alternative courses with the mentally retarded offender: we have ignored his limitations and special needs; or we have sought to tailor traditional criminal law processes to fit them; or we have grouped him with psychopaths, sociopaths, and sex deviates in a kind of conventicle of the outcast and hopeless. What is suggested here is a "fourth way," a way not of rejection and despair, but of acceptance and hope (Allen, 1966).

CONCLUSION: LEGAL RIGHTS OF THE MENTALLY RETARDED

In 1967, the International League of Societies for the Mentally Handicapped convened in Stockholm a symposium of experts from all over the world to consider legislative reform in behalf of the retarded. In the document produced by that distinguished body (Sterner, 1967), the following is the first "general principle":

The mentally retarded person has the same rights as other citizens of the same country, same age, family status, working status, etc., unless a specific determination has been made, by appropriate procedures, that his exercise of some or all of such rights will place his own interests or those of others in undue jeopardy.

Society has for a very long time regarded the mentally retarded as objects of charity instead of as citizens with full rights of citizenship until and unless restricted for good reason and under fair and appropriate procedures.

Among the barriers along the way "from charity to rights" are a myriad of laws, administrative regulations, and practices, many of which were adopted with the most humanitarian of motives but whose effect is to denigrate the citizenship—indeed the humanity—of the retarded: "charitably" to deprive them of the very thing which is most precious to any human being and most essential to his fulfillment. The principle announced in Stockholm is the legal counterpart—and a vital one—of the "normalization principle" which has guided formulation of policies for the handicapped in the Scandinavian countries (Nirje, 1967). The National Association for Retarded Children has called for its full recognition in this country (National Association for Retarded Children, 1968)—it is long overdue.

This has been an era of great civil libertarian decisions by our courts. The Supreme Court of the United States, in *Gideon v. Wainwright* (372 U.S. 335, 1963), affirmed the right of *every* criminal defendant to the effective assistance of counsel (and a few lower courts have begun to apply the same requirement to civil commitment cases); in *Miranda v. State of Arizona* (384 U.S. 486, 1966) it further amplified the right of every citizen to protection of his constitutional right not to be compelled to testify against himself; in *Robinson v. California* (370 U.S. 660, 1962) it declared the imposition of criminal sanctions for the "offense" of narcotics addiction to be "cruel and unusual punishment" proscribed by the Constitution; and in *Kent v. U.S.* (383 ULSL 541, 1966) and *Matter of Gault* (387 U.S. 1, 1967) it applied the due process guaranties of the Constitution to juvenile proceedings, despite the contention that since juvenile courts act "for the welfare of the child" and proceedings before them are denominated "civil" rather than criminal, these fundamental rights are inapplicable. And the United States Court of Appeals for the District of Columbia—often in the forefront of liberal reform—has recently declared (*Rouse v. Cameron,* 373 F. 2d 451, 1966) that one who is hospitalized on the basis of a finding of his need for mental health care has a constitutional right to treatment, and that "Continuing failure to provide suitable and adequate treatment cannot be justified by lack of staff or facilities." The court observed:

Regardless of the statutory authority, involuntary confinement without treatment is "shocking." Indeed, there may be greater need for the protection of the right to treatment for persons committed without the safeguards of civil commitment procedures.

The concept would seem directly pertinent to an evaluation of the kind of warehousing of children that characterizes many of our residential care institutions—what was termed in another chapter in this book the process of "de-habilitation" (see Dybwad, Chap. 25).

The Board of Directors of N.A.R.C. listed the following among the significant rights which must be accorded to the retardate (National Association for Retarded Children, 1968):

The right to choose a place to live, to acquire and dispose of property, to marry, and have children, to be given a fair trial for any alleged offense, the right to engage in leisure time activities and to receive such special training, rehabilitation, guidance, counseling, education, and special education, as may strengthen his ability to exercise these rights with a minimum of abridgement.

To the foregoing one might add: the right to privacy, to freedom of communication, to the assistance of an attorney in any legal proceeding affecting his liberty or substantial rights, to freedom from unnecessary restraint, to job training and placement, to respect for his bodily integrity (the right not to be sterilized, or experimented upon or—for "administrative convenience"—to be kept naked, or tied to a crib, or unnecessarily sedated), and to enjoy all of these rights regardless of his family's financial condition, and, insofar as possible, in his own home and community.

But the "legal rights of the mentally retarded" are in the final analysis a single legal right: the right to equal justice under law—that noble concept first enunciated in Magna Carta, embodied in the Constitution of the United States from its inception, and extended to every state of the Union a century ago by the Fourteenth Amendment to that great document.

If the mentally retarded citizen is to receive equal justice, he must be accorded the following component rights: (1) all the rights of citizenship that he is capable of exercising; (2) the right to such protection, assistance, and restriction in exercising such rights as is necessary and appropriate in light of his limitations; (3) the right to humane and appropriate care and treatment—preferably in his own home and community, but if necessary in a residential care institution—with the objective of enabling him to live as fully, as freely, and as self-sufficiently as possible; and (4) fundamental fairness—due process of law —in the provision and safeguarding of each of the foregoing rights.

The Old Testament enjoins us to ". . . do justice to the afflicted" (Psalms 82:3). The quest for justice is the most demanding task of man; insuring equal justice for the unequal can become its noblest expression.

NOTES

1. The Infant's Lawyer, 1712. The Old Testament puts it even more succinctly: ". . . do justice to the afflicted" (Psalms 82:3).

2. Portions of this chapter were first presented at the First Congress of the International Association of the Scientific Study of Mental Deficiency at Montpellier, France, Sept. 18, 1967; and at the Fourth Congress of the International League of Societies for the Mentally Handicapped at Jerusalem, Israel, Oct. 21, 1968. The author's Montpellier paper appeared in the *American Journal of Orthopsychiatry* (July, 1968), and his Jerusalem paper is scheduled for publication in *Mental Retardation*. Portions of the chapter dealing with the retarded offender first appeared in *Mental Retardation* and in *Federal Probation*.

The empirical studies conducted by the Institute of Law, Psychiatry and Criminology referred to in this chapter are: The Mental Competency Study and the Mentally Retarded and the Law, each of which was a three-year research project supported by grants from the National Institute of Mental Health. The final project report in the first study noted has been published as Allen, R., Ferster, E., and Weihofen, H., *Mental impairment and legal incompetency,* Englewood Cliffs, N. J., Prentice-Hall, Inc., 1968. Publications resulting from the second study are listed in the References section to this chapter.

3. An excellent illustration can be found in the description of the determination of indefinite hospitalization and incompetency in Texas, described in Allen and others (1968*a*, p. 50, *et. seq.*).

4. For example, in this country "mental retardation" is the preferred generic term and "mental deficiency" is regarded as an acceptable synonym; but in England, "mental deficiency" is the preferred generic term and "mental retardation" is used to connote functional impairment to a level below presumed capacity (W.H.O., 1954). And in a recently enacted New Jersey law the term "mental deficiency" is used to indicate a greater degree of impairment than the term "mental retardation," and its application results in a different legal status. (See Allen, The dynamics of interpersonal communication and the law, in Allen et al., 1968*b*).

5. For example, Kanner cites ancient and distinguished authority for each of the following assertions as to the etymology of the term "cretin": that it is a corruption of *Chretien* or Christian ("because due to their simplicity of mind, people so afflicted are incapable of sinning"); that it comes from the root *cretira*, or "creature"; from *creta,* or "chalk" because of the "pale, chalk-like color of the skin" (although, interestingly, in another part of Europe they are referred to as *marrons* because of their dark, chestnut-colored complexion); and that it is a derivation of *cretine,* meaning alluvium ("Is not cretinism endemic in such mountain gorges as are very swampy and exposed to damp air?").

6. That distinction may be of critical importance; for example, some statutes refer to commitment "until recovery" when there is a finding in a criminal case of incompetency to stand trial. For the retardate, for whom "recovery" in the conventional sense of the term is not possible, the result of a literal construction of the statute may well be commitment for life.

7. These views are cited and commented upon in Brown and Courtless (1967; reprinted in Allen et al., 1968*b*).

8. An analysis of why this is so may be found in Allen (1968*b*).

REFERENCES

(Publications based on research conducted by the Institute of Law, Psychiatry and Criminology are indicated by an asterisk.)

* Allen, R. Toward an exceptional offenders court. *Ment. Retard.*, Feb., 1966, *4*, 1.

* ————. Legal norms and practices affecting the mentally deficient. *Amer. J. Orthopsychiat.*, July, 1968, *38*, 4. (*a*)

* ————. The retarded offender: unrecognized in court and untreated in prison. *Fed. Probation*, Sept., 1968, *32*, 3. (*b*)

Allen, R., Ferster, E., and Rubin, J. *Readings in law and psychiatry.* Baltimore, Md.: Johns Hopkins Press, 1968. (*a*)

* Allen, R., Ferster, E., and Weihofen, H. *Mental impairment and legal incompetency.* Englewood Cliffs, N.J.: Prentice-Hall, Inc., 1968. (*b*)

* Brown, B., and Courtless, T. *The mentally retarded offender.* Washington, D.C.: President's Commission on Law Enforcement and Administration of Justice, 1967. Reprinted in Allen et al., 1968*b*.

————. The mentally retarded in penal and correctional institutions. *Amer. J. Psychiat.*, March, 1968, *124*, 9.

Davitz, J. R. (Ed.). *Terminology and concepts in mental retardation.* New York: Teachers College, Columbia University, 1964.

* Ferster, E. Eliminating the unfit—is sterilization the answer? *Ohio State Law J.*, 1966, *27*, 591–633.

Infants' Lawyer, The, 1712.

Kanner. *A history of the care and study of the mentally retarded.* Springfield, Ill.: Charles C Thomas. 1964.

* Levy, R. Protecting the mentally retarded: an empirical study and evaluation of the establishment of state guardianship in Minnesota. 49 *Minn. L. Rev.*, 821–887, 1965.

National Association for Retarded Children. *Policy statements on residential care adopted by the board of directors*, 1968.

* Newman, R. (Ed.). Institutionalization of the mentally retarded: a summary and analysis of state laws governing admission to residential facilities and legal rights and protections of institutionalized patients. New York: National Association for Retarded Children, 1967.

Nirje, B. The normalization principle and its human management implications. In: R. Kugel and W. Wolfensberger (Eds.). *Changing patterns in residential services for the mentally retarded.* Washington, D.C.: President's Committee on Mental Retardation, 1967.

President's Commission on Law Enforcement and Administration of Justice (Crime Commission). *The challenge of crime in a free society.* Washington, D.C.: 1967.

President's Committee on Mental Retardation. *MR68: The edge of change.* Washington, D.C.: 1968.

President's Panel on Mental Retardation. *Report of the task force on law.* Washington, D.C.: 1963.

Sterner (Ed.). *Legislative aspects of mental retardation (Stockholm symposium)*, 1967.

* Silber, D., and Courtless, T. Measures of fantasy aggression among mentally retarded offenders, *Amer. J. Ment. Defic.*, May, 1968, *72*, 6.

* ————. Intellectual classification of the educationally and socially disadvantaged prisoner. *Amer. J. Corrections* (to be published).

Study Commission on Mental Retardation. *Mental retardation and the law.* California: 1964.

World Health Organization. *The mentally subnormal child.* Geneva: 1954.

PART FOUR

Training

: 28 :

Mental Retardation and Child Psychiatry

Jack Tizard

INTRODUCTION

IN England and in most of Europe, the Mental Deficiency Services are part of the Mental Health Services, and the subject of mental defect might therefore be considered to be properly a part of psychiatry.[1] However, the boundaries of mental retardation extend beyond those of psychiatry, just as psychiatry itself includes provinces which are far removed from mental retardation. The overlap between the two subjects is greater in the case of children than in the case of adults since mental retardation is by far the commonest of the severe mental disorders of childhood, whereas schizophrenia and depressive disorders are more prevalent in adult life. But in spite of the fact that mental defect is such an important part of child psychiatry, until recently there has been little contact between those concerned with the mentally retarded and those concerned with children suffering from other kinds of mental handicaps.

In these circumstances, one might have expected that little progress would be made in mental subnormality. Yet this is clearly not the case. During the last thirty years, spectacular progress has been made in the biochemistry and genetics of mental retardation. Other notable advances have been made in our knowledge of diseases of environmental origin. There has been much progress in mapping the epidemiology of mental defect. Finally, since World War II, there has been a revival of interest in the exploration of psychological problems, in the study of methods of teaching, and in finding just how best to employ the mentally retarded and to cope with their problems and those of their families.

I am inclined to believe that during the last thirty to forty years, in spite of the unparalleled expansion in services and some fruitful research, no comparable advances have been made elsewhere in child psychiatry. The same sterile arguments are to be seen in the pages of the journals; the same confusion surrounds our views as to the nature of different kinds of disordered behavior; the same conflicting estimates are made about the prevalence of maladjustment in the child population; and the same disputes take place about the efficacy of different kinds of treatment. Therefore, I propose to contrast the state of knowledge and research in mental subnormality, on the one hand, and in child psychiatry, on the other, and to point out that the methods that have proved so successful in mental subnormality have also been shown to offer the same promise when they have been applied in child psychiatry.

The difference between the two disciplines lies in the fact that whereas scientific methods are standard practice among research workers in mental deficiency, only a few child psychiatrists are interested in posing questions that permit scientific answers. If this is so, one may speculate as to the reason for it, and that I propose to do also.

ADVANCES IN MENTAL SUBNORMALITY

Let us first look at the way in which advances in the field of mental retardation have proceeded, going back to the beginning to do so, and noting the developmental milestones which mark the advances in our knowledge.

First came the recognition of the condition of extreme mental backwardness as something worthy of psychological and medical study. In a way, this was Itard's contribution in 1799 to 1804. He demonstrated that a fool, an idiot with no recognizable human characteristics at all except physical ones, could become a subject for scientific and humane study. Moreover, he opened the way to clinical research in this field by showing the value of the intensive study of a single case. His scientific success and his deep concern with his patient put the subject on the map, and things could never be the same again.

The next advance came very soon afterward. It was a *grading* of mental subnormality in behavioral terms, according to the severity of the handicap. Early in the nineteenth century Esquirol (1845) used language as the principal criterion; an imbecile, he said, is a mental defective who can communicate verbally; idiots can use only a few words and short sentences, or utter monosyllables and grunts, or have no language at all. Later Séguin (1846), wrote that "The primary aim of classification is to attain a gauge of mental activity which shall facilitate learning," and throughout the nineteenth century there was much discussion of how best to divide the mentally subnormal by grade or severity of their mental handicap (Kanner, 1964). Séguin himself was much interested in this problem of measurement of all kinds. He, thus, is credited with the invention of the clinical thermometer; also he wrote a book on clinical thermometry for mothers.

The distinction between idiots, imbeciles, and the feeble-minded (morons) was first made on the basis of subjective impressions and clinical judgment and was much later objectified and quantified by the brilliant work of Binet and Simon, whose invention of the intelligence test opened up a whole new branch of psychological enquiry. Interest in this continues unabated today. The point that I wish to make here is that the classification of mental defect in the terms of severity came well before the differentiation of any clinical types.

Classification by grade, or severity is still of fundamental importance, even today when much more is known about the different diseases which give rise to mental retardation, because of its biological and social significance. Idiots and imbeciles are qualitatively different from the feeble-minded and educationally subnormal and from people of ordinary intelligence. Their handicaps, we now know, are usually brought about by different causes from those which result in educational subnormality; they have a different expectation of life; they are rarely fertile; and they require a different kind of management and services to enable them to develop their potentialities.

Whenever these differences between the grades of mental defect are not recognized, serious mistakes in social policy are made. For example, in 1948 O'Connor and I tested all the so-called feeble-minded patients in a large mental deficiency hospital and showed the average IQ to be over 70 points rather than less than 60. Later we showed and others confirmed that this pattern of test scores was quite typical of the feeble-minded patients who constituted three-fifths of adult defectives in institutions in England. We deduced from our enquiries that the great majority of them were fully employable, and that the main need was for an effective rehabilitation and social training program to enable them to return as quickly as possible to the general community (O'Connor and Tizard, 1956). At that time very little of this sort of thing existed in the mental deficiency service—the patients were treated more or less as imbeciles, given so-called "craft work" or "occupational therapy" to do and little education or social training. All this had the effect of reducing rather than developing their industrial and social potential. When the mental deficiency hospitals changed their training programmes to meet the real needs of their patients, the results were very good indeed, and today the situation in virtually all mental deficiency hospitals and in many local-authority adult training centers is quite different from what it was even fifteen years ago. This change is the more remarkable when one remembers the opposition there was to the suggestion that most of the hospital patients were capable of occupational training rather than raffia work or folding envelopes.

It has already been mentioned that the differentiation of the mentally retarded by diagnosis, or "clinical type" as it is called in mental deficiency practice, came much later than the diagnosis by grade or severity of the handicap. With the exception of cretinism, no differentiations were made by clinical type until Langdon Down gave a clear description of the condition of mongolism in 1866. Down's work is important for two reasons: first, because he described what is numerically the largest clinical group of severely subnormal; secondly because he saw the need for a classification of mental retardation based on etiology. The fact that his own excursions into etiology were ridiculous does not lessen the importance of his achievement. During the last thirty years of the nineteenth century a number of other diseases, mainly degenerative diseases of the central nervous system, were discovered, and knowledge has accumulated steadily over the last century. However, even today, the causes of at least two-thirds of severe mental defect remain obscure, and in about one-half of these cases there are no indications whatsoever in the family history, the mother's environment or pregnancy, or the child's early years which give a clue as to why he should be so backward. Thus, although great progress has been made, we still have a long way to go.

It is easier to see today than it was a century ago that no one form of classification of diseases or conditions will serve all purposes. For educational and administrative purposes, classification by grade is the most important. For many biological and medical purposes, classification by cause is needed.

A third field in which conspicuous advances have been made is in the field of treatment; unfortunately, fewer advances have been made in specific treatment for the diseases which result in mental subnormality than in what has come to be called remedial treatment. Séguin was the real founder of special educational treatment for the mentally handicapped. His main textbook was published in French in 1846, with a revised edition in English in 1870. Séguin had the idea that the mentally subnormal have their minds shut up in imperfect organs, so that little is able to get through the tiny windows of perception for the mind to work upon. He was influenced in his thinking by what was known about the deaf, where language development is clearly stunted and delayed by the failure of the ear to transmit the requisite verbal pabulum for the brain to work upon. Séguin thought that whereas deafness and blindness are due to defects in particular sense organs, mental subnormality is the result of a more general defect in the sensory neurones. He therefore advocated a form of sense training to exercise the mind through the senses, and in one form or another this idea persists right up to the present time. In Tredgold (1949), for example, one can still find exactly the same phrases about stimulating the sensorium through the special sense avenues of sight, hearing, touch, and muscle movement, as were first to be found in Séguin and then repeated by various writers, such as Shuttleworth, Montessori, and others throughout the twentieth century.

At the present time, there are two lines of current research which offer much more promise. One is psychological, concerned with the analysis of specific defects and deficits, which has been pioneered by Luria (1961), Kirk (1958), O'Connor and Hermelin (1963), and others. The second line of approach is an educational and developmental one which attempts to utilize and, where necessary, modify ordinary child development practices, adjusting them to the general developmental level of the mentally retarded. Of course this second approach leaves many questions unanswered about the nature of mental defect, and it is, indeed, complementary to the first. Nonetheless it has a great deal to recommend it from an educational point of view.

I have already mentioned the developments that have taken place as far as the training and employment of adult defectives are concerned. My view is that, as a *research* problem, this matter has now been solved, at least insofar as the twentieth-century industrial society is concerned. We have a very good idea indeed about the potentialities of the mentally retarded, the kinds of things they can be taught to do, and the way to teach them. The great majority can be gainfully and happily employed and can live socially useful and contented lives, given a certain amount of help of a kind that we all know about. That this help is not provided today is due to the inadequacies of our services rather then to a lack of knowledge about what kind of help should be provided.

However, it must be said that in the provision of services a very great deal has been done. The first services to be created were residential institutions, modeled on the pattern of a pedagogical establishment set up near Interlaken in Switzerland in 1839 by Guggenbuhl. The idea of model asylums for the mentally defective caught on, both in this country and in other parts of Europe. Throughout the nineteenth century and the early twentieth century, there was a steady expansion in residential asylum provision. The development of day services came much later, and progress was delayed by World War I, followed by the chronic economic depression in the years that led up to World War II and then by that war itself. Today we are in the middle, or perhaps at the beginning, of a great expansion in what have been called "community" services; many varied and interesting developments are taking place in local health authorities throughout England. The idea of a *local* mental health service is a very significant extension in our thinking about health service. Much experiment along these lines is taking place in the mental illness field, and the weakest feature of our mental deficiency programmes today is that little or no evaluation of the efficacy of different kinds of service has as yet been carried out; indeed, the very idea of an experimental social science still remains to be translated into practice. Nowhere would it be easier to do so than in the field of mental subnormality.

A final way in which progress in mental subnormality has occurred is the field of epidemiology. In this respect mental deficiency has a particularly rich history. As early as 1811, Napoleon ordered a census of cretins to be made in one of the Swiss cantons (Kanner, 1964). Nothing much came of this, but throughout the nineteenth century other attempts were made in various places to determine the frequency of subnormality and the factors that influenced it. However, progress *did* come about during the twentieth century. In 1904, The First Royal Commission ordered a census to be made of the numbers of defectives in various parts of England. The case fact-finding was inadequate, but the data were used for administrative purposes in the framing of policies which led up to and followed the 1913 Mental Deficiency Act. Twenty years later E. O. Lewis (1929), between 1925 and 1929, carried out the most thorough and informative survey which has ever been undertaken in England or any other country. Lewis was able to use intelligence tests to assist him in his grading of severity of mental defect. He also found that, owing to the introduction of extensive services, case-finding, particularly among children, was relatively easy. Finally, he was able to use epidemiologic methods that were, by this time, fairly sophisticated. He presented his data in a form which makes it possible still to interpret them today and see exactly what was done.

Other surveys have been carried out, both before and after World War II; one being undertaken at present by Kushlick in Wessex, England, promises to bring Lewis's findings up to date and to supplement them. Today, also, a National Child Development Study is being undertaken by Drs. Neville Butler and Kelmer Pringle, which holds much promise. In this inquiry, all seventeen thousand children born during the first week of March 1958 are being followed up at intervals to determine their intellectual and physical progress and its relationship to social and environmental circumstances. The study is likely to give definitive information about such factors as the relationship between prematurity, social class, and mental defect, and the outcome of pregnancies in which there have been complications of labor, neonatal asphyxia, or other difficulties in the antenatal, perinatal, or postnatal periods.

Looking at the subject of mental defect as a whole, therefore, we see that research is flourishing. A great deal of biological work is being done, research leading to the discovery and diagnosis of new diseases and to the elucidation of genetic factors that are responsible for specific types of mental retardation. Advances in our understanding of biological and biosocial factors associated with mental and physical handicaps are leading to the introduction of preventive programs and to specific forms of treatment. Great steps have been taken in methods of training and educating the mentally handicapped, finding them work, and fitting them into the community. Much is known about the social factors associated with mental subnormality and the steps that need to be taken in order to reduce the load on the parents and on the community. The epidemiologic picture is being pretty thoroughly drawn. And with the introduction of the so-called "at risk" register, through which babies with adverse factors in the prenatal, perinatal, or postnatal period are being specifically followed up by public health nurses and, where necessary, by pediatricians, public health measures are being taken which are likely to lessen the incidence of some conditions which bring about mental retardation. Likewise, the introduction of special services to deal with handicapped children and their families will enable us to take effective measures to prevent secondary handicaps from developing in children who are at risk because of hereditary factors or adverse circumstances in the prenatal, perinatal, or postnatal periods, or during later infancy or childhood.

CHILD PSYCHIATRY

Let us now examine some aspects of child psychiatry which are not primarily concerned with mental defect—the general psychiatry of childhood if you like. I do not propose to survey the field in any detail; however, it should be clear that our knowledge in general child psychiatry is by no means as complete as it is in mental defect.

Diagnosis

The diagnosis of mental disorder in children is fraught with uncertainty and controversy. There is not even any widely accepted scheme of classification of mental disorder in children, and the situation is so unsatisfactory in this respect that little attempt is made in, for example, the World Health Organization's *International Statistical Classification of Diseases* to cope with child psychiatry (1964).

Secondly, even when a system of classification is adopted, such as the one used in the Underwood *Report on Maladjusted Children* (1955) and in many clinics throughout England, few attempts are made to assess the severity of any condition. In mental deficiency practice, the rating of severity, or grade, of mental defect has proved indispensable. I am sure that estimates of severity would also prove useful in other branches of psychiatry. Yet such things are rarely attempted.

One might ask does all this matter in practice? Yes it does. It means, for example, that in many child guidance clinics all cases go through the same diagnostic procedure, the child and his family all being seen by all members of the team. The majority then get taken on for "treatment," which is, in this case, psychotherapy for the child and counseling for the parents. This is a lengthy business, more often than not terminated by the refusal of the child or his parents to continue with it. Because it all takes so long, almost all child guidance clinics have inordinately long waiting lists. I am told that in one enquiry carried out some years ago among child guidance clinics in London, only Dr. Winnicott's clinic was able to see a child immediately. The rest had waiting lists of from three months to a year or even longer. This is an intolerable situation and one which would not, I suspect, be remedied merely by the proliferation of clinics throughout the country. More realism is needed in our attitude to treatment and to the public health problems of child psychiatry (see, for example, Hunt, 1961; Anderson and Dean, 1956).

The Efficacy of Treatment

These issues raise another question: the efficacy of treatment. Vernon (1964) has recently reviewed the literature, and he concludes (as all who have undertaken this thankless task have concluded):

. . . except in some fairly straightforward instances such as vocational counseling, the effects so far isolated (of psychotherapy and counseling) are still often small or inconsistent, indicating that expert diagnosis and treatment may not, as one would expect, have much more to offer than naive methods. Particularly important . . . is the lack of any demonstrated superiority for deep-oriented methods.

Concern about child psychotherapy, its objectives, and its effects is, of course, very widespread. Scott (1965) discusses some of the main problems in a review of a book containing a comprehensive and representative presentation of fifty-seven contrasting methodological approaches to various aspects of the psychotherapy of children. He writes:

The objective of treatment is variously stated: reduce anxiety to allow new relationships to occur, decrease fear to the point at which "inherent normal ambivalence" can again operate, help the child to assume responsibility for himself, bring him to the level of development appropriate to his age, provide opportunity to play out a forbidden theme, in one contribution the objectives seem to be coextensive with a good system of education. There is a curious reluctance to state the objective as the removal of symptoms. . . . Because of the lack of adequate definition of problems, types and objectives, the processes of treatment do not carry conviction or clarity. Klein recommends immediate interpretation, Anna Freud a preliminary building-up of the "good parents" relationship, Smolden claims good results without too much use of verbal communication. There is remarkably little enquiry into the large number of possible operative factors which might occur when the resources of a clinic are concentrated upon a child. The general complacency is illustrated by one of the contributor's statements: "The scientific world wants to know why we are so sure—the parents only that we are sure." The numerous case reports are literally sprinkled with such phrases as "it became clear that," "explanation seems almost superfluous," "I have good reason to believe," "this clearly represented"; to the reader it is not always so clear.

By no means an unsympathetic critic, Scott dismisses this book (which contains major contributions from all the leading analysts) as of "historical interest," and he concludes by saying that it reveals that the field of psychotherapy is badly in need of scientific appraisal. Few people who are not themselves deeply committed to one or other "school" of psychoanalysis could, I think, disagree with this appraisal.

Epidemiology

The only other aspect of child psychiatry to be discussed here is epidemiology. What is the frequency of mental disorder or maladjustment in children? How many children require the services of the child guidance clinic? What kinds of backgrounds do they come from? What kinds of services do they require? What are the effects of these services upon the incidence or prevalence of maladjustment?

In England since World War II, there have been two official reports published on maladjusted children of school age. The first was the "Report of the Underwood Committee" (1955), which not only failed to answer the question of how many children require treatment for neurotic conditions, but found it impossible to forecast the number of day schools or additional boarding schools likely to be needed for maladjusted pupils during a ten-year period, or to make an estimate of the number of teachers and houseparent staff who would be required. The second official report is the recent Scottish one, with the promising title of "The Ascertainment of Maladjusted Children" (Scottish Education Department, 1964).

Unfortunately, after thirty meetings the committee responsible found it impossible to answer the question they were specifically asked as part of their terms of reference, namely, "the percentage of children of school age likely to be ascertained as needing special educational treatment because of maladjustment."

General Problems

As these examples show, there is a widespread failure to tackle problems of diagnosis and classification and a lack of realism regarding the effectiveness of treatment in child psychiatry. Because of a very proper concern with the uniqueness of the individual we too often fail to see the similarities between one child's problems and another's; also few properly controlled experimental studies are carried out of different patterns of service. We seem unable to come to terms with the public health problems of child psychiatry, either through epidemiologic studies of the prevalence of various kinds of mental disorder, or through studies designed to show the best ways of utilizing the scarce resources of child guidance clinics in the most socially useful way. These failings bring us into disrepute among our colleagues in other branches of medicine and the social sciences.

It is worth asking ourselves the reason for the success of research in the field of mental retardation, as opposed to general child psychiatry. In the first place it is not because in mental defect there has been a striking success in treatment. Mental subnormality is notoriously resistant to curative treatment—indeed, among severely handicapped defectives there is almost always gross structural damage to the brain, and cure in any final sense is impossible. Secondly, the success in research in mental retardation cannot be ascribed to the size of the resources poured into mental deficiency work. In Britain, the numbers engaged in research in mental subnormality have always been small. In 1960, for example, this author carried out an enquiry to find out just how much research was being done on psychological and social problems of mental defect in England and Wales, and at that time the number of fulltime research psychologists engaged on such problems was three. There was, in addition, one medical statistician working on a temporary basis and another engaged in part-time work. There were three or four research students and a few doctors and psychologists who were doing part-time research in the mental deficiency hospitals. In all, the total was probably not more than a dozen to fifteen people (Tizard, 1962).

Thirdly, it is a mistake to believe that in some way the subject of mental subnormality is "easier" than child psychiatry. Other people's problems always look simple, but it has already been pointed out that even such an obvious matter as the recognition of mongolism as a clinical entity did not take place until people had been working with the subnormal for nearly seventy years. Likewise it is only during the last two decades that any serious thought has been given to the possibility that cerebral-palsied children are not all mentally defective; also we are only just beginning to differentiate between autistic children, on the one hand, and the mentally subnormal, on the other.

Fourthly, the productiveness of work in mental subnormality does not come from the fact that some genius—a Darwin or a Sherrington—has opened up a whole new field of work which will keep many generations busy. There *have* been able people working in this field, of course, but on the whole it has not been a fashionable field for research, and it has not attracted many of our brighter sparks.

The reason for the success of so much research in mental subnormality is, perhaps, to be found in the fact that people have posed their questions carefully in a manner which has permitted scientific answers to be given to them. In contrast, the large literature on child psychiatry is mainly clinical. There is a dearth of sustained, professional research and a widespread impatience on the part of clinicians to undergo the discipline which research entails. The very richness and subtlety of the Freudian dialectic, profound though its influence has been on the whole of our thinking, has, I believe, served to impoverish research in child psychiatry. It has led men to believe that they know more than, in fact, they do, and it has prevented them from asking questions to which scientific answers can be given.

What I have said so far about child psychiatry has been almost entirely destructive. Let me, therefore, now try to make amends by drawing attention to work which does seem to me to be likely to produce answers to some of the questions that I have raised. My own biases—an interest in public health aspects of psychiatry, a distrust of the grand theorists, an excessive empiricism perhaps, and a concern with practical matters and the short run—will be evident. To apologize for these biases would be insincere; the question is where do they take us in psychiatry?

RESEARCH IN CHILD PSYCHIATRY

I want to look again at the five aspects of child psychiatry that I have already considered in relation to mental defect: the classification of mental disorders, their severity, the problems of treatment, epidemiology, and aetiology. They are not, of course, the only important aspects of psychiatry, but that they *are* important none will deny. Let us consider them in turn.

Classification

The need for a workable system of classification is clear. It should be equally clear that no system of classification based on typology or supposed aetiology is likely to win general support at the present time. Indeed, if we are to achieve agreement on any system of classification, it must be one which is based on behavioral symptoms, for example the classification used in most child guidance clinics and included in the appendix to the Underwood Report (1955).

My colleague, Michael Rutter (1965), who has clarified my own thinking on this matter enormously, has laid down principles upon which a classification must be based if it is to be useful, and has outlined the way in which an acceptable system of classification might be arrived at. Rutter points out that the diagnostic distinction made in child psychiatry between conduct disorders, on the one hand, and neurotic or nervous disorders, on the other, has in practice been found to be clinically meaningful and to have predictive value. Factor analyses of studies of symptoms nearly always give rise to two factors, one on which antisocial and aggressive traits have high loadings, the other defined by nervous, anxious, and fearful traits. More important, clinicians working in child guidance practices are able to make these distinctions more often than they perhaps realize. Thus a few years ago, when Mulligan, Douglas, and I asked psychiatrists to pick out seriously disturbed children about the age of thirteen who were attending their clinics for treatment and to rate them where possible as presenting a nervous or neurotic disorder, a habit disorder, or a mixed or unclassifiable disorder, they nearly all protested that this could not be done for the majority of cases. However, in fact, they rated over 90 per cent of their patients as presenting either a behavior disorder or a nervous disorder, and only about 5 per cent as having a mixed or unclassifiable disorder. Moreover, in this particular study, as in others, the classification on these lines was found to have predictive value, both as far as the children's subsequent adjustment was concerned and in regard to later delinquency. This finding was not dependent upon the social background of the children or the kind of school that they attended.

There are, of course, other groups of mental disorders which can be clinically differentiated, showing different response to treatment and having different prognoses. Rutter (1965), for example, lists a mixed group, the habit disorders, or as he calls them "developmental disorders," the hyperkinetic syndrome, child psychosis, the mental deficiencies, educational retardation and one or two more which can be clinically differentiated having different ages of onset and different prognoses.

Severity

In mental subnormality classification by grade of defect has been found to be valuable. Unfortunately, virtually no work on similar lines has been done in child psychiatry. Douglas, Mulligan, and I found, as others have done, that a rating of severity of disorder based on the number of symptoms reported by teachers had high predictive value as far as later conduct and also delinquency were concerned. We are at present looking at educational and other social correlates of maladjustment and are hopeful that the data that we have already collected will be found useful here also. The question of severity has not, however, been well studied, and further work is needed before a satisfactory system of grading is devised.

To rate the severity of a disorder, one would have to arrive at scores based on a number of factors: the number and duration of the symptoms, their consequences in terms of the extent to which they affect the child's personal life or happiness, and their impact upon the lives of others. Clearly one would also have to consider some symptoms in a different way from others—encopresis, or attempted suicide, or ungovernable rage which led to serious attacks on other children, if they occur in a child of ten years of age, are in a very different category from wetting the bed, food fads, or a tendency to weep when tired. Only when we have succeeded in devising a rating of the severity of presenting problems will we be able to achieve a system of priorities in child guidance which will enable the child guidance clinics to fulfill their public health function of serving the needs of hard-pressed families who seek their aid.

Treatment

Here, as Leon Eisenberg (1961) says in a significant paper, we confront a paradox. Psychological influences have been shown to be extraordinarily powerful in modifying human behavior at physiological levels; yet proof of the superiority of one treatment method over another, or even of prolonged therapy over brief therapy, has been remarkably elusive. Eisenberg argues that the facts at our disposal compel us to look again at what he calls the "strategic deployment" of the child psychiatrist in preventive psychiatry. Central nervous impairment in the fetus follows upon the malnutrition, inadequate prenatal care, and life stress to which the pregnant mother in the marginal family is subject. The brain of the infant may be further victimized by poor control of infections, injury, and toxins. When young, the child in a marginal family receives less intellectual stimulation and is particularly vulnerable to the deprivation which follows family disintegration. As Eisenberg notes, the child psychiatrist can make a major contribution to mental health by helping to mobilize the community in support of social welfare programs to minimize the sequelae of poverty. He gives many examples of how this can be done: through the prevention and treatment of certain metabolic disorders which in time lead to irreversible brain damage; through public health measures designed to eliminate or control environmental factors which often result in damage to the child; and by affecting changes in child-care practices, particularly among children brought up in public institutions, which result in intellectual and emotional deprivation. Finally, as he points out, there are many studies which show that the effects of short-term treatment are significant in altering the course of psychiatric illness among children suffering from a wide range of disorders. All this suggests to him (and also to me) that a shift in emphasis is required in psychiatric practice toward preventive work, and that in our clinical practice a change is required in the methods used.

Might it not be that the comparative ineffectiveness of long-term therapy, as compared with short-term therapy, arises because too much emphasis is placed on the elucidation of the "mechanisms" which are thought to be responsible for the disorder, while too little attention is paid to the advising of teachers, parents, and other adults, and the child himself as to how to handle his problems. It may be more effective to teach a child who is painfully nervous and shy, for example, a set of manners that will enable him to meet strangers, knowing, at any rate, how to behave toward them, rather than to tease out the reasons for his shyness through a reconstruction of his past history in the hope that this will in some way cure it. Likewise, it may be more effective to offer advice to child-care workers concerned with deprived children or delinquents than to treat the children themselves. My own view is that the role of the expert in many fields of medicine and education is to advise the practitioners, teachers, and parents rather than to treat the patients or pupils. The school inspector's job is not to do remedial teaching. In like manner, the psychiatric social worker might do better to spend a large portion of her time advising and working with her colleagues rather than with her clients; the speech therapists and physiotherapists with the parents and teachers rather than the children; the psychologist with the school teacher rather than with the "subject." It is through education rather than through treatment that the best results are often achieved, but even fifty hours of education spread over the course of a year are an insignificant part of a child's life when set apart from the rest of his experience.

Epidemiology

The Underwood Committee and its Scottish counterpart imply that the problems of measurement are such that it is not possible to estimate the prevalence of psychiatric disorder in children. Is this really the best that we can do? Surely not—for the following reasons:

First, there are available fairly effective and reliable paper-and-pencil questionnaires which can be given to teachers and parents for the purpose of screening out children who present problems that are a cause for concern. In England such questions have been used effectively by Rutter (1965) and Stott (1958), among others. More work along these lines has been carried out in the United States. The extent to which children are reported through the use of any type of screening device will, of course, depend upon a number of factors, including the way in which parents and teachers are approached and briefed and the way in which the questions are posed. On the basis of our present evidence, it seems likely that the great majority of seriously disturbed children can be discovered through the use of screening devices of one sort or another—the main problem is not that of missing large numbers of seriously ill children, but what to do about the ordinary healthy children, the false positives, that are picked up through the use of such devices.

So the question is, having screened out children who are likely to be maladjusted, together with a number of children who are incorrectly selected by our screening procedures, can we decide which children have rightly been selected and which have not? This problem has received rather little attention. Attempts by psychologists to devise batteries of personality tests for this purpose, analogous to intelligence tests for the assessment of intellectual ability, have not proved rewarding. The whole approach seems to be misconceived, and I think it unfortunate that so much time is spent on it. It is more likely that a carefully devised and properly standardized clinical procedure will yield reliable and valid results. Of course, to devise such a procedure is impossible unless we first agree upon a classification of disorders and until suitable criteria are devised by which to assess severity. These tasks should not be insuperable. Where work on these lines has been carried out, the results achieved so far have been encouraging.

Aetiology

We are on much less firm ground in regard to the aetiology of various forms of child maladjustment than we are in regard to the other matters I have mentioned. Some organic conditions are now reasonably well understood. In other conditions, for example, child psychosis, important misconceptions about aetiology, such as the view that child psychosis is caused by faulty rearing, have been shown to be untenable. On the whole, however, the classification of disorders according to supposed aetiology has not made much progress, and personally I find myself unconvinced by the most of what I read on these lines. However, a similar situation exists in subnormality. The literature is strewn with papers purporting to explain the causes of mongolism, from Langdon Down's vaguely formulated racial theory, to the more recent but no better supported views about pituitary dysfunction or maternal shock. The only point to be made in this connection is that classification of disorders by aetiology is important, but not all-important. Advances are likely to be slow, and an inadequate theory about cause may be worse than no theory at all—for example, the classification of mental deficiency into primary and secondary amentia, according to their supposed aetiology, impeded progress in this field for a long time. The words themselves explained nothing, though they appeared to explain everything and left no questions to be asked. One day we will know much more about the cause of maladjustment in children; in the meantime there is much that we can do.

In conclusion, then, I think that although there is a great deal to criticize in contemporary child psychiatry, the situation is not as bad as a hostile critic would picture it. Now that funds for research are becoming more easy to get, we have the opportunity and the duty to begin systematic long-term studies of many aspects of our field. I have already mentioned some of the ones which I think important. Can I add to the list the need for research into the function of the child guidance clinics themselves, the effects of different types of residential schools, hospital in-patient units, and the study of alternative ways of using scarce mental health personnel.

SUMMARY

The mentally subnormal form the largest class of severely disordered children for whom special provision is made in the Mental Health Services. Mental subnormality is thus of great importance to child psychiatry. In spite of this, the subject has been much neglected by child psychologists and psychiatrists working in other fields, and by pediatricians, educationists, and psychiatric social workers.

Research into mental subnormality has suffered from its isolation from other branches of medicine, psychology, and sociology. Nonetheless a great deal has been found out about the epidemiology, causes, and treatment of mental defect. Our knowledge of this field compares very favorably indeed with that of the rest of child psychiatry, where too little attention has been paid to scientific problems.

I have discussed the ways in which advances have been made in mental subnormality. Similar advances are possible elsewhere in child psychiatry, and where systematic research has been carried out it has already proved strikingly successful.

================

NOTE

1. This chapter is adapted from, "Mental subnormality and child psychiatry," published in *J. Child Psychol. Psychiat.,* 1966, *7.* It was given originally as the Chairman's Address to the Association for Child Psychology and Psychiatry on February 10, 1965.

REFERENCES

Anderson, F. N., & Dean, H. C. Some aspects of child guidance intake policy and practice. U.S. Department of Health, Education and Welfare. *Publ. Health Monogr.* Washington, D.C.: 1956, *42.*

Eisenberg, L. The strategic deployment of the child psychiatrist in preventive psychiatry. *J. Child Psychol. Psychiat.,* 1961, *2,* 229–241.

Esquirol, J. E. D. *Mental maladies: A treatise on insanity.* Transl. with additions by E. K. Hunt. Philadelphia: Lea and Blanchard, 1845.

Hunt, R. G. Age, sex and service patterns in a child guidance clinic. *J. Child Psychol. Psychiat.,* 1961, *2,* 185–192.

Itard, J. M. G. *The wild boy of aveyron.* New York: Appleton-Century-Crofts, 1962.

Kanner, L. *A history of the care and study of the mentally retarded.* Springfield, Ill.: Charles C Thomas, 1964.

Kirk, S. A. *Early education of the mentally retarded.* Urbana: University of Illinois Press, 1958.

Lewis, E. O. *Report of the mental deficiency committee,* Part IV. London: H.M.S.O., 1929.

Luria, A. R. *The role of speech in the regulation of normal and abnormal behavior.* Oxford: Pergamon Press, 1961.

O'Connor, N., & Hermelin, B. F. *Speech and thought in severe subnormality.* Oxford: Pergamon Press, 1963.

O'Connor, N., & Tizard, J. *The social problem of mental deficiency.* Oxford: Pergamon Press, 1956.

Rutter, M. Classification and categorization in child psychiatry. *J. Child Psychol. Psychiat.,* 1965, *6,* 71–83.

Scott, P. D. Review of child psychotherapy. In: M. D. Haworth (Ed.). *Brit. J. Psychiat.,* 1065, *3,* 199–200.

Scottish Education Department. *Ascertainment of maladjusted children: Report of the working party appointed by the secretary of state for Scotland.* Edinburgh, 1964.

Séguin, E. *Traitment moral, hygiene et education des idiots et des autres enfants arrieres.* Paris: J. B. Balliere, 1846.

———. *Idiocy and its treatment by the physiological method.* Reprinted, New York: Columbia Teachers College, 1907.

Stott, D. H. *The social adjustment of children: Manual to the Bristol Social Adjustment Scales.* London: University of London Press, 1958.

Tizard, J. Treatment of the mentally subnormal. In: Richter, D. (Ed.). *Aspects of psychiatric research.* London: Oxford University Press, 1962.

Tredgold, A. F. *A text-book of mental deficiency* (7th ed.). London: Bailliere, Tindall & Cox, 1949.

Underwood Committee. *Report of the committee on maladjusted children.* London: H.M.S.O., 1955.

Vernon, P. E. *Personality assessment: A critical survey,* London: Methuen, 1964.

World Health Organization. *International statistical classification of diseases.* Geneva: World Health Organization, 1957.

: 29 :

Experiences of Pregnancy: Some Relationships to the Syndrome of Mental Retardation

Richard L. Cohen

INTRODUCTION

THIS report will focus on the training aspects of a larger research project conducted primarily within the Departments of Obstetrics and Gynecology of two medical schools.[1] The parent study has had two objectives: the exploration of relationships between pregnancy stress and the course of subsequent development in the child; the development of preventive intervention techniques which could be useful to nonpsychiatric personnel working in prenatal clinics and obstetric wards. Although many of the observations which have been made as a result of the early work are reported elsewhere in the literature (Cohen, 1966 *a,b;* Cohen et al., in press), a brief summary of the project will be included in part of this chapter so that the reader will be able to understand more clearly the training procedures.

From the outset, it was the intent of the project staff to evolve both concepts and techniques which would be understandable to personnel who did not have special training in the mental health field. For this reason, a great number of medical and nursing personnel (senior medical students, obstetric residents, pediatric residents, student nurses, obstetric and public health nurses, and others) have been incorporated into the administration of screening instruments, interviewing procedures, and rating scales. Any item which proved to be awkward or obscure to these kinds of personnel has been modified or discarded even though it may have been yielding useful data so far as the research was concerned.

HISTORICAL BACKGROUND OF THE STUDY

The particular significance of this work for the field of mental retardation will be evident to the child psychiatrist or other clinician interested in developmental medicine. In this author's experience in child psychiatry and child development centers, many children have been encountered in whom the chief complaint, as expressed by the parents, was related to concerns about mental retardation, brain damage, or other primary defect; yet in many instances, these conditions could not be demonstrated by careful and repeated clinical evaluation. In other instances, developmental delay in the child appeared to be reactive to a parental image of the child which was "defective." The parental assessment of the child as one in whom normal growth and development could not be expected preceded historically the appearance of substandard performance.

As the pregnancy histories of these children were examined in greater detail, the author was intrigued by the high incidence of events or conditions which the mothers have reported as being so stressful as to interfere with the usual adaptive process of pregnancy (and the immediate care of the neonate). In many instances, these experiences had either been repressed or minimized in their importance so that they had never been revealed to previous interviewers. Several cases of this type have been reported in a previous publication (Cohen, 1966b). The most striking aspect of these situations was that the degree and nature of the stress was only rarely related to the specific characteristics of the internalized fears about the child's welfare or health. Rather, the relationship between the stress and attitudes toward the child were global and diffuse. For instance, one mother handled her ambivalent feelings about her own mother's sudden death due to a ruptured cerebral aneurism (this event occurred during the middle trimester of pregnancy) by developing overriding fears that she would have a defective child.

In addition to the experience of clinical practice, impetus for this study came from several other sources. The author was strongly influenced by the work of Rose (1960) and his colleagues at the Children's Hospital of Philadelphia. In considering maternal reactions to real or fantasied defects in babies, Rose (1961) pointed out that

. . . it appeared that there could be a continuum of damage to the child, depending on the intensity of maternal disturbances and the degree to which they impinged on the child, and depending also on the time period of the child's maturation at which the disturbances were effectively in contact. It seemed likely also that there was very little basic difference in the maternal reaction between those cases in which the mother *perceived* the child as having been damaged in utero consequent to pregnancy complications and those in which the perception of the threat was reinforced by realistic medical opinion in the newborn period. The mothers were not as clearly or greatly in distress, but the avoidance mechanism was almost as pronounced. In simple avoidance patterns, the mothers seemed mystified about their own behavior and were self-accusatory about deficiencies in their love for this infant.

The concept embodied in the above statement is at one and the same time simple and complex. It holds that fantasies about or perception of defect or damage to the infant (or fetus) may be as influential a force upon child-rearing behavior and mother-infant interaction as objectively (medically) determined illness or defect may be.

Even in the presence of real threats to the survival or function of the child, many parents have been observed to harbor an internalized image of the child as one incapable of initiative, self-care, and mastery of new skills. The child is seen as "vulnerable," and both child and parents often express fears of separation and feelings of marked dependency. The considerable interference with growth and learning which is inevitable in such a parent-child constellation has been described by Green and Solnit as the "vulnerable child syndrome."

In another study involving mothers and offspring where there was blood-group incompatibility, Rose (1962) noted that

. . . regardless of objective deficit in the offspring, the mother's perception of the child's viability seemed to have been damaged in the neonatal period. The mothers seemed to continue to view their children as in danger of death and in need of blood at each new phase of development. The mother's child-rearing behavior seemed to have been governed more by this perception of the child as constantly in a state of hazard to survival than by realistic appraisal of the needs of the child for a more diversified environmental experience. It is apparent that the consequences of salvage are not only that many children are affected by sensori-motor integration deficits in their development but that additionally, even those cases showing full clinical recovery have had introduced into their rearing a special bias which disadvantages them more than an average peer group.

When one views these observations against the background of knowledge now emerging in the fields of neonatology, learning theory, ethology, child development and family interaction, the impact is a striking one. The interrelationship of dependency and learning seems an inescapable fact. In a vast array of laboratory studies (Jaffe, 1965; Lehrmann, 1962; Rheingold, 1963; Schneirla, 1963) performed on higher mammals, for instance, it is now being clearly demonstrated that the capacity of offspring to perceive threats in the environment, to cope with change, to learn basic skills and to become an acceptable member of a group are all strongly influenced by the constancy and quality of the nurturance which was experienced during the first weeks and months of life.

The choice of the pregnancy period as an arena for the study, prevention, and management of early disturbances in mother-infant interaction is hardly a new one. Early papers by Hall and Mohr (1933), by Kasanin and Handschin (1941), and by Squier and Dunbar (1946) all emphasized the critical aspects of development for the mother during this period and the need for special care and attention in order to avoid disruptive influences on the subsequent development of the child. For many years, obstetricians and other professional people have been aware of the relationship between the emotional status of the gravid woman and the course and outcome of the pregnancy. A recent review by McDonald (1968) will provide the reader an excellent summary of past work in this particular area. More specifically, many investigators have explored the possible relationship between maternal anxiety or maternal psychopathology and the occurrence of childbirth abnormalities (see particularly Davids and Devault, 1962, and Gunter, 1963). Many retrospective studies have attempted to show a significant relationship between behavior disorders in children and pregnancy and labor abnormalities. Because of the many problems in acquiring reliable retrospective data, these studies are not conclusive. They have yielded much presumptive evidence, however.

DESCRIPTION OF THE PROJECT

In the hope of dealing with some of the technical problems encountered in retrospective studies and with the expectation that whatever research was accomplished would be applied immediately and directly to obstetric and pediatric practice in academic settings, a long-term prospective study was designed. This is being reported upon in other publications (Beitenman et al., in press; Cohen et al., in press; Helper et al., in press). However, a brief summary is appropriate at this point in order to make the training programs more understandable.

To begin with, previous assumptions about what most women found stressful or disturbing during their pregnancies were abandoned. Large numbers of randomly selected pregnant women in a university prenatal clinic were interviewed according to an open-ended, adaptively oriented interview model. Most of these sessions were tape-recorded. The tapes were played several times in order to identify with a patient-centered focus those factors, forces, experiences, and conditions which women reported as subjectively stressful.

Virtually all of the conditions described by women fell into one of four categories: experiences which they interpreted as being evidence of inadequate or distorted preparation for child bearing or child rearing (category I); some adverse previous experience with child bearing or child rearing (for example, multiple abortions, already rearing a disturbed child, and so on) (category II); deficient dependency supports (marital, kinship, social, professional) (category III); the perceived existence of some maternal condition which might be worsened by the pregnant state (category IV).

Using the adaptive model of pregnancy promulgated by Caplan (1960), we also looked for those behavioral cues which would be most likely to serve as presumptive evidence of: failure to accept the pregnancy extending beyond the first trimester (category V); denial of or overreaction to the pregnant state (category VI); failure to show preparatory behavior for the coming baby during the third trimester (category VII).

In effect, we added these three behavioral categories to the stress categories as defined by the women. Although this may appear to be an "apples and oranges" kind of arrangement, the seven indexes provide us with a multilevel screen which picks up most women who see themselves as ill-prepared, or uncared for, or vulnerable to damage by the pregnancy or unduly apprehensive about the welfare of the fetus. Using these categories, the project staff devised a series of fourteen questions (see the Pregnancy Profile Questionnaire in Table 29–1), each one of which was aimed at uncovering the existence of maternal concerns in one of these categories. This screening device went through several revisions both in the content and sequence of questions until we arrived at a format which was syntonic with the verbal habits of professional people and the communication skills of the average clinic population.

A way was devised to introduce the screening device into the routine history-taking for each new patient during the first clinic visit. This was administered by a senior medical student as a part of the usual workup and with no special introduction or preparation to the

TABLE 29–1
Pregnancy Profile Questionnaire

Marital Status____Marriage Date____Race____   (Hospital Identification Plate)
E.D.C.____Para.____Agency____Keeping Baby____

1. How long have you lived in this area? (Category III)

2. How often do you see your mother or other relatives?
   (Category III)

3. What was your reaction when you found out you
   were pregnant? (Category V)

4. (M) Is your husband much help?
   (S) Does the father of the baby know you are pregnant? (Category III)

5. How would you compare the way you feel now with
   before you became pregnant? (Category VI)

6. Are you doing anything to get ready for the baby?
   (Category VII)

7. Have you thought of any names for the baby?
   Boy? Girl? (Category VII)

8. How active is your baby? (Category VI)

9. Has anything happened *in the past* that might cause you to worry about the baby?
   If so what? (Category II)

10. What experience did you have as you were growing up in taking care of younger
    children? (Category I)

11. How do you plan to raise your children that is different from the way you were
    raised? (Category I)

12. Has anything happened *during this pregnancy* that might hurt the baby or cause you
    to lose the pregnancy? (Category II)

13. Do you have any condition that could be made worse by getting
    pregnant? (Category IV)

14. Is there anything else we should know about? (Catchall question)

H.R. for:
1. Inad Prep
2. Adv Exp
3. Supp
4. Health
5. Rej Pr
6. Den O.R.
7. Prep Beh

patient. The administration of the instrument required between ten
and twelve minutes. The student recorded the exact words of the patient in response to each question and without interpretation.

The reliability of the instrument was tested by bringing a large
number of these patients back for intensive interviewing by examiners
who had not had an opportunity to see the Pregnancy Profile Questionnaire. The interviews were rated according to a similar scale by
independent judges, and the results obtained from the screening instrument and the intensive interviewing were compared by statistical

methods. The Pregnancy Profile Questionnaire has demonstrated a very high level of reliability in uncovering the kind of information which was desired for the study.

The Pregnancy Profile Questionnaires were rated daily for new patients by two project staff members. The presence of one high-risk response was deemed sufficient to categorize the pregnancy as "high risk" for developmental outcome in the child. "High risk" was specifically defined as related to the outcome of development in the child rather than to obstetric complications, maternal mental health, and so on. On the basis of these ratings (see Table 29–2), we have con-

TABLE 29-2

Summary of Distribution of Total Population [1]

	KEEPING BABY	NOT KEEPING BABY	UNDECIDED	TOTAL	PER CENT
High risk	633	94	46	773	57.8
Control	443	127	13	583	42.2
Total	1076	221	59	1356	100.0

[1] $N = 1,356$.

cluded that almost 58 per cent of women seen in the clinic should be viewed as high risk for the current pregnancy. As indicated in Table 29–3, almost half (48.7 per cent) of the high-risk responses are related to one of two categories: adverse previous experience in child bearing or child rearing, or deficient dependency supports.

TABLE 29-3

Distribution of High-Risk Responses by Category (by Per Cent)

CATEGORY	PER CENT
I. Inadequate preparation	10.2
II. Adverse previous experience	28.0
III. Support system	20.7
IV. Maternal health	8.2
V. Overt rejection of pregnancy	8.6
VI. Denial or overreaction	10.9
VII. Preparatory behavior	8.3
VIII. Catchall question	5.1
	100.0

Because of the obviously large number of women who could be categorized as high risk using this technique, it became necessary to learn something about how these stresses could be ranked in relation to each other in order to determine which stress factors might be most deleterious. This would permit us then to rank patients in terms of priority for intervention. For this purpose, we devised a modification of the technique of Holmes and Rahe (1967). Using our experience in the prenatal clinic, we devised two lists of life events of possible special significance for adjustment in pregnancy. The first list referred to events which might occur during the pregnancy itself, and the second to events during the developmental years and prior to pregnancy. In each list, one item was selected arbitrarily as an anchor point and given a numerical value of 500. For list 1, the anchor item was "being deserted by husband during pregnancy," and for list 2, the anchor item was "loss of mother before the age of twelve." Six widely varying groups of women were asked to rank the various life events in relation to the arbitrary anchor point. These groups consisted of the women's society of a Unitarian church, the women's board of a Roman Catholic hospital, the women's auxiliary of a chapter of the Junior Chamber of Commerce, the medical secretary's association located on the medical school campus, a class of nursing students in the diploma program of a Roman Catholic hospital, and a group of pregnant women receiving prenatal care in a university hospital obstetric clinic. The groups thus included represented a fairly wide range of religious background, socioeconomic status, age and pregnancy status.

The intergroup correlations for list 1 were all 0.69 or higher, half of them being above 0.85. There appears to be generally good agreement among these groups of women as to which life events occurring *during* pregnancy create the most and the least difficulty in adjustment. While some groups showed equally great agreement for list 2, there the median was 0.78 and one correlation was only 0.54. There would appear to be less agreement regarding the impact of *prepregnancy events,* as might be expected. Again, these patient-centered ratings indicated that the areas of greatest concern to women not only qualitatively but quantitatively during pregnancy have to do with adverse previous experience in child bearing or child rearing and perceptions of deficient dependency supports during the pregnancy. This aspect of the study has been reported in detail in another paper (Helper et al., 1968).

Since the endpoint of the study involves the use of child developmental criteria, we are continuing to apply the adaptive model to the mother and child by using developmental scales in order to ascertain the existence of significant differences between low- and high-risk populations. These will be described in subsequent publications.

The stress ratings which were performed by various groups of women described above would suggest that the screening technique and interviewing procedures are equally applicable to private-practice situations.

APPLICATION TO TRAINING

Three precepts have formed the keystone of our teaching in all disciplines. These are the following.

The Importance of Patient-Centered Perceptions

Professional judgments concerning either the presence or the degree of peril in a given situation are not trustworthy. The introduction of personal bias, the value system of a different socioeconomic status, or even the authoritative information of the physician is not an adequate substitute for the patient's assessment of the degree to which he may be called upon to make internal or environmental adjustments in the face of a given risk. We would not presume to make this judgment for a patient with angina pectoris or a fractured femur. Yet, in the most cavalier fashion, we often tell the patient that he has nothing to worry about in the face of extreme anxiety that is not assuaged by reassurance. Another way to state this precept which medical students have found useful is, "If you have authoritatively reassured the patient one or more times in relation to the presence of a given concern and the apprehension does not disappear, you may automatically assume that you really do not know what the question is."

The Importance of Developmental Outcome and Adaptation as a Basis for Judgment

In essence, this is the converse of the first precept. It holds that the pregnant woman is really in no position to make judgments about the effect of a given stress on her own adjustment or on the baby. The patient will often confuse pain with malfunction, discomfort with illness. Judgments about cardiac function are made by the physician even though the patient's statements concerning the nature of the pain and its location may be quite reliable. Particularly during pregnancy is it unwise for the mother to make judgments about her adaptive function or for the clinician to form premature ideas about this since pregnancy is a developmental crisis for most women—one which involves loosening of the ego-structure and the employment of defenses which she may not customarily use. The amount of healthy regression, introspection, and narcissistic investment which is typical during this period may confuse the beginner and cause him to see illness where it does not exist. It is much more important to base one's judgments concerning the effect of stress on the pregnant woman (and on the baby) on the manner in which they are achieving the developmental tasks of a given period. Mother and baby need to be viewed not only as individuals but as a tight interactional system in which response and counter-response may stimulate healthy growth or some adverse outcome.

The Role of "Prediction" as an Influence on Outcome

This involves the development of awareness that a human being who anticipates a given outcome while he is a part of an interactional system will often act in such a way that he forces, or at least prejudices, the interaction in the direction which he has predicted. Medical students and physicians seem to be aware that if they participate in research, the research must be designed in such a way that bias may not determine outcome. This principle has broad applications to child rearing. It tends to explain, at least in part, why parental perceptions of inadequate endowment in a child may indeed precede substandard performance in the child: that is, it may be a powerful influence in contributing those elements of parental behavior and response which are most likely to elicit substandard performance.

These three concepts, together with the clinical skills which express them in practice, must be mastered before really adequate diagnostic and preventive capacities develop in the trainee. If these are not built in, the trainee seems unable to elicit objective behavioral data on which judgments can be based or, worse yet, lacking the data, he will call into play his own spectrum of biases about pregnancy, "maternal instinct," child-rearing behavior and the nature-nurture controversy. Out of this spectrum, he will then construct some impression from which comes a "cook-book" prescription for the mother. For instance, a mother stated in response to the question "Has anything happened during this pregnancy which might hurt the baby or cause you to lose the pregnancy?" that she had been watching a lot of television lately, had seen several "horror programs," and was wondering whether, as a result of this, she might have a "deformed baby." The medical student was rather amused by this piece of mythology and re-assured the mother in a perfunctory way. Once having experienced this rejection, the mother did not spontaneously bring up the question again. On the next visit, when the student asked how she was feeling, she again expressed concern about the intactness of the fetus. At that, the student was at a loss to understand why she harbored such fear and had to be reminded about her previous statement. He seemed startled that she would cling to such fantasies, especially in the face of his authoritative dismissal of the subject. His scientific orientation to-ward genetics, defectology, and human growth left him with such alien feelings about the mother's fears that he could not enter into her support system. His subsequent ability to develop some real respect for her fear and his ability to get to her true concerns about her moth-ering capacity led to the disclosure that she watched a great deal of television because she was alone so much due to her husband's ab-sences from the home. She was estranged from her parents, felt un-supported and uncared for during the pregnancy, and had become very apprehensive not only about the outcome of the pregnancy itself but her ability to be attentive to the baby's needs. The violence and the macabre movies which she had been watching on television had served both as a trigger and a target for her anxiety.

Although our training programs have been for the most part infor-mal in nature, they have been goal-directed and have attempted to pay the most attention to those personnel whose professional educa-tion may not lead to high levels of psychological sophistication. In ad-dition to the heavy emphasis in the teaching on the three precepts dis-cussed above, we have expected all serious students, whatever their discipline, to learn as much as possible about the normal adaptive processes of pregnancy. Students are especially encouraged to read the work of Caplan (1960) and Bibring and her associates (1961) in this area.

All students are introduced to the theory and the application of the Pregnancy Profile Questionnaire, and its scoring is explained in detail. Students who have sufficient time to spend on interviewing are taught to do the semistructured prenatal interview (Table 29–1). Opportu-nity is provided for tape-recording interviews and for supervisory ses-sions during which material can be discussed and interpreted. Stu-dents are given the opportunity to weigh various stress factors and to decide on priorities of management. Types of intervention techniques are discussed, but most students are not able, because of relatively rapid changes in service assignments, to do much follow-through.

Special emphasis is placed in the assessment on uncovering and understanding attitudes and behavior in the mother (or the father) which, on the basis of our present knowledge, might contribute toward developmental delay and interference with perception or cognitive processes. For the more sophisticated student (and for the general and child psychiatric residents who have also taken part in these programs), there is a more conscious effort on the part of the staff to make understandable the intrapsychic mechanisms which may be operating in the maternal economy and which may make for interference in objective perception of the child's endowment.

For these more advanced trainees, an opportunity is provided to study the formation of the social bond between infant and mother and to learn something about how the mother begins to perceive the child as a discrete and separate object from all others and to assign a reality-based identity to it. Heavy emphasis is placed on the infant as a participant in this process.

Most trainees learn in a relatively brief period of time to identify what effect the stress may be having on the mother's capacity to invest herself in the formation of this primary tie.

APPLICATIONS TO TRAINING: SPECIFIC TRAINEE GROUPS

Most of the preceding has application to the various types of trainees with whom we have worked in the last four years. A few specific comments can be made about each group.

Medical Students

The medical-student program has been described above. More specifically, each new group of senior students were given a one-hour orientation period in their first morning in the clinic. They were instructed on how to introduce the Pregnancy Profile Questionnaire into the history-taking in a natural way. Usually this is done by inserting the questions at a point where the clinician is investigating the current course of the pregnancy and the mother's over-all health history. A member of the child psychiatry staff was physically present in the clinic each morning to meet with the students following completion of the questionnaires, to discuss questions, or, as time permitted, to stimulate discussion. Classes were not held, but rather students were engaged on an informal basis and were encouraged, in some instances, to discuss certain details of the questionnaire with the mother on her next visit. It was interesting to note that students wanted to introduce their own information into the questionnaires. For instance, if a mother had a history of cardiac disease during adolescence but yet responded to the question "Do you have any condition which might be made worse by being pregnant?" with a negative reply, some students could not let the matter go at this but would have to fill in the questionnaire with their own comments. Somehow, if the mother were not concerned, they would have to fight with the urge to make her so.

The questionnaire proved acceptable to almost all students. At this writing, it has been used by over 200 seniors. It appears to be much more acceptable than techniques which apply psychiatric terminology or explore intrapsychic pathology. We resisted the impulse to apply pre- and post-attitude testing to the students in order to attempt to learn more about the effects of this kind of experience. Perhaps this was related to the mistrust of the principal investigator that such attitude changes can really be measured over a six-week period. We nevertheless recognized the need for such objective measures and are attempting to design them.

Obstetric Residents

This has not been an easy group to teach. They seem extremely busy and forever plagued with emergencies, which makes it awkward to attain any kind of continuity in teaching. We have relied more on the osmotic method so far. Conferences with students, with child psychiatry fellows, and with pediatric residents are advertised as "open." Attendance by obstetric residents has been fair to good, but there is a constant expression of healthy caution not only about the validity of the concepts but the applicability to obstetric practice. We have attempted to counter these comments by demonstrating that the ideas involved are not "fancy or far fetched," that there *is* a reliable screening instrument which can be used, that cross-cultural testing indicates that the screening device is probably applicable in private practice, and that the practice of good medicine involves the application of any knowledge which will foster healthy development in the patient. There may be an inherent problem in this training area because most obstetricians are adult-oriented. Their concerns about the outcome of child development generally do not extend beyond the neonatal period.

Pediatric Residents

The original program planned for pediatric residents in this area was not very successful, although it had the strong support of the chairman of the department. The inherent error in the program was that it relied entirely too much on retrospective clinical data which the average pediatric resident was either not skillful enough or not motivated enough to elicit. We attempted to bring young children into a "child development clinic" where problems involving developmental lag or deviation could be concentrated on, apart from the ordinary pressures of pediatric hospital practice. The attempt to teach pediatric residents and students the same concepts which have been discussed above in this kind of setting simply did not have the same impact on the trainees. The pregnancy material seemed cold and distant to them, and they could not make a connection between it and the present status of the child except by a tortuous process of detailed, interactional interviewing. The child psychiatric fellows enjoyed this detective game and had the basic skills to pursue it, but trainees in other specialties did not. It was not until we introduced the training program to pediatrics within the obstetric hospital that it began to evince any degree of excitement in the residents.

Our current program for pediatric residents has its focus during the postnatal period. The emphasis is on learning how to do an initial contact interview with a mother on the obstetric ward, with special attention to the pregnancy experience and to the effect of this experience on her current capacities to form a primary tie to the infant. This is taught in the context of pediatric practice and the use of such information for predicting what areas of child rearing may be at risk for the mother and whether there are any forces operating currently which might tend to blunt her perceptions of the child's natural endowment. Within forty-eight hours postpartum, mothers are interviewed either by a staff member, a child psychiatry fellow, or a pediatric resident. A modification of the prenatal interview (Table 29–1) is used. If the child psychiatry supervisor can be present during the interview, it is discussed immediately thereafter. If he cannot be present, the interview is taped and played at a later time for discussion. The two special modifications which are made in the prenatal interview are: (1) Has the mother's perception of stress forces altered in any way since the termination of the pregnancy and her hospitalization? (2) To what degree can she describe her baby, its reactions, its appearance on a reality base? Can she discuss this in relation to her previous ideas and fantasies about the baby? Does she show the capacity to separate reality perceptions from fantasy?

Some effort is made to teach the pediatric resident how he can reinforce the mother's efforts to attend to the baby's responses and behavioral cues. The interactional system of mother and infant is explained again. The need of the mother to internalize an image of the child which is reality-based is underscored to the resident. Pediatric staff members are involved in this program as their time and interest permits. The chief of pediatrics within the obstetric hospital is an active and continuous participant in the program, however.

Nursing Students and Graduates

The group which seems most accepting and most quickly appreciative of these techniques, in this author's experience, is the nursing profession. The instruction of student nurses has been a more formal effort. Classes and seminars in the normal adaptive process of pregnancy, together with information concerning high-risk situations, have met with enthusiasm and excellent, perceptive questions. At the graduate level, we have conducted orientation programs for obstetric clinic nurses and nurses on the obstetric ward. Several psychiatric nurses working for their master's degrees have participated in the program on a more intensive level, and one has written her thesis on one aspect of it. It may very well be that the most powerful force for intervention during pregnancy and the neonatal period may lie with the nursing profession. Our experience has been that many learn to do the prenatal interviewing quickly and efficiently, and their judgments based on the data are accurate and objective for the most part.

Child Psychiatry Fellows

These trainees have participated in the program both as interviewers for the formal research project and as a part of their didactic-practicum experience in normal human development. All first-year child psychiatry fellows in our training program are required to spend one-half day for ten weeks in the prenatal clinic and four half-days in the neonatal nursery and obstetric ward interviewing randomly selected patients and recording a formulation of the assets and liabilities for subsequent child rearing. In fact, this is their first experience in the didactic program in child development and comes during the first few months of their training. Although the long-range effects of this experience cannot be measured at this point, we believe that it will have a lasting impact on their views about mental retardation and developmental problems in children during their entire careers.

A word about intervention is appropriate here. This chapter cannot focus on this subject as a main theme, but it should be emphasized that the "pitch" with nonpsychiatric personnel is that we are not looking for women with gross mental illness and we are not interested in teaching psychiatric treatment in a prenatal clinic. Rather, we would view the professional person as having an opportunity to counterbalance the variety of stresses which may be operating (both past and present) by entering into the system of dependency supports available to the pregnant woman. With the primagravida, his role may be an educative one in which some effort is made to compensate for deficient experience. With the woman who is terrified about having a deformed baby because of watching horror films, he needs to find his way through her displacements to her own concerns about her adequacy and capacity and assume a more supportive role. To the woman who is simply depleted and overburdened by excessive reality demands, as may often be true with the lower socioeconomic multiparous woman, he may need to call upon available community resources to assist her in coping. These functions are not mysterious. They can be taught and they can be learned fairly and quickly and effectively by students who begin to perceive their role in relation to the pregnant woman (and in relation to all patients) as one involving health promotion and the fostering of developmental progress rather than only the correction of disease.

CONCLUSIONS

It is too early to assess the final results of such training programs at this time. I am not certain that we know *how* to assess them in all parameters. Nevertheless, we feel that it is important to proceed with this kind of training *now* and have little doubt about its value over the long range. It is our conviction that it will reduce significantly the amount of developmental retardation seen in some children because it will permit the professional person to have entree into the mother-infant interaction at a time when intervention is easier and when it assumes an anticipatory instead of a corrective or rehabilitative form.

Research in this area must continue. We cannot optimally teach this kind of information and these skills without more hard data concerning the relationship between interference with pregnancy adaptation and adverse developmental outcome in the child. Certainly, within our own project, we anticipate several years of intensive efforts to follow the development of groups of children of high- and low-risk pregnancies. The ever mounting clinical demand for primary prevention services, however, make it mandatory that we introduce to medical and nursing personnel who have the most intimate and frequent contact with young pregnant women the kinds of insights described in this chapter. Certainly, we in the child psychiatric profession are at a point where we can no longer deal with the large numbers of children being brought to care in which careful history-taking reveals that development was sidetracked at a very early age for obscure or perhaps even indefinable reasons. The reasons need not be obscure and can be definable if care is anticipatory and data-gathering is prospective. Child psychiatry may make its most lasting impact on child health through its investment in the training of medical and paramedical personnel with these goals in mind.

SUMMARY

This chapter deals with a series of training efforts conducted largely on the obstetric services of two large university hospitals. The programs carried out under the aegis of academic sections in child psychiatry focused their attention primarily on nonpsychiatric personnel in obstetrics, pediatrics, and nursing. The particular focus of the training had to do with the assessment of pregnancy stress and its potential influence on maternal perceptions of the infant, maternal capacity to form a primary tie to the infant, and maternal attitudes which would influence expectation for normal growth and development. General and specific aspects of the training are described, together with some observations concerning interventive techniques. In conjunction with this, a parent research study involving pregnancy stress which led to the development of the training program is also described briefly. Possible implications for those professions dealing primarily with the syndrome of mental retardation are also discussed.

━━━━━━━

NOTE

1. This project was begun in 1964 at the University of Nebraska and continued until 1967. In 1968, it was renewed at the University of Pittsburgh (within Magee-Women's Hospital and the Pittsburgh Child Guidance Center) and has continued until the present. At the University of Nebraska, it was supported in part by United States Children's Bureau Grant No. 122–R074. At the University of Pittsburgh, it has been supported in part by funds of the Josephine S. Falk Research Pavillion of the Pittsburg Child Guidance Center.

REFERENCES

Beitenman, E. T., Cohen, R. L., Eaton, L. F., & Helper, M. M. Common concerns during pregnancy as expressed in a prenatal clinic. (In preparation.)

Bibring, G. et al. A study of the psychological processes in pregnancy and of the earliest mother-child relationship. *Psychoanal. Stud. Child*, 1961, *16*, 9–24.

Caplan, G. Emotional implications of pregnancy and influences on family relationships. In: H. C., Stuart & D. G. Prugh (Eds.), *The healthy child*. Cambridge: Harvard University Press, 1960.

Cohen, R. L. Some maladaptive syndromes of pregnancy and the puerperium. *Obstet. Gynecol.*, 1966, *27*, 562–569. (*a*)

————. Pregnancy stress and maternal perceptions of infant endowment. *J. Ment. Subnormal.*, 1966, *12*, 18–23. (*b*)

Cohen, R. L., Beitenman, E. T., Helper, M. M., & Eaton, L. F. The incidence of significant stress as perceived by pregnant women. (In preparation.)

Davids, A., & Devault, S. Maternal anxiety during pregnancy and childbirth abnormalities. *Psychosom. Med.*, 1962, *24*, 464–470.

Green, M., & Solnit, A. J. The vulnerable child syndrome. *Pediatrics*, 1964, *34*, 58–66.

Gunter, L. M. Psychopathology and stress in the life experience of mothers of premature infants. *Amer. J. Obstet. Gunecol.*, 1963, *86*, 333–340.

Hall, D. E., & Mohr, G. J. Prenatal attitudes of primipara: A contribution to the mental hygiene of pregnancy. *Mental Hygiene*, 1933, *17*, 226–234.

Helper, M. M., Cohen, R. L., Beitenman, E. T., & Eaton, L. F. Life events and acceptance of pregnancy. *J. Psychosom. Res.*, 1968, *12:*183.

Holmes, T., & Rahe, R. The social readjustment rating scale. *J. Psychosom. Res.*, 1967, *11*, 213–220.

Joffe, J. Genotype and prenatal and premating stress interact to affect adult behavior in rats. *Science*, 1965, *150*, 1844–1899.

Kasanin, J. & Handschin, S. Psychodynamic factors in illegitimacy. *Amer. J. Orthopsychiat.*, 1941, *11*, 66–84.

Lehrman, D. S. Interaction of hormonal and experimental influences on development of behavior. In: E. L. Bliss (Ed.), *Roots of behavior*. New York: Harper, 1962.

McDonald, R. L. The role of emotional factors in obstetric complications: A review. *Psychosom. Med.*, 1968, *30*, 222–237.

Rheingold, H. L. Maternal behavior in the dog. In: H. Rheingold (Ed.), *Maternal behavior in mammals*. New York: John Wiley & Sons, Inc., 1963.

Rose, J. A. *The source of belief in a child's ability for growth and development in feelings*. New York: Ross Laboratories, 1, *12*, 1960.

————. The prevention of mothering breakdown associated with physical abnormalities of the infant. In: G. Caplan (Ed.), *A prevention of mental disorders in children*. New York: Basic Books, 1961.

————. The factors affecting maternal adaptations in cases of blood group incompatibility between adult and offspring. *Act. Paedopsychiat.*, 1962, *29*, 211.

Schneirla, T. C., Rosenblatt, J. S., & Tobach, E. Maternal behavior in the cat. In: H. Rheingold (Ed.), *Maternal behavior in mammals*. New York: John Wiley & Sons, Inc., 1963.

Squier, R., & Dunbar, F. Emotional factors in the course of pregnancy. *Psychosom. Med.* 1946, *8*, 161–175.

: 30 :

The Training of Pediatricians and Psychiatrists in Mental Retardation

Leon Cytryn

INTRODUCTION

IN the beginning of the nineteenth century, all the pioneers in the field of mental retardation came from within the medical profession.[1] Trailblazers like Itard, Séguin, and Guggenheim provided the leadership in medical matters of diagnosis and treatment and laid the foundation for the educational and training endeavors as well. The end of the nineteenth and the early part of the twentieth century witnessed a gradual withdrawal of interest in the problem of mental retardation on the part of physicians. The early enthusiasm was replaced by a diagnostic and therapeutic nihilism. The isolation of the mentally retarded both from the community and from the mainstream of academic learning deterred most physicians from personal involvement.

A renewed medical interest in mental retardation began in the 1930's and has continued with increased vigor since the end of World War II. In Europe psychiatrists, pediatricians, and neurologists provide the leadership in research and in practical management in close collaboration with the fields of psychology and education. Most of the modern facilities in Europe for the mentally retarded that now serve as models for planners in this country are directed by physicians who usually come from the ranks of pediatrics and child psychiatry (President's Panel on Mental Retardation, 1962*a*).

In the United States we are witnessing a gradually increasing involvement in mental retardation on the part of the medical profession, which is being called on to assume leadership and responsibility in providing marginal help to the mentally retarded. The shortage of physicians well trained in the field of mental retardation has been well publicized in the last few years. The President's Panel on Mental Retardation (1962*b*), The American Medical Association (1965), The American Academy of Pediatrics, and The American Psychiatric Association (1964) have all clearly stated their interest in fostering the training of physicians in this long-neglected field. It is obvious that major inroads on the problem of mental retardation can only be made with the help of a great number of physicians with theoretical knowledge and practical experience in this field.

TRAINING OF MEDICAL STUDENTS

The training of medical students may be regarded as the most essential step in the process of the physician's education in mental retardation. The theoretical training should include human development, biochemistry, genetics, and emotional, educational, and social aspects of mental retardation. The students should also become acquainted with the problems of the community resources and planning, with emphasis on prevention. The practical training is best done during the pediatric clerkship in a diagnostic and treatment clinic or in a residential facility that provides opportunity for observation and participation in medical management, parent counseling, contact with the disciplines, such as psychology and social work, and some interaction with public agencies. In addition to this basic, mandatory program, selected students should be encouraged to explore the field of mental retardation in great depth through participation in research projects and prolonged clerkship in a clinical setting.

TRAINING OF PEDIATRIC RESIDENTS

The education of the future pediatrician may be the most important step toward meeting community needs. The pediatrician is usually the first one to be called upon to deal with the mentally retarded child and his family. His diagnostic skill, awareness of the child's emotional and educational needs, his understanding and support of the family, and his knowledge of available community resources may be of crucial importance in the fate of the child and his overall adjustment. At present most pediatric resident programs involve three years of training. The residents should be exposed to problems of mental retardation throughout this residency, but, of course, the degree and length of their involvement will vary at each stage of their training.

There are many approaches to this problem of training, each suited to the peculiar circumstances in a given setting. The merits of these various approaches have been recently discussed in a comprehensive review by Gardner (1968). The methods recommended in the following passages merely reflect the personal experience of the author, without any claim as to their superiority.

The central core of the training program should be a consultation service for the mentally retarded. This service may be headed by a pediatrician, psychiatrist, or a neurologist, but it must be clearly committed to the multidisciplinary approach to the complexities of mental retardation. Such a consultation service will be able to provide good service to the retarded in any part of the hospital rather than only in a specialized setting. In the past, progress in mental retardation was mainly hampered by its isolation from the mainstream of medical activity. The resulting ignorance of the problem on the part of otherwise competent physicians is a fact that we all deplore. We submit that the present trend toward excessive centralization may possibly make a center for mental retardation a "dumping ground," which could only perpetuate the isolation from the medical community.

Interest in mental retardation can only be secured by clinical involvement of physicians, and not even the most comprehensive theoretical preparation can substitute for it. Such clinical involvement is best provided by allowing the mentally retarded patient to remain a part of the general patient population in each department of the hospital, as needed. This would help to familiarize all members of the hospital staff, especially on the resident level, with practical problems of mental retardation.

The members of the mental retardation consultation clinic should concentrate chiefly on the supervision of the pediatric residents in the out-patient department, well-baby clinic, and on the hospital wards. The residents should maintain the chief responsibility for their retarded patients in the process of diagnosis and treatment and should be guided in their tasks by various team members. When consultation from the departments is requested, the resident should be encouraged whenever possible to participate personally in the consultative process. The members of the consulting team should also arrange periodic case conferences attended by the involved pediatric residents, by other members of the medical staff, as well as by the medical students.

The pediatric residents are expected to follow up personally on the active implementation of the recommendations at these case conferences, which would include parent counseling and interaction with community agencies. As the resident progresses in his training, he is allowed increasingly more independence in his handling of the patients and their families. The variety of cases encountered by the resident in his diagnostic work-ups should be supplemented by a study in-depth of selected representative cases. To this end the resident is encouraged to follow a few cases for at least one year and to serve the involved families as the "primary" physician.

In addition in the last year of his training it is important to introduce the resident to an institution for the mentally retarded in order to acquaint him with some aspects of residential placement and treatment. As a group, the pediatric residents often tend to emphasize the purely "medical" aspects of mental retardation (neurological, metabolic, genetic, and so on) and pay much less attention to the emotional and social problems. It is useful, therefore, to combine the residents' training in a residential setting with their rotation through the department of psychiatry (Cytryn and Milowe, 1966). This allows them to actively utilize their newly acquired knowledge about normal and abnormal human development. The observation of a child in a playroom should be followed by a detailed analysis of various aspects of his behavior, external appearance, and performances. The residents are also urged to become better observers of the parents' interaction with the children and more expert in eliciting the particular historical material which is most likely to be helpful in differential diagnosis. This sharpening of parent interviewing and counseling techniques is best done under the tutelage of an experienced social worker in regularly scheduled conferences. The teaching staff, on the other hand, can help to elucidate for the residents the children's group behavior in the classroom and their specific learning difficulties, as well as the methods frequently utilized to treat them.

TRAINING OF PSYCHIATRIC RESIDENTS

The predominantly psychodynamic orientation of psychiatry in the early part of our century was one of several factors responsible for the present dichotomy between psychiatry and mental retardation. The current major change in psychiatric thinking, which now stresses the interplay between biological, psychological, and cultural factors in the shaping of human personality, permits the reintegration of mental retardation into psychiatry. Psychiatry is now broadly seen as a science concerned with human behavior. This places the psychiatrist in the forefront of preventive and treatment efforts on behalf of the mentally retarded.

As with the pediatric residents, it is important to expose the psychiatric resident to mentally retarded patients throughout his training in addition to the provision of a more concentrated period in a residential facility. The success of this training program, as of those in the foregoing sections, will largely depend on the adequacy and availability of the training supervisors. In the diagnostic and treatment process with retarded patients the residents learn that the normal and deviant behavior of the majority of the mentally retarded shares many features with that of people with normal intellectual endowment. The problems are often similar, except for the timetable of their occurrence. It is important to stress the efficacy in the mildly retarded group of methods applied for the prevention of emotional difficulties in normal children. The detailed study of the mentally retarded will help increase the resident's knowledge of the reciprocal interaction of cognitive and affective factors in the process of learning, and of the biochemical and neurophysiological corollaries to the adaptation of the human organism to stress. The residents are sequentially guided towards differentiating between innate developmental forces and environmental influences.

The study of the theoretical and practical aspects of mental retardation will greatly benefit the psychiatric trainee by offering him the following: unique exercise in interpreting the predominantly nonverbal communication; an opportunity to study the evolution of personality defenses in their primitive forms, which is rarely seen in normal children and adults; and a full appreciation for dramatic interplay of organic and dynamic factors in human behavior. The strong feelings of countertransference, often provoked by working with mentally retarded patients, permits the trainee to identify and come to grips with the regressive forces within himself in the early stage of his career, thus increasing his general therapeutic effectiveness.

The psychiatrist's role as an interdisciplinary coordinator, currently emphasized in psychiatric training, seems especially applicable to the field of mental retardation. The residents should be made aware of the pivotal role of the psychiatrist in the prevention and treatment of mental retardation, as a consultant to other physicians, educators, and rehabilitation programs, and as a direct participant, when indicated, in the treatment, care, and rehabilitation of the retarded. This awareness may be fostered by assignments to other departments or social agencies, such as developmental clinics and mental retardation diagnostic centers, for a period of several months.

GENERAL TRAINING NEEDS

A prolonged rotation in a university-based or affiliated residential center for the mentally retarded was found very effective in increasing the resident's skill and interest in all phases of mental retardation. They may spend as little as one-half day a week, but this should be extended to at least a six month's period. This allows for a gradual absorption of the newly acquired knowledge and for the resolution of conflicts initially present in working with mentally retarded patients, their parents, and with nonmedical personnel. Finally it also allows residents to carry at least one institutionalized child in psychiatric treatment and to observe some definite changes, shifts, and improvement.

Because the moderately and severely retarded children in an institution differ greatly from the mildly retarded, the residents need special preparation for what they will encounter. Several didactic sessions about the nature of these differences may prevent bewilderment on the part of the residents. One may mention such features as low frustration tolerance, low anxiety threshold, autistic tendencies, fear of closeness, and difficulties in communication as distinguishing the more retarded individual. The resident will also learn about methods which are helpful in the general management of these patients. These methods encompass using a very cautious approach so as to avoid overwhelming the child, minimizing any anxiety producing situation, judiciously participating in the child's interpersonal activities (regardless of how bizarre they may be) in an effort to counteract withdrawal tendencies, and using psychotropic drugs, to mention just a few.

The residents also need the opportunity to observe the children in their natural surroundings, in the classroom and dining room, and during recreational activities. Differences in interviewing techniques are best demonstrated in joint interviews by the residents and their supervisor(s). Emphasis is placed on the great need for accurate observation of the nonverbal aspects of the child's behavior, which often offer important clues to the intactness of his central nervous system, the degree of his awareness of, and responsiveness to, people and inanimate objects, and the skill and goal-directness of his performance. The exploration of the emotional aspects should be complemented by a discussion of the organic-intrinsic factors in a given child. This is especially important in the training of the psychiatric residents whose training may overly stress primarily the psychodynamic aspects of behavior. Exposure to a great variety of retarded children with deficits in functioning gradually permits the residents to grasp the global concept of mental retardation and to put the emotional aspects of it in proper perspective. In the treatment process it is helpful for the resident, in addition to seeing his patient(s) on a daily basis, to meet periodically with the parents as well as with the other members of the staff directly involved in the care of the child. In addition, the residents are given experience in conducting diagnostic conferences with a variety of children, some of whom will later be presented at the regularly scheduled staff conferences. Thus an opportunity is afforded to see a wide range of psychiatric and developmental problems that are noted in the mentally retarded, to study some of these problems in considerable depth, and to learn to actively collaborate within the multidisciplinary format of professional activity.

The interdisciplinary staff conferences present certain hazards. There is often distrust on the part of the institutional staff, reinforced by the resident's sometimes indiscriminate use of psychoanalytic terminology, which is frequently alien to many institutional staff members. This necessitates at times active intervention on the part of the supervisor, including the "soft pedaling" of some psychoanalytic speculation, the active translation of psychoanalytic terms into everyday language, and tactful prevention of the monopolizing of the staff conferences by the new residents. The free exchange of ideas and information during these case conferences helps the resident to develop respect for the role of each respective professional group and leads to a recognition of the importance of interdisciplinary cooperation. Participation in selected and supervised parent interviews acquaints the resident with the whole range of problems inherent in dealing with parents of mentally retarded and leads to an attitude of compassion and tolerance toward the parents' seemingly perplexed and often irrational modes of coping with their chronically handicapped family member.

A practical exercise in community leadership may be provided by letting the resident conduct the staff conferences toward the end of his rotation period. This new role challenges the resident's ability to bring together the various disciplines, with their often conflicting points of view, into a smoothly operating unit. This should be supplemented by discussions of the social aspects of mental retardation, such as the quantity and quality of existing community resources, the role of the physician in educating the public, and lending active support to community efforts in this neglected field.

DIDACTIC PROGRAM NEEDS

There are many approaches to structuring and organizing a teaching program in mental retardation. Because of the multidimensional nature of the problem, one has to attempt to cover a variety of topics in basic and clinical medicine, sociology, psychology, and education—disciplines which may not necessarily be interrelated except for their relevance to mental retardation. The error commonly committed is to present the material in a disjointed and loose fashion which overwhelms the trainee and seldom leaves a lasting imprint. A more cohesive approach would be to group the topics according to their disciplines. Medical basic sciences, for instance, would include neuropathological, biochemical, and genetic aspects of mental retardation. General background information in mental retardation would include definition and classification, epidemiology, and history of the field. Medical clinical sciences should be given a broad coverage and would include a variety of diagnostic avenues: pediatric, neurological, and psychiatric dimensions of the various syndromes which produce the symptom of mental retardation. Clinical prevention should be divided into primary, secondary, and tertiary considerations according to accepted public health criteria, and will necessarily touch upon almost any medical specialty.

Psychiatric aspects should include the personality development of the mentally retarded child and adolescent, the prevention and treatment of emotional hazards, and the basic principles of parent counseling (Paine and Cytryn, 1965). Psychological evaluation may be conveniently added here. Community problems would encompass cultural deprivation, community resources, and modern trends in special education and institutional care for the retarded.

This didactic material is offered in the form of lectures or seminars and is preferably illustrated by clinical demonstrations. Because of its magnitude, it should be spaced over a period of several years rather than crammed into a short training period. The emphasis of each aspect of such didactic training programs in mental retardation must vary with the trainee's stage of training and primary interests. For example, the basic sciences will naturally be most appropriate to the medical students in their preclinical years, while during the clinical years the problems of diagnosis, prevention, and treatment must be stressed. The pediatric resident will naturally focus on the clinical medical problems and he has to be "sold" on the emotional and social aspects. The reverse is true of the psychiatric residents.

CONCLUSION

The foregoing discussion suggests general practical and theoretical lines of preparation for future pediatricians and psychiatrists in the field of mental retardation. The specific implementation of these broad principles of training will depend on several factors, such as availability of sufficient numbers of specialists with the interest and expertise in mental retardation. Another factor of overriding importance is the availability of university- or hospital-based diagnostic and treatment facilities, as well as an affiliated institution for the retarded. Regardless of the particular circumstances and orientation in a given medical school, the success of the training program will largely depend, in this author's opinion, on the presence of a coordinating team with a primary interest in mental retardation. Such a team will help to cut across specialty lines and above all will provide for the trainee a model for the comfortable integration of diverse pieces of knowledge and experience into a cohesive, multidisciplinary approach to the complex problems of mental retardation.

NOTE

1. Some of the material in this presentation was developed in collaboration with Reginald S. Lourie.

REFERENCES

American Medical Association. *Mental retardation—a handbook for the primary physician.* 1965.

American Psychiatric Association. *Career training in child psychiatry.* 1964.

Cytryn, L., & Milowe, I. D. Development of a training program in mental retardation for psychiatric and pediatric residents. *Ment. Retard.,* 1966, *4,* 5–10.

Gardner, G. Training and education of physicians in the field of mental retardation. *Clin. Proc. Child. Hosp.,* 1968, *24,* 1–14.

Paine, R. S., & Cytryn, L. Counseling parents of mentally retarded children. *Clin. Proc. Child. Hosp.,* 1965, *21,* 4–12.

President's Panel on Mental Retardation. *Report of the mission to Denmark and Sweden.* U.S. Department of Health, Education, and Welfare. Washington, D.C.: U.S. Government Printing Office, 1962. (*a*)

President's Panel on Mental Retardation. *National action of combat mental retardation.* Washington, D.C.: U.S. Government Printing Office, 1962. (*b*)

PART FIVE

======

Research Viewpoints

: 31 :

Facilitation of Psychiatric Research
in Mental Retardation

Wolf Wolfensberger

TENSION SYSTEMS BETWEEN RESEARCH
AND CLINICAL PRACTICE

I once called upon a mental retardation clinic in a psychiatric setting
to collaborate with a research project and asked to have parents of
the retarded children seen at that clinic sent down one floor to a research area so that a certain questionnaire could be administered to
them by research workers.[1] The clinic staff appeared to be quite
threatened by this research intrusion, and they cooperated only reluctantly and with much resistance. Soon the conviction spread among
clinic personnel that the research questionnaire had a very upsetting
effect upon the parents, and that the parents were very difficult to
work with after the researchers "got done" with them. Even transient
practicum students in the fields of social work and psychology who
did supervised work in the clinic were indoctrinated in this belief and,
expecting to see upset parents, they saw upset parents and attributed
this upset to the researchers' meddling. The researchers, on the other
hand, noticed that most parents came to them in an already highly agitated state, particularly after they had been subjected to several hours
of interviewing by several people, sometimes including psychiatric residents with a strong psychoanalytic orientation. When I mentioned this
observation to the clinic staff at one of their staff meetings, the response was one of perplexity, followed by tension release in the form
of embarrassed exhilarity. Apparently the clinicians had never considered this alternative interpretation of the situation.

It is a well-documented observation that in virtually every human
endeavor and in every age there has existed a state of tension between
forces of change and forces of continuity. This has been true of politics, industry, art, and many other fields. It is also true in human man-

663

agement areas. Human management is here defined as "entry by persons or agencies in sanctioned capacities into the lives of others, purportedly for the benefit of the latter or of some social system such as family, community, or society." Human management areas thus include, among others, education, correction, psychology, public relations, rehabilitation, social work, and psychiatry. Examples of agencies engaged primarily in human management services are schools, other educational and training facilities, jails and camps, social service and personnel agencies, residential facilities for the disordered or handicapped, and psychiatric clinics.

Despite the overwhelming reality of the transiency of human affairs, much of man's behavior is governed by human management and other social organizations that "bear the culture" (Fairweather, 1967), and that emphasize continuity and status quo. In contrast, one of the more change-oriented activities of man is research, much of which is designed to do something better, faster, cheaper, or more efficiently. And here, a key dilemma emerges. On the one hand, we all want to do things better, faster, cheaper, and more efficiently, and research is the means to accomplish this; but on the other hand, who wants to admit that he is currently doing things poorly, slowly, expensively, and inefficiently?

Thus, we see states of tension between administrators of social organizations and their subordinate practitioners, on the one hand, and forces of change such as social rebels, protestors, hippies, and researchers, on the other. This tension can be perceived, expressed, explained, rationalized, or denied in many ways. In this chapter, I first want to point out four areas of difficulties that contribute to or express this tension in human management agencies: the threat of change; the alien mode of the researcher's functioning; the clinician's perception of the researcher's personality; and the ambiguous role and status of the researcher. I will then discuss specific administrative implications that various decisions regarding research will have in such agencies.

The Threat of Change

A bureaucratic organization can be an efficient producer but tends to be a poor innovator (Thompson, 1965). We can see this principle in the operation of our bluest blue-chip industries, some of which make major adjustments only in response to great threats from without, rather than to the prodding of the more flexible and imaginative minds from within. Human management agencies, especially if engaged in a "helping" role, may see themselves so overrun by demands for "obviously necessary" services that they allow no time for the work that should underlie policy modification (Zweig and Antisdel, 1968). Industrial and helping organizations share one problem: they may develop high organizational control in order to maximize efficiency, but such control has been shown to be inimical to innovation and research utilization (for example, Miller, 1967; Rosner, 1968). Agencies or persons committed to a status quo or a very slow process of change will be threatened by anything or anyone overtly or covertly challenging "institutionalized" practices or thinking. "Operational programs are often highly entrenched activities based upon a large collection of inadequately tested assumptions and defended by staff and field personnel with strong vested interests in the continuation of the program as it is" (Suchman, 1967, p. 142). This description is not far off the mark in regard to many psychiatric practices involving mental retardation.

To the degree that research is, or is perceived to be, a challenge to prevailing practices and thought, it will evoke all those defensive maneuvers of which threatened humans are capable. The "amplitude" of such defensive behavior can be expected to be directly proportional to the degree of perceived threat.

Research is especially likely to be threatening when it performs an evaluative function, that is, when it attempts to evaluate the validity, quality, and effectiveness of ongoing practices (Fairweather, 1967; Rodman and Kolodny, 1964; Suchman, 1967). In industry, this could mean that the research department continually seeks ways to increase the efficiency of the production process, while the production department sees research and change as disruptive of the continuity of operations and as implying that current operations are inefficient. In human management agencies, an analogous situation may exist, and agency personnel, particularly "helping" oriented clinicians, often see research as disruptive or as casting disparagement on prevailing efforts.

To many clinicians, because of training or experience, research is so negatively affect-laden that they perceive it as threatening even when it is not evaluative or even applied. It is not surprising that such a perception is likely to result in distortions of reality. For instance, Rodman and Kolodny (1964) documented a case where social scientists entered a social service agency with the clearly, publicly, and repeatedly stated goal of exploring possible areas of research. Despite this very clear-cut definition, a large proportion of service staff indicated on a questionnaire that they perceived the researchers' role as being one of *evaluation*. Accentuating the threat potential of the researcher is the fact that researchers *can* evaluate practice and practitioners, while practitioners can only rarely evaluate research and researchers and have rarely been trained in the shaping of human management policy.

With so many occasions to feel threatened, it should not be surprising if many practitioners perceive an objective investigation as a hostile attack (Wilensky and Lebeaux, 1958) or develop a variety of defenses.

One line of defense is a dogmatic assertion that clients will object to recording and monitoring devices necessary for certain types of research. Mitchell and Mudd (1957), however, found that in one study clinicians in a counseling agency had projected their own uneasiness onto their clients who, it turned out, were quite willing to be monitored. The clinicians were also found to be wrong in predicting how clients would respond to various ways of being asked to serve as research subjects. Interestingly, as in other studies, the more advanced the clinician was professionally, the more resistant he was both in regard to research specifically and to change generally.

A powerful and time-honored line of defense is available to clinicians such as psychiatrists who are trained in observing human dynamics (Rodman and Kolodny, 1964). They can explain the researcher's behavior as expressions and projections of his own personality, which makes it easier to also dismiss his findings. This is a particularly effective technique when employed on clinically naive researchers who, in their turn, are likely to be profoundly threatened by psychodynamic interpretations of what they considered to be coldly objective and scientific research behavior. While dynamic interpretations of this nature may have occasional validity, Rodman and Kolodny point out that the clinicians involved are more likely to be trained to observe the functioning of persons than that of social organizations.

A third, more recent, line of defense is that research violates the rights of the subject. Whether or not it does, however, depends on many factors. This problem has been discussed elsewhere (Wolfensberger, 1967).

The Alien Mode of the Researcher's Functioning

Some practitioners have been trained in the methods of research, and some researchers are competent clinical practitioners. However, many practitioners and researchers live in worlds alien to each other (Luszki, 1957; Usdane, 1967) or lead professional lives that differ sharply in certain characteristics.

First of all, practitioners are sometimes unaware of even the most fundamental correlates of research operations.[2] For instance, I knew of one institution for the mentally retarded that was most eager to achieve a close relationship with a university and attract university researchers to conduct research at the institution. However, the superintendent was taken aback when it was pointed out to him that the record system of the institution was so inadequate that researchers did not care to make use of the available subject population. One researcher spent several days going through the records to identify likely subjects and then gave up in disgust because of lack of relevant information. Even though this particular institution had plenty of resources, there was too much inertia to affect a change in the record system.

To cite another experience, I once acted in a consulting role to a group of behavioral scientists at a university which was considering the establishment of a mental retardation research center. In discussing a large and long-range research program, the question arose whether the plans should include provision for a residential center to which retarded persons could be admitted in order to be included in certain research studies. The alternative was to rely on existing state institutions for research cooperation. To help decide this question, a nationwide survey of the research atmosphere of state institutions for the retarded was conducted (Wolfensberger and Committee for Behavioral Research and Training in Retardation, 1965). This survey disclosed that while the superintendents of such institutions were almost universally "for research," many of them lacked knowledge of the practical implications of such research, and some were unwilling to tolerate even the slightest inconveniences in support of research. A similar discontinuity between verbalized and real support for research in the same type of institution was noted by Tarjan (1965). Baumeister (1967), in another survey of state institutions for the retarded, found that superintendents placed very little weight on the research function of psychologists, even though psychologists are usually the most research-oriented and research-trained professionals in such institutions.

Secondly, many practitioners lack understanding of the researcher's way of going about his work. Practitioners tend to have a tightly organized schedule of meetings, interviews, and appointments, whereas even the hardest-working researcher may not have definite times at which specific things must be done. This may result in the practitioner viewing the researcher as a playboy or parasite, a perception obviously not conducive to good relationships. The problem is well illustrated in an example given by Rodman and Kolodny (1964, p. 174):

> Social worker: "I wonder when you would have time to get together with me?" Researcher: "Well I am free on Tuesday afternoon, or anytime Wednesday or Thursday would be okay." Social worker: "Boy, that's quite a schedule; you're really living the life of a lotus-eater!"

Thirdly, many human management practices are derived from theory, dogma, or mere tradition. If a human management practitioner began to question every management practice not anchored to adequate empirical evidence, he would probably be immobilized. Thus, a measure of dogmatism or indifference to empiricism is adaptive to the practitioner, and the skeptical and ever-questioning attitude which researchers have generally been trained to assume is likely to be irritating to the practitioner (Fairweather, 1967; Rodman and Kolodny, 1964).

Fourthly, clinicians may perceive their problems to be of such a nature or complexity as not to be reducible to a researchable form (Blenkner, 1950a, p. 57):

> There seems to be in some quarters an irrational belief that to crystallize one's concepts and hunches and test them in the crucible of scientific evidence is somehow to vitiate them, as though the magic would go out of one if he were to know what he is about.

The Clinician's Perception of the Researcher's Personality

To many practitioners, the researcher is an unfeeling, depersonalizing monster who cannot see the human being behind the statistic. The very fact that the researcher may focus upon groups of "subjects" rather than upon single "individuals" as the clinician does may lead the clinician to view the researcher as dehumanizing. Even when the researcher's subject matter is people, he may spend very little time in their presence: others may collect the data for him, and research planning, data processing, and reporting of results may require vastly more time than data collection. Even worse, the researcher may not only be remote from his subjects, but he may not even spend much time with other professionals or scientists.

The Ambiguous Role and Status
of the Researcher

The researcher in a service-oriented agency may have an ambiguous status and an ill-understood role. There are a number of reasons for this. I have already mentioned that the researcher's mode of functioning may be alien to the clinician. Many helping agencies do not have, and perhaps have never had, a research (or perhaps even evaluation) function carried on as part of the agency's official, sanctioned operation. In consequence, many practitioners lack clear concepts as to what the researcher's proper place, role, and status within their agency might be.

Probably as a result of the way helping agencies function, many clinicians see the work of agency members as falling into an administrator-practitioner dichotomy. To the clinician's perplexity, the researcher may not fit into either of these two categories. As a result, the clinician has no real role concept for the researcher, which adds to the clinician's ambivalence and uncertainty.

As Rodman and Kolodny (1964) point out, role and status definitions of the researcher can be affected by certain characteristics, almost of a demographic nature, which frequently distinguish research and service personnel. For instance, research workers are often younger than practitioners, and while they may have less clinical training and experience, they often have had more formal academic education. Such phenomena make for status inconsistency which, in turn, has been shown in numerous studies to be correlated with instabilities in relationships and functions.

Rodman and Kolodny (1964) also point out that role and status uncertainties will give research a marginal position in an agency. The marginality is underlined by the fact that research is considered a luxury item in most helping agencies and is the first function threatened when there is any kind of financial squeeze. Rodman and Kolodny illustrate how a researcher's marginality is often symbolized in the terms practitioners use in addressing the researcher or in referring to his activities. For example, practitioners may address the researcher good-humoredly as "doctor" or "professor," knowing full well that the researcher has neither patients nor pupils; the researcher may be said to "have his head in the clouds" or to "live in an ivory tower." All these analogies have overtones which suggest a marginality of functioning.

The common administrative practice of isolating and encapsulating the research function of a helping agency both contributes to the marginality of the research function and may also be a result of it. Furthermore, it is a successful device in preventing research from affecting the status quo (Thompson, 1965).

The researcher's inconsistent status and unclear role may lead him to feel isolated, without support, and unessential to the agency. As far as the structure of an organization is concerned, he is the "marginal man." Even when he tries to insure himself against the uncertainties of his position by demanding a relatively high salary, practitioners, even when aware of the uncertainty of the research position involved, resent it.

I want to draw on another personal experience that illustrates the lack of definition of the researcher's functioning in the minds of practitioners and administrators. Some years ago I assumed the position of Director of Research and Training in an institution for the retarded. I was amazed, indeed, bewildered, to discover that my perception of my role and of myself as a researcher-scientist was greatly at variance with the perceptions many members of the staff had of the role they thought I should play. Some members of the clinical staff had absolutely no idea whatever of the nature of research, the mode of functioning of the researcher, and the practical implications of research operations within an institution. At its extreme, this attitude was reflected in the surprise of some staff members that I needed a good deal of clerical help. Some staff members perceived the role of the researcher as being primarily that of a resource person to clinical staff, looking to him for help in identifying literature relevant to specific clinical problems. Interestingly, while I was asked to help with bibliographic material on clinical problems, I was not expected to interpret how research and frontier thinking might affect the actual clinical practices of the institution. Such interpretation was seen as trespassing upon the chain of communication of clinical operations.

Most significantly, some of my fellow professionals perceived the role of the researcher within this type of agency as being primarily that of a person who writes applications for federal grants and who thereby brings vast sums of money to the institution (see also Andrew, 1967 on this point). To these individuals, the nature and quality of an idea and its grant embodiment seemed to matter very little as long as it resulted in money.

I conclude this discussion of tensions between research and practice by quoting Rodman and Kolodny's (1964, p. 171) elegant understatement: "It is well known that problems arise when a social science researcher enters a clinical agency or some other professional setting."

ADMINISTRATIVE DECISIONS
ABOUT RESEARCH

I will not attempt to cover all sides and aspects of the research-practice interaction. A wealth of publications have appeared on this topic. Above, I have tried to describe some tension systems between research and practice. Below, I will discuss certain important items agency administrators (that is, the holders of administrative power) should consider in making decisions about supporting and using research within their agencies.

Most of us do what we do because we are told to; because it has been done that way by others around us or by those who went before us; or because we are driven to it by external events or by unconscious forces within us. Most people cannot state the real reasons for much of their behavior or cannot explain it in terms of broad principles and conceptualizations. To the degree that they fail to do so, they are slaves rather than masters of their behavior and cannot control or change, and therefore improve, their world.

I have come to believe that one of the most important things one can bring to one's functioning is awareness. In professional work, it is important to consciously and honestly define to oneself one's attitudes and orientations, one's beliefs, and the theoretical concepts and assumptions that underlie one's actions. This holds for the topic of this chapter.

Instead of being driven to repeat meaningless cliches, administrators of human management agencies such as psychiatric settings need to define their roles and interests, bring to awareness certain relevant attitudes and values, and make a number of key decisions about research after a cold-eyed look at the implications of these decisions and after weighing certain facts and alternatives.

These decisions will probably fall into three broad categories: whether to start or support intra-agency research; what kind of intra-agency research to support, if any, and how; whether to tolerate or support intra-agency research by extra-agency personnel.

I will now discuss the points that should be brought to full awareness if administrative decisions regarding research are to be made in an adaptive and successful fashion.

Considerations in the Decision to Start or Support Intra-Agency Research

I have discussed earlier the inherent nature of the tension between forces of continuity and forces of change. To the degree that administration is identified with continuity and the preservation of functioning of a human management agency, research and administration must, almost by their very nature and definition, be in a certain state of conflict and tension. Contrary to widespread belief, *there is absolutely nothing wrong about such tension if it is constantly kept in awareness, understood, and handled in a constructive fashion.*

It is here that our educational system has failed us. We have been taught that change took place in the past. We have been taught to use the products of these changes. We may even have been taught to be specialists in bringing about change. However, our educational system has not taught these things with great awareness or as a major objective; it has not taught us to be aware of and comfortable with the relentless process of change; and it has not prepared us for the pace of change required in this age. It has given us a poor conceptualization of the nature of change and failed to provide us with conscious strategies to deal with it as a process. This is true at all levels of education, from grade school through the doctorate and beyond. This is frightening when one considers that we are undergoing the most rapid and extensive changes in the history of mankind, and that the pace of this change apparently is still accelerating.

However, I predict that education for change will soon change, and that in the future one of the most significant trends in education generally will be a sensitization of students to the *process,* rather than the content, of change in man's knowledge and functioning.

To return, however, to the present and to our topic, the implication is that one of the most important tasks for the administrator is to explore his attitudes toward innovation in his own professional functioning. This, of course, does not mean that he should ask himself whether he is "for innovation," because he undoubtedly is, just like he is "for research." What is meant is whether he is *really* for innovation.

Likert and Lippitt (1953) identified conditions that must exist before people are ready to utilize the methods and findings of science. One of these ingredients is problem sensitivity; that is, there must be awareness of shortcomings and problems in prevailing practices. Another ingredient is an "image of potentiality," that is, a belief that there are better ways of doing things. These two conditions are probably complementary; if one truly wants to improve things, one should first perceive and admit the existence in one's field or agency of inadequacies, archaisms and anachronisms, lack of validity of theories and procedures, and inefficient, perhaps invalid, and even harmful practices.

The tension between administration and research could be greatly reduced if it were possible for administrators to adopt consciously a certain conceptualization of the nature of human practices. This is the concept that by definition, practices carried out by the mainstream of a particular field of endeavor are outdated. While we may not always know which of a number of trends at the frontiers of a field will become the mainstream practice of tomorrow, we do know that one or a number of them will. If one then truly embraces the realization that one's current practices are almost certain to be outdated already, and that they will have to change sooner or later anyway, then one's attitudes toward innovation are likely to be adaptive ones.[3]

The second most important question to be explored is the administrator's attitudes toward research generally, toward research in his field specifically, and toward specific types of research, whether in his field or out. If research or researchers bother the administrator, he should say so, at least to himself. This of course, may be difficult to do since belief "in research" has been sanctified to the point where it becomes virtually impossible for a person to publicly take the stand that he is against research. In fact, it is almost impossible for a professional to admit to himself privately that he is against research even when he really is because such a thought is so forbidden and unacceptable that it must be repressed. Alone or together, such unconscious attitudes and lack of understanding of research can result in the "yes-no phenomenon" (Fairweather, 1967): yes, the agency fullheartedly believes in the importance of research and is willing to do anything it can to further it; no, unfortunately there is neither money, space, time, or resources to make the specific project under discussion feasible at this time. Another way of putting it is "research, yes, but not here now."

In addition to his various attitudes toward research, the administrator should explore his beliefs about what research can and cannot do in his area and what problems, if any, he believes to be soluble by means of research. All of these self-examinations may help to determine whether there exists what Likert and Lippitt (1953) have identified as a third crucial precondition for the utilization of science: a general experimental attitude toward innovation.

The task of third-highest importance is to identify what problems the administrator can tolerate to see investigated. Slocum (1956; see also Andrew, 1967) points out that the staff of human management agencies usually subscribes to certain beliefs and practices which have become "sanctified" as far as a particular agency is concerned. Slocum calls these sanctified beliefs and practices "agency mores" and advises researchers to avoid them as topics for study. While such advice is prudent, I feel that agencies and their administrators should exert constant effort to identify and verbalize consciously what their agency mores are. The administrator can then decide more readily whether he and the staff can truly tolerate research that touches upon these mores. Chances are that they cannot, and it would then be adaptive to rule out, consciously, research that bears upon these mores.

Since research, by its very nature, is likely to introduce tension and conflict into a human management agency, the administrator should ask himself whether he and his agency can tolerate tension, controversy, and dissent. An administrator who is a strong repressor or leveler or who cannot tolerate conflict would be a fool to encourage research.

Relevant to all four points above is the administrator's readiness to deal with the ethos and personality of researchers. The creative researcher, like creative persons generally, is likely to be a divergent thinker and doer: ". . . the creative scientist is almost by definition, a nonconformist" (Marshak, 1966, p. 1523). The researcher may be divergent and nonconforming not only in regard to a specific research problem, but also in regard to his professional functioning generally, and even in regard to this entire life style. Only too often, administrators expect the researcher to be a divergent conformist or a nonconforming converger.[4]

A related problem arises from the fact that researchers strongly identify themselves with academia. Consequently, they expect to function in an atmosphere of academic tradition, whether they are employed by a university or not. ". . . Now the conditions of intellectual freedom are regarded as inalienable rights and are strongly sustained by the tradition of academic freedom, which is accepted without reservation by the leading American universities" (Marshak, 1966, p. 1523).

It follows from the above that to the degree to which the researcher is creative and free, he is more likely than the average agency professional to think the unthinkable, say the unsayable, and embrace the unembraceable.

When an administrator decides to support research, he should make a conscious commitment to the researcher. He should be prepared, in principle, to defend the researcher's right to be different. Again, an administrator who does not want to run the risk of having his agency associated with controversy, or who cannot tolerate conflict, would be wise not to establish a research operation.

"Good sound research . . . is expensive and . . . administrators, for the most part, have not been realistic in facing this or in helping agency boards to face it" (Blenkner, 1950*b,* p. 104). Professionals not trained in or experienced with research may lack all notion of the financial, time, manpower, equipment, and space demands of research in general; or they may lack an appreciation of the demands of a particular research project they would like to see done. Sometimes, even a researcher in one discipline will have distorted notions of the cost requirements of research in another discipline.

Research relevant to human management is frequently of a long-term nature. This calls for continuity of agency support. A change in agency policy during the last month of a five-year research project might destroy the value of the entire five years' work. One could make a strong argument that waste of research time is even more tragic than waste of practitioner time: competent researchers are probably much scarcer than competent clinicians; and while the work of practitioners is likely to increase for many years in utility, the most precious commodity of the researcher, namely, his originality and creativity, is believed to decline relatively early in his career: "And creative persons are by definition impatient persons. Time is their most important commodity" (Shakow, 1968, p. 92).

A phenomenon of more recent years has been the administrator who would like to develop a research operation but does not have, or does not want to spend, the money, and who therefore decides that the research operation should be developed entirely by means of federal grants. There have been many instances where such grants, perhaps even very large ones, were actually obtained under such conditions, sometimes with the help of consultants and part-time or short-term researchers (Andrew, 1967; Luszki, 1957). The history of such research is frequently sad: many such projects were never properly completed (the completion of a final report not withstanding); if completed, the research was typically poorly conducted; often, no publication (other than the project report) resulted from the research; and the agency may have enriched itself (with office equipment, and so on) from the grant, no matter how calamitous the project turned out to be. Considerable wrong-doing, falsehood, and deceit has surrounded projects of this nature. In many cases, agencies desired the prestige and other benefits of research without being willing or capable to "pay the price," that is, accept the implications of a research commitment.

Generally, a human management agency should not apply for extra-agency research funds until it has established a firm intra-agency research base, including financial continuity and administrative and research skills. Where cost-benefit considerations are paramount, federal granting agencies might do better to increase the support of established research operations than to fund research in agencies with part-time, itinerant, or nonexistent research bases.

In committing intra-agency research support, the administrator should be aware that while service support can be expected to show results, research may not "pay off." Even applied research, from which administrators may expect relevant pay-off, may lead to dead ends.

If development of intra-agency research is contemplated with intent to apply the findings to agency operations, then the size and organization of the agency must be considered. Glaser and Marks (1966) found largeness to be a deterrent to change and suggested that administrators may have to be prepared to reorganize their agencies so as to bring about increased internal differentiation if they want to see the findings of research leading to innovation. Other writers have shown how the degree of organizational control can affect the conduct and utilization of research (for example, Miller, 1967) and the process of innovation (for example, Rosner, 1968).

If serious about research and innovation, higher-level administrators must be prepared to dismiss, displace, or demote intermediate- and lower-level administrators who appear to be incapable either of carrying out research-related policies or of instituting the innovations suggested by research. How is an agency to be innovative if its leaders lack imagination, the capability of recognizing opportunities, and the enthusiasm to inspire creativity among the staff?

The Decision as to the Kind of Research to Support and How

It is quite possible that an examination of the above questions may reveal a favorable background for research within an agency, but that the administrator may fail to carry his consciousness-expanding one level further regarding the realities of the implications of implementation. He now needs to explore the following issues.

Likert and Lippitt (1953) indicate that even when agencies have decided to turn to research to solve their problems, this may not necessarily imply a broad acceptance of scientific methods and findings. For example, it is possible that the scientific knowledge the agency seeks already exists, but that from ignorance of the generality of principles, or from defensiveness, the agency may insist on conducting research within its own boundaries to validate the more general findings of science for its own operation. Likert and Lippitt call these attempts at treating each problem as an isolated research challenge "firefighting research." Specific problems are too numerous and their piecemeal solution is either too costly or outright impossible because the underlying conditions giving rise to specific problems have not been attacked. One more area in which the administrator's ability to act with awareness is of crucial importance is his readiness to recognize difficult-to-face ultimate causes of proximate effects.

What is to be the role definition of the researcher? A number of roles are conceivable and are played by persons who are identified, or identify themselves, as researchers. Such roles include: the researcher-scientist who is laboratory-oriented; the research-administrator who knows research but does little of it himself, and instead facilitates the research of others; the empire builder who pursues the development of a large and well-known operation; the grantsman who brings in the money and who is often also an empire builder; the resource person who knows a lot about a lot of things, who can identify names, studies, references, and so on, for agency staff, but who may not be productive in other output functions; the college professor or scientist-interpreter who is primarily a teacher and who advises the agency practitioners but does not necessarily do research himself (see Likert and Lippitt, 1953, for a definition of this role). (In certain settings, this person may also function as a master clinician who consults agency staff but does not render clinical services directly or for service's sake—the ideologue or thinker-innovator who does little formal research but who has the gift of expanding the frontiers of knowledge by theorizing, integrating, and so on, or by astute clinical observation. Freud and Montessori constitute examples of this type of "researcher".)

Obviously, some of these roles overlap, but rarely will one person be able to play several of them simultaneously and well. Each of these roles is legitimate, but the administrator should clearly define the rank order in which he values these roles and communicate these values to a researcher prior to employment. A mismatch between an administrator's role definition and the researcher's self-image and competencies can only lead to costly disappointment for both parties.

Another key decision on the implementation level is which discipline or focus of research to establish. In psychiatric settings dealing with mental retardation, research usually falls into one of few broad categories, some of the more common ones being medical sciences, sociobehavioral sciences, and administration. A helping agency embarking on research can rarely support a research effort in more than one broad area if at least one research team is to be of critical size, if the research is to be well-focused, and if senior investigators from different discipline groupings lack a strong urge to work on the same focus.

In deciding upon the area to be selected, administrators should ask themselves two questions: One question concerns the atmosphere and human management model that prevails in the agency. If this model is primarily a medical one, medical research is more likely to flourish than sociobehavioral research. If it is developmentally oriented, behavioral research is more appropriate. If concerned with the management of groups or organizations, a sociological focus may be optimal.

There is a very problematic question as to which aspect of mental retardation is most appropriate for psychiatric research. Here we run into fundamental questions about the identity and role of psychiatry which go far beyond the scope of this chapter. Psychiatry is one of a number of interrelated human management professions. In many human management settings, representatives from several different disciplines may engage in functions that overlap with, or are even identical to, those a psychiatrist might exercise. Table 31–1 lists some such areas of overlap in retardation.

TABLE 31–1

Areas of Overlap between Psychiatry and Other Disciplines in Mental Retardation

FUNCTIONS THAT MIGHT BE PERFORMED BY A TYPICAL PSYCHIATRIST	PROFESSIONALS WHO FREQUENTLY PERFORM THE SAME FUNCTION
The retarded person:	
Diagnosis of etiological syndromes	Pediatrician
Assessment of infant development	Pediatrician, pediatric neurologist
Assessment of intelligence	Psychologist
Assessment of personality	Psychologist
Pharmacological therapies	General practicioner, pediatrician, internist
The family of the retarded:	
Assessment of family functioning	Social worker, psychologist
Education	Nurse, social worker, psychologist
Counseling	Social worker, psychologist
Psychotherapy	Social worker, psychologist
Administration	Numerous disciplines

There is no reason why psychiatrists might not perform a research study that might also be performed by a nonpsychiatrist. However, it is very difficult to identify a specific activity in regard to mental retardation in which the psychiatrist possesses a unique skill. Thus, there is a problem as to the most appropriate research focus of psychiatry in mental retardation.

I propose that one of the potentially most unique as well as promising areas of psychiatric research relative to retardation is psychopharmacology. Here, the medical and the behavioral training of the psychiatrist potentially converge to an apex of competence least likely to be shared by other disciplines. I say "potentially," because sophisticated members of other medical specialties may be as skilled in this area as those psychiatrists who fail to hone and maintain their knowledge in it.

Formerly, psychoactive drugs were used mostly as medications and in order to treat conditions of disease. The area of psychopharmacology is gaining in importance as psychoactive drugs are being used increasingly for nonmedical purposes—not to correct what is defective but to enhance what is well, or at least to purportedly enhance what is purportedly well. It is no longer unreasonable to conjecture that drugs may some day improve normal intellectual functioning or development, or diminish subnormal functioning or development; this possibility makes the area of psychopharmacological research a particularly poignant one for a psychiatrist. (This issue and its research implications are discussed in more detail in Chapters 13 to 16 of this book.)

The second question that administrators should ask themselves is what kind of disciplines they are comfortable with. For example, the previously mentioned survey of the United States state institutions for the mentally retarded (Wolfensberger and Committee for Behavioral Research and Training in Retardation, 1965) disclosed that there are superintendents who hold intensely negative attitudes toward psychologists and behavioral research. Obviously, such a superintendent would not be comfortable with a behavioral research focus, nor would behavioral researchers be comfortable with him. The important thing is to be honest about one's attitudes; whether these be based on fact or not, or whether one believes them to be based on facts or not does not really matter. What does matter in making the decision is the nature of these attitudes, and an administrator is wise in not encouraging research in an area which calls for the substantial presence of members of a discipline toward whom he has negative or strongly conflicted attitudes.

A common error is made by indiscriminate idolization of interdisciplinary research. To be interdisciplinary is as sacred as to be "for research." The pitfalls and problems of interdisciplinary research have been discussed in the literature (for example, Bronfenbrenner and Devereux, 1952; Caudill and Roberts, 1951; Eaton, 1951; Fairweather, 1967; Luszki, 1957; Russell Sage Foundation, 1959, 1960; Simmons and Davis, 1957; Suchman, 1967; Wohl, 1955).[5] It has been stated repeatedly that such research, when it develops, almost always develops on the basis of chance relationships between researchers rather than by design, and that such teams are difficult to assemble but easy to disrupt (Greenberg, 1967). "Some of the more ardent zealots for such intellectual collaboration have indulged themselves so freely in the term that they have succeeded in exasperating much friendly feeling for the principle by their unquenchable, and seemingly ill-founded cheerfulness" (Wohl, 1955, p. 374). Wohl goes on to describe attempts at establishing interdisciplinary research ventures as having ". . . short, gay and expensive careers . . . ," and he sees such research as being ". . . a task for a self-elected few . . ." (*Ibid.,* p. 376).

Interdisciplinary research is to be distinguished from multidisciplinary research where several disciplines work *parallel* to each other in the same setting, rather than *with* each other on the same problem. Even multidisciplinary research has a halo, and some administrators make the mistake of thinly scattering their available resources across a wide range of disciplines, rather than supporting one or two disciplines in each depth. I know one multidisciplinary research center in mental retardation where there may be as many as fifteen doctoral-level researchers from about ten disciplines at the same time. Several of these researchers have had to engage in clerical and technical-level work or have had to pay typists out of their own pockets all because of the obsession of the administration of the agency with being multidisciplinary rather than with being productive. I suggest that prior to adding new disciplines to their senior research staff, administrators would do best to expand the clerical-technical support base of their productive researchers or monodisciplinary research teams until increases in support no longer result in proportionate increases in productivity. To paraphrase Swinburne:

> Spend support while you can
> On the productive man
> Not merely on
> The multidisciplinary one.

The orientation of the research must also be defined. There are three options: basic research, applied research, and a special type of applied research, namely, evaluative research. The administrator needs to bring to awareness what implications and obligations these options carry.

A commitment to basic research implies a hands-off attitude on the part of the administrator who must, in effect, buy the researcher rather than the research. In contrast, a focus upon applied research usually permits the administrator to define the researcher's task more sharply. However, if it is intended that research is to be applied to the agency's own operation, then a very definite implication arises in regard to the agency's personnel and employment practices in the service area. If the research is, indeed, to be useful to the agency, the service personnel will have to be oriented toward change, innovation, and the utilization of science. This principle is often ignored, which usually seems to result in waste and conflict that could have been avoided. An effective measure is to hire only science-oriented practitioners, or to define the agency-oriented nature of the research to prospective staff prior to employment and frequently thereafter. It is much easier to define agency policies from the first when prospective staff still have flexible expectancies, than to redefine it later after expectancies have solidified.

The decision to conduct evaluative research on human management practices carries with it, in most cases, a particularly high likelihood of generation of tension and conflict, and therefore implies a strong commitment to tolerate such tensions and conflict and to be oriented toward meaningful changes and innovations in agency operations. An administrator who cannot handle or afford conflict or who is not change-oriented is usually well-advised not to encourage evaluative research.

If the administrator is sincere in his intent to utilize the findings of agency-oriented applied or evaluative research, he will have to create certain conditions that maximize the likelihood that the research will, in fact, be used. These conditions include the following:

1. Likert and Lippitt (1953) observed that applied or evaluative research is almost impossible to carry out if the research team is administratively subordinate to the person who heads the operations to which the research applies. Some agencies handle this problem in an extreme way by encapsulating the research operation so much that it has little likelihood of having impacts and effects upon agency operations. Likert and Lippitt recommend the compromise of placing the

research team administratively under the man who heads the man who heads the operation to be researched or affected by the research.[6] Thus, the placement of the research function within the administrative structure of the agency should be done with a deliberate rationale which is consistent with one's intended use of the research.

2. The research operation must be defined as being prestigious. Instead of being subtly ridiculed or belittled, research and researchers should be lionized. The administration's support of the research project should be expressed frequently, overtly, and in terms of those symbols that have clear meaning within agencies. For example, within some agencies, the status of a staff member is measured by size and location of his office, the size of his desk, presence of curtains or carpets, or even whether he has a private toilet. No matter how ridiculous and nonfunctional these symbols may be, if they are real and important within an agency, then they should be manipulated consciously rather than haphazardly.

Aside from the importance of increasing receptivity for research by strengthening the researcher's image, a related consideration is of importance. In research-oriented settings such as universities, status and rewards are tied to research productivity where it exists. In human management agencies, however, research productivity or importance may not be recognized or valued because of its perceived lack of relevance to the agency (Connecticut State Department of Health, 1966, p. 188). Thus, while agency practitioners may be presented with many, perhaps daily, reinforcing events (for example, correct clinical predictions, successful case close-out, interesting human incidents, and so on), much research is of a nature that leaves the researcher starved for reinforcements. In fact, he may experience only a few significant reinforcements per year. A researcher may therefore leave or be tempted to pursue activities which detract from his research productivity but increase his reinforcements. On this account alone it is advisable to give thought to possible ways of increasing the strength and frequency of reinforcements for the researcher.

Status, rewards, and relevance of researchers can also be enhanced by appointing respected practitioners as research consultants (Usdane, 1967) and by establishing research conditions similar to those found in universities (Connecticut State Department of Health, 1966, p. 188; Marshak, 1966). Other relevant aspects of the reward system of science and its stabilizing effects on scientific careers are reviewed by Merton (1968).

3. Opportunities for two-way, face-to-face communication between researchers and those potentially affected by the research should be

facilitated (Glaser and Marks, 1966). This type of communication has been found to be more effective in research feedback than certain alternatives, such as written reports or one-way, face-to-face communication.

There is some sentiment that a helping agency engaged in research should engage in both basic and applied research (see Hart, 1965). I disagree with this blanket recommendation. Most senior investigators will, at least for years at a time, prefer to do one or the other, but not both types of research. Furthermore, not many good researchers are capable of directing both types of research effectively and simultaneously. This means that a balanced program may require two research teams or distinct efforts, which implies one of two things.

One implication is that there will be great temptation to spread available money over two research efforts, rather than to concentrate it on one. Such spreading is glamorous but, like many glamorous things, frequently sinful. It has been an obstacle to the development of hierarchical research teams of "critical size" which can attack long-standing problems in depth and perhaps solve them. In the medical sciences, the concept of hierarchically organized research teams has been well established and accepted, but administrators have had a hard time seeing the need for the same type of research organization in the sociobehavioral sciences. In consequence, a tremendous amount of behavioral manpower and training has been wasted on technical and even clerical tasks and has been dissipated on piece-meal projects. Ordinarily, skilled researchers should not have to do routine procedures that can be carried out by less-expensive personnel; they should not have to engage in clerical tasks; and they should not have to write what they could dictate more efficiently. I consider wider acceptance of the concept of the hierarchical research manpower structure one of the most critical problems in the sociobehavioral sciences.

The second implication is that more money is needed to support multiple research teams adequately. If such money can be obtained in legitimate ways and without diluting the research effort, then a balanced program is attractive.

4. Administrators must not only be prepared to permit divergent thinking, but to reward innovative ideas, whether these are actually accepted or not. The generation of innovative ideas must be encouraged at all levels of the organization, even from the consumers of helping services (Glaser and Marks, 1966). Here, helping agencies, especially in retardation, have lacked competition and have therefore been less sensitive to their customers than industry, business, or to some extent even private practitioners. For example, I know one re-

tardation clinic that conducted an extensive follow-up of its clients and solicited suggestions for improvement of its services. Several good and important suggestions were submitted. Because of inertia, not one of these was implemented.

There are other facilitating mechanisms that are more under the researcher's control than the administrator's. As such, they fall outside the purview of this chapter.

A cold reality to be faced on the implementation level of decision making is that the administrator cannot have everything. Alternatives must be weighed, some things must be sacrificed, and decisions and commitments must be made.

The Decision to Tolerate or Support
Intra-Agency Research by Extra-Agency Personnel

In this section I am not attempting to discuss the advantages and disadvantages of having agency or nonagency staff conduct research for an agency. This problem has been well explored by others, such as Likert and Lippitt (1953). My concern is still with the bringing to full awareness of important implications of various courses of action.

An agency that already has a well-established research operation may be capable of granting substantial support to extra-agency researchers without incurring major inconveniences. Important factors would probably be the degree to which the visiting researchers are engaged in the same type of research (that is, basic, applied, or evaluative) as the agency researchers, and the degree to which the agency has defined its focus of research. It is thus possible that research collaboration may not call for major decisions. Such major decisions are in order, however, if the agency lacks a well-established research operation of its own.

Many agencies that are not in a good situation to aspire to major research conduct could readily create those conditions which would encourage researchers from other agencies to come and utilize facilities, subjects, and data on a project-by-project basis as needed. This is not a glamorous role, but for many agencies it is a highly useful and realistic one.

If this view is accepted, what, then, can an agency do to become an attractive research resource? A number of measures are of importance.

1. The higher the quality of an agency's human management operation and the more up-to-date it is, the more attractive it becomes to

researchers. Quality of operations commands respect, and, if they can help it, researchers will avoid agencies they do not respect.

2. Certain types of agency operations are especially important to researchers. These include operations concerned with data collection and management. Thus, researchers will be interested in data descriptive of the consumers of the agency's services. Such data include demographic characteristics of the clients as can often be collected with little difficulty during the "intake" phase of the management process.

3. Even to have the services and the data is not enough. There also must exist a good system of recording and keeping these data so that they are accessible. Thus, a good record system is of major importance in research facilitation.

4. A visiting researcher is a guest. He may be ignorant of the functioning of the agency, unfamiliar with the agency personnel and personnel structure, and perhaps inconvenienced by commuting to the agency. In sum, when he shows up, he may be pretty helpless. He will appreciate being treated hospitably and being made to feel like a wanted staff member rather than a merely tolerated nuisance. He is likely to want to return for future projects if he meets with certain amenities, such as the following: administrative readiness to bear up with the inconvenience created by his research project; an orientation of staff and employees that is cooperative and courteous; invitations to speak to the staff formally; invitations to meet the staff socially; suitable and comfortable research space; parking space; janitor service in his research area; and cheerful assistance in gaining access to the agency's clients.

An agency that has some modest funds which it *could* expend on research may well make a greater contribution to research by investing this money in a record system and operations that will facilitate research, instead of conducting research itself. Also, an agency that definitely plans to develop a research operation in the future should ascertain that its operations and record system are adequate. Such an agency may be well advised to have a lead-in period of several years during which the groundwork in quality of operations and record-keeping can be laid with the help of consultants.

The comments in this section probably have their greatest relevance to residential services such as institutions for the retarded. Although the research potential of institutions has been extolled for over a hundred years, relatively little research has actually been performed by institution workers on institution residents, and few institutions have maintained research efforts of note over respectable periods of time (see the history of United States public institutions for the retarded by Wolfensberger, 1969a). Also, as documented previously (Baumeister, 1967; Wolfensberger and Committee for Behavioral Research and Training in Retardation, 1965), institutions generally do not have atmospheres conducive to behavioral research—or perhaps to research generally—which may explain their relatively low research output.

However, the convenience of performing research on captive populations has seduced many noninstitution researchers into conducting their studies on institution residents. Since institution residents are a highly select group, not representative of the retarded generally, this has resulted in many worthless or even misleading conclusions. For example, from 1890 until recently, there was widespread belief that the retarded were a menace to society and should be segregated in institutions. To a major extent, this belief grew from studies of highly select institutional populations. More recently, the extensive work by Zigler (see summaries, 1966a, 1966b) has demonstrated rather convincingly that significant behavioral attributes of institution residents that had been believed to be correlates of retardation were really correlates of institutional deprivation. The researcher here must be careful not to conclude that behavioral deprivation will only affect behavioral measures. Even biometric, biochemical, and similar aspects may be affected by selection patterns and by experiential deprivation. Thus, researchers are well advised not to use institution residents as research subjects unless aspects related to institutional factors are actually part of the study design, or unless the institutionalization variable has definitely been shown not to be a relevant dimension.

CONCLUSION

In the physical sciences and even in engineering, research will almost invariably precede change. In contrast, the most crucial human management decisions are made with little or no research backing; indeed, such decisions are often inconsistent with existing research findings. The reasons for this phenomenon are historical, political, emotional, and administrative. However, we are now awakening to the fact that as a society we must define priorities and choices, and that we must learn to control social changes rather than have them control and perhaps even destroy us. To control social change, we must modify our approach to human management research (Wolfensberger, 1969b).

In this chapter, I have attempted to describe certain systems of tension existing within human management agencies between the forces of change and those of continuity. Also, the practical longrange but often hidden implications of these tensions have been explored, especially as they bear upon the capability of psychiatric settings to facilitate or conduct research relevant to mental retardation.

———

NOTES

1. The writing of this paper, supported by United States Public Health Service Grant No. HD 00370 from the National Institute of Child Health and Human Development, is based on an address to superintendents of state institutions for the mentally retarded, convened by the Western Interstate Commission for Higher Education, Las Vegas, December 6–7, 1967. The author thanks *Rehabilitation Literature* for permission to reprint excerpts of an earlier and briefer version of this paper.

2. A most spectacular recent example of what can happen when a service-oriented agency embarks without adequate awareness and commitment upon research was documented by Boffey (1967). The report describes the conflict-ridden and almost tragicomedic entry of the American Medical Association into the field of research. Nobel laureate Sir John Eccles, one of the A.M.A. lab heads, was reported to have described A.M.A. personnel as follows: "With the best will in the world, those men cannot understand what is involved in setting up a scientific laboratory. . . ." "They don't understand what we prima donnas in science are like" (p. 1656). Numerous other examples of, or references to, conflict and failure of research or innovation in service-oriented agencies are found in the other bibliographic items cited.

3. There is a vast body of literature on change and innovation in social organizations: for example, Ogburn (1950) discusses cultural change generally, and Spalding (1958) discusses planned change in agencies and organizations; the issues surrounding decisions to base social action on research are well-covered by Wilkins (1965); Fairweather (1967) provides an excellent text, from the theoretical to the procedural level, on orderly experimental social innovation; and Suchman (1967) authored a guide on evaluative research on social and public action programs. Other relevant works include Aiken and Hage (1968), Argyris (1960), Burns and Stalker (1961), and O'Connell (1968).

4. In the aforementioned A.M.A. research debacle (Boffey, 1967), one source of consternation for A.M.A. personnel was the fact that researchers sometimes showed up in sandals and turtleneck sweaters, and that they wanted to work at odd hours.

5. A fascinating psychoanalytic interpretation of research, especially of the interdisciplinary type, is provided by Redlich and Brody (1955).

6. Unfortunately, this leaves the higher levels of administrative process of agencies relatively unresearched (Levinson and Gallagher, 1964).

REFERENCES

Aiken, M., & Hage, J. *The relationship between organizational factors and the acceptance of new rehabilitation programs in mental retardation.* (Project report, Department of Sociology, University of Wisconsin.) Madison, Wis.: University of Wisconsin, 1968. (Mimeographed.)

Andrew, G. Some observations on management problems in applied social research. *Amer. Sociol.,* 1967, *2*, 84–92.

Argyris, C. *Understanding organizational behavior.* Homewood, Ill.: Dorsey Press, 1960.

Baumeister, A. A. A survey of the role of psychologists in public institutions for the mentally retarded. *Ment. Retard.,* 1967, *5*(1), 2–5.

Blenkner, M. Obstacles to evaluative research in casework: Part I. *Soc. Casework,* 1950, *31,* 54–60. (*a*)

————. Obstacles to evaluative research in casework: Part II. *Soc. Casework,* 1950, *31,* 97–105. (*b*)

Boffey, P. M. A.M.A. research institute: Trouble on the road to "Utopia." *Science,* 1967, *158,* 1653–1658.

Bronfenbrenner, U., & Deveraux, E. C. Interdisciplinary planning for team research on constructive community behavior. *Hum. Relat.,* 1952, *5,* 187–203.

Burns, T., & Stalker, G. M. *The management of innovation.* London: Tavistock Publications, 1961.

Caudill, W., & Roberts, B. Pitfalls in the organization of interdisciplinary research. *Hum. Organ.,* 1951, *10,* 12–15.

Connecticut State Department of Health. *Miles to go: Report of the mental retardation planning project.* Hartford, Conn., 1966.

Eaton, J. W. Social processes of professional teamwork. *Amer. Sociol. Rev.,* 1951, *16,* 707–713.

Fairweather, G. W. *Methods for experimental social innovation.* New York: John Wiley & Sons, Inc., 1967.

Glaser, E. M., & Marks, J. B. Putting research to use. *Rehabil. Rec.,* 1966, 7(6), 6–10.

Greenberg, D. S. *The politics of pure science.* New York: New American Library, 1967.

Hart, E. (Ed.) *Role of the residential institution in mental retardation research.* New York: National Association for Retarded Children, 1965.

Levinson, D. J., & Gallagher, E. B. *Patienthood in the mental hospital.* Boston: Houghton Mifflin, 1964.

Likert, R., & Lippitt, R. The utilization of social science. In: L. Festinger & D. Katz (Eds.), *Research methods in the behavioral sciences.* New York: Dryden Press, 1953, pp. 581–646.

Luszki, M. B. Team research in social science: Major consequences of a growing trend. *Hum. Organ.,* 1957, *16,* 21–24.

Marshak, R. E. Basic research in the university and industrial laboratory. *Science,* 1966, *154,* 1521–1524.

Merton, R. K. The Matthew effect in science. *Science,* 1968, *159,* 56–63.

Miller, G. A. Professionals in bureaucracy: Alienation among industrial scientists and engineers. *Amer. Sociol. Rev.,* 1967, *32,* 755–768.

Mitchell, H. E., & Mudd, E. H. Anxieties associated with the conduct of research in a clinical setting. *Amer. J. Orthopsychiat.,* 1957, *27,* 310–323.

O'Connell, J. J. *Managing organizational innovation.* Homewood, Ill.: Irwin-Dorsey Press, 1968.

Ogburn, W. F. *Social change with respect to culture and original nature.* New York: The Viking Press, 1950.

Redlich, F. C., & Brody, E. B. Emotional problems of interdisciplinary research in psychiatry. *Psychiatry,* 1955, *18,* 233–239.

Rodman, H., & Kolodny, R. Organizational strains in the researcher-practitioner relationship. *Hum. Organ.,* 1964, *23,* 171–182.

Rosner, M. M. Administrative controls and innovation. *Behav. Sci.,* 1968, *13,* 36–43.

Russell Sage Foundation. *Annual report 1958–1959.* New York, 1959.

————. *Annual report 1959–1960.* New York, 1960.

Shakow, D. On the rewards (and, alas, frustrations) of public service. *Amer. Psychologist,* 1968, *23,* 87–96.

Simmons, O. G., & Davis, J. A. Interdisciplinary collaboration in mental illness research. *Amer. J. Sociol.,* 1957, *63,* 297–303.

Slocum, W. L. Sociological research for action agencies: Some guides and hazards. *Rural Sociol.,* 1956, *21,* 196–199.

Spalding, W. B. (Ed.) *The dynamics of planned change.* New York: Harcourt, Brace & World, Inc., 1958.

Suchman, E. A. *Evaluative research: Principles and practice in public service and social action programs.* New York: Russell Sage Foundation, 1967.

Tarjan, G. Facilitation of research through administration. In E. Hart (Ed.), *Role of the residential institution in mental retardation research.* New York: National Association for Retarded Children, 1965, pp. 28–38.

Thompson, V. A. Bureaucracy and innovation. *Admin. Sci. Quart.,* 1965, *10*(1), 1–20.

Usdane, W. M. Vocational rehabilitation research information: Problems and progress in dissemination and utilization. *Rehabil. Lit.,* 1967, *28,* 66–72; 94.

Wilensky, H. L., & Lebeaux, C. N. *Industrial society and social welfare.* New York: Russell Sage Foundation, 1958.

Wilkins, L. T. *Social deviance: Social policy, action, and research.* Englewood Cliffs, N.J.: Prentice-Hall, Inc., 1965.

Wohl, R. R. Some observations on the social organization of interdisciplinary social science research. *Soc. Forces,* 1955, *33,* 374–383.

Wolfensberger, W., & Committee for Behavioral Research and Training in Retardation. Administrative obstacles to behavioral research as perceived by administrators and research psychologist. *Ment. Retard.,* 1965, *3*(6), 7–12.

————. Ethical issues in research with human subjects. *Science,* 1967, *155,* 47–51.

————. The origin and nature of our institutional models. In: R. Kugel & W. Wolfensberger (Eds.), *Changing patterns in residential services for the mentally retarded.* Washington, D.C.: President's Committee on Mental Retardation, 1969, pp. 59–171. (*a*)

————. A new approach to decision-making in human management. In: R. Kugel & W. Wolfensberger (Eds.), *Changing patterns in residential services for the mentally retarded.* Washington, D.C.: President's Committee on Mental Retardation, 1969, pp. 367–381. (*b*)

Zigler, E. Mental retardation: Current issues and approaches. In: L. W. Hoffman & M. L. Hoffman (Eds.) *Review of Child Development Research,* Vol. 2. New York: Russell Sage Foundation, 1966, pp. 107–168. (*a*)

————. Research on personality structure in the retardate. In N. R. Ellis (Ed.), *International review of research in mental retardation,* Vol. 1. New York: Academic Press, 1966, pp. 77–108. (*b*)

Zweig, F. M., & Antisdel, A. E. Children, civil liberties, and community policy change. *Children,* 1968, *15,* 2–6.

: 32 :

The Research Challenge of Delineating Psychiatric Syndromes in Mental Retardation

Frank J. Menolascino

INTRODUCTION

AS has been amply illustrated in the preceding chapters of this book, psychiatric emphasis has changed from attempts at differentiation between emotional disturbance and mental retardation to active explorations of the interaction of both of these disorders and of how to intervene therapeutically in a positive fashion. In this chapter, I shall initially review our experiences with a clinical sample of 256 children who were both emotionally disturbed and mentally retarded,[1] review treatment dimensions therein, and then discuss some research challenges that confront the psychiatrist in his ongoing attempts to provide more effective services for emotionally disturbed mentally retarded children.

CLINICAL SAMPLE

In an effort to underscore some of the recurrent psychiatric research challenges in mental retardation, I will review some of my own clinical experiences in this area. Chess (see Chapter 2) has reviewed a similar group of emotionally disturbed mentally retarded children. The clinical sample to be presented in this chapter is thus intended to focus the reader's attention on the research issues to be discussed in the third part of this chapter.

Since 1958 there has been an active, multi-disciplinary mental retardation out-patient clinic at the University of Nebraska College of Medicine. Primary attention has been given to the evaluation of young children who had been suspected of manifesting symptoms of mental retardation by a variety of referral sources. From 1958 to mid-1966 a total of 1,025 young children were thoroughly evaluated (including individual psychiatric examinations). The presence and type of emotional disturbance in any given child was formally diagnosed during a case conference wherein the psychiatric examination findings were considered part of the overall clinical findings. A previous report on this clinic's activities reviewed our diagnostic methods, social-cultural population characteristics, and associated findings (Menolascino, 1965a).

The sample of 256 emotionally disturbed and mentally retarded youngsters (from the total group of 1,025 who had been evaluated) contained 153 boys and 103 girls. The age range was from 1.6 years to 14.2 years with the mean being 8.2 years for the boys and 7.8 years for the girls.

The frequency and types of emotional disturbances found in this sample[2] of children are presented in Table 32–1. The diagnosis of an emotional disturbance was based on an individual psychiatric examination of each child (Haworth and Menolascino, 1967), psychological evaluation, and family assessment, all within the total context of the remaining pediatric, neurological, and laboratory (including electroencephalography) findings on each child when discussed at case conference.

These 256 children presented a perplexing number of types of clinical findings. The group tested both the diagnostic acumen of our clinical team and the ability of the team members to communicate freely and interdigitate their respective clinical impressions and treatment recommendations.

The four most frequently noted behavioral reactions in this sample of emotionally disturbed mentally retarded children will be reviewed; treatment and management considerations will be stressed.

Chronic Brain Syndromes with Behavioral Psychotic Reactions (and Mental Retardation)

Descriptive and Management Aspects

The 177 children in these two categories (chronic brain syndrome with behavioral reaction, chronic brain syndrome with psychotic reaction) displayed similar types of emotional disturbances which were differentiated primarily on the basis of the degree of the emotional disturbance noted and the associated family interactional dynamics. The descriptive behavioral symptom clusters, noted in these two categories, have been recently discussed in much detail (Menolascino, 1968).

TABLE 32-1

Psychiatric Aspects: Emotionally Disturbed and Mentally Retarded Children

A.A.M.D. CATEGORY [1]	CBS [2] WITH BEHAVIORAL REACTIONS	CBS WITH PSYCHOTIC REACTIONS	FUNCTIONAL PSYCHOSES	PERSONALITY DISORDERS	ADJUSTMENT REACTION	PSYCHIATRIC DISORDER NFS
I. Infection	11	0	0	0	3	1
II. Intoxication	6	0	0	0	0	0
III. Trauma or physical agents	20	3	0	0	4	2
IV. Disorder of metabolism, growth, or nutrition	0	0	0	0	0	0
V. New growth	2	0	0	0	0	0
VI. Unknown prenatal influence	28	3	1	1	7	3
VII. Unknown or uncertain cause with structural reaction manifest	64	17	4	1	19	8
VIII. Unknown or uncertain cause with functional reaction manifest	3	20	3	2	25	1
Sub-Totals	134	43	8	4	58	15

(N = 256)   Total: 262 [3]

[1] The etiological classification and definition of mental retardation employed were those of the American Association on Mental Deficiency (1961).
[2] The psychiatric diagnostic entities are consistent with the nomenclature of the American Psychiatric Association (1952).
[3] The "mixed" clinical pictures (e.g., a child with a Chronic Brain Syndrome, with associated behavioral reaction and an adjustment reaction) resulted in more final diagnoses (262) than the number of children (256).

Management considerations initially demanded a treatment ledger sheet of these children's specific assets and deficits. This ledger was shared with the child's parents at the time of interpretation of our findings. Clarification of the parents' understanding of the child's multiple needs and their level of past expectation from him consistently led to mutual augmentation of treatment recommendations.

Functional Psychoses[3] and Mental Retardation

Descriptive and Management Aspects

The presence of a functional psychosis in a child who is functioning at a subnormal intellectual level has long been problematical as to etiological, diagnostic, and associated treatment considerations (see Part One–B of this book). The occurrence of schizophrenic reactions in children with Down's Syndrome (Menolascino, 1965*b*) clearly illustrates the development and presence of a functional psychosis in a child with distinct neuropathological determinants.[4]

The management approach to this group of children with primary mental retardation and an associated functional psychoses was accomplished in an in-patient setting. The global quality of the child's multiple deficits in ego functioning was further studied, and an attempt was made to conceptualize the ego functions that were particularly disturbed in each patient, in conjunction with the possible etiological factors. Once the pattern of ego disturbances had been delineated, it was time to plan specific treatment strategies and tactics (for example, support to intact ego functions, personal incorporation of therapist, testing of reality determinants in a sequential fashion, and so on) for improving the child's overall pattern of personality functioning. Since similar treatment approaches have been described in the literature (for example, Alpert, 1965), we shall only stress the corollary need for special educational dimensions in such comprehensive treatment approaches.

Adjustment Reactions of Childhood

Descriptive and Management Aspects

The thirty-nine children noted in this group were very complex from a diagnostic-descriptive viewpoint since all of them presented multi-dimensional problems in adaptation. The symptomatic clusters of obstinancy, enuresis, temper tantrums, disobedience, and masturbation were commonly noted against a background of much free-floating anxiety, cognitive developmental delays, mild language retardation, and frequently associated physical or special sensory handicaps. Further, the impact of each parent's emotional health status on their child, the effects of the interactional family factors, and situational crisis features were frequently noted. A frequent form of adverse child-parent interactional problem noted in this group occurred when chronic parental dissension (especially with rejection overtures) had produced anxiety and confusion in the child with subsequent feelings of massive insecurity. Thus, the parental psychopathology seemed most frequently to be based on two major factors: their reaction to their child's atypical or abnormal developmental attainments; and the communication patterns and personality characteristics of the parents themselves.

Management considerations in this group of children necessitated a modified psychotherapeutic technique for the child and his parents. These modifications had to be inserted because of the child's intellectual handicap, the frequent accompaniment of concretistic thinking, and associated limitations in how he actually perceived his interpersonal environment as to perceptual-psychological considerations. Family counseling was of major importance. Alterations in family attitudes (with encouragement toward more healthy, constructive, and consistent expectations for and from their child) and decrease in the anxiety levels in mother and father tended to provide sufficient support to allow the child to improve in his overall adjustment. Where there was major family psychopathology and poor motivation to involve themselves in collateral treatment, we have noted that enrollment in a therapeutic nursery school can at least provide the child with a partially corrective emotional-educational set of experiences.

Psychiatric Disturbances—Not Further Specified

Descriptive and Management Aspects

This group of eleven children displayed frequent periods of general irritability against a personality backdrop of passivity, inflexibility, and personality immaturity. All of this group of children were in the moderate range of mental retardation. These particular behavioral components seemed most closely associated with the child's delayed intellectual development and contained many of the personality characteristics of young mentally retarded children described by Webster (see Chapter 1 of this book).

This was our "wastebasket category" since the behavioral picture of these children was only mildly atypical for their given mental age and only minimally negative family interactional forces were noted. Here we noted the behavioral ingredients of possibly more structured psychiatric disturbances in the future. For example, they represented behavioral characteristics from which a future adjustment reaction of childhood might easily arise if the currently tenuous family interactional patterns became less cognizant or empathetic of the child's developmental handicaps and associated emotional needs.

Management considerations in this last group of children tended to hinge on adequate transmission of diagnostic findings to the parents and subsequent help in altering their previous expectations of and from the child. Since realignment of parental expectations from their child tended to lead to more realistic parental demands upon the child (in keeping with his developmental level), these treatment considerations have embodied the principles of secondary prevention in psychiatry (Caplan, 1964).

In summary, the foregoing brief overview of a rather large clinical sample of children who were both emotionally disturbed and mentally retarded stresses what the clinician usually observes in this area of endeavor. Yet the reader may note that the diagnostic system utilized in this clinical sample is different from that utilized by Chess in Chapter 2. Also, the treatment modalities utilized in this clinical sample do not embrace the wide range of treatment possibilities noted in Part Two of this volume.

I shall now explore some of the general and specific research dimensions that may have eventuated in these discrepant approaches to diagnosis and treatment in the psychiatric aspects of mental retardation.

SELECTED CLINICAL RESEARCH DIMENSIONS

General

As in other areas of medicine, diagnosis and treatment must be individualized in terms of the child, his presenting symptomatology, and the psycho-social family milieu. Concerning the psychiatric aspects of mental retardation, this medical maxim becomes clinically more difficult to apply because of the wide etiological umbrella of mental retardation, the frequently associated multiple handicaps, the rapidly changing psycho-social needs of the developing child, and the complexity of family interactional patterns. The experimental factors may also mask, modify, or exaggerate the underlying patho-physiological processes in some of these children. For example, the quality and quantity of early mothering, the parental handling of developmental crisis situations, the social-cultural factors, the family's initial and long range reaction and adjustment to their child's chronic disabilities, the effect of overt distortions of bodily appearance on the child's self-image, and the timing of the etiological insult in relation to the stage of physical growth and psychosexual adjustment—any or all of these factors may determine the child's future level of adjustment more than the intrinsic factors that are present. These considerations again caution one against singular hypotheses as to etiology and treatment.

Our team has come to refer to this group of children with distinct clinical indices of both mental retardation and emotional disorder as "mixed cases" since they do present signs and symptoms of multiple disorders. For example, in the children who manifested chronic brain syndromes with associated behavioral reactions, we frequently noted combined clinical findings of an underlying cerebral dysfunction process with associated physical, neurological, intellectual, and emotional symptoms. We view these particular complex disturbances as representing a chronic brain syndrome with associated adaptive emotional problems secondary to the underlying cerebral disorder or reactive to the interpersonal environment. These children have forcibly focused our attention on such problems as: reformulation of the behavioral aspects of a chronic brain syndrome in early childhood; the ever-widening spectrum of causative factors noted in the autistic reactions of childhood, and relative interpretations of the interactive role played by family psychopathology in both the evolution and maintenance of a given child's emotional problems.

It would appear that treatment approaches must address themselves first to the global nature of the child's personal-social interactional problems, and only secondarily focus on specific handicaps such as a seizure disorder, motor dysfunction, or speech and language delay. The types of emotional disturbances noted in our sample of retarded children are not unduly different from those reported in the nonretarded emotionally disturbed child population. Indeed, current models of psychiatric care are efficacious for these emotionally disturbed mentally retarded children if some of the previously noted treatment modifications are utilized. It is my opinion that the most important aspect of a successful treatment approach to these particular groups of children and their parents is the use of multiple treatment modalities such as supportive play therapy (with focus on nonverbal aspects), psychotropic medications, family counseling, aid in seeking community resources, and last, sequential follow-through visits to assure the continuity of needed services. Needless to say, this management approach is not new. However, I am continually impressed by the negative results of the frequent singular diagnostic treatment approaches to these children in the past. It appears that these children with chronic multiple handicaps and a propensity to emotional disorganization are too commonly treated in a symptom-to-symptom temporal time sequence, rather than with a total approach which focuses flexibly on the multi-level physical, emotional, educational, social, and family needs on a long-range basis.

Many of these behavioral disorders can be helped by widely differing treatment methods and approaches. This is not surprising when we consider that they are the outcome of a multi-factorial complex of forces which suggest that the equilibrium is likely to be positively altered by modifying any of a number of factors. Selective inattention to the multiple diagnostic-treatment challenges that these children commonly present can lead to faulty diagnosis and incomplete treatment. These considerations were particularly pertinent to our previously reviewed group of mentally retarded children with concomitant adjustment reactions of childhood, since this particular emotional disturbance is, by definition, a transitory disorder. The psychotherapeutic approach to these children differs from traditional approaches since the total picture is not self-limiting after treatment. The child remains with a chronic adaptive handicap (lower social-adaptive and intellectual ability) and parental treatment considerations have to include guidance as to the location of available special educational facilities and realistic future developmental expectations. The clinician must be fully appreciative of the mixed etiologies that are frequently present since mixed prognoses are also in order in these instances. We would like to underscore this point since in the past we had commonly had the treatment experience (and expectations) that psychotherapeutic procedures would result in the "evaporation" of the associated findings of mental retardation in these children.

Future clinical research in the evaluation and treatment of young children who display both emotional disturbance and mental retardation must attempt to elucidate further guidelines as to the types and modifications of personality development in these young children with multiple handicaps. We also need more basic information on possible impairments in their mechanisms for handling conflicts (for example, are they able to fantasize adequately? Are the psychosexual stages of early personality development also atypical because of the associated cognitive defects?, and so on). Such research may suggest that mental retardation imposes limitations for personality maturation above and beyond the emotional consequences of social nonacceptance.

In summary, the combination of possible intrinsic limitations that may blur attempts at valid descriptive diagnostic attempts, multiple nonspecific treatment approaches that are commonly utilized with this group of children, and specific treatment-management guidelines that are also necessary, highlights a conceptual research dilemma for the psychiatrist. This lack of distinct correlations between etiology, psychiatric diagnosis, and resultant treatment-management guidelines in the psychiatric aspects of mental retardation is a specific psychiatric research challenge to which we now turn.

Specific

A specific major research problem in the psychiatric aspects of mental retardation is suggested by the similarity of the treatment-management considerations that are currently utilized for both the children discussed in this chapter and in the population of emotionally disturbed, nonmentally retarded children. Such similarity suggests that our current diagnostic approaches may not be very specific for treatment implications. This diagnostic-treatment problem epitomizes one of the major conceptual problems that presents a real dilemma to the psychiatrist in mental retardation. This was previously noted in the brief discussion of the American Psychiatric Association nomenclatural problems involved in the etiological designation of an "organic brain syndrome (of unknown etiology) with associated psychotic reaction and mental retardation." More often than not, the psychiatrist in mental retardation must deal with descriptive diagnoses since etiological determinants are so often elusive. However, nomenclatural systems currently available (American Psychiatric Association [1968]; and the American Association on Mental Deficiency [1961]) literally demand classification by etiology, whereas treatment-management techniques are usually based on behavioral and social descriptive criteria. The problem here is a conflict between an etiological classification versus a clinical descriptive treatment orientation, and the associated currently unresolved question as to whether there are any truly significant relationships between them. Since I feel that this is a major stumbling block to future advances in this area of clinical endeavor, I would like to discuss this matter further and suggest a research strategy that may help clarify this problem.

Although any system of classification is arbitrary, there are three areas of classification systems that continually recur: etiology, description, and treatment prognosis. I will illustrate the problem of effective utilization of these three ingredients of classification systems by referring to the field of mental retardation. The application of descriptive criteria in the field of mental retardation has clarified *treatment-prognoses* rather clearly—without having to be unduly concerned with etiology. For example, the descriptive term "trainable retarded" describes specific intellectual and social-adaptive levels of functioning and specific guidelines for treatment (such as special education for the retarded) and prognosis (for example, limitations in adult expectations as to vocational abilities and social autonomy). However, when a mentally retarded child (of unknown etiology) is noted to also be emotionally disturbed, the previously noted focus on the descriptive aspect of classification is too often ignored in delineating what the current treatment needs and prognostic expectations encompass. Instead, undue focus is placed on the question, "Is he really emotionally disturbed or is he really mentally retarded?" Too often this "obsession" with etiology places undue focus on etiology, with resultant distortions of treatment and prognostic considerations.

Some examples of this recurring professional diagnostic posture in the psychiatric aspects of mental retardation follow. A school age mentally retarded child is referred from a special education class because of neurotic symptomatology; his mother also has prominent symptoms. The child and mother are engaged in psychotherapy and their mutual emotional status improves. However, the child is still observed to be functioning at a retarded level. Accordingly, the closing case diagnosis is "Mental retardation secondary to emotional disturbance." In this instance, undue focus on presumed etiology seemingly precludes the descriptive assessment of multiple or interacting disorders (mental retardation and emotional disturbance). A four-year-old boy is referred because of obstinacy and frequent temper tantrums; his parents are perplexed by his behavior and only minimally invested in his ongoing child care. Psychiatric examination reveals an adjustment reaction of childhood, general intellectual functioning in the mildly retarded range, a borderline abnormal electroencephalogram, and an isolated Babinski response. Psychotropic medications and anti-convulsant medications are prescribed; the case closing diagnosis is "Chronic brain syndrome with behavioral reaction," and the parents are counseled on how to manage their "brain damaged" son. Here etiological prejudgment has reduced a multiple disorder to a unitary disorder. Descriptive assessment would have suggested one, two (or more) diagnoses and a specifically tailored treatment regime which focused on varying prognoses for each of his disorders (for example, mental retardation [indeed psychotherapy may well have altered his

ability to utilize his native endowment], adjustment reaction of childhood, possible minimal cerebral dysfunction, family psychotherapy,
and so on). A quiet, withdrawn five-year-old-boy who has stereotyped
hand movements, no formal language, is accompanied by his anxious
mother for developmental assessment. His general uncooperativeness
precludes thorough assessment, and diagnostic focus shifts to his
overly anxious mother. His general clinical picture is termed "autism," and the presence of marked maternal psychopathology even-
tuates in an etiological diagnosis of "Early Infantile Autism" or
"childhood psychosis." Intensive inpatient treatment is recommended
for the child and individual psychotherapy for the mother. Here the
etiological implications lead to the unwarranted conceptual jump to
treatment-prognostic considerations without ample attention to the
descriptive range of diagnostic findings in the autistic reactions of
childhood.

Briefly, the classification ingredients of etiology, description, and
treatment-prognosis are not comparable or juxtaposable. Tizard (see
Chapter 28 of this book) has underscored this particular area of conceptual confusion as a major obstacle to further advances in the field
of child psychiatry. These considerations are of extreme importance
to the apparent lack of major differences in the specific treatment programs that we have utilized in our own currently reported sample of
emotionally disturbed mentally retarded children.

Similarly, the conceptual confusion embodied in the etiology-de-
scription, syndromic treatment-management paradox just reviewed ex-
tends to the clinical overlaps between mental retardation, "brain injury," emotional disturbance and sensory handicaps. The current
clinical descriptive-syndromic approaches to autism (see Menolascino
in Chapter 5) also exemplify this conceptual confusion. On the treatment side, the relative noncoexistence of relationships between treatment and etiology—descriptive syndromic dimensions is illustrated by
the widely divergent treatment approaches noted in Part Two of this
book (especially in the chapters by Lott and Gardner). Those considerations shed some light on the common clinical postures exemplified
by statements such as, "If the child is autistic, then psychoanalysis will
be of benefit to him," or conversely, "Psychoanalytic psychotherapy is
not of value in autistic children, therefore it will not help this autistic
child."

Rather than bring forth hollow research challenges, I would like to
describe an anterospective research project which would test some of
these etiological-descriptive-treatment quandaries. Figure 32–1 illustrates the general design of this particular research.

In brief, this research design could match on a three dimensional model, the elements of descriptive diagnostic aspects (with scaling of each symptom); suspected etiological determinants; and a variety of interventive treatment techniques. This research design would allow for the ongoing study of individual symptoms or syndromes, different presumed etiologies, and a number of the commonly utilized treatment and management approaches. For example, many of the descriptive-diagnostic symptoms of infantile autism reviewed in Part One—B of this book can be listed as "present," "absent," "irrelevant," or "uncertain" in regards to their presence in a given child. Similarly the presumed etiology (psychosocial, intrinsic, combined etiologies) can be listed for any given grouping of descriptive symptoms under study. The paradigm could be extended to a four-dimensional model, as noted in Figure 32–1, with focus on different etiological-descriptive-treatment dimensions. Finally, the foregoing dimensions can also be selectively studied as to their responses to a variety of treatment and management interventions such as child analysis techniques, family therapy, behavioral therapy, and so forth.

Such a three-dimensional research design can review objectively

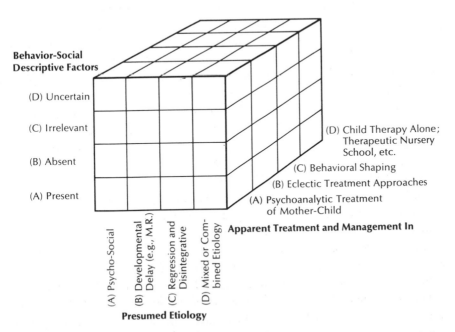

FIGURE 32–1 *A Suggested Research Approach to Infantile Autism* (*Homogeneous / Heterogeneous Populations*)

whether there are significant relationships between current etiological, descriptive-diagnostic, and treatment-prognostic approaches to infantile autism. Many current clinical views of this disorder may be clarified by using this suggested research approach. These conceptual re-examinations and possible clarifications may encompass the objective validation of some diagnostic models in the approach to childhood psychosis that stress primarily treatment accessibility and amendability (as in Anthony, 1958). If these current purported diagnostic-therapeutic relationships are correct, then perhaps we are unduly stressing irrelevant etiological dimensions. Some of the past treatment-prognostic models for infantile autism have essentially resulted in therapeutic impasses wherein the child's autistic features are resolved—yet the child remains at a primitive developmental stage (suggesting the dilemma previously noted by Dr. Creak: Were the autistic-psychotic features a secondary process? Or did the destructive inroads of a psychotic process forever disrupt future developmental potentials?). The two horns of this dilemma can be further illustrated by the report of Alpert (1957) concerning the end result of developmentally arrested (but no longer psychotic!) former psychotic children following extensive psychoanalytical child therapy, versus the rather remarkable treatment results from reinforcement therapy (for example, Lovaas, 1966) wherein similar children have apparently experienced both a remission of their overt psychotic features and developmental progression. Accordingly, these considerations strongly suggest that some of the methods of treatment, in the three-dimensional research paradigm, may possibly be shown to outweigh etiological and descriptive diagnostic indices. Finally, the revaluations of our current professional postures in this perplexing area may challenge all of us to utilize more rigid research methodology rather than the impressionistic postures that our own selective experiences and professional observations so forcibly impose upon us.

This research design would allow for ongoing study of individual symptoms and syndromes, different presumed etiologies, and a number of the commonly utilized treatment and management approaches. Indeed, this research approach to the diagnosis and treatment of emotional disturbance in the mentally retarded may well call for a basic re-examination of both the current models of treatment, and the orientation of those who can most effectively provide such treatment services. As noted in other chapters of this book, many of these challenges for wider utilization of psychiatric principles concerning personality functioning and child care in the field of mental retardation are currently being explored.

SUMMARY

In summary, the foregoing considerations imply that psychiatric disorders in young mentally retarded children are relatively frequent occurrences and may differ qualitatively from what is noted in non-mentally retarded children. I would underscore the urgent need to evolve more specific methods of treatment for these large groups of chronically handicapped young children. The psychiatric clinical research approach to treatment and management aspects of emotional disturbances in mentally retarded children has been largely neglected. Yet it is apparent that the need for such clinical research does not vanish as the IQ drops below 70. The increasing realization that the mentally retarded child has a personality as well as an intelligence quotient is likely to be accompanied by further positive clinical research developments in this area of professional endeavor.

NOTES

1. This investigation was supported by Public Health Service Research Grants MH–08767 from the National Institute of Mental Health and HD–00370 from the National Institute of Child Health and Human Development.

2. All of the children in this study were noted (on full multi-disciplinary team initial evaluations and follow-up evaluations) to be mentally retarded. Accordingly, not included in this sample are the children who had primary emotional disturbances presented with the "facade" of mental retardation (Menolascino, 1966*b*).

3. Children from our total sample who had indices of a primary childhood psychosis are not included in this chapter. We have discussed the diagnostic and treatment-prognosis dimensions of our experiences with such children elsewhere (Eaton & Menolascino, 1967).

4. The writer is aware of the contradictions and problems inherent in the concurrent utilization of the American Psychiatric Association (1968) and American Association on Mental Deficiency (1961) nomenclatural systems in the assignment of patients in this particular diagnostic category. Admittedly, the children listed in the bottom horizontal column of Table 31–1 frequently display no clear-cut physical or neurological signs of an organic brain syndrome in childhood (Ingram, 1963) and at times this becomes a rather arbitrary clinical categorization. In our sample, the impressions of a chronic brain syndrome were gleaned from the retrospective review of the personal and clinical histories, the findings by other members of the multi-disciplinary team, and our past experiences in following up similar sub-samples of such children. These diagnostic difficulties are compounded when one concurrently utilizes the A.A.M.D. nomenclatural system (A.A.M.D., 1961, p. 39), since Category VIII stresses ". . . due to uncertain (or presumed psychologic) causes with the functional reaction alone manifest." The clinician is cautioned, "No case is to be classified in this division except after exhaustive medical evaluation." However, if such

precautions are taken, and the child is noted to be mentally retarded with the above noted clinical-historical indices but of "uncertain cause" with a superimposed emotional disturbance—then what? Lastly, it has been our most consistent experience that young children who display mental retardation due to presumed psychological cause (for example, the facade of mental retardation (Menolascino, 1966b) present quite different initial diagnostic findings and follow-up (post-treatment) results.

This diagnostic issue becomes even more difficult when dealing with a child who had indices of mental retardation which "exhaustive medical examination suggests is of uncertain cause (as to etiology) and has a superimposed functional psychosis (for example, propf-schizophrenia). Creak (1963) splendidly reviews this diagnostic quandry—replete with eight cases which underwent post-mortem study. Though such post-mortem findings (and the associated general impression that A.A.M.D. Category VII "should" have been utilized) are helpful after-the-fact guidelines, they hardly comfort the clinician in the current clinical encounter. These diagnostic issues suggest the need for further refinement in both the clinical-diagnostic and etiological nomenclatural approaches to this topic. A suggested research paradigm that may further illuminate these issues is elaborated upon in the section on specific Selected Clinical Research Dimensions of this chapter.

REFERENCES

Alpert, A. A special therapeutic technique for certain developmental disorders in pre-latency children. *Amer. J. Orthopsychiat.*, 1957, *27, 256—270.*

———. Institue on programs for children without families: Introductory remarks. *J. Amer. Acad. Child Psychiat.*, 1965, *4,* 163–167. (a)

———. Children without families: Comments. *J. Amer. Acad. Child Psychiat.*, 1965, *4,* 272–278. (b)

American Association on Mental Deficiency. *Standard nomenclature of diseases and operations* (5th Ed.), E. T. Thompson (Ed.). New York: Blakiston Division, McGraw, 1961.

American Psychiatric Association. American Psychiatric Association: Diagnostic and Statistical Manual of Mental Disorders (2nd Ed.). Washington, D.C.: A.P.A., 1968.

Anthony, J. An experimental approach to the psychopathology of childhood autism. *Brit. J. Med. Psychol.*, 1958, *31*, 211–225.

Caplan, G. Principles of preventative psychiatry. New York: Basic Books, 1964, pp. 89–112.

Chess, S. Treatment of the emotional problems of the retarded child and his family. In W. A. Fraenker (Ed.), *First Brooklyn Medical Conference on Mental Retardation.* New York: Assoc. for the Help of Retarded Children, 1966, pp. 25–36.

Creak, E. M. Schizophrenia in early childhood. *Acta Paedopsychiat.* (Basel), 1963, *30,* 42–47.

Eaton, L., & Menolascino, F. J. Psychotic reactions of childhood: Experiences of a mental retardation clinic: Follow-up study. *Amer. J. Orthopsychiat.*, 1967, *37,* 521–529.

Haworth, M., & Menolascino, F. J. Video-tape observations of disturbed young children. *J. Clin. Psychol.*, 1967, *23,* 135–140.

Heber, R. A manual on terminology and classification in mental retardation. *Amer. J. Ment. Defic.*, Monogr. Suppl., 1954, *64.*

Ingram, T. Chronic brain syndromes in childhood other than cerebral palsy, epilepsy, and mental defect. In R. MacKeith and M. Bos (eds.), *Minimal cerebral dysfunction.* London: Heinemann Med. Books, Ltd., 1963, pp. 10–17.

Lanzkron, J. The concept of propf-schizophrenia and its prognosis. *Amer. J. Ment. Defic.*, 1957, *61,* 544–547.

Lovaas, O. T., Berberich. J. P. & Perloff, B. F. Acquisition of imitative speech by schizophrenic children. *Science,* 1966, *151,* 705–707.

Menolascino, F. J. Emotional disturbance and mental retardation. *Amer. J. Ment. Defic.,* 1965, *70,* 248–256. (a)

―――. Psychiatric aspects of mongolism. *Amer. J. Ment. Defic.*, 1965, *69*, 653–660. (*b*)

―――. Autistic reactions in early childhood: Differential diagnostic considerations. *J. Child Psychol. & Psychiat.*, 1966, *6*, 203–218. (*a*)

―――. The facade of mental retardation: Its challenge to child psychiatry. *Amer. J. Psychiat.*, 1966, *122*, 1227–1235. (*b*)

―――. Mental retardation and comprehensive training in psychiatry. *Amer. J. Psychiat.*, 1967, *124*, 459–466.

―――. Emotional disturbances in mentally retarded children: Diagnostic and treatment aspects. *Arch. Gen. Psychiat.*, 1968, *19*, 455–464.

Rank, B. Adaptation of the psychoanalytic technique for the treatment of young children with atypical development. *Amer. J. Orthopsychiat.*, 1949, *19*, 130–139.

PART SIX

A Perspective

Psychiatry's Past, Current and Future Role in Mental Retardation

Frank J. Menolascino

FOR the past decade or so, enlightened citizens, government officials, and professional groups throughout the nation have come to recognize the need for a substantial improvement in services for the mentally retarded and their families. Although mental retardation should be a concern for all health professions, it presents a variety of problems that invite the special participation of modern social psychiatry for their resolution.

Initially, this chapter will review some historical data recalling the central position which nineteenth-century psychiatry occupied in the initiation and development of systems of care, training, and education of the mentally retarded. Following this review of the evolution of psychiatric involvement with and attitudes toward the mentally retarded, I shall focus on some current perspectives and then discuss possible future guidelines for promoting psychiatry's renaissance in mental retardation.

THE EVOLUTION OF PSYCHIATRY'S PARTICIPATION IN MENTAL RETARDATION[1]

Perspective on the Past

The Remote Past

Prior to the modern age one can hardly speak of the history of psychiatry in mental retardation since the early history of mental retardation is shared by all professions. Readers who are particularly interested in the early historical aspects will find much relevant material in Cranefield (1966), Kanner (1964), and Zilboorg and Henry (1941). Although mental retardation or any identifiable description of it does not appear in the medical writings of antiquity, it is highly probable that the occasional severely retarded individual who survived beyond infancy in those times was thought to have some form of mental illness. Except for Hippocrates and a few of his contemporaries, the physicians of antiquity and of the first seventeen or eighteen centuries of the Christian era had but little or no interest in mental illness and the forms in which it occurred. The nature of the mind was considered to be the province of philosophers, and the care and cure of "madmen" was delegated to the Church and its bishops and priests. On the one hand, the Church inspired some very benevolent approaches to the retarded such as refuges, alms houses, and so forth. For instance, in Geel, Belgium, the entire town was a religiously motivated, sheltered community setting for the mentally handicapped. Yet, during the Middle Ages, the other extreme of service to the retarded has also been recorded. Thus, the retarded were often used as objects of ridicule such as court fools and jesters, and they were occasionally viewed as "possessed" and subjected to exorcism and torture.

Medicine had to wait hundreds of years, almost until the latter part of the eighteenth century, before it could involve itself with mental illness without being looked upon as an intruder by philosophers and theologians. Even near the end of the eighteenth century, Immanuel Kant violently opposed any move to involve medicine in the nature of psychopathology. The retarded apparently shared with the mentally ill the onus of being regarded as social outcasts, and they were indiscriminately segregated along with criminals and other social misfits. While a number of often perceptive observations about the retarded were made during the Middle Ages and the Enlightenment, these did not generate significant or generalized interest in mental retardation, nor concern about the retardate and his needs as a human being. These matters lay dormant for another 125 years.

The first modern reference to mental retardation as such appeared in medical writings of the early years of the seventeenth century when Paracelsus described "Cretinous Idiocy" and its frequency in the Alps (1616). This was some 2,000 years after Hippocrates had tried to dispel that belief that madness—and retardation—was a mysterious manifestation of some supernatural phenomenon, such as demonological possession.

An Enlightened Awakening

At the dawn of the nineteenth century, Jean-Marc Gaspard Itard (1801), a pupil of the famous Parisian psychiatrist Philippe Pinel, published a report on his five-year project of "educating the mind" of Victor, known as the "Wild Boy of Aveyron." Victor was, in all probability, a severely retarded child who had been abandoned by his family. Itard's report sparked the beginnings of widespread scientific and professional concern with "idiocy" (mental retardation) as a problem in biology, sociology, and education.

Itard's project arose out of his rewarding efforts in the education of the deaf, his commitment to the Cartesian theory of the mind as a *tabula rasa,* his dedication to John Locke's maxim that "nothing can produce that which it does not contain," and his conviction that Victor's mind could be educated by a system of sensory input and habit training. His work clearly illustrated what a highly structured and creative educational approach to the retarded could accomplish. Itard's monograph *De l'Education d'un Homme Sauvage* revealed his recognition of the significance of motivation, needs, and transference in his work with Victor. Much of his effort, too, was directed toward fostering what we would today call ego development and the strengthening of ego controls through the use of identification. Itard's monograph might also be called the first detailed published report on dynamic psychotherapy.

In the United States, even as late as the mid-nineteenth century, the care of the mentally ill and the mentally retarded was at a shockingly low level. Dorothea Dix in her report to the Congress of the United States in 1848 stated that she had seen ". . . more than 9,000 idiots, epileptics, and insane in the United States, destitute of appropriate care and protection, bound with galling chains, lacerated with ropes, scourged with rods and terrified beneath storms of execration and cruel blows; now subject to jibes and scorn and torturing tricks; now abandoned to the most outrageous violations" (Zilboorg, 1941). Obviously, the shift of responsibility for the care of the mentally ill from the Church to the "body politic" had not wrought any striking reforms. Indeed, it was this very set of deplorable conditions that were later to propel the work of Seguin and Howe into prominence as a humanely relevant posture toward the retarded.

Edouard Séguin's book *The Moral Treatment, Hygiene and Education of Idiots and Other Backward Children* (1846), a landmark in the literature on mental retardation, is based on the self-same principles of psychotherapy that guide today's psychiatrist in his therapeutic endeavors . Séguin, a Parisian neuro-psychiatrist and also a specialist in education of deaf mutes, was inspired by Itard's reported work with Victor. All modern training and education of the mentally retarded is based on the principles laid down by Séguin in the first half of the nineteenth century. Séguin's book sparked widespread recognition of idiocy and his systematic approach to the "education of the idiot."

Under the leadership of Samuel G. Howe, a Boston neuro-psychiatrist specializing in the education of deaf mutes, Séguin's inspired system was introduced to American psychiatry in the mid-nineteenth century when Howe became the director of the first state-supported school for idiots in South Boston, Massachusetts. At about the same time, for political reasons, Séguin fled France and, with Howe's encouragement, came to the United States. From then on (about 1850), until his death in 1881, he was active in assisting nineteenth-century American psychiatry to establish schools for "idiots and other feeble-minded persons" and residential centers for their humane care.

In the second half of the nineteenth century, psychiatry began to involve itself with some of the more basic issues of retardation. Griesinger (1860), of Berlin, espoused psychogenic causology in retardation; in his textbook on *Mental Pathology and Therapeutics,* he wrote;

There are cases where the mental development remains stationary from want of external impulse—from extreme neglect and inattention—associations with other dements, unfavorable outward relations, etc. Finally, in certain cases the mentality does not progress, because in weakly children there exists such an excessive degree of emotional irritability of timidity and fear, that a state of passionate excitement is awakened by every attempt at mental influence, even by any lively sensorial impression, so that development of the normal process of perception is rendered impossible. Although few of the latter cases originally belong to the idiotic states, still they have the same practically important result: arrest of mental development.

The American Association on Mental Deficiency was founded in 1876. All of its charter members were psychiatrists. They and many other psychiatrists who followed in their footsteps were dedicated to the proposition that through the application of psychotherapeutic principles and dynamically oriented education "idiotic" and "imbecile" children could be substantially improved—a fact that has been rediscovered only very recently!

However, in the last half of the nineteenth century, another fateful trend was developing. Within ten years or so after Virchow published his treatise on *The Cellular Theory of Disease* (1858), the Parisian School of Psychiatry and Neurology turned its attention to the basic nature of idiocy and imbecility. The Parisian School, while describing mental illness and mental retardation in psychological and behavioristic terminology, firmly adhered to the thesis that the ultimate nature of these conditions lay in some form of cerebral histo-pathology. Before the end of the nineteenth century, Bourneville (1893) and his co-workers seemingly had established that most of idiocy was an expression of some form of brain pathology or was associated with neurological disease; unfortunately this view predominates to the present day and is expressed in a variety of "defect theories" [2] which assume that the symptom of mental retardation is *always* a manifestation of distinct and fixed central nervous system pathology. This conceptualization implies a distinct limitation on the learning and adaptive ability of the retarded person which, because of damaged internal mechanisms, was seen as beyond the scope of extrinsic manipulation. We shall note how this particular conceptualization played a dominant part in shifting the interests and role of the psychiatrist from one of positive therapeutic intervention to that of the custodial gatekeeper. The "defect position" conceptualization was also utilized in the late nineteenth century to "explain" some occasional manifestations associated with mild mental retardation that were being increasingly recognized. One particular area drew a great deal of attention: maladaptive social behavior. Most retarded individuals with such problems were identified in adolescence and came to the "idiot asylums" as social misfits, neglected children, or both. Self-evident limitation in the "learning of letters" in conjunction with social failure prompted the English psychiatrists initially to term these individuals as "moral imbeciles." For all practical purposes, Goddard later equated social imbecility with his definition of the "moron" and attributed the condition to heredity.

As the twentieth century approached, the findings of Bourneville and his co-workers had become widely known and accepted. The reality of brain pathology in idiocy had a sobering effect upon the optimism and enthusiasm for "educating the minds of idiots," and in only a few years, custodial care for the moderately and severely retarded had practically replaced all remedial efforts in their behalf. As Wolfensberger (1969) has documented, the initial professional view of "making the deviant undeviant" (1850–1880) was slowly to undergo change during the following twenty years. During this transitional period, though, a spirit of benevolence and purpose continued to permeate the professional approaches toward the retarded until the advent of the "defect position" and its dim view of the prognosis of retardation became an increasingly more prominent professional rationale and mission.

The ascendancy of the "defect position" in professional thinking not only dimmed hopes for the education of the retarded but also drastically altered the transitional period's emphasis—from sheltering the retarded from society to protecting society from the retarded. Concomitantly, the residue of benevolence toward the retarded faded away.

In summary, borne along on the crest of a dawning social conscience, the nineteenth century saw the discovery of mental retardation as a "condition in which the intellectual faculties have never developed sufficiently"; it witnessed the introduction and vigorous pursuit of a rational plan for "educating the minds of idiots"; and for about 100 years, psychiatry had a well-established and well-documented role of pre-eminent leadership in promoting the best interests of the mentally retarded. Also, much that is accounted today as "new developments" in the care, training, and education of the mentally retarded had been anticipated with sophisticated skill by and under the leadership of many nineteenth-century psychiatrists. However, while new forms and aspects of mental retardation were identified, and while the nature of many types of retardation was discovered, classified, and demonstrated, this increasing concentration on neuropathology and its accompanying professional commitment to the "defect position" as the *sine qua non* of mental retardation also began to dim the previous therapeutic enthusiasm of the psychiatrist. Thus, in the span of but twenty years (1880–1900), the professional role of the psychiatrist underwent a profound and lasting change, from the enlightened "educateur" to the behavioral pathologist whose major activities were identifying, segregating, and isolating the "deviants."

The Tragic Interlude

At the end of the nineteenth century, societal trends coalesced into a tragic interlude that left a lasting imprint on psychiatric involvement in the field of mental retardation. The tragic interlude occurred in a time span of only about twenty years (1900–1920), but it produced a radical shift of psychiatric interest away from mental retardation. Concomitant changes in societal views of the retarded ushered in institutional models of care focusing on protecting society from the "deviant" who was isolated in low-budget institutions that placed a premium on labor as a major means of institutional support. Unfortunately, this new role was not only less challenging than the previously noted optimism and enthusiasm for treating the retarded, but it also increasingly allied the psychiatrist in mental retardation with penology. This phenomenon is underlined by the fact that the National Conference on Charities and Corrections became a major vehicle for the transaction of professional affairs in mental retardation at this time. These trends began a half century or more of "bench-sitting" and "wheel-chair ambulation" for the moderately and severely retarded in most of our institutions throughout the United States and the historical period of the "retarded as a menace."

Three crucial developments, operating in a symbiotic relationship, each with the other, administered the coup-de-grace to the challenge of mental retardation for the psychiatric profession in the United States: (1) The appearance of the Binet Test on the American scene in 1908; (2) Brill's introduction of psychoanalysis to American psychiatry in the same year; and (3) Goddard's 1912 publication of his monograph on *The Kallikak Family*. Let us explore how these developments operated to alienate psychiatric interest from mental retardation.

Almost overnight the Binet Test and its subsequent modifications gained acceptance as a crucial diagnostic technique for mental deficiency. It soon came to be used, too, as the one and only guide for educational programs and even for the prognosis of social effectiveness. The psychiatric approach was replaced by the mental test approach, and the professional services of the psychiatrist became expendable. The discovery of vast numbers of "morons in our midst" through the use of mental tests soon became a matter of widespread concern, especially because so many morons appeared to be social misfits. That it was mostly the "social misfits" that came under scrutiny was overlooked, and the conclusion was drawn that all morons were social problems, or potentially so. This gave rise to the catch phrase, "the menace of the feebleminded" (for example, Barr, 1915). Goddard was not alone in sounding the "eugenic alarm." Others such as Davenport, Fernald, and Crookshank also contributed to the growing consensus which, in time, included four distinct conclusions: (1) there were more retarded persons in our society than people realized; (2) the mentally retarded accounted for virtually all of the current social ills; (3) heredity was the major cause of mental retardation; and (4) since the decadent retarded appeared to reproduce faster than nonretarded citizens, society would soon be destroyed unless drastic measures were taken.

While these concepts about mental retardation were jelling, American psychiatry was rapidly assimilating the dynamic concepts of psychoanalysis into psychiatric evaluation and treatment. Psychotherapeutic efforts with the psychoneuroses served to entice psychiatrists away from allegedly prosaic and purposeless activities in mental retardation, and Itard's psychopedagogical efforts with Victor were forgotten.

The "menace of the feebleminded" and the sounding of the "eugenic alarm," together with the notion "once feebleminded, always feebleminded," led to the advocacy of immediate institutionalization for all mental retardates, wherever and whenever identified, and the policy of keeping them "out of circulation" at least for the duration of their reproductive years. This alone was enough to repel most psychiatrists motivated by an ambition to rehabilitate persons with mental handicaps or to cure and ameliorate mental disabilities.

The tragic interlude stimulated major financial commitments on a national scale to the construction of ever larger institutions in which to incarcerate the "dangerous" retardate. From the early twentieth century until 1960, the institutional leitmotif became "protect society from the deviant." In rapid succession, restrictive marriage and sterilization laws and life-long segregation ("warehousing") of retardates in inexpensive institutions produced what Vail (1966) has aptly described as "dehumanization." The role of the psychiatrist became that of jailer, and the professional-societal expectations left little room for the humane and supportive care models that had so typified the earlier role of the psychiatrist in mental retardation. At that time, the major journal in this field was entitled "The Journal of Psycho-asthenics," a title which implied a "constitutional inferiority" in its prime focus toward the retarded.

A close review of this period (1900–1960) clearly reveals that professionals literally led the field into a wilderness. The arguments brought forth to support mass sterilization, enforced labor, and inexpensive warehousing by the leading "defectologists" of that era could be viewed as unfortunate events, if this hindsight did not directly conflict with the persisting results of their labors. For example, as noted by Wolfensberger (1969), the period from 1925 to the present has been typified by a loss of the rationales for the prevailing institutional practices but a continuity of momentum for the practices that evolved from these outdated professional rationales. The pictorial overview entitled *Christmas in Purgatory* by Blatt and Kaplan (1966), coupled with a recent report of the President's Committee on Mental Retardation (Kugel and Wolfensberger, 1969), documents this aimless continuity of momentum in pictures and words.

I have stressed the institutional aspect of the psychiatrist's recent history in the field of mental retardation because, as we shall note, it may hold the key to a new renaissance of psychiatric involvement. New rationales are direly needed, and the wave of humanism that typifies our society's current posture toward the handicapped can provide multiple challenges for the psychiatrist to invest (or reinvest) his intellectual, empathic, and global therapeutic skills in an area which genuinely needs him.

In summary, mental retardation attracted the interest and participation of the psychiatric profession throughout the nineteenth century and for the first decade or so of the twentieth century. But by 1920, the interests of psychiatry and other mental health disciplines in the mentally retarded had begun to deteriorate. From then until now, mental retardation and the mentally retarded has occupied only a peripheral position in psychiatric teaching, training, and practice.

Perspectives on the Present

Stereotyped Psychiatric Views of the Retarded

In the foregoing, I have reviewed some of the extraordinary historical events which led to psychiatry's relative withdrawal from the field of mental retardation. This withdrawal and the historical events that led up to it have resulted in a number of stereotyped views or blindspots that psychiatrists characteristically exhibit when they must deal with the retarded. Briefly, these blindspots are: uncritical acceptance of mental age as an adequate description of a person; treatment nihilism that is usually based on lack of program knowledge and a myopic view of conceivable or even available program alternatives; and excessive focus on the severely retarded and their families, in contrast to the mildly retarded. I shall now elaborate on each of these stereotyped views in some detail.

The Mental Age Myth

The psychometric mental age as an overall description is still all too often utilized to pigeonhole mentally retarded persons. This stereotype can be altered by realistic study of these individuals and of how they actually experience the world around them. A number of recent works by professionals, laymen, parents and siblings of the retarded, and even the retarded themselves provide an insight into the phenomenological world of the retarded. For example, a recent book by Edgerton, entitled *The Cloak of Competency* (1968), well illustrates the wide range of adjustment styles of the adult retardate and dispels the common professional stereotype of the passively compliant and socially-vocationally inept individual in our contemporary society. Similarly, the recent autobiography (Hunt, 1967) of an adult with Down's Syndrome, *The World of Nigel Hunt,* affords the reader an opportunity to get "under the skin" of a human being who has an adaptive problem which we choose to call mental retardation. Though Nigel employs grammatical construction quite typical of a third or fourth grader, the word fluency and range of topics which he covers are quite beyond that. They quickly attune the reader to the fact that this young man has a rich interpersonal world and feelings, hopes, aspirations (and a wide range of other interests) that go beyond the usual stereotype of "moderate mental retardation" or "mental age of seven years," of the individual with Down's Syndrome as a "slobbering idiot."

The mental age myth is also operative in considering the socioeconomic context in which the retardate is examined. A mildly retarded lad who is seen in the company of his low socioeconomic status parents is too often termed "cultural-familial" mental retardation. Yet a similar youth from a higher socioeconomic grouping is apt to be diagnosed as "minimal cerebral dysfunction," and his low mental age is ignored or interpreted to represent a spurious assessment in view of the accompanying neurological findings. In these two instances, the myth of mental age reflects a negative bias on the part of the examiner toward the value system of the retardate from a low socioeconomic class and strong professional conjectures as to the relative efficacy of psychotherapy for the retarded. That this negative attitudinal bias is not limited to psychiatrists is illustrated by recent educational reports which strongly suggest that the "track system" for educating the retarded from low socioeconomic groups may reflect the myth of fixed mental age and its associated low expectancy set for the mentally retarded student.

Thus, the mental age myth, with all of its trappings of fixed intellectual functioning and developmental expectancy, has given rise to a companion myth about the value of any psychiatric treatment for those declared "unchangeable." As noted by Lott in Chapter 10 of this book, the myth that the intelligence quotient determines an individual's capability and ability to partake in and benefit from psychotherapy is often implicit in current psychiatric practice. Similarly, Bernstein (1969) reports the surprise and subsequently changed attitudes on the part of psychiatric trainees who had been given an opportunity to relate to the retarded on a protracted basis.

All of these considerations strongly suggest that the mental age myth will only be destroyed when the professional is able fully to view and appreciate the recently rediscovered social-adaptive potential of the retardate. This demands an individualized assessment of the retardate's global function in the worlds of family, peer group, school or work demands, and a new look at him as a person-in-the-world, in contrast to the mental age label that attempts to predict academic adjustment rather than life adjustment potentials. Thus, the mental age myth has permeated both professional and institutional postures toward the retarded. Interestingly, a re-examination of this entire topic may suggest that we return to the "pre-IQ tester," with strong focus on individualized assessments in a variety of performance-eliciting life settings.

Preoccupation with Severe Retardation

There are eight times as many mildly retarded as moderately, severely, and profoundly retarded combined. Because their problems are more educational, psychological, and habilitative in nature rather than medical, the mildly retarded have less in common with the more severely retarded than with normal children. Nevertheless, the majority of psychiatric attention—especially that motivating institutional services—appears to focus on the more severely retarded. This unbalanced distribution of psychiatric help is based upon the current orientation held by many human management professionals that such services must remain correlated with interaction between socioeconomic class structure and degree of mental retardation. The contemporary selection process for psychiatric treatment strongly reflects the successful push for services by the National Association for Retarded Children which is largely a middle-class movement. Indeed, in some states (for example, Ohio), there is mandatory legislation for special services for its moderately retarded citizens—but not for the mildly retarded. Though the mildly retarded within their usual low socioeconomic grouping are commonly referred to as the "invisible retarded," this designation may go beyond the respective life styles of the retardates therein and reflect a distinct negative bias on the part of the psychiatrist not to "see" their need for services.

The vast number of the mildly retarded will manage fairly well in our society, given some aid and guidance from other members of the family, from neighbors and friends, and from society via its agencies and special services. The members of this large group will acquire sufficient reading, writing, and arithmetic, and if provided with vocational training and guidance, they will be able to obtain and hold unskilled, semi-skilled, and occasionally even skilled jobs. If they have adequate emotional support and guidance, it is highly probable that they will not be social misfits. Most will marry, and most of these will bring up families. The long term follow-up studies of community-based mentally retarded individuals by Kennedy (1966) and Baller,

Charles, and Miller (1966) are forceful reminders of what the retarded *can* do!

As noted by Chess in Chapter 2 of this volume, a significant percentage of mildly retarded children have adjustment problems which contribute significantly to their learning difficulties and with which they need help. The primary psychopathological features of the retarded (reviewed by Webster in Chapter 1), their poor self-image, and their unfavorable competitive position in the world around them make them especially prone to anxiety. Interventive psychiatric care thus becomes a crucial ingredient in providing adequate services for a large number of mentally retarded children. Without psychiatric care, secondary emotional disturbances may well preclude the inclusion of these children in ongoing developmental special education programs during childhood. In adults, emotional disturbance or personality dysfunction often disrupts vocational training and job placement. The importance of obtaining necessary psychiatric services for emotionally complicated instances of mental retardation again stresses the incongruent nihilistic treatment posture adopted by many contemporary psychiatrists.

In this regard I would point out that the psychiatrist has usually viewed or treated a very selected sample of retardates, those who have emotional disturbances. What about the 70 per cent who are not emotionally disturbed (Menolascino, 1965, 1966)? Unfortunately, I suspect that the average psychiatrist's training and clinical experiences tend to generalize his selected experiences into an expectation of disturbed behavior in all or most of the retarded, just as the selected samples of severely retarded children usually seen by pediatricians has led to generalizations reflecting their selectivity. For example, in the past, pediatricians have rarely seen the age range and socioeconomic class that is commonly associated with mild mental retardation. This has led some prominent pediatricians to seriously question whether this very large group of individuals even exists.

Retarded children thrive in selected community settings; this is particularly true of those with retarded speech and language development. There is much evidence to show that speech and language develop earlier and more completely in retarded children when they reside at home and attend developmental day care centers and community schools, instead of residing in institutions. Similarly, these children display greater development when they reside in small residential units with high staffing ratios and flexible treatment regimens, in contrast to residence in large, overcrowded, and understaffed facilities where care and training is "institution-centered" rather than "child-centered."

In conclusion, the overemphasis on severe mental retardation has not only produced a distorted view of psychiatric dimensions of the mentally retarded, but has also failed to focus psychiatric effort where it is quantitatively, socially, and programmatically more desperately needed: the mildly retarded.

Treatment Nihilism and Lack of Program Knowledge

Treatment nihilism flowing from stereotyped psychiatric concepts regarding mental retardation is well illustrated in the usual lack of knowledge among psychiatrists concerning the therapeutic possibilities and necessary programmatic components of meaningful programs for the retarded (Berstein, 1968). For example, the 1969 revision of the nomenclatural system of the American Psychiatric Association has attempted to stress mental retardation as a primary diagnosis. The new A.P.A. nomenclature also utilizes the descriptive levels of mild-moderate-severe-profound retardation introduced by the American Association on Mental Deficiency. This is in sharp contrast to the old A.P.A. nomenclatural system that referred to an IQ under 50 as "severe"—and the hopelessness it implied for the large and extremely heterogeneous group of the retarded thus lumped together. Under the older nomenclatural wastebasket of "chronic brain syndrome," the overriding focus on chronicity, implied irreversibility, and associated therapeutic nihilism (for example, "custodial care") was enough to dishearten even the most empathic psychiatrist. The negative attitudinal postures toward treatment and rehabilitation of the retarded (for example, "You can't fight the genes," "Little if any change with treatment—it's all rather hopeless," and so on) that were literally grafted on a generation of psychiatrists are incongruent with dynamic contemporary approaches to other major chronic disorders (such as, cancer, heart, and strokes).

The blunt fact is that few psychiatrists are conversant with the dramatic vistas in vocational rehabilitation (Gunzberg, 1960; O'Connor, 1965) and residential programming (Tizard, 1964; Kugel and Wolfensberger, 1969) that have been fully documented. The significance of the actual implementation of these programmatic components, as in the Scandinavian facilities for the retarded, are frequently not grasped or ignored. I have heard colleagues comment most vociferously in a negative vein on both of these topics, for example: "Vocational training successes occur in 'atypical' or undiagnosed retardates"; or "Tizard's Brooklands film gave me the impression that it was a small pilot project which had ideal staffing patterns and, like so many pilot programs, it isn't really applicable to the problems at large." I am stressing this lack of understanding of modern service concepts and systems because I feel that it has led directly to administrative situations wherein the psychiatrist continues to defend the tragic models of care which Blatt and Dybwad have so eloquently discussed in Chapters 24 and 25. To implement the enlightened programming suggested by Potter in Chapter 26 of this volume, we must actively utilize the new concepts and programs in the field of mental retardation.

However, we may first have to admit that Blatt's "purgatories" do exist! The writer has personally visited over one-fourth of the state-supported residential facilities for the retarded in the United States. Typically, I have noted the antitheses of the positive effects that the new conceptual-programmatic views can produce in all, even the profoundly, retarded. Every large institution for the retarded that I have visited has units where ambulatory young adult and middle-aged moderately and severely retarded individuals regularly embark on a schedule of futility in their daily lives.

In such units, residents are awakened en masse very early in the morning so that night attendants can line them up and get them toileted before hustling them down to a barren dining room in which they are seated on benches before lengthy tables. They are placed in close proximity to the sloppy mess in their steel or unbreakable plastic plates and are only given large spoons because *we* surely "know" that they cannot be trusted with forks and knives. They are encouraged to eat as quickly as possible, or they are fed at a rapid pace so that they can be dispatched to the day room. Once in the day room, they are again seated on benches or chairs and allowed the grand pleasure of viewing TV or simply one another until mid-morning. About 10 A.M. (in the summertime), they are hustled out to a large fenced area, commonly termed the "play area," so that they can partake of the clean fresh air which Guggenbühl so eloquently described as beneficial to the human organism. In the "play yard" they wander around aimlessly; stereotyped behavior is commonplace; and the attendants busy themselves maintaining a watch for the "hole-diggers," the "excessive" masturbators (there *is* a degree of distinction!), and anyone subject to overt seizures. This same routine—appropriate for the separation and temporary maintenance of cattle at a livestock yard—is repeated in the afternoons. In winter, the residents may not get outdoors for months; in some institutions they do not go outside from one year to the next.

The more severely retarded are typically housed in buildings on the periphery of the institutional grounds because they emit unpleasant noises and odors, because of their generally disheveled appearances, and because of all the associated facets which do not make for a very good "public relations image" to visitors. Thus, the term "back-ward" is not a figurative expression, but a literal reality. These "back-wards" are usually thinly staffed; in my experience, a typical staff ratio may be two attendants per one hundred patients per eight hour shift, with the staff coverage ratio diminishing as day wears on into night.

Why did I feel it necessary to discuss this fairly typical pattern for fellow professionals who surely know it all too well? Because we continue to fail to stress that active use of available program knowledge for the moderately and severely retarded individuals who enter our institutions can completely change these terrible patterns which reinforce a prison or barnyard-like structure and perpetuate an environment devoid of respect for the human dignity of the retarded. For example, a severely retarded ambulatory young adult who works on even the simplest industrial task in a sheltered workshop (on the institution grounds or, even better, off them) is constructively occupied; is preparing himself for placement in the community (or in a hostel in the community); is viewed by others more positively; has a more positive self-image than he did formerly; and contributes to society. Today, such an individual would most probably live in one of the Scandinavian countries. The same retardate living in a public institution for the retarded in the United States probably would be wandering around out in the "play yard," exhibiting stereotypic hand movements, mumbling to himself, perhaps digging aimlessly at the ground or himself, and performing no purposeful activity whatsoever. After all, we *know* that he is too stupid to perform any useful activity and that he cannot be trained for such tasks, and even if he were trained, his memory would not retain his instructions long enough to make the time spent in teaching him profitable, and so on.

We must stress not only the vocational habilitation and rehabilitation potentials that are available, but also those very dimensions that are of such importance to politicians and state legislative budgetary committee members. Specifically, we must reassess the high rate of tranquilizer drug usage in current institutional programs (see Lipman, Chapter 15 in this volume), the high rate of furniture and physical plant destruction, and the high frequency of bizarre, "autistic" primitive behaviors which are too frequently and erroneously accepted as part and parcel of the syndrome of severe retardation. It is difficult to rid oneself of this particular stereotype unless one sees *quality* programming on a large *quantitative* scale, as in Scandinavia, and finds how little "autistic" behavior is exhibited in such environments. I saw hardly any of this behavior in Scandinavia, although I was specifically looking for it. As other visitors to Scandinavia also have observed, the focus on a truly total therapeutic milieu, embodying the most advanced programmatic knowledge and competence, coupled with positive attitudes of the child care worker (as a "teacher," rather than as an attendant), have changed the dehumanization, therapeutic nihilism, and isolation from which such behavior so commonly springs into one of "normalization" (Nirje, 1969). Such programming also has major implications with regard to how parents view their retarded children, and their role vis-á-vis an institutionalized child. Once their child has become behaviorally quiescent by being taught a more purposeful role and function in life via meaningful education-vocational programming, the parents are more eager to visit him regularly, to take him home for visits, and to assist in the eventual transition to hostel placement or even community habilitation.

I have stressed the seeking of alternatives to the current handling of problems and issues in mental retardation. The current myopic professional view of treatment for the moderately and severely retarded ambulatory adult commonly consists of high doses of tranquilizers, selective restraint, isolation, and an attitude of "leave him alone—or he'll slug you. If he's quiet, we've done our job." I am fully aware of the present state of the art in institutional care as it commonly pertains to the severely retarded; it typically views any alternative programs as "utter insanity" because of the stereotyped views of what the retarded *can't* do, which are more prevalent than convictions regarding what they *can* do; low budgets are a chronic problem—and scapegoat—and there is a rampant lack of professional awareness concerning new program knowledge and competence. The "low budget" argument is rather embarrassing when one notes that the *per diem* at some of our inadequate public institutions is higher than the pro-rated *per diem* of some of the Scandinavian facilities or even of some outstanding private facilities in the United States. Also, the spectre of "politics" and "national health systems" are commonly advanced to belittle the Scandinavian comparisons. Yet the writer knows of no instance wherein a cost-service benefit ratio approach has been applied to assess realistically these differing political-societal postures to programmatic approaches for the retarded.

Could it be that we do not want to look squarely at the national disgrace of our residential facilities for the retarded? Have we unconsciously or otherwise accepted the previously noted historical "loss of rationales" and acquiesced to an aimless continuity of momentum? Or can the psychiatrist come to grips with his historical heritage from the past, learn, and then implement the available alternatives of programmatic excellence both in the institutional and community setting? So often it appears that the psychiatrist involved in institutional administration escapes from confrontation with his treatment nihilism by entering the realm of administration. Thus, rather than actively dealing with the problem, he "sits on top" and administrates the continuity of the aimless momentum from a distance. As previously noted, there *are* available treatment programs that disavow treatment nihilism. To embrace this "new deal" for the retarded becomes a major opportunity and challenge for the psychiatrist.

Many of the contributors to this volume have defined a challenge to psychiatry by offering specific guideposts for a road to a new professional relevance in mental retardation. For example, we may implement this needed change by pilot programs for residential or community based retardates (in different geographic regions of the United States) so that the message would come directly home to professionals as a pattern of currently available services that offer an excellent alternative for both individual retardates and those who are entrusted to help maximize their developmental potentials. I almost said "entrusted with their care" and thus realize how ingrained this particular posture of "caring" for the "poor retarded" actually is in all of us!

Manpower Trends

Manpower needs remain a major problem in the delivery of mental retardation services. I shall approach this subject by reviewing its historical context and then focusing on methods and models for realistically initiating viable alternatives for filling manpower voids.

In a paper presented at the 1927 annual meeting of the American Psychiatric Association, Howard Potter called mental retardation the "Cinderella of Psychiatry." In his presidential address before the American Association on Mental Deficiency in 1933, he emphasized the need for "a well-structured, dynamically-oriented, professional training program in mental deficiency." Potter is one of a very small group of psychiatrists who have consistently and persistently urged a greater participation of psychiatry in mental retardation. Indeed, his has been one of the few voices crying in the psychiatric wilderness of mental retardation.

Walter Barton, in an editorial in the October 1961 issue of the *American Journal of Psychiatry,* wrote:

Psychiatrists as a group are disinterested in mental retardation. Many have no more accurate knowledge about the retarded than the layman does. Training centers seldom provide serious field study. If questioned, most psychiatrists would agree that mental retardation is a sub-specialty in their area of responsibility and then disqualify themselves. Should we be concerned that psychiatry as a profession is unable to meet its responsibilities? Or, after a long, hard look, should we admit our mistake, say this is not our field, and bow out? Are there other alternative actions that are appropriate and desirable?

The American Psychiatric Association's Section on Mental Deficiency, which was replaced many years ago by a Section on Child Psychiatry, has not been reactivated. The report of the Joint Commission on Mental Illness (1960), in which the American Psychiatric Association was heavily involved, largely ignored mental retardation. Further, the Council of the American Psychiatric Association has periodically issued "Position Statements" concerning the special interest of psychiatry in mental retardation. The first such "Position Statement" was issued in 1963 (Council of American Psychiatric Association, 1963). Potter (1965) has discussed some of the incongruent aspects of this particular "Position Statement" regarding organized psychiatry's involvement on the national scene in the needs of the mentally retarded. At that time, the indices of psychiatry's involvement in mental retardation were listed as follows. Some many years ago the American Psychiatric Association had a section on Mental Deficiency. It has been replaced by a Section of Child Psychiatry. In the last six volumes of the *American Journal of Psychiatry* (through 1968) there were but twelve articles on mental retardation. Psychiatrists represented but 6.2 per cent of the 1968 membership of the American Association on Mental Deficiency. Forty years ago they accounted for 43 per cent. Of one hundred and six state schools and hospitals for the mentally retarded in the United States in 1968, only forty-four were administered by physicians who are members of the American Psychiatric Association. Less than 1 per cent of the board-certified psychiatrists in the United States are attached to the staffs of state residential facilities for the retarded, and nearly half of these are on a relatively inactive consultancy basis.

With such apathy emanating from a group of professionals who had been charged traditionally with providing psychiatric services to the retarded, it is surprising that the organized protest from the consumer of these services did not jell until the recent past. The National Association for Retarded Children, initiated in 1952, started as a protest-inspired movement largely because of psychiatry's laissez-faire attitude about mental retardation. For years, parents of retarded children had fruitlessly searched psychiatrists' offices, child guidance clinics, and general psychiatric clinics for helpful counsel and constructive advice. For example, in 1961, only 5.5 per cent of the patients seen in 1,100 psychiatric clinics were retarded, and the only service rendered to 90 per cent of these was a brief diagnostic work-up (Chandler, Norman, and Bahn, 1962). General psychiatric out-patient services and, in particular, out-patient as well as in-patient services in child psychiatry, with only a few exceptions, continue to deny mentally retarded children and their parents those professional services that they so sorely need.

Today, when there is an urgent need for active participation of mental health personnel in the field of mental retardation, the United States has only a handful of psychiatrists, clinical psychologists, and psychiatric social workers prepared to respond to the demands and opportunities of implementing the mental health aspects of a national program of action for the mentally retarded. According to the President's Panel on Mental Retardation (1962), trained personnel is in even shorter supply today than forty years ago. At both the community and institutional levels, if one combines the needs, there is an alarming gap between supply and demand for mental health personnel to work with the mentally retarded.

Just what ideally should be the role of the psychiatrist in mental retardation? As I have noted, much of his historical role in the field has been supplanted by changes both in the fields of mental retardation and psychiatry. Stripped of his cherished professional "standbys" (the diagnostic interview, assessment of intellectual functioning, and so forth), he has apparently slipped into the role (albeit uncomfortably) of clinical and institutional "gatekeeper," whereas his clinical skills in mental retardation have not been embellished or extended by concurrent trends in general psychiatry. The previously noted manpower elements underscore the current status of ideological perplexity and practical disengagement (both conceptually and in service involvements) of psychiatry in the area of mental retardation. Ideologically, the psychiatrist has adopted (or supported) the medical model of management in retardation wherein too frequently he has become an administrator of a clinic or a gatekeeper at an institution. This overemphasis on an administrative role is rather ironic in view of the great professional challenge to understand the entire psycho-biological unit that is presented by the retarded individual. In other words, focus on administration—with its concern for control at all levels—has currently gained precedence over the study of individual or collective dimensions of mental retardation. As noted, this appears to be a result of the past overconcern with therapeutic hopelessness and resultant custodial approaches to the "untreatables."

With its nihilistic conceptual approach and its physical disengagement from the field, it comes as no surprise that psychiatry has been relegated to a voluntarily (and also an involuntarily) diminishing role in the planning and administration of both community programs and residential facilities for the retarded. The current trend toward more lay administrators has demanded a hard new look at the necessary training and individual personality variables that are needed to operate mental retardation programs or facilities. Despite the historical-professional fact that administration of mental retardation programs was once the sole prerogative of the psychiatrist, this lingering bias is no longer tenable. What is tenable is a renaissance of the psychiatrist as an enlightened purveyor of human services, and Potter's guidelines in this volume for this particular professional role delineation can be an excellent "administrators bible."

As Vail (1966) has noted, dealing with a captive population and the tendency for "total" institutions to develop dehumanizing practices present major problems of philosophy and overall conceptualization. Have we actively given rise to some of the current "road-blocks" (see Dybwad, Chapter 25) that stand in the way of a renaissance of residential service to the retarded? Have we been too busy defending positions in which we no longer have a true investment, while, at the same time, misusing the public, professional, and political power associated with such roles? For example, many private facilities have been operated quite adequately, and will undoubtedly continue to do so, by individuals who are not psychiatrists or in the related mental health disciplines. Can we learn to "share the wealth" and become truly multi-disciplinary as requested by Blatt in Chapter 24, or at least to let other professional movements and groups grow to fill the administrative and service voids we have stepped out of?

The psychiatrist's current identity crisis in mental retardation was thoroughly reviewed during the round-table discussion at the 1969 national meeting of the American Psychiatric Association (Miami Beach, Florida) entitled: "The Psychiatrist and Mental Retardation: Divorce, Separation, or Re-Marriage?" This discussion was a contemporary version of the problems alluded to in the first part of this chapter. It evaluated the questions so succinctly asked of organized psychiatry by Barton in 1961. For example, shall we continue to fight the movement toward increasing lay administration of mental retardation programs? Would such a professional posture be of any real value to the persons we are privileged to serve? When will we appreciate and accept that we are not needed in a central role in many ongoing current treatment approaches to mental retardation?

It was the consensus of this round-table discussion that the recent role of psychiatry in mental retardation could be best summarized as a "flirtation." The participants concurred that a new refocusing of involvement would have to build upon the past model of psychiatric excellence and leadership and stress the modern treatment approaches in psychiatry training programs. This new role would have to more actively involve the "consumers": the retardate, his parents (for example, The National Association for Retarded Children), and the community. Such re-emphasis would require that some cherished professional blindspots and postures be altered drastically.

As Wolfensberger noted in Chapter 31 of this volume, psychiatry's medical role in mental retardation overlaps heavily with that of administrators, mental health specialists, educators, pediatricians, practitioners in general medicine, neurologists, geneticists, and pharmacologists. The psychiatrist has functioned actively (past and present) in all of these possible medical or medical science roles in mental retardation—except surgery. Yet this very diffuseness of involvement adds to rather than clarifies the identity and specific role of the psychiatrist in mental retardation.

We have to remind ourselves that diagnosis and treatment are the core of the specialty of psychiatry—not research and administration. Further, as noted by Bolian (1968) in discussing the role of the child psychiatrist on the usual multi-disciplinary mental retardation team, there is very little that is *specific* (exclusive or inclusive) to the role of the psychiatrist in mental retardation. Yet, in mental retardation there are many roles that—both currently and in the future—can truly utilize the skills of the psychiatrist in a meaningful manner.

Since many of the diagnostic and treatment needs in mental retardation can be provided by others in the mental health, medical, and para-medical fields, I believe we must broaden our discussion to include other human management personnel, rather than persevering in the "psychiatrist alone" posture of the past. Such a shift gives full cognizance to the efforts of our colleagues in the fields of child development, education, nursing, psychology, social work, and vocational rehabilitation. Lest I unfairly castigate psychiatry in its need to truly delineate its future role in the field of mental retardation, it should be noted that other professionals have similar identity problems. Unification of attitude and training experiences regarding mental retardation are necessary in virtually all professional fields. For example, though pediatrics has recently taken an active role in mental retardation (via the university-affiliated Mental Retardation Centers), there are relatively few developmentally oriented pediatricians who are strongly identified in the field of mental retardation. Concentrating almost exclusively on the medical and neurological needs of the young child, pediatrics has aimed at only a limited portion of the needed diagnostic-treatment-management services for the retarded. Just as the retarded do grow into adults, and thus limit the range of involvement of the pediatrician, so does the psychiatrist have built-in "limits" that delineate his role.

Virtually every professional group that is currently involved in mental retardation has had its "heyday" in the field. One wonders if this alternation of leadership does not reflect the attitudinal and social values of both society and of the professionals themselves. If this conjecture is correct, then we may be "beating a straw horse" in regard to professional one-up-manship. We could more profitably utilize our energies to explore current societal and professional expectancy sets for the retarded, study them closely, and gear our current professional training programs to erase these blindspots. The next section will explore some possible ramifications of this new deployment of psychiatric energies as we look to the future.

A LOOK INTO THE FUTURE

In a recent book entitled *The Future as History,* Heilbroner (1960) warned that the rapidity of change in the world of ideas makes all groups and persons in our society prone to temporal obsolescence. Psychiatry has the opportunity to alter positively its recent professional estrangement from mental retardation if it will realistically view its current attitudinal blindspots and minimal involvement. To do otherwise would be tantamount to continuing to prevent psychiatry from showing what it can do!

Within the confines of mental retardation, the present gives some indication of psychiatry's future involvement. In global terms, the psychiatrist may become a coordinating and motivating force behind and with other human management personnel, actively utilizing and working with those who have differing types of training. In the perspective of the greater picture of public health and preventive medicine (for example, community psychiatry), this coordinating role may be one of the most helpful and effective future postures for the psychiatrist. Its effectiveness within mental retardation has been assured by the very conditions of the field: most instances of mental retardation have no known etiology, very little can be "cured," it is very expensive to treat mental retardation institutionally, and most of it could be prevented with means now available to our society. These conditions call for a diagnostic and treatment process for mental retardation that is distinctly different than that found in other patterns of medical care.

For example, curative medicine is usually associated with a diagnostic process that is primarily of a negative feedback character. That is, diagnosis leads to treatment that is determined by survival rates, complication rates, and functional loss or gain. The desirable regimes are continued; less effective ones are not. In mental retardation, the relationships between the diagnostic process and treatment are not so easily formulated. The fact that these relationships remain difficult to answer and implement does not remove their importance. We must be willing to place trust in the integrity of the individual professional to treat the disabled as an individual. I do not mean to imply that this is not now the case, or even that the professional's integrity is not responding to responsibility. On the contrary, I mean that the diagnostic process as seen in the care of the mentally retarded is quite different from those which are utilized in traditional (curative) medicine.

My term for the difference is "feedforward." The diagnostic treatment process in mental retardation is qualitatively different in that "feedforward" encompasses enlightened training, leadership, optimism, a commitment to optimizing human fulfillment, and above all, it is a creative, rather than curative, process. The artist uses "feedforward" to endow his medium with the ability to provide others with a meaningful experience. In the use of "feedforward" via the diagnostic process, and its conclusion—treatment—the clinician distinguishes himself as an applied scientist. The clinician caring for the mentally retarded individual requires "feedforward" to be truly effective in his ongoing efforts to embellish the retardate's life.

I have attempted to place the diagnostic and treatment processes necessary in mental retardation in the light of our times. The mentally retarded individual requires a diagnostic process and set of treatment transactions that are apparently unique. Furthermore, as previously noted, there is historical and contemporary evidence to indicate that this clinical process can serve as a most effective means of optimizing the environmental conditions for the individual. The ability of the individual to find fulfillment in our world is severely challenged by the conditions of our era. The necessary diagnostic and treatment ingredients in mental retardation should epitomize all of these elements that characterize a humanistic approach which can both avoid temporal obsolescence and provide quality to survive our era and lead health care into the future. Yet the foregoing remarks may sound like a muted clarion call unless a *specific* set of recommendations are brought forth to alter both the current identity and man-power problems of psychiatry.

In essence, the history of psychiatry's involvement clearly reveals that it has stepped out of an active role in mental retardation. Now, psychiatry must allow other mental health personnel to fill this void. Though its own role may be a realistically modest one, it carries with it a corollary of encouraging others into activity and prominence in the field. Accordingly, I will review future role delineations of the psychiatrist in mental retardation, suggesting three major roles; and I will suggest a mechanism for training that will produce future psychiatrists who can truly embrace these proposed roles.

Future Psychiatric Roles in Mental Retardation

First, the psychiatrist can function as a "generalist" in mental retardation, as described by the older title of "defectologist," wherein the clinical aspects of etiology and description as they bear upon the diagnostic and treatment-management aspects of mental retardation become his major professional forte. His specific role would be to correlate and interpret the diagnostic findings of a multi-disciplinary team into meaningful therapeutic prescriptions. In this role—either as a resource person, a private practitioner, or a team coordinator—he can represent a bastion of applied knowledge for clinical approaches to the retarded. Many of the mental retardation clinics in the United States were initiated by psychiatrists, both in the past and again in the late 1950's. Despite the well-documented drawbacks of "the Holy Trinity" approach (psychiatrist, psychologist, social worker), these clinics are a viable entity which can be made more effective, by infusion of the training elements outlined later in this chapter.

Second, *special interest areas* of mental retardation can be a major focus of the psychiatrist in mental retardation. Special interest areas which are complex and challenging enough to embrace his full-time efforts encompass topics such as psychopharmacology, both as an adjunct to symptomatic management and possibly as memory and learning agents, as noted in Part Two–B of this volume. Competence in the area of management of families of the retarded represents a pressing need for psychiatric involvement (see Part Two–D of this volume). Another special area is the study and treatment of the emotional dimensions and disturbances that are often noted in the retarded (see Parts One and Two of this volume). This has been a most neglected area of psychiatric involvement and can quickly resolve both the identity crisis and urge to be of therapeutic help of the psychiatrist.

Third, the psychiatrist can firmly embrace the new treatment model within the burgeoning community psychiatry programs as noted by Coda in Chapter 22 of this volume. An interesting re-integrational model for community psychiatry and mental retardation was suggested by Stedman (1966). He noted that the child psychiatry clinic movement, despite its recent difficulties in meeting community mental health needs, could be redirected and challenged to meet the needs of retarded children. Since the staff and facilities to provide mental health services for retarded children already exist in these clinics, Stedman suggests that such clinics can be actively utilized if the personnel will only "think mental retardation." Similarly, the evolving community mental health centers can be programmed for meeting the needs of the retardate at all age levels. Family services, diagnostic, educational, and rehabilitation areas could be coordinated in their developmental and community functions by an information and referral center that plans, coordinates, and often directs the full circle of services that is required. This last function, coordination, consultation, information, and direction, can well be a primary mission of the child and adult psychiatry clinics in mental retardation. There are few substitutes for this approach and fewer alternative systems the community can turn to in order to meet its needs unless it creates a new system for specialized mental retardation centers. As Stedman noted, such a new system would be costly, duplicative, and uneconomical.

It would appear that we here in the United States are literally over-concerned about the distinct delineation of professional roles, in mental retardation as elsewhere. Perhaps we should take a long look at the various roles ("identity equivalents") of the European psychiatrist in mental retardation. The professional title of "neuro-psychiatrist" is commonly utilized by European psychiatrists who specialize in mental retardation and often encompasses both generalist and special area involvement in the field. Professionals with combined pediatric and child psychiatry training are also frequently encountered in mental retardation programs in Europe. Similarly, one finds European psychiatrists as combined educator-regional program directors. The European psychiatrist has also truly accepted the challenge of the multi-disciplinary administrative role concept, as in the Danish system where the regional residential facilities for the retarded are jointly administered by a physician, a business administrator, an educator, and a social worker. It is clear that the European psychiatrist has carved out a wide range of psychiatric roles and identities in mental retardation from specific to generic.

Other future possible roles for the psychiatrist must be viewed against the backdrop of personal professional interests and organizational changes in the field of mental retardation. Thus, there are many possible alternatives and positive resolutions to the identity crisis of the contemporary (and future) psychiatrist in the field. However, the above noted considerations strongly suggest that all professionals who are interested in mental retardation must work together to bridge the professional gaps between the currently available meager service patterns and programs. Indeed, the overwhelming needs for services in mental retardation makes it extremely unlikely that any professional group could become the "prima donna" in mental retardation—even if it wanted to. Yet every professional group can strive to change the interest, expectations, and general range of knowledge of the behavioral aspects of mental retardation.

Accordingly, I shall focus on training as the major ingredient necessary for basic change in the current and future goals of psychiatric involvement in mental retardation. Lest the reader consider that I have sidestepped a "real" approach to future guidelines in this area, I would like to remind him that it has been this very element of professional training activity (since the initial "push" by the National Association for Retarded Children in the 1950's), that has produced the ever increasing number of all professionals who have become active in the field of mental retardation. Coupled with the new reconceptualizations of service, training, and research (as noted throughout this book) that must be tackled by future trainees, this very element of training may hold the key to helping the Cinderella of Mental Retardation to more quickly find her Prince to take her out of the current professional wilderness.

Training for Relevant Involvement in Mental Retardation

If the psychiatrist in mental retardation is to embrace a modest, but realistic role, then specific diagnostic and treatment issues in mental retardation must be included in his training program. Further, a focus on attitudinal modification toward the chronically handicapped must be intertwined throughout the teaching experience. Indeed this very attitudinal modification will aid the trainee to be a better psychiatrist, whether or not he ever treats a retarded individual in his future professional career.

Diagnosis

The broad diagnostic demands of mental retardation can be very effectively utilized to offer mental health personnel excellent training opportunities to integrate the ingredients of their formal training. As noted throughout this book, the multiple streams of interest in mental retardation both encompass and extend many areas of long-standing psychiatric involvement. For example, formal training and guided experiences in the cytogenetic, biochemical, metabolic, and neurological aspects of mental retardation can broaden the trainee's understanding of the most complex interrelated factors that are often involved in the genesis of even the most easily recognized conditions associated with mental retardation, such as mongolism or phenylketonuria. Such training experiences will underscore the necessity for thinking in terms of multi-factorial etiological models and the interaction of dynamic processes. For example, it is always possible that the emotionally disturbed, retarded, deaf child is emotionally disturbed and retarded because he is deaf. Thus, retarded intellectual functioning, emotional disturbance, and the neurologic manifestations of central nervous system impairment and dysfunction can all be viewed as contributors to a particular child's developmental problems.

Guidance in the actual assessment of both the quantitative and qualitative aspects of a retarded individual's intellectual functioning provides firsthand appreciation of the diagnostic methods available, as well as an awareness of the limitations of these methods at various ages, particularly when special handicapping conditions are present (see Bialer in Chapter 3 of this volume). Evaluating the intellectual potential of a retardate then becomes much more than simply assessing the global level of intellectual functioning. The presence and role of a host of multiple handicaps and other specific cognitive or conceptual deficits also need to be determined and appreciated. Furthermore, these deficits must be differentiated from the disorganizing effects of anxiety or concomitant emotional disorder, and from cultural and ethnic factors. The important dimension of social-adaptive behavior can also be underscored by utilizing the newly available scales for its assessment.

Such rich and challenging experiences which are common in mental retardation can prepare the trainee to be more effective and sophisticated in other potential areas of future professional activity. They can help him to avoid far too common unitary (symptom-oriented) viewpoints on the etiology of behavioral disorders, and aid him to think more in terms of multi-dimensional and complex etiological and management systems. These experiences can also introduce him to some of the methodological problems in current psychiatric research programs in this area (see Part Two—B and Part Five in this volume).

The trainee can have the opportunity to view the personality development of a child within the context of the often varied and kaleidoscopic manifestations of physical, neurologic, and psychiatric disorders occurring during infancy and childhood. As reviewed by Webster and Chess (see Chapters 1 and 2 of this volume), these dimensions can often significantly alter or modify the normal sequences of personality differentiation and maturation. The perplexing problems associated with the psychotic reactions in childhood (see Part One—B of this volume) present an excellent opportunity to both study and appreciate the problem of personality regression versus developmental fixations and primitive behavior. The trainee can also obtain invaluable insight into the adult counterparts of impaired cerebral functioning: the acute and chronic brain syndromes and their frequently similar clinical manifestations. Further, personality immaturity and simplicity of psychic functioning can be distinguished from regressive phenomena and the clinical subtype of "inadequate personality" in other areas of mental health activity.

The inclusion of mental retardation in the trainee's program provides opportunity for modification of attitudes toward other or all types of chronically ill children and adults. He may learn to respect the diagnostic considerations that lead to realistic treatment guidelines, to appreciate and empathize with a person's multiple limitations and the associated adjustments of his family, and to work actively with them in a positive fashion. This attitudinal change leaves little room for certain professional rationalizations that can lead to negative treatment and prognostic postures.

Treatment-Management

The trainee can learn that comprehensive treatment of mentally retarded individuals necessitates multiple approaches that must be flexible enough to adapt to a variety of changing developmental needs. The multiplicity of available management techniques and modalities for the mentally retarded (as illustrated in Part Two of this volume), and acceptance of the challenge of long-term planning (via a close liaison with the family) are essential for both positive therapeutic intervention and the prevention of unnecessary handicaps in the mentally retarded person. Although Tizard, Cohen, and Cytryn (see Part Four of this volume) have elaborated the conceptual and programmatic aspects of such training in mental retardation, we will review some further specific training experiences which can help to provide effective treatment that focuses on the maximization of developmental potential.

The trainee must learn techniques for transmitting and interpreting the diagnostic findings to the parents, since this is the first step in the administration of any therapeutic-habilitative program for the child and his parents. Solomons (in Chapter 19 of this volume) has reviewed this crucial area of initial parental-professional transactions in counseling parents of the mentally retarded. Supervised experiences therein can orient the trainee to the issues and problems that are unique to this group of parents. Educational exposure to counseling families of the retarded will remind the trainee rather forcibly that not all family psychopathology reflects earlier stages of conflict-induced fixation in the respective parent's development. A resident can appreciate these particular parent-child constellations as unique only if he has had the opportunity to fully evaluate their problems in adaptation and observe specifically tailored therapeutic approaches. Wolfensberger and Menolascino, and Frederick and Mackinnon, in Chapters 20 and 21 of this volume, have discussed the need for professional attitudinal changes toward parents of the retarded, as well as specific management regimens that can be initiated. Feeling comfortable and helpful in discussing and guiding the mother of a retarded child in such mundane, but important reality problems as toilet training, the psychiatric trainee increases his variety of techniques for making a successful entry into the family. Guidance in providing such parents with specific management skills which enable them to live more comfortably with their child can provide the trainee with direct experience in how to intercede positively into the child-parent interactional unit. Both the attitudinal and methodological treatment issues in a combined behavioral-developmental management approach for the retarded individual and his family must be specifically reviewed and considered with the trainee. Additionally, the trainee will understand all families better, since experience with parents of the retarded will allow him to more easily identify reality-based crises in family dynamics from more diverse origins.

In Chapter 10 of this volume, Lott stressed that the necessity for high intellectual endowment has been overemphasized as a pre-requisite for psychotherapy of the emotionally disturbed mentally retarded individual. Nevertheless, appreciation of the retarded child's problems in interpersonal adjustment, which are often associated with his intellectual and social adaptive problems, can lead to more empathic and realistic psychotherapeutic approaches. Psychotherapeutic efforts with mentally retarded children must often focus heavily on play therapy with emphasis on nonverbal techniques. Also, in some of these children, uncovering techniques, with their possible aftermath of heightening management difficulties, may have to be supplanted by therapeutic-educational approaches which place a premium on behavioral control and the acquisition by training of socially acceptable modes of behavior (see Gardner, Chapter 11 in this volume).

A wide spectrum of pharmacological agents may be necessary in increasing, decreasing, or maintaining the level of arousal and motor overactivity, convulsive thresholds, and general emotional status of mentally retarded individuals (see Freeman, Chapter 13 of this volume). For example, experience with the hyperkinetic behavioral syndrome so commonly seen after postnatal infections, and with quasiepileptic behavior disturbances, can familiarize the resident with a wide range of drugs that may well benefit these and other children with similar behavioral syndromes but diverse etiologies. Experiences with diligent drug combination and dosage selection in the management of behavior, without jeopardizing the child's profitable participation in ongoing educational programs, will be most valuable in the trainee's professional preparation. Part Two–B of this volume provides an overview of both the challenges and frequently occurring professional quandaries in this exciting clinical area.

Relevance to Consumer Needs

With the increasing emphasis on community psychiatry, mental health personnel of the future will undoubtedly find themselves not only thrust into positions where they give direct services to mentally retarded individuals, but they will also be called upon to coordinate the efforts of other resources and agencies which render such services. The current blossoming of community service programs for the retarded, and the parental push for more, faster, and better treatment, emphasize the need to introduce the trainee to the wide gamut of community services and facilities available and guide him in the selective utilization therein. I believe that this aspect of training must go beyond the superficial call for "community awareness" experiences. On the immediate horizon are growing national consumer demands for direct service involvement of professionals at the front lines of community health programs. The evolving Child Care Coordinating Committees (Sugarman, 1969) and the clarity of the recommendations of the Joint Commission on Mental Health in Children (1969) are unmistakable signposts. We must actively orient and involve the trainee in rising to meet these challenges—rather than letting him slide into the "golden ghetto" posture of academia, clinic, or private practice. Thus, involvement in modern management of mentally retarded persons can sensitize the trainee to emerging treatment and habilitative programs applicable to the emotionally disturbed. While service patterns in mental retardation and mental health tend to go hand in hand, there presently appears to be relatively greater movement in the field of mental retardation. Manifestations of this phenomenon are seen in the dynamic evolution of new service ideologies and rationales, the previously noted move toward new community service patterns for the mentally retarded, and the present proliferation of research. A number of contributors to this book have focused on these important topics (see Parts Two, Three, Four, and Five of this volume). Mental health practitioners can profit from these trends. For example, the growing emphasis in the field of mental retardation on behavioral shaping techniques and programs may offer broad treatment possibilities. As noted by Gardner, in Chapter 11 of this volume, research in many areas of behavioral modification, especially for children whose intellectual development is affected by emotional conflicts, is directly applicable to psychiatric services.

Our current national approaches to mental retardation may well benefit from close review and adoption of some European service patterns. In our country, a diagnosis of mental retardation often excludes the child from the spectrum of available child-care and educational services. By contrast, in European approaches, the same diagnosis often stimulates treatment avenues which strongly focus on educational placement and active case work with the family. Education is stressed as an integral part of these treatment approaches, rather than the far-too-frequently separated treatment and educational plans for the retarded in our country. Since community and institutional service programs for the retarded are currently undergoing creative transitions, we owe it to the trainee to help him become fully cognizant of these new frontiers. For example, one principle which is gaining much attention and acceptance in mental retardation is the principle of normalization, especially as formulated and implemented in Scandinavia (Nirje, 1969). This principle, although having its origin in mental retardation, has equal relevance to mental health services as well as to many other human management areas. In barest outline, the normalization principle implies that a deviant person be treated in every possible way as a nondeviant; this includes helping him not to be deviant and presenting and interpreting him to others so that he will not be perceived as deviant. Application of this principle to current mental health practices would underscore the need for home-like treatment centers rather than institutions, community settings in contrast to remote geographical settings, utilization of community recreational facilities, such as recreation departments, rather than hospital-based services. Study trips to geographical areas that have implemented such programs (for example, Scandinavia, Connecticut) can help him see the new model in action, rather than only being told or reading about them. Perhaps we should even aim at placing some of our trainees for three-month periods into outstanding service programs abroad.

These considerations can enlighten the trainee on current and possible future changes in the mental health field. They give him a global and positive view of management-habilitative approaches and an appreciation of the dynamic continuity of both past and current professional attempts to serve the mentally retarded. Guided training experiences in meeting the broad treatment and habilitative needs of the retarded child and adult can serve as a model for providing similar comprehensive services to any individual with complex or chronic problems. Lastly, utilizing the training format reviewed herein, the trainee will have been shown how the traditional psychiatric treatment approach can be extended to capitalize on the treatment skills and services of other human management colleagues; in this way he will also have learned how to effectively utilize all the treatment and rehabilitative resources of the family and community to truly aid either the individual or societal challenges posed by the symptom of mental retardation.

CONCLUSION

The recent policy statement of the American Psychiatric Association on mental retardation (1966) succinctly documented the need for more activity and leadership in this area of professional involvement. Yet the phenomenon of meager manpower in mental retardation is not peculiar just to psychiatry—it typifies all mental health and allied professionals. In a historical review of conceptual treatment-management models for the retarded, Wolfensberger (1969) noted that between the period of the "eugenic alarm" and the early 1960's, no new treatment-management models had emerged. Looking at it in this manner, the "Purgatories" of residential facilities and the "road-blocks" that stem from administrative fiat become symptoms of conceptual confusion, programmatic bewilderment, and professional uncertainty about both the general field of mental retardation and the lack of a distinct ongoing challenge with which psychiatrists could identify. Many of the contributors to this book have gone beyond the mere description of manpower shortages to the even more important systemic points of redefinition of professional goals and roles in program revamping, and the needed realignment of societal and professional expectations that would be more consistent with our current zeitgeist of equal opportunity for all of our citizens whether handicapped or not.

It is truly remarkable how mental health personnel have singularly avoided the opportunities for applying to mental retardation our knowledge and skills in child development, personality dynamics, and multi-disciplinary team approaches. In regard to psychiatry—and with due respect to professional, social, and political changes that have occurred—it is my opinion that psychiatry's low decline from its previous leadership status in mental retardation stems from narrow visions of what the psychiatrist could contribute, negative attitudinal postures toward treatment that led to static and custodial expectations for the retarded, and a general disinterest in learning, teaching, and utilizing the specialized skills and techniques that were so readily available. Implementation of the recent American Psychiatric Association Policy Statement, reinforced by the writers who have shared their experiences and thoughts with us in this volume, can lead to the active fulfillment of these opportunities and challenges both for mental health personnel and the retarded individuals whom we are privileged to serve.

Training in modern approaches to mental retardation can prepare mental health personnel for a better understanding and functioning in the ever-changing social-cultural-political demands for their services. Whether they relish it or not, they will be cast in the "expert" role in areas in which their skills are deemed necessary. The current kaleidoscopic involvement of mental health personnel in a wide array of mental retardation service settings, as noted throughout this volume, is an example of this trend. Cast in such roles, but without the needed training, experiences, or attitudes to function effectively therein, they may too easily think (or hope!) that they indeed are experts. Structured training exposures to both the general and psychiatric aspects of mental retardation can materially aid future mental health trainees to prepare more realistically for the many professional expectations that will be placed upon them in the ongoing renaissance of professional reinvolvement in the area of mental retardation.

In closing, I would like to state once again that it is my hope that the contributors to this volume, by providing specific and up-to-date information on many facets of the psychiatric aspects of mental retardation, will stimulate both the current and future cadres of mental health professionals toward the active implementation of needed mental health services for our mentally retarded fellow citizens.

N O T E

1. The author is indebted to Dr. Howard W. Potter for much of the material used in the section on Historical Perspectives in Mental Retardation which was taken from his unpublished lecture notes.

2. This conceptualization implies that the symptom of mental retardation is always a manifestation of distinct and fixed central nervous system pathology (of known or unknown etiology.) Even if one does entertain such a defect position, which the writer does not, it should be noted that severe mental retardation is usually due to static neuropathology, which usually does not improve, nor does it get worse. More importantly, we would stress that the severely retarded child continues to develop, and a more important professional consideration is attention to the actual abilities of the patient and how they can be programmed, developed, and generally embellished so as to improve his social-adaptive capabilities.

R E F E R E N C E S

American Association on Mental Deficiency. Membership Lists, 1964, 1601 W. Broad Street, Columbus, Ohio.
————. Director of Institutions, 1964, 1601 W. Broad Street, Columbus, Ohio.
American Journal of Psychiatry. New York, July 1958–June 1964, Vols. 115–120.
American Psychiatric Association. Psychiatry and mental retardation (official actions). *American Journal of Psychiatry*, 1966, *122*, 1302–1314.
Bakwin, H. Loneliness in infants. *Am. J. Dis. Child.*, 1942, *63*, 30–40.
Baller, W. R., Charles, D. C., & Miller, E. L. *Mid-life attainment of the mentally retarded: a longitude study*. Lincoln, Nebraska: University of Nebraska, 1966.
Barton, W. E. The psychiatrist's responsibility for mental retardation. *American Journal of Psychiatry*, 1961, *118*, 362–363.
Bigelow, N. Irremedial (Editorial). *Psychiat. Quart. Supple.*, 1953, *27*, 297–301.
Blatt, B., & Kaplan, F. *Christmas in Purgatory*. Boston: Allyn & Bacon, 1966.
Boggs, E. M., & Jervis, G. A. Care and management of the mentally retarded. In Arieti, S. (Ed.), *American Handbook of Psychiatry*. New York: Basic Books, 1966, *3*, 30–36.
Bolian, G. C. The child psychiatrist and the mental retardation "team." *Arch Gen. Psychiat.*, 1968, *18*, 360–369.
Bourneville, D. Recherches sur l'idiotie. *Recherches cliniques et therapeutiques sur l'hysterie et l'idiotie*. Paris: Bureau du Progress Medical, 1893.
Brill, A. A. *Freud's contribution to psychiatry*. New York: Norton, 1944.
Brodbeck, A., & Irwin, O. The speech behavior of infants without families. *Child Development*, 1946, *17*, 145–146.

Camp, B., & Waite, T. Report of four cases of mental deficiency on parole. *Am. Ass'n. Study of Feebleminded*, 1932, *37*, 381–395.

Chandler, C., Norman, V., & Bahn, A. The mentally deficient in out-patient psychiatric clinics. *Amer. J. Ment. Defic.*, 1962, *67*, 218–226.

Clark, L. P. *The nature and treatment of amentia.* Baltimore: W. Wood, 1933.

Clark, A. D. B. Genetic and environmental studies of intelligence. In A. M. Clarke & A. D. B. Clark (Eds.), *Mental deficiency: The changing outlook* (Revised Ed.). New York: Free Press, 1965, pp. 92–137.

Clarke, A. M. & Clark, A. D. B. *Mental deficiency: The changing outlook.* Glencoe, Ill.: The Free Press, 1958.

Council of American Psychiatric Association. *A Position Statement.* Washington, D.C.: American Psychiatric Association, 1963.

Davenport, C. *Heredity in relation to eugenics.* New York: Holt, 1911.

Davies, S. *Social control of the mentally deficient.* New York: Crowell, 1930.

Eveloff, H. H. Psychopharmacologic agents in child psychiatry. *Arch. Gen. Psychiat.*, 1966, *14*, 472–481.

Goddard, H. *The Kallikak family.* New York: Macmillan, 1912.

Goldfarb, W. Effects of psychological deprivation in infancy and subsequent stimulation. *Amer. J. Psychiat.*, 1945, *102*, 18–33.

Goldstein, H. Social and occupational adjustment. In H. A. Stevens & R. Heber (Eds.), *Mental retardation: a review of research.* Chicago: University of Chicago Press, 1964, pp. 214–258.

Griesinger, W. *Mental pathology and therapeutics* (2nd ed.). London: New Sydenham Society, 1860.

Guskin, S. L. & Spicker, H. H. Educational research in mental retardation. In N. R. Ellis (Ed.), *International review of research in mental retardation.* New York: Academic Press, 1968, pp. 217–278.

Haywood, H. C. & Tapp, J. T. Experience and the development of adaptive behavior. In N. R. Ellis (Ed.), *International review of research in mental retardation.* New York: Academic Press, 1966, *1*, 109–151.

Heilbroner, R. L. *The future as history.* New York: Harper, 1960.

Hunt, J. McV. *Intelligence and experience.* New York: Ronald Press, 1961.

———. Intrinsic motivation and its role in psychological development. In D. Levine (Ed.), *Nebraska Symposium on Motivation.* Lincoln, Nebraska: University of Nebraska Press, 1965, pp. 189–282.

Itard, J. *The Wild Boy of Aveyron.* 1801 (Translation). New York: Century, 1932.

Joint Commission on Mental Illness and Health. *Action for Mental Health.* New York: Basic Books, 1960.

Kennedy, R. *A Connecticut community revisisted: A study of the social adjustment of a group of mentally deficient adults in 1948 and 1960.* Hartford, Conn.: Connecticut State Department of Health, 1966.

Kirk, S. *Early education of the mentally retarded.* Urbana, Ill.: University of Illinois Press, 1958.

Kirman, B. Mentally handicapped persons. *Brit. Med. J.*, 1968, *4*, 687–690.

Kugel, R., & Wolfensberger, W. (Eds.). *Changing patterns in residential services for the mentally retarded.* Washington: U.S. Government Printing Office, 1969.

Levy, R. Effects of institutional versus boarding home care on a group of infants. *J. Personal.*, 1947, *15*, 233–241.

McCandless, B. R. Relation of environmental factors to intellectual functioning. In H. A. Stevens & R. Heber (Eds.), *Mental Retardation: A review of research.* Chicago: University of Chicago Press, 1964, pp. 175–213.

McKay, B. A study of IQ changes in a group of girls paroled from a state school for mental defectives. *Amer. J. Ment. Defic.*, 1942, *46*, 496–500.

Menolascino, F. J. Emotional disturbance and mental retardation. *Amer. J. Ment. Defic.*, 1965, *70* (2), 248–256.

———. The façade of mental retardation: its challenge to child psychiatry. *Amer. J. Psychiat.*, 1966, *122*, 1227–1235.

Morel, B. *Traite des degererescenses physiques, intellectuelles et morales de l'espece humaine.* Paris: Beulliere, 1857.

National Association for Retarded Children. 286 Park Avenue, S., New York, N.Y.

O'Connor, N. The successful employment of the mentally handicapped. In L. T. Hilliard & B. H. Kirman (eds.), *Mental deficiency* (2nd ed.). London: J. & A. Churchill, 1965, pp. 642–674.

Potter, H. W. Personality in the mental defective with a method for its evaluation. *Ment. Hyg.,* 1922, *6,* 487–497.

———. Mental deficiency and the psychiatrist. *Amer. J. Psychiat.,* 1927, *83,* 691–698.

———. The needs of mentally retarded children for child psychiatry services. *J. Amer. Acad. Child Psychiat.,* 1965, *3,* 352–374.

———. A commentary on the American Psychiatric Association's action program for psychiatry in mental retardation. *Psychiatric News,* 1966.

President's Panel on Mental Retardation. *A proposed program for national action to combat mental retardation.* Washington, D.C.: Government Printing Office, 1962.

Rheingold, H. Mental and social development of infants in relation to the number of other infants in the boarding home. *Amer. J. Orthopsychiat.,* 1933, *3,* 41–45.

Ribble, M. *The rights of infants: Early psychological needs and their satisfaction.* New York: Columbia University Press, 1943.

Sarason, S., & Gladwin, T. Psychological and cultural problems in mental subnormality: A review of research. *Genetic Psychology Monograph,* 1958, *57,* 1–284.

Séguin, E. *The moral treatment, hygiene and education of idiots and other backward children.* New York: Columbia University Press, 1846.

Simonsen, K. M. *Examination of children from children's homes and day nurseries by the Buhler-Hetzer Development Tests.* Copenhagen: University of Copenhagen, Faculty of Medicine, 1947.

Skeels, H. M. *Adult status of children with contrasting early life experiences.* (Monograph). Society for Research and Child Development, vol. 31 (3). Chicago: University of Chicago Press, 1966.

Spitz, R., & Wolf, K. Anaclitic depression. An inquiry into the genesis of psychiatric conditions in early childhood. *The Psychoanalytic Study of the Child,* 1946, *2,* 313–342. International University Press, New York.

Stedman, D. J. The child psychiatric clinic and the mentally retarded child. Presented to the American Association of Psychiatric Clinics for Children, 1966 Meeting, April 13th, 1966, San Francisco.

Tizard, J. *Community services for the mentally handicapped.* Oxford University Press, 1964.

Willis, T. *De anima brutorum.* Translated by S. Pordage. London: Dring, Harper & Leigh, 1683.

Vail, D. J. Dehumanization and the institutional career, Springfield, Ill.: Charles C Thomas, 1966.

Wolfensberger, W. The origin and nature of our institutional models. In R. Kugel & Wolfensberger (Eds.), *Changing patterns in residential services for the mentally retarded.* Washington: U.S. Government Printing Office, 1969, pp. 59–171.

Index

Abbott, P., 312
Abel, T. M., 233
Abraham, W., 483
Ackerman, N. W., 9
Adams, M. E., 429
Adamson, W. C., 306, 394, 395
adolescent stage, 236, 237
adolescents, and group therapy, 435–440
affect unavailability, 128, 129, 134
Afflech, D. C., 277
aggression, 8, 37, 38, 63
Aid to Dependent Children, 16
Akim, Keith, 245
Albini, J. L., 231, 239
Alderton, H. R., 312, 339
Aldrich, C. A., 479
Aldrich, K. C., 107
Alexander, T., 327
Alexandris, A., 312, 326
Allen, Frederick, 436
Allen, M., 312, 394
Allen, P., 263
Allen, Richard C., 585, 587, 591, 594, 598, 600, 601, 605, 607, 611
Alpert, A. A., 693, 702
Alvarez, W. C., 238
American Academy of Pediatrics, 652
American Association on Mental Deficiency (A.A.M.D.), 6, 10, 45, 68, 70, 72, 85, 193, 211, 244, 467, 572, 575, 576, 698, 712, 721, 725
American Medical Association (A.M.A.), 399, 652
A.M.A. Council on Drugs, 310, 311, 317, 320, 321, 322, 332
American Psychiatric Association (A.P.A.), 11, 45, 193, 554, 652, 698, 721, 725, 726, 728, 740, 741
anal stage, 236, 237
Anastasi, A., 117
Anderson, F. N., 622

Andrew, G., 670, 674, 675
Andrews, E., 155
anencephaly, 91, 132
Angle, C. R., 304
Anthony, E. James, 229, 230
Anthony, J., 117, 701
Antisdel, A. E., 665
Apert-Park-Powers syndrome, 98, 103, 104, 105
aphasia, 92, 98–100, 127, 128, 141, 246
Appel, J. B., 266
Arnold, D. G., 321
Asatoor, A. M., 330
Asperger, Hans, 6
Association for Research in Nervous and Mental Disease, 402
Astin, A. W., 336, 394, 416
Astrachan, M., 233
Atkinson, R. M., 332
attention span, 63
autism, 8, 22, 26, 28, 33, 40–41, 43, 50, 55, 62, 64, 69, 74, 75, 93–94, 97, 99, 110, 148, 149–150, 235, 280, 283, 379, 449, 625, 700, 701; central nervous system intactness, 121, 122, 132; in child psychiatry, 132; in childhood schizophrenia, 116, 124, 126–127, 157, 172–174, 188; cretinism, 618; definitions, 116–117, 141–142; developmental approach, 121–122; etiology, 116, 117–118, 121, 124, 131–132; family effects, 136; language, 117, 123, 125, 126–127, 130–132, 144–145, 149; overemphasis on, 132; personality development, 131–132; and psychosis, 120–127, 143–144; sociocultural, 121; as unique syndrome, 115–116, 120; see also schizophrenia, childhood
autoeroticism, 31

Axline, V. M., 233, 277
Azrin, N. H., 263

babbling, 130
Babcock, S. D., 337
Babinski reflex, 102
Bachrach, A. J., 272
Badham, J. N., 312
Baer, D. M., 255, 256
Bahn, A., 727
Bair, H. V., 306
Baldwin, R., 305, 312
Ball, T. S., 269
Baller, W. R., 719
Barancik, M., 305, 312
Barkauskas, A., 312
Barker, J. C., 331
Barker, P., 316
Barker, R. G., 82, 83, 84, 85
Barnes, K. A., 312
Barnet, C., 560
Baroff, G. S., 251, 263, 264, 268
Barr, M. W., 220, 713
Barsa, J. A., 320
Barsch, R. H., 277
Barton, Walter E., 725, 727
Baum, M. H., 477
Baumeister, A. A., 191, 299, 300,
    667, 686
Bayley Infant Scale, 336
Bazelon, M., 336
Beaudry, P., 309
Beck, H. L., 244
Beck, H. S., 291
Becker, H., 107
Beddie, A., 476
Beecher, H. K., 297, 298
Begab, M., 423, 428, 430
behavior disorders, 6, 7, 56, 58,
    59–60, 61, 62, 63–64
behavior modification, 85; behavior
    analysis, 253–254; electric shock,
    263, 264, 265; extinction, 258,
    259–262, 268, 271; punishment
    procedures, 254, 256, 258–259,
    262–265, 270, 271; reinforcement
    procedures, 268–272; successive-
    approximation technique, 270;
    theory of, 252–257; time-out pro-
    cedures, 265–268, 271; schizo-
    phrenia, 253
Beier, D. C., 70, 75
Beitenman, Edward T., 527–542, 638
Beley, A. P. L., 192

Bell, A., 327
Bellak, L., 125
Bellevue Psychiatric Hospital, 149,
    150, 151, 152, 153, 155, 157, 173,
    174, 175, 177, 179, 180, 182, 183,
    185, 186, 187
Belmont, L., 402
Benda, C. E., 19, 116, 129, 193, 307,
    537
Bender, L., 8, 94, 96, 117, 142, 149,
    150, 153, 155, 157, 159, 162, 170,
    174, 177, 178, 180, 320, 324, 332,
    337
Benedek, T., 207
Bensberg, G. J., 269
Bensberg, G., 560
Benton, A. L., 70, 71, 72
Bergin, J. T. F., 308
Bergman, A. B., 304
Bergman, P., 117
Berlin, I. N., 297
Berman, H. H., 335
Berman, P. W., 291
Bernstein, Norman R., 91–114,
    435–454, 718, 721
Berry, K., 305
Berthiaume, M., 316
Bessman, S. P., 337
Bettleheim, B., 122
Betz, B., 448
Bialer, Irv, 68, 69, 70, 71, 75, 77, 78,
    83, 735
Bibring, E., 437
Bibring, G., 643
Bijou, S. W., 251, 254, 270, 271
Bills, Robert F., 233
Billy, J. H., 244, 245
Binet, A., 617
Binet test, 715
biochemistry, and learning, 342
Birch, H. G., 74, 75, 291, 402
Birnbrauer, J. S., 251, 254, 261, 270,
    271
birth injury, 36
Black, D. B., 338
Blackman, L. S., 405
Blackwood, R. O., 258, 269
Blatt, Burton, 7, 542–552, 575, 576,
    716, 722, 728
Blenkner, M., 668, 675
Bleuler, E., 116, 141
blindness, 619
Blom, G. E. D., 109
Blos, P., 447
Blumberg, E., 308

Boatman, M. J., 297
Bolian, G. C., 729
borderline children, 237
Bornstein, B., 277
Boston Preschool Retarded Children's
    Program, 12
Bourne, Harold, 109, 110
Bourneville, D., 713
Bowen, M., 324
Bowlby, J., 108, 117
Bowling, E., 339
Bowman, P. W., 308
Boyer, L. B., 117
Bradley, C., 324
brain damage (*see* chronic brain syn-
    drome)
Brain, R., 100
Brengelmann, J. C., 79
Breuer, J., 107
Brill, A. A., 715
bronchiectasis, 122
Bronfenbrenner, U., 680
Brown, B., 601, 604, 605, 607
Brown, Dorothy, 276–293
Bruner, J., 110, 117, 136
Buchanan, D. S., 304
Bucher, B., 251, 261, 263, 265
Buck, P., 483
Buckley, P., 301, 308, 321, 327
Burgemeister, B. B., 327, 336
Burk, H. W., 316
Burks, H. F., 324, 325
Burns, J. T., 400
Burton, A., 231
Butler, Neville, 620
Butterfield, E. C., 77, 78

Caldwell, T. E., 79
Call, J., 97
Calverly, J. R., 326
Cameron, H. C., 205, 206
Cameron, I. A., 315
Cantor, G. N., 70, 111
Caplan, G., 202, 528, 529, 637, 643,
    695
Cappon, D., 155
Carter, C. H., 207, 304, 308, 311,
    330, 333
Cass, L. J., 298
Castner, C. W., 308
Cattell Infant Intelligence Scale, 13,
    282, 284
Caudill, W., 680
central nervous system (CNS) pathol-
    ogy, 5, 59, 70, 72, 74, 75, 76, 121,
    147; *see also* chronic brain syn-
    drome
cerebral dysfunction (*see* chronic
    brain syndrome)
cerebral palsy, 24, 407, 468, 469, 471,
    625
Cerebral Palsy Center, Seattle, 424
Cewen, E. L., 233
Champelli, J., 339
Chandler, C., 727
Charles, D. C., 473, 719
Chase, M. E., 231
Chesler, M. A., 81
Chess, S., 9, 10, 46, 47, 55, 60, 61,
    64, 200, 238, 690, 695, 720, 736
Chidester, L., 9, 277
Chien, C. P., 304
Child Care Coordinating Committee,
    738
child-care workers, 529–530
child development, and drug treat-
    ment, 342, 343
child psychiatry and mental retarda-
    tion, 92, 111, 112, 276–292; au-
    tism, 132; basic precepts, 641–644;
    child psychosis, 198–200, 630;
    classification by cause, 618–619;
    classification by grade of defect,
    627–628; classification of mental
    disorders, 626–627; clinical ap-
    proach, 625–626; in community
    mental health programs, 733,
    738–740; Connecticut, 740; defect
    theories, 713, 714; diagnosis, 622;
    diagnosis-compulsion, 481; early
    history of field, 709–711; edu-
    cational-vocational programming,
    721–725; epidemiology of malad-
    justment, 624, 629–630; etiology,
    630–631; in Europe, 721, 724,
    733–734, 739–740; family manage-
    ment, 482–483; feedforward, 731;
    future psychiatric roles, 732–734;
    identity equivalents of psychiatrists,
    733; manpower, 727–728; mental
    age myth, 717–719; mental test ap-
    proach, 715; multidisciplinary team
    approach, 733–734; normalization,
    724, 739–740; overemphasis on se-
    vere retardation, 719–721; pilot
    training program, 641–649; preg-
    nancy adaptation and development
    of child, 631–641, 642; Pregnancy
    Profile questionnaire, 637–639,
    643, 644; professional apathy to re-

child psychiatry (*cont'd*)
 tardation, 725–727; psychiatric
  training, 735–736, 736–738, 740,
  741; psychiatrist as generalist, 732;
  psychoanalysis, 623, 626, 715–716;
  psychopharmacology, 732, 738;
  psychotherapy, 622–623, 717–719;
  retardates as menace, 714–716; retardation and emotional disturbance, 720; role of psychiatrists,
  728–730; special interest areas,
  732–733; training, of medical students, 644–645, 652; training, of
  nurses, 647; training, of obstetric
  residents, 645; training, of pediatric
  residents, 646–647, 652–654; training, of psychiatric residents,
  647–648, 655–656; treatment,
  628–629; typical institutional care,
  722–723
children, and drug therapy, 343–353
Children's Medical Center, Boston, 13
choreoathetosis, 127, 133
chronic brain syndrome, 4, 5, 6, 8, 9,
  11, 16, 17, 18, 20, 21, 29, 33, 37,
  46, 49, 50, 51, 65, 66, 100–103,
  109, 111, 125, 131, 171, 291, 369,
  468–469, 591, 620, 691–693, 696,
  721, 733
chronic mourning, parental, 476
chronic sorrow, 477, 496
Clarinda, S. R., 308
Clark, E. T., 81
Clark, L. P., 8
Clarke, A. D., 70, 233
Clarke, A. M., 70, 233
Clausen, J., 327
Clements, S., 468
Clements, S. D., 291
Close, Henry T., 227
Cobb, D., 277
Coda, Evis, 507–526, 733
Cohen, P., 422, 429
Cohen, P. C., 477
Cohen, Richard L., 633–651, 737
Cole, J. O., 295, 298, 330
Collins, D. T., 220
Collipp, P. J., 335
Colodny, Dorothy, 245, 368–386
Committee on Mental Retardation of
 the Group for the Advancement of
 Psychiatry, 9
community care: child psychiatry,
  733, 738–740; child psychosis,
  522–523; crisis assistance, 515–
517; day-care centers, 523–524;
 diagnostic services, 512–514; en-
 abling legislation, 507–508; goals,
 508; group programs, 518–520;
 mother's groups, 520; psychotherapy, 511–512; psychotic retarded,
 522–523; speech therapy, 519–
 520; treatment services, 514–515
Connecticut, 600, 740
Connecticut State Department of
 Health, 682
Connell, P. H., 316
Conners, C. K., 325, 327, 395
Conrad, W. G., 325
constitutional origin, 72
convulsive disorders, 17, 36, 38, 50,
  63, 106, 132, 133, 147, 316, 323,
  334–335, 370, 372; and childhood
  schizophrenia, 167, 174, 176; drug
  treatment, 167, 334–335, 370,
  372
convulsive therapy, 173, 174, 175,
  177, 178, 179, 183, 184, 186, 263,
  264, 265
Cook, Virginia, 33
Copeland, R., 394, 396
Corless, J. D., 304
Corsini, R., 439
Cottington, F., 324
countertransference, 448–449, 450,
  452–453
Court, J. H., 315
Courtless, T., 601, 604, 605, 607
Cowen, M. A., 303
Craft, M., 300, 301, 308, 319, 320,
  394, 395
Crane, G. E., 304, 316
craniostenosis, 105
Creager, R. O., 328
Creak, E. M., 703
Creak, Mildred, 116, 117, 126, 127,
  140–149
cretinism, 24, 91, 335, 369, 618, 620,
  710
crimes of violence, and retardates,
  603–604
criminality, 69
Cromwell, R. L., 77, 78
Crowley, Francis J., 231
Cummings, S. T., 425
Curry, S. H., 303
Curtis, L. T., 79
Cutler, M., 324
cytogenic subgroups, in Down's syn-
 drome, 191, 193

Cytryn, Leon, 56, 133, 651–660, 737
Cytryn, S. H., 309, 320

Dabbous, I. A., 304
Dalton, J., 477
dance therapy, 232
Daneel, A. B., 313
Darling, H. G., 310
Daudet, G., 317
Davenport, C., 713
David, L., 327
Davids, A., 636
Davies, T. S., 331
Davis, J. A., 680
Davis, J. M., 295
Davis, K. V., 312
deafness, 141, 146, 238, 246, 618, 619, 711
Dean, H. C., 622
decathexis, 34–35, 50
decision theory, 468, 488
Dehnel, L. L., 315
delinquency, 69
delinquents, retarded, 596–597
DeMartino, M. E., 9
dementia praecox, 116, 157
Denhoff, E., 324, 460
Denmark, 556, 558, 560, 564, 567, 568–569, 573, 733–734
Dentler, R. A., 79, 80
Denton, L. R., 231
deprivation, 30, 31–33, 35, 50
Deutsch, Albert, 561
Devault, S., 636
development stages, 236–237, 404–405
Devereux, E. C., 680
Dexter, L. A., 108, 109, 450
diagnosis-compulsion, 481
diagnosis-treatment problem, 698–700
Dietze, H. J., 314
differential diagnosis, 58–61, 72–74, 85, 145–146, 238
DiMascio, A., 297, 304
Dinello, F. A., 339
Dinitz, S., 231, 239
disability, vs. handicap, 82
distractibility, 63
Ditman, K. S., 332, 339
Dix, Dorothea, 711
Domino, G., 192
Donoghue, E. C., 195
Doris, J., 238, 244

dosage, of drugs, 389–390, 391, 410–413
double-blind studies, 298
Dougan, H. T., 319
Doughty, R., 263, 268
Down, Langdon, 618, 630
Down's syndrome, 18, 19–20, 25, 32–33, 34–35, 36, 41, 63, 202, 335, 336, 404, 456, 558, 618, 625, 630, 693, 715–716, 733; cytogenic subgroups, 191, 193; diagnostic stigmata, 193–194; EEG findings, 192, 193, 194, 201; and emotional disturbance, 201–202; institutional admissions, 196–198; institution-alization, 590; and parents, 478, 479, 480, 481; Prince Charming stereotype, 192, 196; psychiatric disturbances, 198–200; sample population, 192–193, 195–196
Drake, M. E., 337
Draw-a-Person test, 602
Dreikurs, R., 439
drug combinations, 340
drug-experience interaction, 405–413
drug therapy and research, 63, 167, 235, 311, 399–402, 512, 531, 697; absorption rates, 410; amphet-amines, 404; brain damage, 369; child development, 342–343; choice of subjects, 407–410; cler-gymen's attitudes, 384; consent of subjects, 413; cretinism, 335, 369; criteria of change, 296; and devel-opmental stages, 404–405; diagnos-tic homogeneity, 416–417; direct-action theory, 400; distribution of scores, 414–415; dosages, 389–390, 391, 410–413; double-blind studies, 298; Down's syndrome, 404, 335, 336; drug combinations, 340; drug-experience interaction, 405–413; duration of administration, 391; EEG findings, 325, 334; energizing theory, 400; enuresis, 333, 334, 339–340, 351; environment and drug effects, 405–407; evaluation of treatment, 382; family attitudes, 379–381; as field for psychiatric research, 379–380; Gilles de la Tourette's syndrome, 316, 317; glu-tamic acid, 178, 226–337, 369, 400, 401, 404, 406, 411, 416, 417; guidelines to drug use, with children, 343–353, hypothyroidism, 401; in-

drug therapy and research (*cont'd*)
tellectual ability, 343; intelligence-
enhancing drugs, 399–419; IQ,
306, 312, 315, 324, 325, 327, 328,
334, 335, 336, 339; IQ and mental
growth rate, 402, 405, 407–410;
magic bullet theory, 399–400,
404, 415; magnesium pemoline, 400,
402; and mental retardation, 368–
370, 378; methodology of drug studies, 295–300, 340–341; metrazol,
407, 413; minimal cerebral dysfunction, 369; model experimental design, 411–413; moral implications,
373–375; objections to, 371–373,
374; on outpatient basis, 379; parental attitudes, 381–382; patients'
attitudes, 384–386; phenylketenuria
(P.K.U.), 369, 370, 406; placebo
effects, 297–298, 377, 394–395,
403, 406, 411, 417; pseudoretardation, 369; psychedelic drugs, 373;
as psychiatric research field, 732,
738; psychoanalytic viewpoints,
375–378; reading ability, 327; regression effect, 299; replacement
theories, 401; research personnel,
418–419; in residential facilities,
387–397; with retarded children,
299–300; sample size, 414; schizophrenia, 311, 393, 396; seizures,
334–335, 370, 372; siccacell therapy, 338; side-effects, 302, 410,
411; study samples, 296; stuttering,
339–340; teachers' attitudes, 383–
384; therapists' attitudes, 383; tics,
351; in total treatment, 343; triple-
blind studies, 298; tranquilizers, 170,
173, 178, 186, 187, 245, 294, 302–
318, 318–322, 342, 370, 387–
396, 723, 724; unblocking theory,
400, 401; *see also* psychopharmacology
Dunbar, F., 636
Durling, D., 306, 308
Dyamond, R. F., 246
Dybwad, Gunnar, 108, 489, 552, 558,
560, 561, 562, 575, 576, 609, 722,
728
Dye, H. B. A., 277
dystonia, 133

Eaton, J. W., 483, 484, 680
Eaton. L., 75, 115, 124
echolalia, 130, 149, 167, 183, 283

Eddy, E., 205, 206
Edgerton, R. B., 84, 715
educable, 460, 465
Edwards, A. E., 414
Edwards, G., 334
EEG findings, 13, 106, 186, 192, 193,
194, 201, 284, 285, 286, 287, 288,
290, 325, 334, 462, 463
Effron, A. S., 318
Effron, D. H., 302
Efron, H. Y., 81
Efron, R. E., 81
ego structure, 8, 9, 22–26, 27, 28, 31,
32, 33, 37, 39, 41, 50, 55, 92, 98,
110, 148, 237, 437, 438, 451, 452,
693, 711
Eisenberg, L., 6, 109, 167, 179, 230,
309, 322, 324, 325, 328, 343, 395,
628
Ekstein, R., 117
electric convulsive treatment, 173,
174, 177, 178, 179, 183, 184, 186,
263, 264, 265
emergence, 148
emotional development, 4, 5, 6, 9, 10,
12, 13, 17, 19, 20, 22–23, 27, 30,
31–41, 41–44, 49–52, 55–61,
63–64
emotional disturbance, 39, 50, 57–58,
68–74, 92, 93, 115–120, 494–495,
691–695, 720; in Down's syndrome, 201–202; vs. retardation,
493–494, 495
encopresis, 628
enuresis, 333, 334, 339–340, 351,
516, 693
epidemiology, of maladjustment in
children, 620, 624, 629–630
Epstein, H., 477
erethism, 6
Erikson, E., 238
eroticism, 33–34
Escalona, S. K., 117
Esen, F. M., 306, 308
Esquirol, J. E. D., 616
Europe, mental retardation services,
556, 558, 560, 564, 567, 568–569,
573, 608, 721, 724, 733–734,
739–740
Eveloff, H. H., 301, 327
Eysenck, H. J., 251, 253
exceptional offenders court, 605–607
extinction, 258, 259–262, 268, 271
extrapyramidal symptoms (EPS), 303,
304, 311, 315, 316, 317

Fabrega, H., Jr., 424
Fairweather, G. W., 664, 665, 668, 674, 680
familial retardation, 15, 16, 18, 19, 92, 279, 537, 718
family, and autism, 136; and drug therapy, 379–381; group therapy, 422–424; therapy of, 499, 501
Farber, B., 424, 430, 477, 478, 483, 571
Fareta, G., 159, 308, 320, 332
feedforward, 731
Ferster, C. B., 266
Ferster, E., 596
Filotto, J., 315
Fine, M. J., 79, 81
Fine, R. H., 310
finger painting, 232
Finley, K. H., 129
Fish, B., 162, 301, 304, 307, 309, 310, 312, 313, 318, 319, 322, 323, 324, 334, 341, 344, 391
Fish, C. H., 339
Fishberg, M., 155
Fisher, G. W., 339
Fisher, S., 295
Food and Drug Administration (FDA), 332, 395, 413
Frank, H. F., 193
Frank, J. P., 483
Frankenstein, C., 71
Fraser, I. A., 316
Frederick, Barbara S., 493–503, 737
Frederik, W. S., 298
Freed, H., 301, 306, 307, 309, 310, 312, 320
Freedman, A. M., 162, 177, 307, 318, 320, 324
Freeman, H., 340
Freeman, M., 232
Freeman, R. D., 245, 294, 296, 301, 369, 394, 400, 404, 474, 738
Freud, Anna, 110, 236, 237, 623, 677
Freud, S., 107, 232
Friedman, E., 231
Friedman, S., 332
Friend, D. G., 330
Frignito, N., 310, 320
Frommer, E. A., 331
Fuller, J. L., 343
Fuller, P. R., 257
Furst, W., 331

Gaddini, E., 205, 206, 207, 211
Gaddini, R. O. B., 205, 206, 207, 211

Gadson, E. J., 336
Galambos, M., 321
Gallant, D. M., 317
Gant, W., 483
Garcia, B., 117, 136
Gardner, G., 653, 700, 738, 739
Gardner, William I., 250–275, 329
Gardos, G., 321
Garfield, S. L., 277, 307, 394, 395
Garner, A., 93, 94
Garrard, S. D., 92
Gatski, R. L., 307
Geiger, L. A., 305
Gelfand, D. M., 251, 256
Gelfand, S., 329
Geller, S. J., 327
genitality, 237
Gerle, B., 315
Gerritsen, T., 401
Giannini, M. J., 319
Gibby, R. G., 75
Gibson, D., 193, 309
Giles, D. K., 263, 269, 270
Gilles de la Tourette's syndrome, 312, 316, 317
Gillie, A. K., 311
Gillies, S., 145
Gilman, A., 323
Gilmour, S. J. G., 331
Girard, J., 71
Girardeau, F. L., 262, 269, 270
Gittelman, M., 74, 75
Gladstone, R., 79
glandular therapy, 178
Glaser, E. M., 676, 683
Glaser, K., 64
Glasser, G. H., 109
glutamic acid (GA), 178, 336–337, 369, 394, 400, 401, 404, 406, 411, 416, 417
Goddard, H., 713, 715
Goffman, E., 109, 449
Goldberg, B., 75, 290
Goldberg, S. C., 393, 396
Goldfarb, W., 109, 117, 136, 141, 142
Goldstein, H., 401
Goldstein, K., 117
Gombas, G. M., 305
Gonzalez, R., 339
Goodman, L. S., 233, 323, 477
Gorlow, L., 79
Gorton, C. E., 251, 269
Gozun, C., 308
Grad, J. R., 479

Graham, F. K., 291
Graham, R., 235
Grant, Q. R., 301, 394
Green, E., 324
Green, M., 635
Greenacre, P., 207
Greenberg, D. S., 680
Greenberg, I. M., 334
Greiner, A. C., 305
Grewel, F., 71
Griesinger, W., 712
Group for the Advancement of Psychiatry, 45, 461
group counseling, 484, 487
group therapy, 233, 245, 422–435, 435–440, 518–520; adolescents and group therapy, 435–440; countertransference, 448–449, 450, 452–453; ego structure, 451, 452; family effects, 422–424; fantasies, 442–443; fathers' attitudes, 429–430, 441–443; leadership roles, 443–446; mother-child relations, 425, 443; reinforcement techniques, 434; sexuality, 427, 431, 441–442, 444, 446–447, 451
Grugett, A. E., 155, 162
Grunberg, F., 117
Grunebaum, H., 449
guardianship, of retardates, 598–601
Guey, J., 334
Guggenbühl, 619, 722
Gunter, L. M., 536
Gunzburg, H. C., 437, 721
Gupta, J. M., 304
Gurevich, Saul, 180
Guskin, S., 81
Guthrie, G. M., 79
Guy, W., 298

Hackett, E., 315
Hagopian, V., 305
Haka, K. K., 424
Hall, D. E., 636
Hamilton, J., 260, 263, 267
Handschin, S., 636
Hanlon, T. E., 313
Harlow, H., 122
Harman, C., 314
Hart, E., 683
Hartlage, L. C., 307, 395
Hartmann, D. P., 251, 256
Hassibi, S., 61
Haworth, Mary, 133, 192, 691
Haywood, H. C., 78

Heath, S. R., 277
Heaton-Ward, W. A., 320, 331
hebephrenia, 147, 175
Heber, R., 6, 7, 43, 68, 69, 70, 71, 72, 76, 211
Heilbroner, R. L., 728
Heimlich, E. P., 232
Heiser, K. F., 231, 235, 239, 277
Heller's disease, 172, 179
Helper, M. M., 307, 394, 395, 636, 640
Henderson, R. A., 483
Hendriksen, K., 263, 268
Heninger, G., 303
Herbert, M., 291
heredity, and childhood schizophrenia, 157–159, 171–172, 174, 176, 178, 179, 181
Hermelin, B. F., 619
Herold, W., 306
Herrmann, J., 318
Hertzig, M. E., 74
Hesbacher, P. T., 296
Heuyer, G., 71
Hilliard, L. T., 104
Himwich, H. E., 308, 309
Hinton, G., 75
histamine treatment, 179
Hoch, P. H., 150, 304
Hoddinott, B. A., 312
Hoffer, A., 298
Hoffman, J. L., 484
Hollis, J. H., 251, 269
Hollister, L. E., 304, 305, 312, 317, 330
Holmes, T., 640
Holt, K. S., 423, 424, 426, 430, 479
Holtz, W. C., 263
Hood, D. E., 233
Hope, J. M., 303
Horenstein, S., 306, 394
Hormuth, R. P., 484
Hornsby, L. D., 297
House, M., 401
Houze, M., 336
Howe, Samuel G., 711, 712
Huff, F. W., 343
Hull, C. L., 252
human management, defined, 664; *see also* research in human management agencies
Hundziak, M., 269
Hunt, B. R., 394
Hunt, J. McV., 717
Hunt, P. V., 311

Hunt, R. G., 622
Hunter, H., 310, 394
Hurler's disease, 34
Hurst, J. G., 79
Hutt, M. L., 75
hydrocephalus, 171, 172
hyperkinesis, 101
hypomotility, 63
hypothyroidism, 401
hypotonia, 95, 102, 143

idiocy, 711, 712, 713, 714
imaginary playmates, 126
incurability, 72
Ingram, T. S., 117
Inouye, E., 338
Insel, J., 325
Institute of Law, Psychiatry, and Criminology, 586, 588, 594, 601, 602
Institute for Mental Studies, Vineland, 239
institutionalization, 471–473, 501, 589–591
insulin-shock treatment, 175, 178, 179
intellectual development, 167–171, 173
intelligence-enhancing drugs, 399–419
intelligence quotient (IQ), 4, 5, 9, 14, 16, 17, 18, 19, 57, 59, 61, 65, 68–69, 79, 95, 104, 108, 174, 177, 179, 183, 184, 186, 215, 231, 240, 242, 243, 244–245, 271, 277, 282, 286, 287, 288, 289, 306, 312, 315, 324, 325, 327, 328, 334, 335, 336, 339, 343, 418, 450, 453, 589, 593, 597, 601, 602–603, 606, 617, 721; concept of, 466–467; mental age myth, 717–719; mental growth rate, 402, 405, 407–410; mental test approach to retardation, 715
International League of Societies for the Mentally Handicapped, 586, 607
invisible retardates, 108
islets of ability, 145
Ison, M. G., 308
Itard, J. M. G., 581, 616, 651, 710, 711, 716

Jacobs, R., 316
Jacobson, L., 60
Jaffe, J., 636
Jaffe, Norma, 276–293
James Jackson Putnam Children's Center, 38

James, William, 111
Jancar, J. A., 320
Jaquith, W. L., 309
Jaros, E., 171
Jenner, W., 146
Jensen, O., 315
Jervis, G., 8
Jews, and childhood schizophrenia, 153, 155, 176, 179, 181
Johnston, A. H., 306
Joiner, L. M., 80
Joint Commission on Mental Health in Children, 739
Joint Commission on Mental Illness, 726
Jonas, A. D., 334
Jones, D., 301
Joynes, T., 311
Jubenville, C. P., 277
Junker, K. S., 483

Kalish, H. I., 251
Kallman, F. J., 157
Kamm, I., 302, 312
Kanfer, F., 253
Kanner, L., 6, 8, 28, 57, 91, 94, 108, 111, 112, 115, 116, 117, 120, 141, 147, 149, 155, 167, 172, 176, 179, 183, 191, 206, 207, 208, 294, 617, 620, 709
Kant, I., 709
Kaplan, F., 716
Kaplan, S., 277
Karacan, I., 310
Karelitz, S., 8
Kasanin, J., 636
Katz, B. E., 320
Katz, M. M., 295
Kaufman, M., 333
Keele, D. K., 310
Kees, W., 232
Kennedy Child Study Center, Los Angeles, 495, 511, 523, 524, 525; organization and programs, 509–511
Kennedy, John F., 552, 553, 573, 585
Kennedy, R., 719
Kennedy, R. J. R., 473
Kenny, T. J., 305, 312
Kent, L. R., 339
Kerr, Nancy, 255, 269
Kessler, J. W., 92, 291
Kinross-Wright, J., 303, 304, 305, 308, 313
Kirk, S. A., 7, 277, 619

Kirkham, J. E., Jr., 313
Kirkpatrick, B. B., 334
Kirman, B. H., 104, 401
Klein, D. F., 334
Klein, M., 441
Klerman, G. L., 297
Kline, N. S., 304
Klingman, W. O., 328
Klotz, M., 313
Knight, R. M., 232
Knobel, M., 328
Koch, R., 299
Koch, Robert, 146
Koestler, Arthur, 402
Kolodny, R., 665, 666, 668, 669, 670
Koppitz, E. M., 291
Kordas, S. K., 315
Korner, M., 110
Korsch, B., 457
Kosman, M. E., 323
Kozinn, P. J., 304
Kraft, I. A., 301, 320, 333, 352
Krakowski, A. J., 321, 333
Kramm, E. R., 480, 483
Krasner, L., 251, 252, 257
Kratter, F. E., 71
Krech, D., 402, 407, 413, 418
Krupanidhi, I., 331
Kugel, R. B., 327, 714, 719
Kugelmass, I. N., 301, 320, 336
Kuhlman test, 277
Kurland, A. A., 297, 339
Kurlander, LeRoy F., 245, 368–386
Kurtis, L. B., 333
Kysar, J. E., 238

lability, 63
Laird, D. M., 309
Lane, G. G., 394
Langley Porter Neuropsychiatric Institute, 10, 56
language, and autism, 117, 123, 125, 126–127, 130–132, 133, 144–145, 149; development, 41, 50, 61, 62, 98–100, 104, 110, 167, 718
Lanzkron, J., 200
Lasky, J. J., 393
latency stage, 236, 237
Laties, V. G., 324
Laufer, M. W., 323, 324, 325, 329
LaVeck, G. D., 301, 308, 310, 327, 328
law, and mental retardation: background, 585–586; basic rights of retardates, 609–610; California, 587–588, 600; Connecticut, 600; guardianship, 598–601; institutionalization, 589–591; the IQ, 589, 593, 597, 601, 602–603; involuntary sterilization, 595–596; legal incompetency, 591; Louisiana, 599; Maryland, 600; Massachusetts, 600; Michigan, 600; Minnesota, 600; mongolism, 590; New Jersey, 594, 599; New York, 600; Ohio, 719; proposed exceptional offenders court, 605–607; protective services, 600–601; retarded delinquents, 596–597; retardates and crimes of violence, 603–604; retardates in prison population, 601–607; rights of institutionalized retardates, 591–596; in Scandinavian countries, 608; Supreme Court decisions, 608–609; terminology, 587–589; Washington state statutes, 600
Lawler, J., 254, 270, 271
Lebeaux, C. N., 666
Lecuyer, R., 192
Leff, R., 251
Leger, Y. A., 312
Lehrmann, D. S., 636
Leland, H., 233
Lesch-Nyhan syndrome, 337
Lesser, L. E., 305
Letchworth Village, 157
LeVann, L. J., 312, 316, 327
Lever, R. F., 117
Levy, D., 236
Levy, J. M., 327
Levy, R., 600
Lewinian field theory, 82, 83–84, 85, 86
Lewis, E. O., 620
Lewis, I., 298
Liberman, R. A., 295, 296, 297
libido, 8
Likert, R., 673, 677, 681, 684
Lindholm, O., 311
Lindquist, E. F., 414
Lindsley. O. R., 269
Lingren, R. H., 78
Lipman, Ronald S., 245, 296, 387–398, 721
Lippitt, R., 673, 677, 681, 684
Lipton, R., 109
Litchfield, H. R., 319, 320

Livingston, S., 334
locus of control, 78
Logan, H., 483
logotherapy, 484
Logothetis, J., 305
Logue, D. S., 337
Lombard, J. P., 336
Lorraine-type dwarfism, 175
loss reactions, 38–39, 51
Lott, George M., 227–250, 700, 718, 737
Lourie, R. S., 56, 207, 322, 328
Louttit, R. T., 301, 338, 400, 401
Lovaas, O. E., 251, 253, 256, 260, 261, 263, 265, 701
Lovejoy, F. H., Jr., 304
Low, N. L., 318
Lowery, L. G., 107
Lucas, A. R., 312, 313, 316, 333
Luckey, R. E., 265
Lundell, F., 312, 326
Luria, A. R., 619
Luszki, M. B., 667, 675, 680
Lytton, G. J., 328

McAfee, R. O., 79
MacAulay, B. D., 269
MacColl, K., 306
McConnell, T. R., Jr., 325
McCray, W. E., 314
McDaniel, M. W., 257
McDermott, J. F., 326
McDermott, W. H., 232
McDonald, E. T., 480
McDonald, R. L., 636
McGough, J. L., 329
McIntire, M., 193
McIntosh, J. S., 305
McIntyre, M. S., 304
McKenzie, M. E., 318
Mackinnon, Marjorie C., 493–503, 737
Mackler, B., 79, 80
McLaughlin, B. E., 310
Madsen, H., 311
magic-bullet theory, 399–400, 404, 415
Mahler-Schoenberger, M., 8, 33
Maisner, E. Q., 233
Makita, K., 71
Malitz, S., 304, 330, 332, 334
Malzberg, B., 155
Mandel, A., 305, 312

Mandelbaum, A., 422
Marasciullo, D. L., 79
Markenson, D. J., 71
Marks, J. B., 676, 683
Marmor, J., 374
Marshak, R. E., 674, 682
Marshall, J. H. L., 303
Martin, C. H., 306
Martin, W. C., 303
Martz, E. W., 277
Marzani, C., 75
Masland, R. L., 7
Mattson, R. H., 326
Max, P., 290
Mead, M., 402
Mebane, J. C., 327
medical students, and child psychiatry training, 644–645, 652
Meier, C. W., 343
Mellinger, T. J., 312
menace, of feeblemindedness, 576–577, 714–716
meningitis, postnatal, 36
Menninger, C. F., 9
Menninger, K. A., 9, 277
Menolascino, Frank J., 10, 11, 46, 75, 91–114, 115–140, 150, 191–204, 205–223, 316, 399–421, 475–493, 530, 538, 690–705, 709–744
mental-age myth, 717–719
mental deficiency (*see* mental retardation)
Mental Deficiency Act, 1913, 620
mental retardation: absolute, 91, 105, 101, 108, 110; abstraction. 50; adjustment reactions, 82–85, 693–694, 697; aggression, 8, 37, 38, 63; apparent, 91, 92–97, 108, 111; autoeroticism, 31; behavior disorders, 6, 7, 56, 57, 58, 59–60, 61, 62, 63–64; behavioral characteristics, 132–135; classification by cause, 618–619; classification by grade of severity, 59–60, 616–618, 622, 627–628; as clinical developmental syndrome, 4, 5, 12, 13, 20, 21–30, 41, 44, 49, 50, 51; compulsive traits, 28, 29, 34, 39; deficit theories, 713–714; defined, 68–69; deprivation, 30, 31–33, 35, 50; developmental history, 59; developmental patterns, 4, 22, 42–44, 50, 95–97; diagnostic-treatment prob-

mental retardation (*con't*)
lem, 622, 731; differential diagnosis, 58–61, 72–74, 85, 145–146, 238; drug therapy, 299–300, 368–370, 378; early history of professional interest, 709–712; early psychiatric intervention, 276–292; educable, 460, 465; emotional development, 4, 5, 6, 9, 10, 12, 13, 17, 19, 20, 22–23, 27, 30, 31–41, 41–44, 49–52, 55–62, 64–67; ego-structure, 8, 9, 22–23, 25–26, 27, 28, 31, 32, 33, 37, 39, 41, 50, 55, 92, 98, 110, 148, 237, 437, 438, 451, 452, 693, 711; emotional disturbance, 36, 50, 57–58, 68–74, 92, 93, 494–495, 691–695; emotionally disturbed parents (EDP's), 35, 50; emotions, simplicity of, 27, 43, 50, 56, 133; epidemiology, 620, 624, 629–630; etiology, 4, 5, 15, 17–18, 70, 72, 73, 75–76, 85–86, 92, 98, 104, 109, 618, 630–631, 698–699, 701, 735; in Europe, 556, 558, 560, 564, 567, 568–569, 573, 608, 721, 724, 733–734, 739, 740; external-internal factors, 93, 110; familial cases, 15, 16, 18, 19, 92, 279, 537, 716; fathers' attitudes, 429–430, 441–443, 500; fears, 38, 51, 63; immaturity, 40, 51, 55, 69; impulsive behavior, 36–37, 39, 51; infantilization, 35–36, 40, 50, 55; inflexibility, 26–27, 28, 29, 39, 43, 50, 56; inhibitions, 38, 51; intellectual functions, 4, 5, 6, 20, 21, 41–42, 47, 50, 56, 69; language development, 41, 50, 61, 62, 718; maturation, 96, 97; medical diagnosis, 17–19, 20, 50, 96; mother-child relation, 5, 8, 11, 19, 23, 25–26, 29, 30–33, 34–35, 39, 40, 96, 205, 207, 208, 221, 425, 443, 539–540; motivation, 99; multidisciplinary team approach, 455–456, 473–474; narcissism, 7–8; negativism, 28, 34, 51; neurotic disturbances, 69; organicity, 151, 155, 157, 159, 162, 171–74, 175–178, 280, 290, 291; overemphasis on severe, 719–721; overstimulation, 50; parent-child relations, 19, 34–36, 37, 41, 50; parent counseling, 65–66, 67, 97, 101, 102, 103, 104, 105, 106, 455–475, 694, 697; passivity, 27, 43, 50, 56; perseveration, 28, 61; physiological retardation, 19–20; play patterns, 9, 11, 41, 50, 61, 134; precocious sociability, 40; primary psychopathology, 6, 13, 14, 17, 21–30, 31, 35, 36, 37, 39, 41, 43, 44, 45, 50, 64; in prison population, 601–607; problem solving, 41–42, 50; pseudoretardation, 5, 8, 10, 30, 33, 142, 150; psychogenesis of, 5, 69, 74, 92, 94, 109, 276–277; psychosocial factors, 69; regression, 40, 51; relative, 91–92, 98–107, 108, 111; repetitiousness, 26, 28, 29, 31, 39, 43, 50, 55–56; retardates as social menace, 576–577, 714–716; schizophrenia, 9, 46, 61, 69, 74–75, 132, 430; school phobia, 230; secondary influences, 30–41, 45, 50–51; self-concept, 78–79, 129; shyness, 38; social adaptation, 4, 13, 69; social work, 557; sociocultural factors, 136, 148; specific learning difficulty, 4, 22, 42; symbol formation, 41, 50; temperament, 60–61, 65; terminological difficulties, 44–48; trainables, 460, 465, 589; training, of adults, 617–618, 619; typical institutional care, 721–723; unique features of, 4; vocalization, 8
Mental Retardation Centers, 730
Mental Retardation Facilities and Community Mental Health Construction Act, 507
mental tests, and retardation, 715
Merini, A., 79
Merlet, L., 79, 80
Merrill, M. A., 100, 107
Merrill-Palmer test, 13
Merton, R. K., 682
metabolic disorders, 18, 41
metrasol convulsive treatment, 173, 174, 175, 177
Meyerson, L., 82, 83, 253, 269
Midtown Manhattan study, 136
Miksztal, M. W., 307
Miller, E. L., 719
Miller, G. A., 665, 676
Milowe, I. D., 654
Milton, R., 331
Minge, M. R., 269
minimal cerebral dysfunction (*see* chronic brain syndrome)
Mitchell, A. C., 308

Mitchell, H. E., 666
Mohr, G. J., 636
Molitch, M., 324
Molling, P. A., 309
mongolism (*see* Down's syndrome)
Moore, J. W., 394, 395
moron, 713, 715
Morris, J. V., 324
Moskowitz, H., 324
mother-child relations, 5, 8, 11, 19, 23, 25–26, 29, 30–33, 34–36, 39, 40, 96, 205, 207, 208, 221, 425, 443, 539–540
motivational variables, 76–78, 84, 86
motivator-hygiene, 78
Mowatt, Marian H., 422–435
Mowrer, O. H., 212, 219
Mudd, E. H., 666
Muffly, R., 394
multidisciplinary team approach, 455–456, 473–474, 534–535, 680–681, 733–734
Munday, L., 231, 233
Murphy, M. M., 232
muscolorus deformans, 127
music therapy, 232
mutism, 99, 100, 132, 144, 149, 167, 184
Myers, G. G., 318

narcissism, 7–8
Nash, H., 295
National Association for Retarded Children (N.A.R.C.), 494, 572, 591–592, 599, 608, 609, 719, 729, 734
National Institute of Mental Health, 393
Nebraska Psychiatric Institute, 10, 115
negativism, 28, 34, 39, 51
Neham, S., 232
neuroleptics, 318
neuropathology, 72, 74
Neuropsychiatric Institute, U.C.L.A., 495
neurotic behavior disorders, 63, 64, 66
Newcombe, D. S., 337
Newman, R., 588
Nirje, B., 489, 608, 724, 739
Niswander, G. D., 310
Noble, R. C., 319
normalization, 724, 739–740
Norman, V., 727

Normanly, J., 71
novelty shock, parental, 478–481, 487, 489
nurses, training, 647
nursing, therapeutic, 220–221

obsessive thought, 63
obstetric residents, training, 645
O'Connor, N., 450, 617, 619, 719
oedipal stage, 236, 237
Oettinger, L., 312, 314, 327, 328
O'German, G., 116
Ogle, W. A., 231
oligophrenic racism, 547
Olshansky, S., 432, 472, 477
Oltman, J. E., 332
Operation Headstart, 16, 112
operant conditioning, 252, 557; *see also* behavior modification
Opscig, S. J., 110
oral stage, 236, 237
organicity, 151, 155, 157, 159, 162, 171–174, 175–178, 280, 290, 291
Orr, D. W., 448
orthomolecular psychiatry, 402
Osmond, H., 476
Oster, J., 193
Otis Quick Scoring test, 603
Overall, J. E., 296, 330
overdependence, 63
Owens, C., 477
Ozehosky, R. J., 81

Paine, R. S., 133, 658
Pandemonium, 548–551
Papageorgis, D., 70
Paracelsus, 708
Paraschi, G., 75
Paredes, A., 296, 319
parents, and mental retardation: assessment of child, 489–490; chronic mourning, 476; chronic sorrow, 477, 496; congregational support, 484–485; counseling, 65–66, 67, 97, 101, 102, 103, 104, 105, 106, 455–475, 694, 697; decision theory, 486, 488; diagnosis, 467–470; Down's syndrome, 478, 479, 480, 481; and drug therapy, 381–382; emotional disturbance vs. retardation, 493–494, 495; emotionally disturbed, 35, 50; emotional problems, 469–470; existential management, 484; family attitudes, 498–499; family physician's role,

parents (*con't*)
457–458; family therapy, 499–501;
father's role, 500; group counseling,
484, 487; infantilization, 35–36,
40, 50, 55; institutional placement,
471–473, 501; IQ concept, 466–
467; interpretation interview, 463–
470; management defined, 475–476;
minimal cerebral dysfunction, 468–
469; multidisciplinary team approach, 455–456, 473–474; novelty shock. 478–481, 487, 489; psychiatric management, 482–483;
and psychiatric social worker, 493–
501; psychoanalysis, 476–477; psychologist's role, 457–458; reality
stress, 478, 481–483, 487, 489;
relations with child, 19, 34–36, 37,
41, 50; religious counseling, 484,
487; role organization crisis, 478:
shoppers, 497–498, 510; special
education, 458–460: stages in management, 486–489; tragic crisis,
478; treatment guidelines, 470–474;
trainable vs. educable, 460, 465;
value conflicts, 478, 483–486, 487,
489; work-up of case, 462–463
Parnicky, J. J., 483
Pasamanick, B., 334
Patterson, G. R., 256, 258, 268, 269
Pauker, J. D., 84
Pauling, Linus, 402
Pavlov, I. P., 252
Pearson, G. H. J., 9
Pearson, P. H., 509, 558
Pecheux, M. G., 79
pediatric residents, training, 646–647,
652–654
Pedrini, D. T., 528
Peifer, C., 306, 307
Pellet, J., 317
Pelton, R. B., 417
Penrose, L., 104
Peppel, H. H., 311
Perron, R., 79
Perry, S. E., 235, 239, 448
personality, of mental retardates: anx-
iety, 76–77; assessment of, 84–85;
attitudes of others, 81; autism, 131–
132; awareness of success/failure,
77–78; conceptions of other people,
79–80; development of, 4, 7, 10,
51, 56, 68, 76–82, 93, 133–135,
147, 236; disability vs. handicap,
82; ecological approach, 84–85, 86;

motivational variables, 76–78, 84,
86; new situations, 83, 86; phenomenological variables, 78–82, 84, 86;
projected self-percept, 81–82; and
self-concept, 78–79
Peterson, L. R., 268, 473
Peterson, R. F., 268
phallic stage, 237
phenobarbital, 106
phenomenological variables, 78–82,
84, 86
phenothiazine, 167
phenylketenouria (PKU), 369, 370,
401, 406, 456, 473
placebo effects, 277, 294–395, 403,
406, 411, 417
play interview, 133
play patterns, 9, 11, 41, 50, 61, 134
play therapy, 94, 185, 233, 236, 696,
738
Philips, I., 10, 46, 56, 244, 300,
450
Phillips, V. P., 107
Piaget, J., 121–122, 129, 130
Pilkington, T. L., 308, 314, 332
Pincus, J. H., 109
Pinel, Philippe, 576, 710
Pinsky, R. H., 297
Piuck, C. L., 319
pleuriglandular syndrome, 175
Polatin, J., 150
Pollack, M., 75, 117, 170
Pond, D. A., 117
Porteus Maze test, 307
Potter, H. W., 7–8, 111, 200, 234,
239, 473, 527, 575–584, 722, 725,
726, 728
Poussaint, A. F., 339
Pratt, J. P., 317
preadolescent stage, 237
precocities, among childhood schizo-
phrenics, 167, 172, 177, 179, 182,
183
Pregelj, S., 312
pregnancy adaptation, and develop-
ment of child, 631–641, 642
pregnancy pathology, and childhood
schizophrenia, 159–162, 175–176,
181–182
Pregnancy Profile questionnaire, 637–
639, 643, 644
prepsychotic, 237
President's Commission on Law Enforcement and Administration of
Justice, 605, 607

President's Committee on Mental Retardation, 527, 552, 572, 604, 716
President's Panel on Mental Retardation, 6, 456, 552, 572, 573, 585, 590, 592, 593, 596, 603, 651, 652, 727
Price, S. A., 338
primary stage, 236
Prince Charming stereotype, 192, 196
Pringle, Kelmer, 620
prison population, retardates in, 601–607
protective services, 600–601
Provence, S., 109
pseudodefectiveness, 142
pseudofeeblemindedness, 70, 72, 111–112
pseudoimbecility, 33
pseudoneurotic, 150
pseudopsychopathic, 150
pseudoretardation, 5, 8, 10, 30, 33, 40, 57, 70–72, 85, 111–112, 132, 142, 150, 235, 244, 369
psychedelic drugs, 373
psychiatric residents, training, 647–648, 655–656
psychiatric social worker, 493–501
psychoanalytic approaches, to mental retardation, 6, 7–8, 21, 476–477, 623, 626, 657, 666, 700, 701, 715–716; developmental stages, 236–237; drug therapy, 375–378; vs. psychotherapy, 228, 244
psychodrama, 233, 245
psychogenesis, of retardation, 5, 69, 74, 92, 94, 109, 276–277
psychologist, role of, 457–458, 532, 556–557
psychoneurosis, 176
psychopathology, primary, 6, 13, 14, 17, 21–30, 31, 35, 36, 37, 39, 41, 43, 44, 45, 50, 51, 64
psychopharmacology, and mental retardation: acetophenazine, 310–311; Actomol, 331; allopurinol, 337; amitriptyline, 333; amphetamines, 323–326, 395, 404; anticonvulsants, 302, 334–335; antidepressants, 329–334; antihistamines, 302, 395; Atarax, 319; Aventyl, 333; Azacyclonol, 319; barbiturates, 322–323; benactyzine, 322; Benadryl, 318, 319–320, 395; benperidol, 317; benzchlorpropamide, 338; Benzedrine, 323; benzodiazeprines, 321–322; benzquinamide, 319; biochemistry, and learning, 342; bovine brain hydrate, 338; buclizine, 319; butaperazine, 311; buthrophenones, 315–318; captodiame, 318–319; carphenazine, 311; Catron, 331; celastrus paniculata seeds, 338; chlorprothixene, 395; chlordiazeposide, 321; chorionic gonadotrophen, 335–336; chlorpromazine, 305–307, 313, 387, 388, 389–391, 394, 395–396, 397; chlorprothixene, 314; Clopenthixol, 315; Compazine, 308; Covatin, 318; Cylert, 329, 402; cypenamine, 339; Dartal, 309; Deaner, 327; deanol, 327, 369; Deprol, 322, 388; Desaxyn, 323; desipramine, 333; Dexedrine, 323; dextroamphetamine, 391, 392, 395; diazepam, 321; Dilantin, 106; diol derivatives, substituted, 320–321; diphenhydromine, 318; diphenylmethane derivatives, 318–320; dixyrazine, 311; ectylurea, 322; Elavil, 333; emylcamate, 322; Ensidon, 334; Equanil, 320; Esucos, 311; etptamine, 331; Eutonyl, 332; 5-hydroxytryptophan, 336; fluphenazine, 310, 313; Frenactil, 317; Frenquel, 319; gamma-hydroxybutyric acid, 337; glutamic acid, 336–337, 369, 394; Haldol, 315; haloperidol, 315–317, 350; hormones, 335–336; hydroxyzine, 319; hypnotics, 302, 322–323; iminobibenzyl, 332–334; imipramine, 332–333; iproniazid, 330; isocarboxazid, 330; Largactil, 305; Levanil, 322; Librium, 321, 391; lithium salts, 337; LSD-25, 337; Lybatran, 320; magnesium pemoline, 329, 369, 400, 402; Majeptil, 311; Marplan, 330; Marsalid, 330; mebanazine, 331; Mellaril, 312, 388; mepazine, 311, 313; mephenesin, 320; meprobamate, 320; Meretran, 328; Methedrine, 323; methophenazine, 311; methyphenidate, 327–328, 395; metrazol, 407, 413; Metrazol, 329; Metronol, 311; Miltown, 320; Mogadon, 322; molindone, 318; monoamine oxidase inhibitors, 330–332; Monase, 331; Mysoline, 106; Nardil, 331; Navanne, 314; neostigmine, 338; Neulactil, 313; Neulepit, 313; nialimide, 331; Ni-

psychopharmacology (*cont'd*)
amid, 331; nitrzepam, 322; Norpramin, 333; nortriptyline, 333; Norstyn, 322; opipramol, 334; Oxazepam, 321–322; oxypertine, 311; Pacatal, 311; pargyline, 332; Parnate, 331; pentylenetetrazol, 329; Permitil, 310; perphenazine, 309, 313; Pertofrane, 333; phenaglycodol, 321; phenelzine, 331; pheniprazine, 331; phenothiazine, 167, 302–313, 388, 389, 394, 395; piperacetazine, 313; piperazine phenothiazines, 395; pipradrol, 328–329; placebo effects, 297–298; prochlorperazine, 308–309, 313; Proketazine, 311; Prolixin, 310; Promazine, 307–308, 313; propericiazine, 313; prothipendyl, 318; protriptyline, 333; Prozine, 308; Quantril, 319; Quide, 313; Rajotte, 311; Randolectil, 311; Rauwolfia alkaloids, 313–314; Repoise, 311; Reserpine, 313; Ritalin, 327, 395; Ro 5-4556, 322; sedatives, 302, 322–323; Serax, 321; Softran, 319; Solacen, 320; Sordinal, 315; Sparine, 307, 391; Stelazine, 309, 344, 391, 395; Stemetil, 308; stimulants, 302, 323–329, 341; Striatran, 322; Suavitil, 322; Surmontil, 334; Suvren, 318; Taractan, 314, 395; terminology, 301–302; thalidomide, 372; thioridazine, 312, 313, 388, 389, 390–391, 394, 397; thiopropazate, 313; thioproperazine, 311; thiothixene, 314–315; thioxanthenes, 314–315; Thorazine, 305–306, 388, 389; Tindal, 310; Tofranil, 331; Tolnate, 318; Tolserol, 320; tranquilizers, major, 302–318, 342, 370; tranquilizers, minor, 302, 318–322; tranylcypromine, 331; Trelmar, 320; Triavil, 388; trifluoperazine, 309, 313, 395; trifluperidol, 317; triflupromazine, 308, 313; Trilafon, 309; Trimidone, 106; trimipramine, 334; Triperidol, 317; tybamate, 320; Ultran, 321; Valium, 321, 391; Vesprin, 308; Vistaril, 319; vitamins, 336; Vivactil, 333; *see also* drug therapy and research
psychosis, childhood, 8, 11, 17, 18, 21, 28, 36, 38, 40–41, 49, 51, 61, 63, 64, 65, 66, 69, 74, 75, 92, 96–97, 121, 127, 146–147, 522–523, 630, 693; and autism, 120–127, 143–144; characteristics, 142–144; classification, 135–136; diagnosis of, 128–130; as a syndrome, 124–127
psychotherapy, 6, 8, 13, 14, 17, 21–30, 31, 35, 36, 39, 41, 42, 43, 44, 45, 50; with childhood schizophrenics, 180, 183; in community programs, 511–512; defined, 227–231; development stages, psychoanalytic, 236–237; differential diagnosis, 238; eclectic methods, 244–245; external / internal conflicts, 237–238; group, 233, 245, 422–423, 435–440, 518–520; personality development, 236; vs. psychoanalysis, 228, 244; reading disability, 238; relationship therapy, 232–234; *see also* psychosis, childhood
punishment procedures, 254, 256, 258–259, 262–265, 270, 271
Putnam, M., 8

Quay, H. C., 296
Quigley, W. A., 272

Rake, R., 640
Ramsay, G., 433
Ranier School, 271
Rank, B., 8, 37, 121
Rapaport, J., 174, 333
Rappaport, S., 8, 37, 277
reactive behavior disorders, 63–64, 66
Read, T. E., 72
reading, 238, 327
reality stress, parental, 478, 481–483, 487, 489
Reed, E. W., 107
regression, 40, 51
regression effect, 299
reinforcement learning theories, 252, 268–272, 434
reinforcement therapy, 434, 701
Reiser, D. E., 96
Reiss, M., 335
relationship therapy, 232–234
religious counseling, 484, 487
Rembolt, R. R., 455
remedial education, 233, 246
remedial reading, 245
Renard, P., 315

research, 3-dimensional research model, 700–702

research, in human management agencies: agency mores, 674; autism, 700; basic vs. applied, 683; diagnostic-treatment problem, 698–701; etiology, 698–699, 701; evaluative, 665–666, 682–683; by extra-agency personnel, 684–687; financing, 675–676; human management defined, 664; innovation, 673, 677, 684; institutional residents as subjects, 686–687; interdisciplinary vs. multidisciplinary, 680–681; kinds of research, 677–684; practitioners vs. researchers, 666–668; psychiatric, 678–680; psychoanalysis, 701; psychopharmacology, 679–680; reinforcement of researchers, 682–683; role and status of researchers, 669–671; starting intra-agency research, 672–677; threat of change, 664–666

residential care: administration, 575, 577–579; architecture, 562, 563–571; Arkansas, 562; California, 553, 558; case-seminar consultation, 528–529, 535–536; child-care workers, 529–530; Connecticut, 562, 571; costs, 723; daily living, 582–584; Denmark, 556, 564, 567, 568–569, 573; drug use, 387–396; in Europe, 556, 558, 560, 564, 567, 568–569, 573, 608, 721, 723, 734–736, 739–740; diagnosis, 579–580; educational programs, 557; educational therapist, 531; goals, 578–579, 581–582; history of, 575–577; housing units, 563–564; institutional management, 556–557, 559–562; legal status of residents, 561, 591–596; medical model, 554–555, 558, 559, 560, 575, 727–728; Netherlands, 567; New York, 553, 554; nurse's role, 530–531; physician's role, 531–532; professional attitudes, 557–559; psychologist's role, 532, 556–557; social worker's role, 532–533, 557; state expenditures for, 553–554; Supreme Court rulings, 561; team coordination, 534–535; vocational rehabilitation, 533

retardates, in prison population, 601–607; as social menace, 576–577, 714–716

Rettig, J. H., 306

revascularization, 401

Rheingold, H. L., 636

Rice, H. K., 257

Richardson, S. O., 71, 555, 559

Richmond, J. B., 92, 205, 206

Rimland, B., 74, 115, 116, 117, 135, 155, 159

Ringness, T. A., 79

Risley, T., 263, 264

Roberts, B., 680

Robinault, I., 460

Robinson, H. B., 6, 7

Robinson, J. T., 311

Robinson, N. M., 6, 7

Rocklin, G., 39

Rodman, H., 665, 666, 668, 669, 670

Rogers, A. C., 107

Rogers, C. R., 232, 233, 246

Rogers, D. E., 483

Rogers, L. L., 417

role-organization crisis, parental, 478

Rood Method of Sensory Stimulation, 519

Roos, P., 269, 477

Rorschach test, 185

Rose, J. A., 634, 635

Rosen, E., 232

Rosenblum, S., 301, 306, 308

Rosenthal, R., 60, 295

Rosewell, H. G., 310

Rosner, M. M., 665, 676

Ross, A. O., 422

Ross, S., 336, 394, 416

Roswell-Harris, D., 318

Roth, P., 157

Rothman, R., 233

Rubella syndrome, 498

Rudnik, R., 122

Rudy, L. H., 306, 308, 311, 319, 320

Ruesch, J., 232

rumination syndrome: defined, 205–206; IQ, 215; interventive therapeutic nursing, 220–221; mother-child relation, 205, 207, 208, 221; treatment, 207–212, 214–219

Russell Sage Foundation, 680

Rutter, Michael, 74, 75, 131, 200, 235, 626, 627, 630

Ryckman, D. B., 483

Sackler, M. D., 179
Salzman, M. M., 334
Santostefano, S., 84
Sarason, S., 450
Sarvis, M. A., 8, 117, 136
Sarwer-Foner, G. J., 244
Saslow, G., 253
Satanove, A., 305
Saunders, J. B. de C. M., 374
Saunders, J. C., 320, 331
Scandinavia, 560, 608, 721, 724, 739, 740
Schacter, F. F., 238
Schain, R. J., 74, 117, 120
Schilder's disease, 147, 172
schizophrenia, childhood, 9, 46, 61, 62, 69, 74–75, 94–96, 121, 142, 311, 430; with adult social adjustment, 180–187; autism, 116, 124, 126–127, 157, 172–174, 188; behavior modification, 253; Bellevue study population, 151–156, 187–188; congenital defects, 162–167; defined, 150; drug therapy, 186, 187, 311, 393, 396; EEG findings, 186; heredity, 157–159, 171–172, 174, 176, 178, 179, 181; infantile illness, 162–167; intellectual development, 167–171, 173; IQ, 177, 179, 183, 184, 186; language development, 167; vs. mental retardation, 142, 430; with organic factors, 174, 175–178; organicity, 151, 155, 157, 159, 162, 171–174; without organicity, 178–180; play therapy, 185; precocities, 167, 172, 177, 179, 182, 183; pregnancy pathology, 159–162, 175–176, 181–182; psychotherapy, 180, 183; seizures, 162–167, 174, 176; sex ratios, 158–159; as syndrome, 126–127; tranquilizers, 186, 187; treatment, 173, 174–175, 177–178, 179–180, 183–184
Schlicht, J., 245
Schmidt, M., 317
Schmuttermeier, E., 71
Schneirla, T. C., 636
school phobia, 230
Schulman, J. L., 308
Scott, P. D., 623
Scott, W. C. M., 241, 244, 245
Segal, L. J., 319
Séguin, Edouard, 576, 616, 617, 618, 619, 651, 711, 712

seizures (*see* convulsive disorders)
self-concept, 78–79, 129
self-injurious behavior (SIB), 263, 365
self-percept, 81–82
sexuality, 441–442, 427, 431, 444, 446–447, 451
Shakespeare, R. A., 195
Shakow, D., 675
Shapiro, A. K., 316, 403, 415, 449
Sharman, George, 559
Shaw, C. R., 56, 308, 394
Sherwin, A. C., 335
shopping, parental, 497–498, 510
side effects, 302, 410, 411
Silberstein, R. M., 310
Simmons, J. G., 337
Simmons, O. G., 680
Simon, T., 617
Simonds, R., 312
Skeels, H. M., 8, 277
Skinner, B. F., 252
Slavson, S. R., 438
Slivkin, Stanley E., 435–454
Sloan, W., 277
Sloane, H. N., Jr., 251, 269
Slocum, W. L., 674
Smith, B., 555
Smith, D., 233
Smith, E. H., 339
Smith, J. R., 79
Soblen, R. A., 331
social worker, role of, 532–533, 557
sociopathy, 69
Soddy, K., 6, 104, 117
Solnit, A. J., 238, 244, 422, 476, 479, 653
Solomons, Gerald, 324, 455–475, 737
Soper, H., 75
Southern Regional Education Board, 560
special education, 458–460
specific learning difficulty, 4, 22, 41
speech therapy, 99, 104, 233, 243, 278, 519–520
Spencer, D. A., 338
Spencer, S. M., 294
Spitz, R., 8, 39, 108, 117, 207
Splitter, S. R., 333, 334
Spradlin, J., 262, 269, 270
Sprague, R. L., 312, 325, 326, 328, 340, 342
Sprogis, G. R., 306
Squier, R., 636
Stacey, C. E., 9

Stanford-Binet test, 13, 95, 167, 184, 186, 277, 282, 284, 288, 417
Stark, M. H., 422, 476, 479
Stedman, D. J., 733
Stephenson, G. M., 310, 394
sterilization, involuntary, 595–596
Sternfeld, L., 472
Sternlicht, M., 232, 234, 239, 433, 438
Stevens, H., 6, 7
Stevenson, H. W., 85, 232
Stirling County study, 136
Stone, M. M., 402
Stone, N. D., 483
Stott, D. H., 630
Stout, L., 483
Strauss, A. A., 468
Strauss syndrome, 468
Strazzula, M., 277
Striefel, S., 254
stuttering, 339–340
subnormality (*see* mental retardation)
Suchman, E. A., 665, 680
Sugerman, A. A., 318, 738
Sullivan, J. P., 324
superego, 237
symptomatic therapy, 109
Szasz, T., 374
Szurek, S. A., 117, 136

Tansley, A. E., 319
Tarachow, S., 228, 229
Tarjan, G., 234, 238, 239, 306, 395, 667
Tate, B. G., 251, 263, 264, 268
Taylor, Edith Meyer, 13
team approach, 455–456, 473–474, 534–535, 680–681, 733–734
Terman, L. M., 100
Thal, N., 331
thalidomide, 372
Thematic Apperception Test (TAT), 185, 602
Thomas, A., 60
Thompson, V. A., 664, 670
Thorne, D. C., 230, 231, 238, 244
Thurston, J. R., 477
tics, 351
Tisza, V. B., 477
Tizard, J., 46, 148, 277, 450, 479, 559, 615–632, 700, 721, 737
Towne, R. C., 80
tragic crisis, parental, 478
trainable, 460, 465, 589
tranquilizers, 170, 173, 178, 186, 187, 245, 294, 301–318, 318–322, 342, 370, 387–396, 723, 724
treatment, 64–67, 85, 96, 109, 111, 146–148, 173, 174–175, 177–178, 179–180, 183–184, 207–212, 214–319, 514–515, 628–629, 693–702
treatment evaluation, in drug therapy, 382
Tredgold, R. F., 6, 104, 117, 619
triple-blind studies, 298
tuberous scherosis, 147
Turkel, H., 401
Turner, W. J., 334

Ucer, E., 322
Uhlenhuth, E. J., 320
Ullman, L. P., 251, 252, 257
Umbarger, B., 406
Underwood Committee, 624, 626, 629
Unna, K. R., 323
Usdane, W. M., 667, 683
Usdin, E., 302

Vail, David J., 558, 559, 716, 728
Vale of Siddem, 107, 112
value conflicts, parental, 478, 483, 486, 487, 489
Van den Horst, A. P. J. M., 71
Van Riper, C., 328
Vernon, P. E., 622
Veterans Administration, 393
Vineland Social Maturity Scale, 13, 59, 277
Virchow, R., 712
Vogel, W., 336–337, 400, 401, 411
Von Bracken, H., 80, 82
vulnerable child syndrome, 635

Waisman, H. A., 401
Waites, L., 310
Walker, C. F., 334
Walker, N. R., 192
Wanderer, Z. W., 232
Wapner, I., 335
Wardell, D. W., 394
Wartel, R., 313
Waskowitz, C. H., 479
Watkins, J. G., 244
Watson, L. S., Jr., 254, 256, 261, 263, 265, 266, 269, 270
Weber, H., 231
Webster, Thomas G., 3, 11, 12, 46, 55, 97, 110, 121, 126, 133, 192,

Webster, Thomas G. (*cont'd*)
202, 208, 219, 290, 449, 695, 720, 736
Wechsler, D., 171
Wechsler Bellevue Scale for. Adults, 167
Wechsler Intelligence Scale for Children (WISC), 167, 185, 417, 602
Weil, R. J., 483, 484
Weiland, I. H., 122
Weir, T. W. H., 313
Weiner, H., 263
Weingold, J. T., 484
Weinstein, E., 429
Weiss, B., 324
Weiss, D., 429
Weiss, G., 307, 326, 395
Wenar, C., 94, 195
Werry, J. S., 238, 296, 307, 312, 322, 326, 328, 341, 350, 394
West, R., 117
Wheeler, E. M., 422
Whipple, B., 109
Whitehorn, J. C., 448
Whitehouse, F. A., 246
Wiener, H., 304
Wiesen, A. E., 256, 263, 265, 266, 269
Wilber, R. C., 277
Wilcott, R. C., 394
Wild Boy of Aveyron, 711
Wilensky, H. L., 666
Williams, E. J., 333
Williams, J., 191, 245
Wing, J. K., 116, 141, 142
Winn, D., 314
Witmer, Helen, 437
Wohl, R. R., 680
Wolberg, L. R., 451

Wolf, S., 297, 298
Wolf, M. M., 251, 256, 258, 259, 260, 263, 266, 269, 270
Wolfensberger, Wolf, 75, 81, 399–421, 475, 476, 481, 483, 489, 524, 554, 663, 666, 667, 686, 713, 716, 721, 737, 740
Wolff, K. M., 117
Wolfson, I. N., 306
Wolpe, 246, 251
Wolpert, A., 298, 314, 315
Woodward, Katharine F., 9, 38, 46, 233, 276–293
Woody, R. H., 244, 245
Work, H. H., 291
World Health Organization, 6, 622
Wortis, J., 200, 202
Wright, H. F., 85
Wright, Margaret M., 134, 196, 205–223, 530
Wright, W. B., 319
Wylie, R. C., 78

Yannet, H., 74, 117, 120, 399
Yarden, P. E., 305
Yuwiler, A., 329

Zigler, E., 59–60, 78, 98, 109, 299, 499, 686
Zimmerman, F. T., 327, 336, 401, 416
Zrull, J. P., 296, 321, 325
Zubeck, J. P., 327
Zubin, J., 295, 303
Zuk, G. H., 483, 484
Zukin, P., 321
Zweig, F. M., 665
Zwerling, I., 479